D1395209

MINOR SURGERY

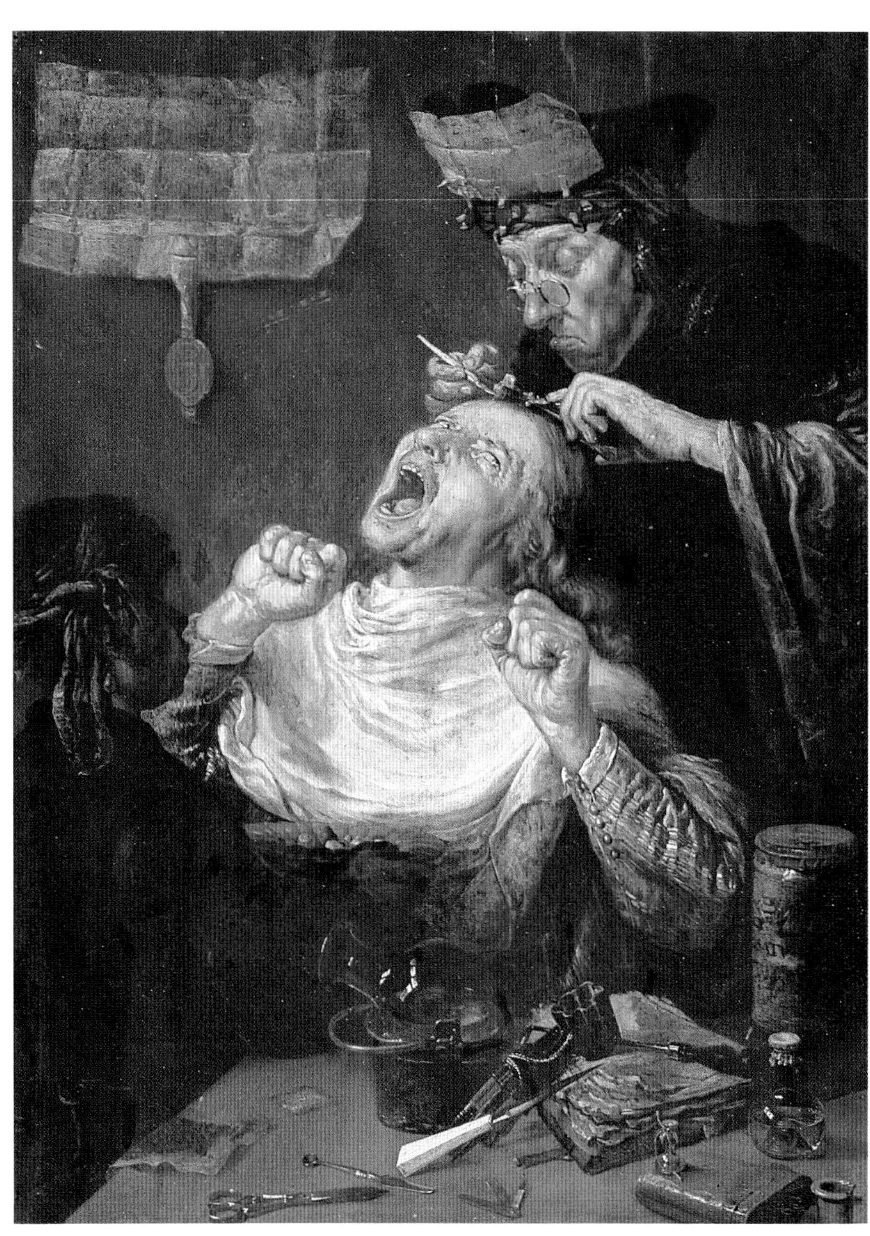

'The extraction of the stone'. Painting by Jan de Bray (17th century). Museum Boymans – van Beuningen, Rotterdam. (Photograph: Wellcome Institute Library, London.)

MINOR SURGERY

A TEXT AND ATLAS

THIRD EDITION

John Stuart Brown
OStJ, MB, BS(Hons), MRCS, LRCP
FRCGP, DCH, D(Obst)RCOG, AKC

General Medical Practitioner
Thornhills Medical Group, Larkfield, Aylesford, Kent

WITH A FOREWORD BY PROFESSOR SIR ROBERT SHIELDS

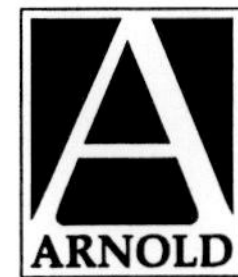

A member of the Hodder Headline Group
LONDON • SYDNEY • AUCKLAND
Copublished in the USA by
Oxford University Press, Inc., New York

First edition published in Great Britain in 1986
Second edition 1992
Third edition 1997
Reprinted 1999 by Arnold, a member of the Hodder Headline Group,
338 Euston Road, London NW1 3BH

http://www.arnoldpublishers.com

Co-published in the USA by
Oxford University Press Inc.,
198 Madison Avenue, New York, NY10016
Oxford is a registered trademark of Oxford University Press

©1986, 1992, 1997 J. S. Brown (except Chapter 44)
Chapter 44 © Patrick Dando

All rights reserved. No part of this publication may be reproduced or transmitted in any form or by any means, electronically or mechanically, including photocopying, recording or any information storage or retrieval system, without either prior permission in writing from the publisher or a licence permitting restricted copying. In the United Kingdom such licences are issued by the Copyright Licensing Agency: 90 Tottenham Court Road, London W1P 9HE.

Whilst the advice and information in this book are believed to be true and accurate at the date of going to press, neither the authors nor the publisher can accept any legal responsibility or liability for any errors or omissions that may be made. In particular (but without limiting the generality of the preceding disclaimer) every effort has been made to check drug dosages; however, it is still possible that errors have been missed. Furthermore, dosage schedules are constantly being revised and new side-effects recognized. For these reasons the reader is strongly urged to consult the drug companies' printed instructions before administering any of the drugs recommended in this book.

British Library Cataloguing in Publication Data
A catalogue record for this book is available from the British Library

Library of Congress Cataloging-in-Publication Data
A catalog record for this book is available from the Library of Congress

ISBN 0 412 75060 0

2 3 4 5 6 7 8 9 10

Designed by Geoffrey Wadsley
Typeset in 10.25pt Galliard
Printed and bound in Hong Kong

To Anne

Contents

Acknowledgements

The first edition of this book was based on a series of articles on minor surgery in the *Pulse* reference section, 1984, and my grateful thanks are due to the staff of *Pulse* who gave me so much help and advice, and in particular to Cynthia Clarke for her medical illustrations, Philip Fraser-Betts and Paul Thorpe for many of the photographs.

To Mrs Vaux and Mrs Harrison, state registered chiropodists in Maidstone, my grateful thanks for their tuition on the method of treating ingrowing toe-nails.

My thanks are also due to Mr W. Keith Yeates for allowing me to use his slides illustrating vasectomy in the first and second editions and to his widow Mrs J. Yeates for her permission to use the slides in this section; also to Dr Philip Hopkins for his advice on liquid nitrogen cryosurgery.

The new chapter on histological appearance of various skin lesions was made possible with the help I received from Dr R. J. Cairns who allowed me to use his slides of skin lesions, and Dr Trevor Telfer who personally made the photomicrographs of all the histological specimens and gave me invaluable advice. To both of them, I extend my sincere thanks.

Chapter 44 on medicolegal aspects of minor surgery is based on the booklet of the same title by Dr Patrick Dando of the Medical Defence Union Ltd and I am extremely grateful to him for his help. Copyright in the material is retained by the Medical Defence Union Ltd.

Mr Maurice Frohm showed me the technique for stab avulsions for varicose veins and I am grateful to him for his advice.

I am very grateful to my partners, and to all the nurses who have worked with us at Larkfield and given so much help and advice, also to all our receptionists and staff for all their help.

I am especially grateful to Mrs Sylvia Smith, practice manager of the Thornhills Medical Group for over 25 years for her invaluable help in typing, reading, and correcting the manuscripts for the first and second editions, a task which she did meticulously.

Finally, a special word of thanks to my wife, Anne, who has given me so much help throughout all the preparation of all three editions, and without whose assistance it would not have been possible.

J.S.B.

Preface to the third edition

Further changes and additional procedures have been included in the third edition of *Minor Surgery – A Text and Atlas* to reflect improved techniques and also to take account of those doctors who wish to undertake more complex minor surgical operations.

In the first edition decompression of the carpal tunnel and release of trigger finger were included, but because of the risks of intravenous regional block anaesthesia they were omitted from the second edition. They have been reintroduced, together with stab avulsion of varicose veins and excision of ganglion, in a separate new section on 'Advanced minor surgery' and, instead of intravenous regional block, a much safer technique is described.

In Chapter 50 there is a more comprehensive collection of patient information leaflets reflecting the growing awareness of the importance of giving patients as much information about their operation as possible.

Finally, there is now a completely new section of radio-surgery, a technique which is widely used in America and other parts of the world and which is gaining in popularity in this country.

Preface to the second edition

With the introduction of the new NHS contract, general practitioners in the UK are now being actively encouraged to undertake more of their own minor operations.

This has been reflected in the second edition of *Minor Surgery – A Text and Atlas* by enlarging the sections on joint and peri-articular injections, hormone replacement therapy, alternative methods of treating ingrowing toe-nails and a greatly expanded section on cryotherapy which undoubtedly has an important place in minor surgery outside hospital practice.

New sections on histological appearances of common skin lesions are included, together with colour photographs of those frequently encountered.

Finally, there is a new chapter on the medicolegal implications of minor surgery in general practice in the UK; this should help to allay many fears some doctors have about doing their own surgery. It also offers very helpful guidelines on ways of avoiding problems and of ensuring a good outcome and a satisfied patient.

Preface to the first edition

This book provides an illustrated step-by-step guide to minor surgery. It covers all minor surgical conditions and treatments encountered by the author over 25 years in general practice.

The selection of suitable instruments and equipment is described, followed by methods of instrument sterilization, skin preparation, choice of incisions and a comprehensive description of methods of anaesthesia, including intravenous regional anaesthesia, nerve blocks and infiltration anaesthesia.

Wound closure and the use of different suture materials are described, together with a section on the timing of suture removal to obtain the neatest scars. Follow-up and statistical analysis of the types of operation feasible in general practice are covered.

Individual minor surgical procedures are then described with illustrations. The practitioner is taken through each operation, commencing with simple injection techniques, through excision of cysts, biopsies, ingrowing toe-nails and varicose veins to more complex minor operations including decompression of the carpal tunnel, release of trigger finger and excision of ganglion.

Finally, simple diagnostic procedures such as proctoscopy, sigmoidoscopy and biopsy are described.

This volume provides a valuable reference book for all general medical practitioners, both in practice and in training.

Although all the operations described can be performed under general or local anaesthesia, the author has described local anaesthetic techniques almost exclusively.

Foreword

In the National Health Service, there is an increasing trend towards the provision of treatment in the primary care setting. As part of this trend, two of the most remarkable changes in surgery, in the last decade, have been the reduction in the time that a patient spends in hospital after a major operation and the increasing number of operative procedures undertaken in general practice. As a result, patients can look forward to having their treatment from doctors whom they know and in whom they have confidence, in familiar surroundings near to home. In addition, long waiting lists for outpatient consultation and inpatient treatment, and the risk of cancelled admissions, can be avoided.

However, patients will quite properly insist that operations in general practice must be to the same high standard as that delivered by a hospital surgeon. Unfortunately, undergraduate medical education and postgraduate training programmes do not prepare the general practitioner to cope with the increasing trend to minor surgery in general practice. It has been left to the enthusiasm of many general practitioners to acquire their skills in an *ad hoc* manner. Such training has often been incomplete and haphazard.

Conventional text books of surgery are often short in detailed descriptions of operative procedures and atlases of operations contain much that is irrelevant. Fortunately, for the benefit of those who wish to embark upon minor surgery in general practice, or, indeed, the young trainee surgeon who seeks details of procedures that he, or she, may be called upon to carry out in a day-case surgery unit, this book provides all the necessary detail. The successful contribution, which this book has made to this important and expanding field of surgery, is manifested by the fact that it has now gone to a third edition within a decade. The book introduces the general practitioner and the trainee surgeon to safe and sound operative techniques and stresses the importance of undertaking minor surgery in a safe environment. The surgeons, whether in hospital or in general practice, who follow the principles and details described in this book, will ensure that their patients are provided with the higher standards of minor surgery.

Professor Sir Robert Shields, DL, MD, DSc, PRCSEd, FRCSEng, FRCPSGlas, FRCPE (Hons), FACS (Hon), FCS (SA) (Hon), FCSHK (Hon), FRCSI (Hon), Professor of Surgery, Royal Liverpool University Hospital, President Royal College of Surgeons of Edinburgh.

Part One :

Basic techniques

1

Introduction

If thou examinest a man having a gaping wound in his head, penetrating to the bone, thou shouldst lay thy hand upon it and thou shouldst palpate his wound. If thou findest his skull uninjured thou shouldst say regarding him 'an ailment which I will treat'

Edwin Smith, Surgical Papyrus, 3000–2500 BC

All doctors have seen many minor operations performed, and as medical students, resident house-surgeons and trainee general practitioners have performed many of them personally. Before the advent of the National Health Service in the United Kingdom, most family doctors undertook their own minor surgery – lancing boils and abscesses, excising cysts, and suturing lacerations. Some had contracts with the local hospitals and performed all their own minor surgery, together with many major surgical procedure. Patients expected their family doctors to operate, and family doctors themselves expected to undertake most minor surgical procedures – including delivering babies at home, and even 'tonsillectomies on the kitchen table'!

In recent years, there has been a gradual move away from general practitioner minor surgery – family doctors in hospitals have been replaced by specialist consultant colleagues, fewer general practitioners are now undertaking their own minor surgery, preferring instead to refer the majority of their patients with such conditions to hospital. Inevitably, as this trend increased, hospital surgical waiting lists increased.

In many instances, because the patient realizes his or her condition is not serious and knows that there are long delays, he or she may not even consult the family doctor, preferring to keep the 'cyst' or 'mole' or 'veins'. In recent years, however, there has been a renewed interest by general medical practitioners in minor surgery; with training now taking up to ten years, and many doctors moving into purpose-built premises complete with treatment rooms, and working with attached community nurses or practice nurses, many now feel they would like to undertake their own minor operations again. This has been welcomed by the patients, who now find they can receive treatment for their minor lesions promptly, in familiar surroundings, and done by a doctor they know well, with follow-up by the nurses they know already.

Because of the great variety of minor surgical procedures, there is a good chance that doctors will never have seen some of them actually performed, and if they wish to learn the techniques they may have to refer to 12 or more specialized textbooks of surgery. For example, a GP would need to consult a surgical instrument catalogue for the choice of instruments, equipment firms for sterilizers, tables and lights, textbooks on

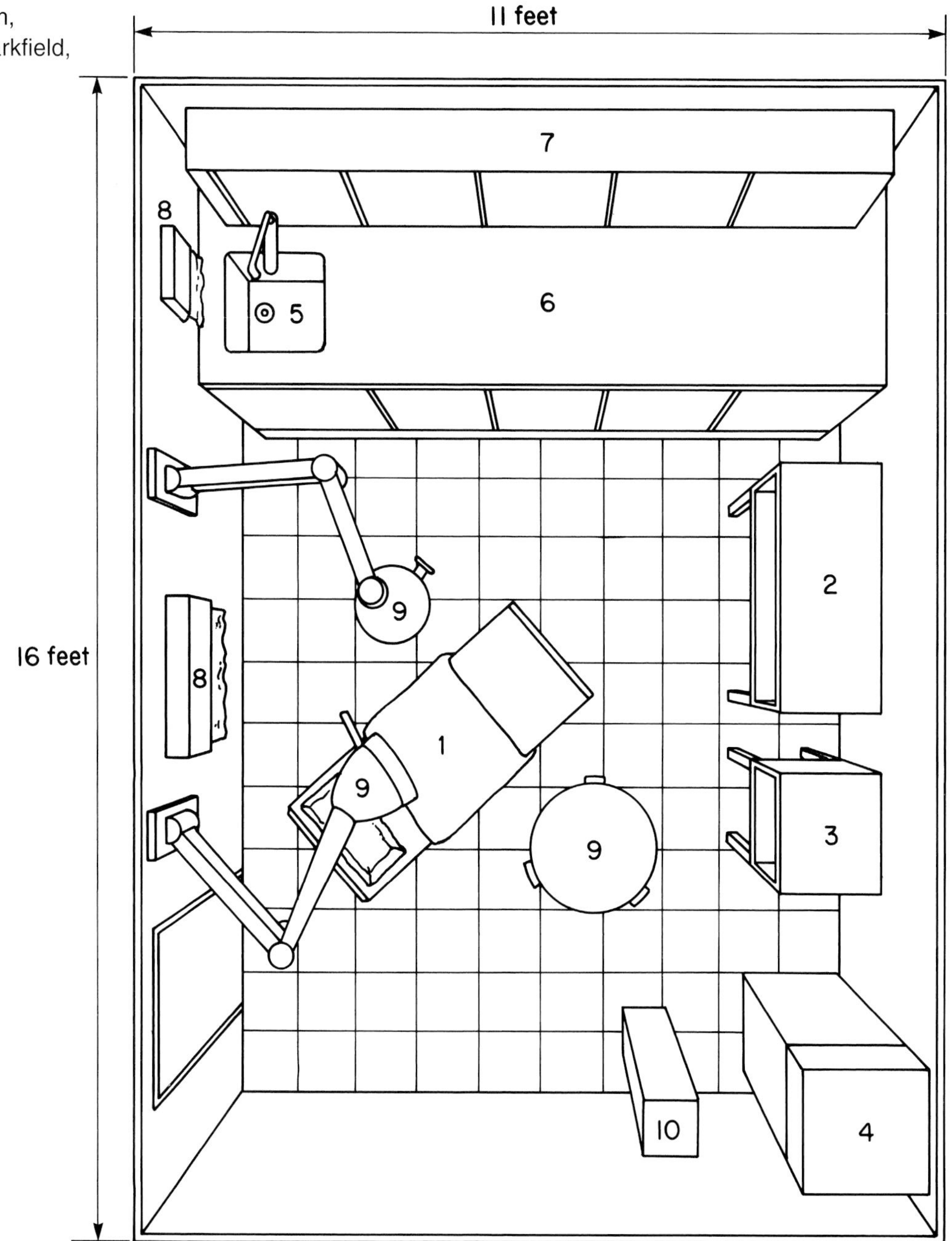

Fig. 1.1 The treatment room, Thornhills Medical Group, Larkfield, Kent.
Key:
1. Operating theatre table
2. Dressing trolley
3. Dressing trolley
4. Instrument cupboard
5. Handwash-basin
6. Work surface
7. Storage cupboards
8. Paper towel dispenser
9. Lights
10. Wastebin.

general surgery for the excision of sebaceous cysts, and reference books on ophthalmic surgery for the treatment of meibomian cysts.

Removal of intradermal naevi might be found in a textbook of dermatology or general surgery, whereas intra-articular steroid injections might be found in books on rheumatology, general medicine or orthopaedics. Proctoscopy, sigmoidoscopy and the injection of haemorrhoids could be covered in three separate textbooks, while the treatment of ingrowing toenails might be included in books on general surgery, orthopaedics, dermatology and chiropody! Skin tumours and their management would be found in specialist books on oncology, dermatology, general surgery, plastic surgery and even lasers in medicine, while injection of the carpal tunnel

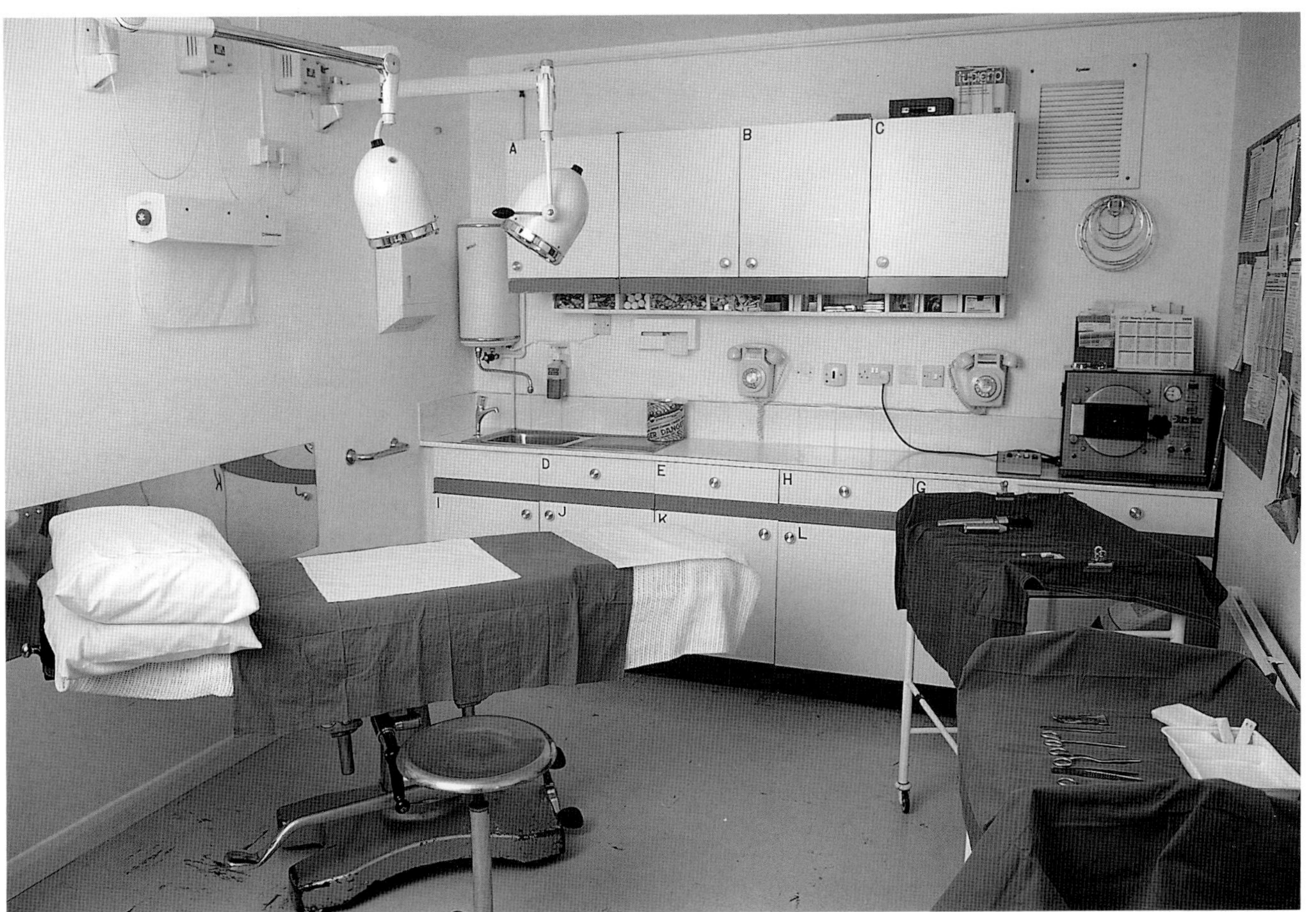

Fig. 1.2 The treatment room, Thornhills Medical Group, Larkfield, Kent.

would be included in books on rheumatology, neurology, physical medicine or general surgery. Practitioners wishing to learn the technique of cryotherapy might have difficulty knowing which specialized textbook to consult, as they would if they wished to sterilize instruments or equipment. Thus, although each procedure may correctly be classified as minor surgery, nevertheless the term embraces many different specialities, and hence the reason for this book: it is an attempt to bring together under one cover all the minor operations and practical surgical procedures that general practitioners might wish to perform themselves.

With a few exceptions, all the minor operations described can be performed single-handed by the practitioner or with the assistance of an 'unscrubbed' nurse.

The techniques described and the instruments used are those which the author has found most suitable over 35 years performing more than 15 000 minor operations personally. The choice of firms supplying instruments and equipment is always difficult as there are many excellent firms both in the United Kingdom and America; thus only a representative sample has been included in the book, mainly of suppliers the author has used himself.

1.1 SCOPE AND LIMITATIONS OF MINOR SURGERY

All the minor operations described in this book are well within the capability of any general medical practitioner, house-surgeon, casualty officer or trainee general practitioner as well as the specialist. Some require the purchase of a special item of equipment such as an electrocautery, others require a special instrument, for example chalazion ring forceps for meibomian cysts. Above all, practitioners must satisfy themselves that they can safely carry out any particular surgical procedure before attempting it. Thus it may be helpful, as well as referring to texts and photographs, to watch a procedure being performed by a colleague and obtain expert tuition before embarking on it.

As experience grows, so the number and variety of minor operations attempted will increase, and the final decision of what to attempt, and what not to attempt will rest entirely with the doctor. A single-handed practitioner will be inadvised to attempt any operation involving intravenous

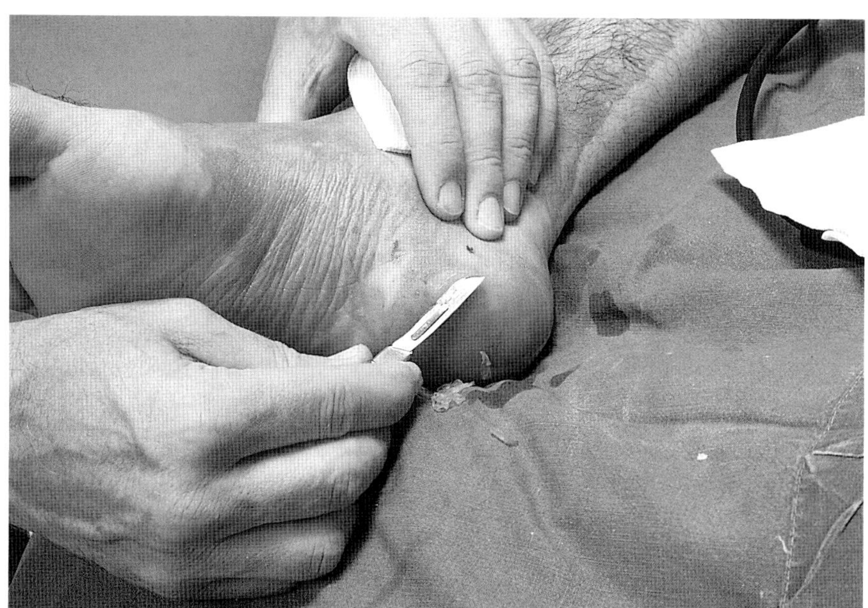

Fig. 1.3 In the past it was not considered necessary to wear gloves for some procedures, but it is now recommended that gloves be worn for all minor operations.

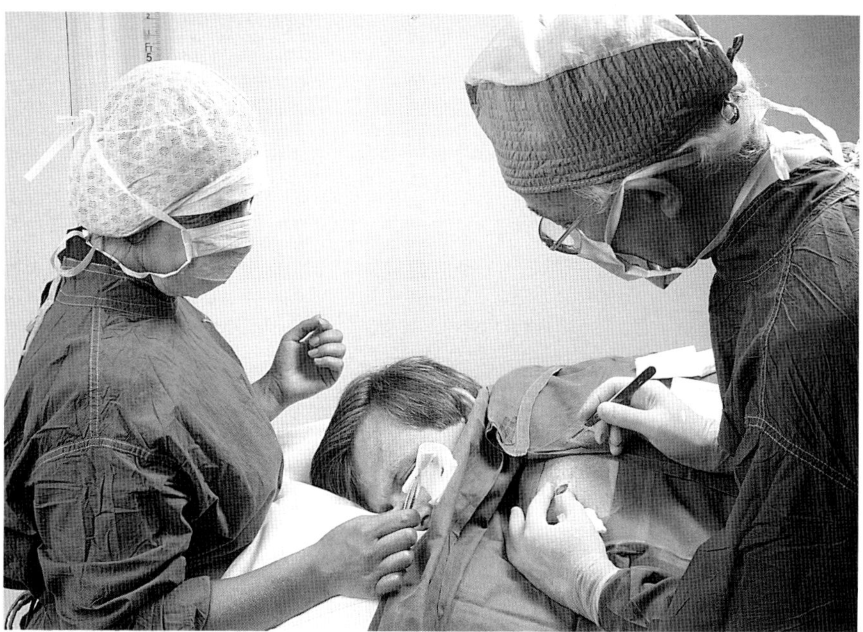

Fig. 1.4 For others, such as excision of lipoma, opening joints, or vasectomy, sterile gloves and gowns may be used, together with masks.

regional anaesthesia, where an assistant is mandatory, and although the majority of operations described can safely be performed single handed, nevertheless, if an assistant such as a nurse or colleague can be available, it helps both the patient and operator considerably. For this reason, if the doctor contemplates undertaking minor surgery to any extent, it is a good idea at the outset to reserve a time for an operating session or 'list'; this may be daily, weekly, or once a month depending on numbers and circumstances. General anaesthesia has not been included in this book as it was assumed most general practitioners would not have adequate recovery beds and facilities in the average GP surgery. However, all the procedures described can easily be performed very safely and comfortably using local anaesthetic techniques.

Where the patient can have a short rest afterwards and transport can be arranged, there are very few minor operations which cannot readily be performed in the general practitioner's consulting or treatment room. Where the patient is too ill (e.g. malignant ascites) or too handicapped (e.g. confined entirely to bed) it may be preferable to bring the equipment and instruments to the patient's home rather than bringing the patient to the doctor's premises, and in this respect, minor surgery lends itself admirably.

1.2 ADVANTAGES AND DISADVANTAGES

There are considerable advantages where the patient's doctor undertakes minor surgery (see Table 1.1). First, the patient and doctor are already well known to each other, and this immediately allays much anxiety, particularly with very young patients. Secondly, there is saving of time both for the patient and the hospital; the patient can generally choose a convenient time and the hospital, by not seeing the patient, can offer the time saved to another patient. Thirdly, there are considerable financial savings, particularly to the hospital budget. It has been shown that one general practitioner performing only a few minor operations per week can save the local hospital a significant amount [1, 2] and that, on average, it is 15 times cheaper to perform the same operation in general practice compared with hospital. Fourthly, there is a continuity of care; the doctor performing the

Table 1.1 Advantages of GP minor surgery

1. Staff already known to patient
2. Saving of time for patient and hospital
3. Financial savings to local hospital
4. Continuity of care
5. Less infection
6. Greater job satisfaction
7. Greater efficiency
8. Offering a better service
9. Rapid biopsy and histology results
10. Greater patient satisfaction

Table 1.2 Disadvantages of GP minor surgery

1. Lack of suitable training
2. Lack of suitable equipment and premises
3. The risk of missing serious pathology
4. Allocating sufficient time
5. Worry should complications occur (with mediolegal implications)
6. Financial disincentives

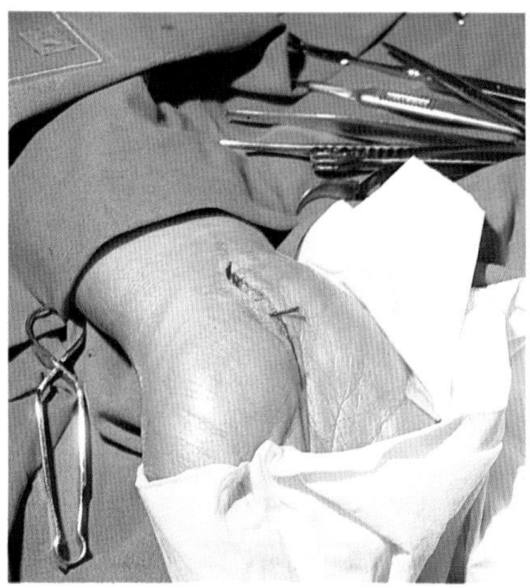

Fig. 1.5 Sterile drapes, either paper or linen, will ensure less risk of infection.

operation is the same doctor who initially saw the patient – the nurse assisting at the operation is likewise already known to the patient, and is the same nurse who will remove any sutures and undertake any further follow-up, and, when the patient is ready to return to school or work, it is the very same doctor who will check all is well and discharge the patient.

Cross-infection outside hospital is much less of a problem than inside hospital, commonly less than 1 or 2%. Among other advantages could be included greater job satisfaction, greater efficiency, offering a better service, rapid biopsy and histology results, and greater patient satisfaction.

Offset against these many advantages are a few disadvantages (Table 1.2). Some of the most commonly voiced worries are lack of suitable training, lack of suitable equipment and premises, the risk of missing serious pathology, worry about medicolegal implications should complications occur, and finding sufficient time. However, the advantages greatly outweigh any disadvantages, and rarely does one find a doctor who has started to undertake surgery thinking of abandoning it.

1.3 ORGANIZATION WITHIN THE PRACTICE

Some procedures such as injection of tennis elbow, golfer's elbow, carpal tunnel and the like, take so little time that it is usually preferable to perform these at the time of the initial consultation. Similarly, if the electrocautery and an ampoule of local anaesthetic are available easily, small skin tags, papillomata and warts and naevi may all be dealt with in less than five minutes.

Where any number are to be done, or where it is likely to take longer than the initial consultation appointment time, it is easier and preferable to set aside a certain time each week, and to make a minor operations 'list' at which the practice nurse and/or an assistant can help. With a little experience the doctor will soon know how long each procedure takes, and will be able to offer appropriate appointments accordingly.

Accurate records of all operations performed should be kept, together with any drugs used, and types of sutures and dressings; a register of operations enables the doctor to analyse his or her work and produce an annual breakdown of the type of work being done (Chapter 20).

Many 'elementary' procedures are described in this book, and lists of instruments are often repeated throughout the book. This is a deliberate policy to avoid the reader having to refer back to several previous sections.

2

Instruments

When thou meetest a tumour that has attacked a vessel ... say 'I will treat the disease with the knife, poultice it with fat, and burn it with fire so that it bleeds not too much'.

Ebers Papyrus, 1500 BC

2.1 CHOICE OF INSTRUMENTS

Every doctor has a favourite selection of instruments; what suits one surgeon does not always suit another. One practitioner may prefer small, fine toothed delicate instruments whereas another is happier with larger instruments. However, certain basic sets of instruments seem to be generally popular, and the following are included as being the most commonly used by the author (Fig. 2.1).

1 size 3 scalpel handle
scalpel blades 15, 10, 11
5 in. toothed dissecting forceps (Treves) (12.7 cm)
5 in. standard (sharp/sharp) stitch scissors (12.7 cm)
5 in. straight artery forceps (Halstead) (12.7 cm)
5¼ in. Kilner needle holder (13.3 cm)

These five instruments plus scalpel blades form the nucleus of most minor operating sets; they can be used for simple suturing of lacerations and excision of most dermal lesions. Where the practitioner intends building up various instrument packs to be sterilized by the CSSD (Central Sterile Supplies Department) several such basic packs should be made up.

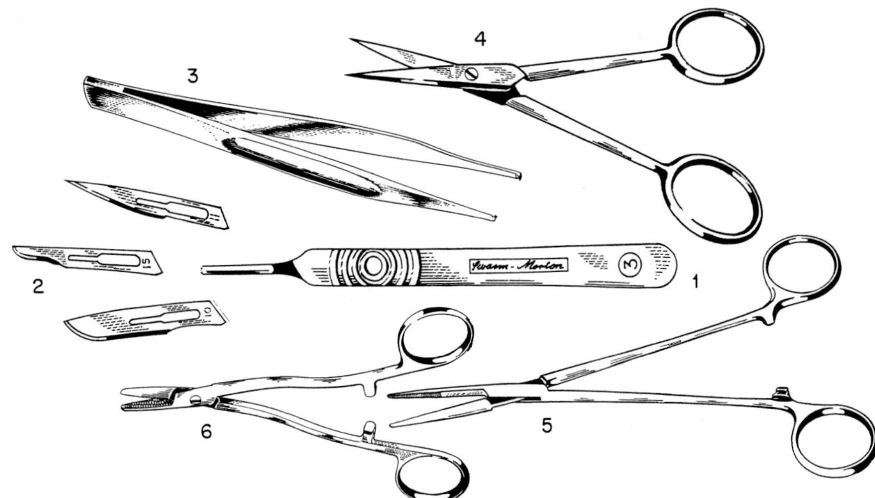

Fig. 2.1 A basic instrument pack.
1. Scalpel handle, size 3
2. Scalpel blades, sizes 10, 11 and 15
3. 5 in. (12.7 cm) toothed dissecting forceps
4. 5 in. (12.7 cm) standard stitch scissors, pointed
5. 5 in. (12.7 cm) straight artery forceps (Halstead's)
6. 5¼ in. (13.3 cm) Kilner needle holder.

Next to the scalpel, the needle holder will be the most frequently used instrument during a doctor's working life in minor surgery; it is, therefore, worth spending relatively more on this instrument in order to have the best quality available. In particular, it is essential to check the jaws to ensure that they not only hold the finest needle accurately, but more importantly hold the finest suture without slipping or traumatizing. Nothing is more frustrating than trying to tie a knot in 6/0 monofilament nylon only to find the suture material slipping through the jaws of the needle holder.

The Gillies combined needle holder and scissors is a very popular instrument, although it sometimes takes practice to learn the technique of using it. Where the surgeon is working with limited assistance, the Gillies can be used as a needle holder, to tie the knot, and to cut the suture, all without having to change instruments.

The next most useful instruments are the sharp-spoon Volkmann curette and electrocautery, which between them enable the practitioner to remove most warts, verrucae, papillomata, granulomata, keratoses, and similar intradermal lesions. The curette is generally easy to choose, depending on the doctor's preference, but selection of an electrocautery can be difficult as there are many excellent models on the market (Chapters 3 and 16).

Where smaller instruments are required for fine surgery, Adson's $4^{3}/_{4}$ in. (12 cm) toothed dissecting forceps are ideal, together with a pair of Iris scissors, fine $4^{1}/_{2}$ in. (11.4 cm) straight or curved. Similarly, the fine 5 in. (12.7 cm) Halstead mosquito forceps, curved or straight, are most useful instruments.

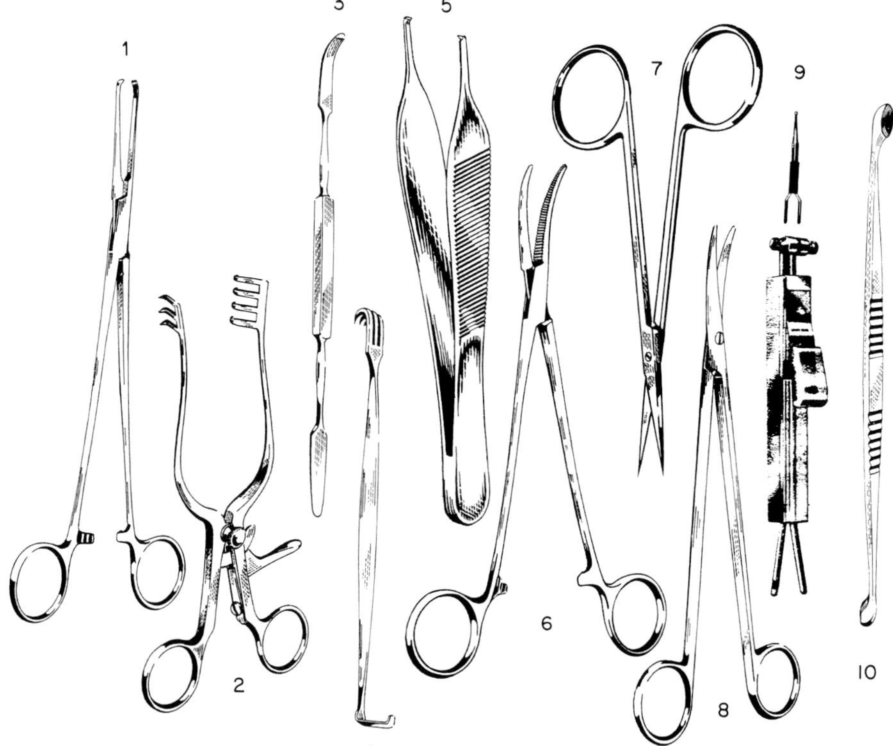

Fig. 2.2 Some of the most commonly used instruments in addition to the basic set.

1. Allis tissue forceps 3 × 4 teeth 6 in. (15.2 cm)
2. Self-retaining retractor (Kocher's thyroid or equivalent)
3. McDonald's double-ended dissector $7^{1}/_{2}$ in. (19 cm)
4. Retractor: double-ended Kilner Senn Miller 6 in. (15.2 cm) (so-called cat's paw retractor)
5. Adson's toothed dissecting forceps $4^{3}/_{4}$ in. (12 cm)
6. 5 in. (12.7 cm) curved fine artery forceps (Halstead's mosquito)
7. Iris scissors, straight, $4^{1}/_{2}$ in. (11.4 cm)
8. Curved 7 in. (17.8 cm) McIndoe's scissors
9. Electrocautery burner and handle (Mark Hovell's)
10. Volkmann double-ended sharp spoon curette

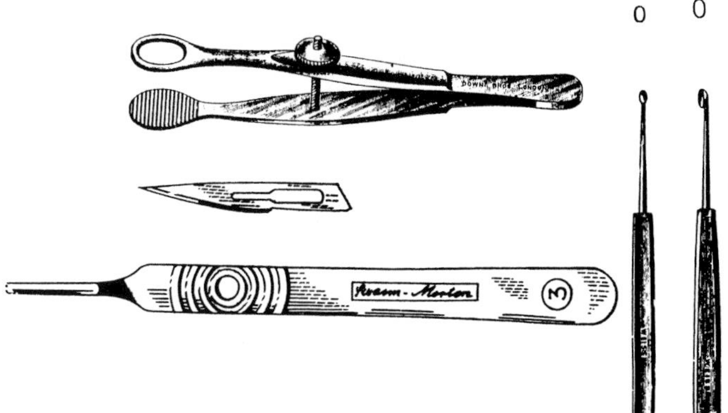

Fig. 2.3 Instruments required for incision and curette of meibomian cyst (chalazion).

Sebaceous cysts and lipomata can be nicely dissected using a pair of curved 7in. (17.8cm) McIndoe scissors which may also double up for cutting the threads of intra-uterine contraceptive devices after they have been inserted (Fig. 2.2).

At some stage, the practitioner will need some small retractors: these may be either self-retaining such as the Kocher's thyroid retractor, West Weitlander $5^{1}/_{2}$in. (14cm), or the baby Kilner/Dickson Wright spring self-retaining retractor, or single/double retractors which will need to be held by an assistant. Of these, the Gillies skin hooks $6^{1}/_{2}$in. (16.5cm) are popular, as are the double-ended Kilner Senn Miller 6in. (15.2cm) (so called cat's paw retractors).

To complete the list of small general instruments is the McDonald's double-ended $7^{1}/_{2}$in. (19cm) dissector, which is extremely versatile and useful for many minor procedures.

All doctors regularly see patients suffering from meibomian cysts (chalazion); normally such patients would need to be referred to an ophthalmic surgeon, but the treatment of incision and curettage is so simple and quick that it can be one of the most rewarding conditions to treat, provided the practitioner has the necessary instruments. These comprise a pair of chalazion ring forceps, a small chalazion curette, no. 3 scalpel handle with the pointed no. 11 blade, together with syringe and needle for administering local anaesthetic (Fig. 2.3).

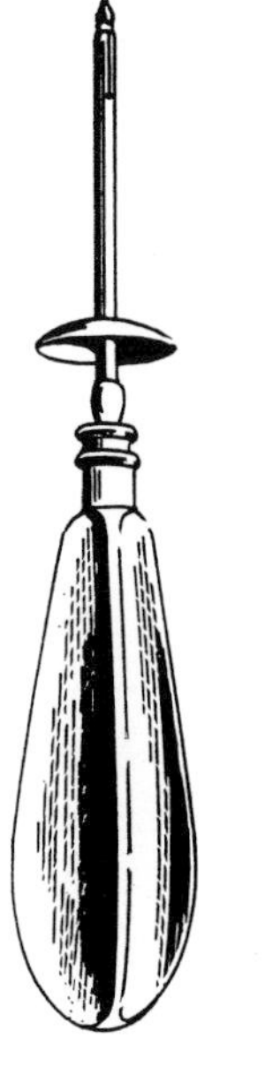

Fig. 2.4 Trocar and cannula used for draining abdominal ascites.

Another valuable instrument, although not used as frequently as the above, is the abdominal trocar and cannula for draining abdominal ascites. More recently with the introduction of plastic intravenous cannulae, a less traumatic aspiration may be obtained by the use of one of these instead. In general practice the commonest cause of ascites is inoperable malignant disease, and great relief, albeit temporary, can be offered by the judicious tapping of ascitic fluid when symptoms of pressure become distressing (Fig. 2.4).

As the treatment of haemorrhoids is included in the textbook, a choice of proctoscope, sigmoidoscope and haemorrhoid injection syringe should be considered. There are many different sigmoidoscopes and proctoscopes on the market with a variety of methods of illumination and magnification, some disposable, some non-disposable, and costs vary considerably. Where a practitioner is considering purchasing such instruments, it is often helpful to ask the advice of the local general surgeon and ask for a demonstration.

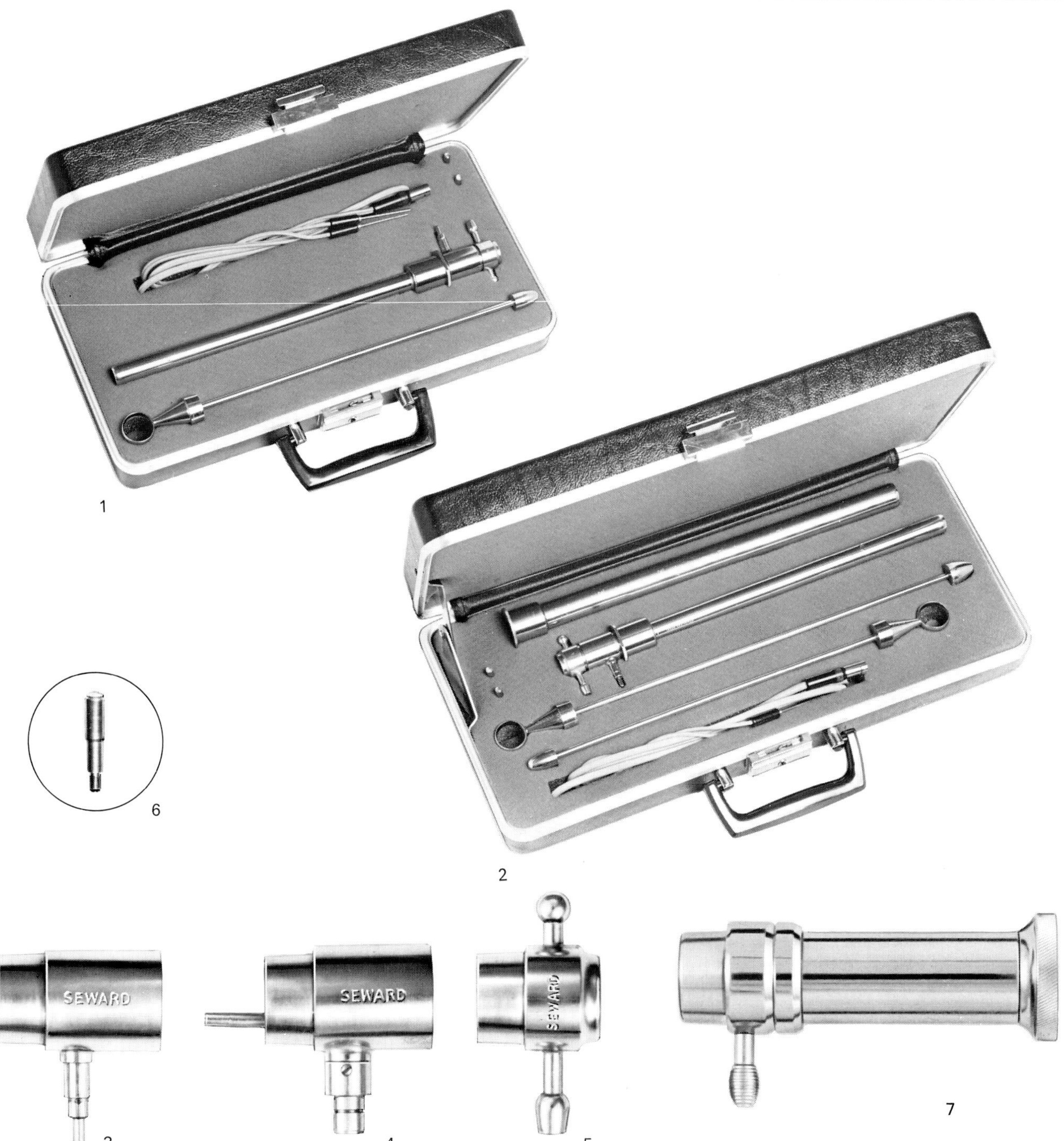

Fig. 2.5 The Lloyd-Davies stainless steel rigid sigmoidoscope.

1. Adult size 250 mm × 15 mm
2. Adult size 300 mm × 20 mm
3. 3.5 V lighting chamber
4. Fibre-optic lighting chamber
5. Inflation window
6. 3.5 V tungsten-filament bulb
7. Telescopic attachment (×1.5 magnification) (Seward Medical, London).

The Lloyd-Davies stainless steel sigmoidoscope has been in use for many years and is a popular, virtually indestructible instrument. Illumination can be by fibre-optic cable, filament bulb, or tungsten or quartz halogen lamp; they are rigid, reasonably priced and interchangeable (Fig. 2.5). More recently, flexible, fibre-optic sigmoidoscopes have been marketed, but the cost is still high, and probably outside the price range of the average practitioner. However, the illumination and view are excellent and more of the sigmoid colon can be visualized than with the rigid instrument.

Naunton Morgan's proctoscope is ideal for the general practitioner. As with the sigmoidoscope, illumination may be from either a fibre-optic

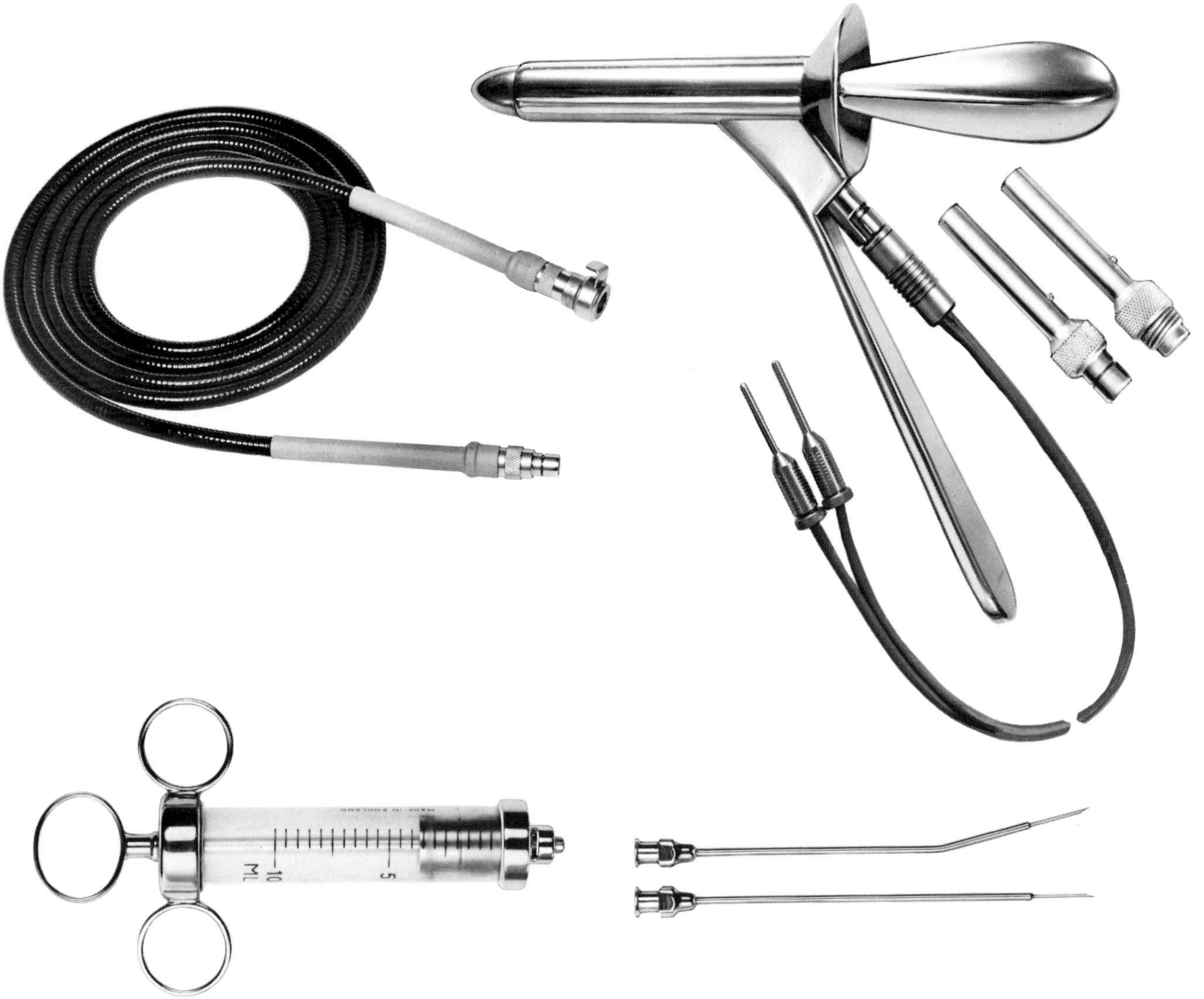

Fig. 2.6 St. Mark's Hospital pattern proctoscope with Gabriel's haemorrhoid injection syringe and needles. Illumination by tungsten filament 3.5 V bulb, or fibre-optic cable and light (Seward Medical, London).

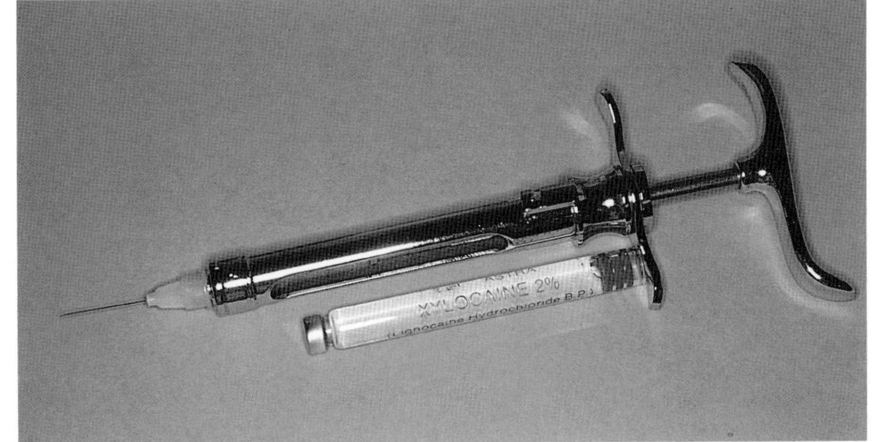

Fig. 2.7 Dental syringe with cartridges of local anaesthetic and 30 swg needles; ideal both for children and for digital nerve blocks (Nova Instruments)

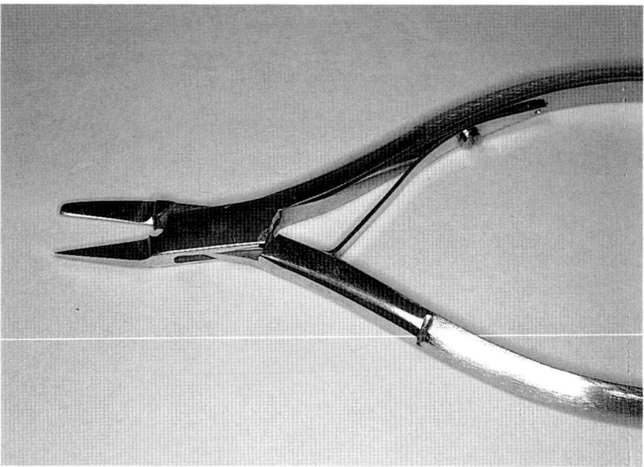

Fig. 2.8 Thwaites nail nipper (English pattern, Nova Instruments).

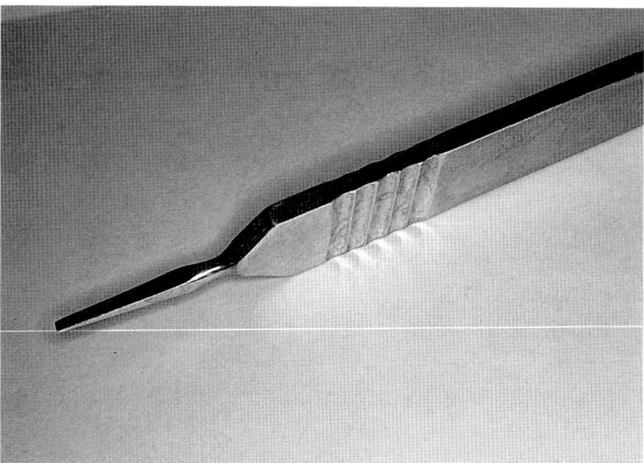

Fig. 2.9 Nail chisel (Nova Instruments).

cable or filament bulb. It is an excellent instrument to use if the practitioner contemplates injecting haemorrhoids. For this latter procedure, a Gabriel's haemorrhoid syringe is used. It has the advantage of good finger control, although many simpler disposable haemorrhoid syringes have now been introduced with Luer-lock fittings to prevent the needle being expelled under pressure (Fig. 2.6).

As all the operations described in this book are performed under local anaesthesia, it is important that this be made as discomfort-free as possible.

To this end, the finest possible needle should be used for infiltration anaesthesia, and there is no better needle to use than the 30 swg (0.3 mm) needle mounted on a dental syringe loaded with a cartridge of local anaesthetic. If the injection is given slowly and gently, it can be virtually painless – a point greatly appreciated by the younger patients! (Fig. 2.7).

Where larger volumes of local anaesthetic need to be injected, the initial 'bleb' or 'weal' can still be raised with the dental syringe and needle. Larger needles merely traumatize the tissues, cause unnecessary pain, delay healing and increase the risks of infection.

Finally, before leaving this section on the choice of instruments, mention must be made of two invaluable instruments in the surgical treatment of ingrowing toe-nails, these are the nail chisel and the Thwaites nail nipper (Figs 2.8 and 2.9). With these two instruments plus a pair of straight artery forceps the practitioner can offer a treatment for ingrowing toe-nails which carries a 99% cure rate! (Chapter 30).

2.2 INSTRUMENT AND EQUIPMENT MANUFACTURERS (Appendix A)

The list given at the end of this book is far from comprehensive; it includes all the firms which the author has used during the past 35 years; however, each practitioner will have his or her own favourite suppliers, and it is certainly worth 'shopping around' for the 'best buy'. All the items of equipment and surgical instruments described in this book can be obtained from firms included in this list.

2.3 SOURCES OF SUPPLY

To build and equip a minor operating theatre using all new materials and instruments could be prohibitively expensive for most general practitioners, particularly as they are unlikely to be able to recoup much of the expenditure either from grants, item-of-service payments or patients' fees.

However, by making careful enquiries and contacting various agencies, a very acceptable treatment room can be equipped for a fraction of what it would cost new. Major items such as operating theatre tables, trolleys, sterilizers and lights may often be obtained from the local Hospital Supplies Officer who knows of obsolete items of equipment no longer required by the hospital. They may often be purchased for a nominal sum, and although classified as 'obsolete' as far as the hospital is concerned, may prove to be exactly what is needed in a small minor operating room.

Often equipment has been purchased for use in hospital, only to be superseded by an improved model after several years; the original is then relegated to the stores, yet is still perfectly serviceable. Similarly, it is worth contacting large surgical equipment manufacturers to see if they have any reconditioned, obsolete, or demonstration models available at a reduced price. Medical representatives from these firms are always most helpful if they can see what is needed, and it is always worth contacting them, usually through the Operating Room Supervisor or Theatre Sister at the nearest hospital.

Charitable organizations will often be prepared to raise money and purchase a piece of equipment, particularly if they can see the benefits which will accrue locally if an improved surgical service is offered.

Finally when all else fails, it is still possible to advertise for equipment and instruments in the various journals and weekly magazines, and be successful.

2.4 ADVANTAGES OF INSTRUMENT PACKS

Where a doctor is performing a regular number of minor operations and particularly if the CSSD (Central Sterile Supplies Department) facilities can be used, there is much to commend compiling a number of 'instrument packs'. For example, suture pack, ingrowing toe-nail pack, meibomian cyst pack, abdominal paracentesis pack, etc. In this way, just the instruments which are required are sterilized and used in a more efficient way. Individual packs may be sterilized and kept for future use, as well as being available for use both at the surgery or in the patient's home. It is also easier to check the contents of each pack at the end of each operation to ensure no instruments have been lost. Unfortunately the smaller autoclaves are not suitable for instrument packs as they do not have a vacuum cycle and will therefore not dry the instruments, so the practitioner will normally have to rely on a hospital autoclave, or failing this a hot-air oven.

The following instrument packs will be found to be most useful for the general practitioner undertaking minor surgery.

2.4.1 Basic suture pack (Fig. 2.10)

1 scalpel handle size 3
1 Kilner needle holder $5^1/_4$in. (13.3 cm)
1 stitch scissors, pointed, 5 in. (12.7 cm)
1 toothed dissecting forceps 5 in. (12.7 cm)
1 straight artery forceps 5 in. (12.7 cm)
1 scalpel blade size 10
1 sterile Prolene suture. Ref. Ethicon WB020T
(1.5 metric) with curved cutting needle 26 mm.

2.4.2 Meibomian cyst pack (Fig. 2.11)

1 pair chalazion ring forceps
1 scalpel handle size 3
1 pair iris scissors, curved $4^1/_2$in. (11.4 cm)
1 chalazion curette
1 scalpel blade size 11
1 sterile eye pad and bandage
sterile gauze swabs.

2.4.3 Abdominal paracentesis pack

1 scalpel handle size 3
1 scalpel blade size 15
1 trocar and cannula or intravenous cannula
connecting tubing and screw clip
sterile gauze swabs.

2.4.4 Ingrowing toe-nail pack

1 scalpel handle size 3
1 scalpel blade size 15
1 pair artery forceps, straight 5 in. (12.7 cm)
1 pair stitch scissors, sharp/sharp 5 in. (12.7 cm) or Thwaites nailnipper (English pattern) $5^1/_8$in. (13 cm) (Nova Instruments)
1 nail chisel (Nova Instruments)
1 Volkmann sharp-spoon curette
2 wooden applicators with cotton wool
sterile gauze swabs.

2.4.5 Minor operations pack (Fig. 2.12)

1 pair Rampley sponge forceps $9^1/_2$in. (24.1 cm)
2 Mayo towel clips
3 Dunhill artery forceps 5 in. (12.7 cm)
3 Halstead mosquito forceps straight 5 in. (12.7 cm)
3 Halstead mosquito forceps curved 5 in. (12.7 cm)
2 Allis tissue forceps 6 in. (15.2 cm)
1 McDonald's dissector

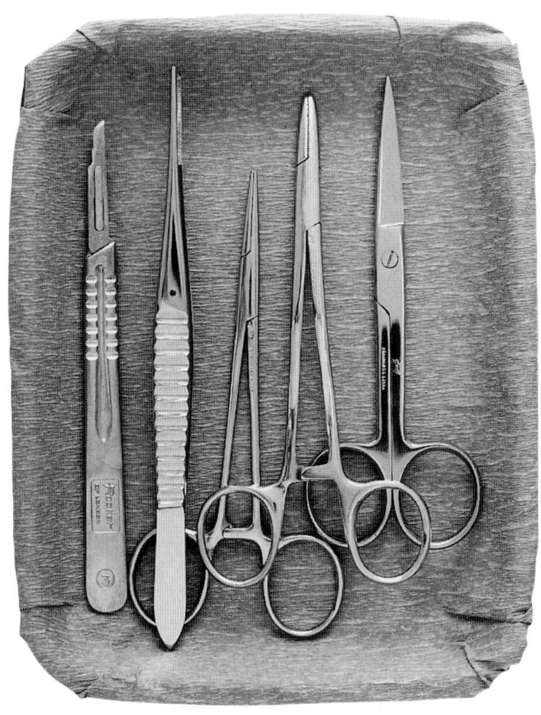

Fig. 2.10 Basic instrument set, ready for autoclaving (Rocket of London Ltd).

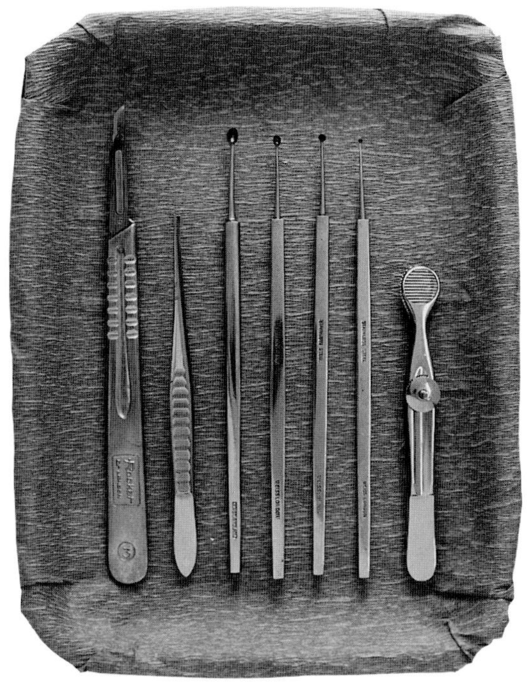

Fig. 2.11 Meibomian cyst pack, ready for autoclaving (Rocket of London Ltd).

1 McIndoe dissecting forceps 6 in. (15.2 cm)
1 Gillies dissecting forceps 6 in. (15.2 cm)
1 McIndoe's scissors, curved 7 in. (17.8 cm)
1 Mayo scissors straight $5^1/_2$ in. (14 cm)
2 Gillies skin hooks
2 Kilner, double-ended retractors
1 Volkmann scoop
1 Kilner needle holder
1 scalpel handle size 3
scalpel blades 10 and 15
sterile drapes, gauze swabs,
1 sterile Prolene suture. Ref. Ethicon W 8020T (1.5 metric) with curved cutting needle 26mm.

Certain manufacturers make comprehensive instrument packs in stainless steel containers ready for immediate autoclaving (Fig. 2.13).

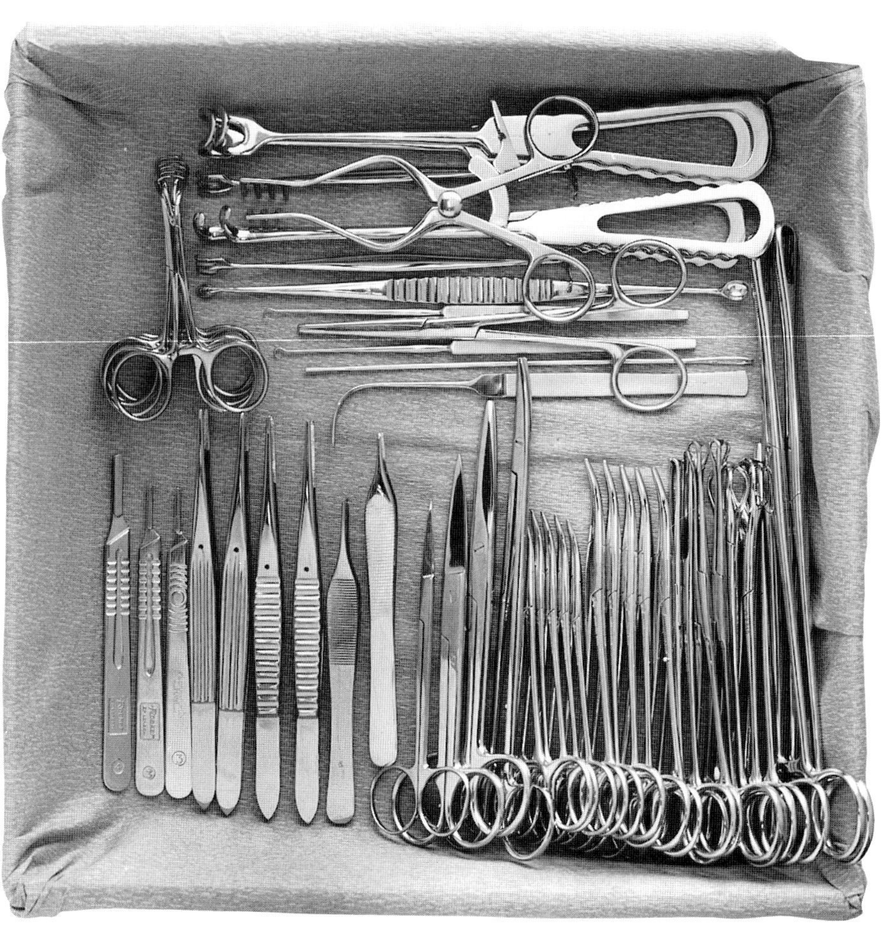

Fig. 2.12 A comprehensive minor operation set of instruments, in tray, ready for autoclaving (Rocket of London Ltd).

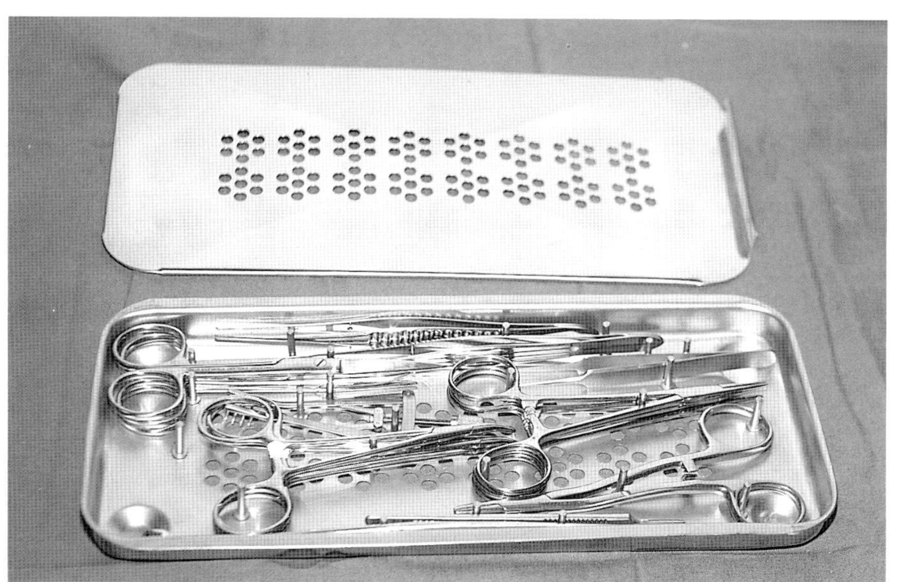

Fig. 2.13 General minor surgical set in stainless steel case which may be autoclaved for immediate use (Chas Thackray Ltd).

3

The minor operating theatre

There are two kinds of light, the common and the artificial – the common is not at our disposal – the artificial is at our disposal

Hippocrates, 460–377 BC

The physical dimensions of the treatment room will ultimately decide what equipment can be accommodated, thus the smallest room compatible with reasonable operating conditions would have a floor area of 140 square feet (13 square metres) and in most cases, the larger the room, the better the facilities. It should be emphasized that a separate operating room is not an essential prerequisite; indeed, many minor surgical procedures described in this book may be performed in the doctor's consulting room using the examination couch as an operating table, and an anglepoise lamp fitted with a reflecting spotlight as the source of illumination. Where presterilized instrument packs are used, the standard of asepsis can be extremely high.

However, there is no doubt that where a purpose-built treatment room is available, a much more satisfactory service can be offered to the patient; not only can all the instrument packs be assembled in readiness, but sterilizers, resuscitation equipment, trolleys, illumination and recovery facilities can also be prepared.

In general practice this room has the advantage that it can double as a nurse's treatment room, chiropody clinic, examination or recovery room, and immunization or family-planning clinic, so the maximum use can always be made of the facilities.

3.1 FIXTURES AND FITTINGS

Fitted cupboards and a good working surface are essential. Wall-mounted cupboards can be used if space is at a premium; these are used to store instrument packs, dressings, bandages, suture materials, equipment such as sphygmomanometers, electrocauteries, etc., as well as resuscitation equipment.

A glass-fronted instrument cupboard, although not essential, makes selection of instruments and drugs very much easier, and this too can be permanently fixed to the wall. One X-ray viewing box is a relatively inexpensive item and if not used for viewing X-ray films, can still be used for viewing colour transparencies. Sufficient hooks for coats should be provided and a separate clothes locker would be even better.

A good quality, stainless steel hand wash-basin is essential, with hot and cold running water, preferably with an elbow operated mixer tap, and an antiseptic/soap dispenser fitted above. Waste disposal is usually by means of bins with plastic liners (Figs 3.1, 3.2 and 3.3).

Disposable paper hand towels and paper sheets are becoming more popular. Several of the large paper manufacturers produce wall-mounted dispensers and holders for the rolls of paper; likewise disposal bags and

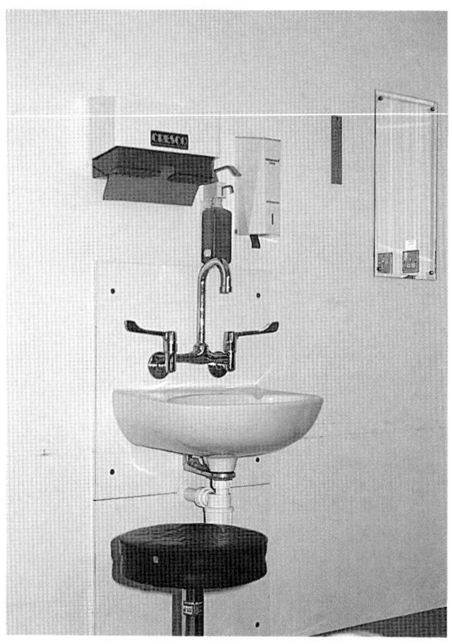

Fig. 3.1 Elbow-operated mixer-taps help to avoid cross-infection.

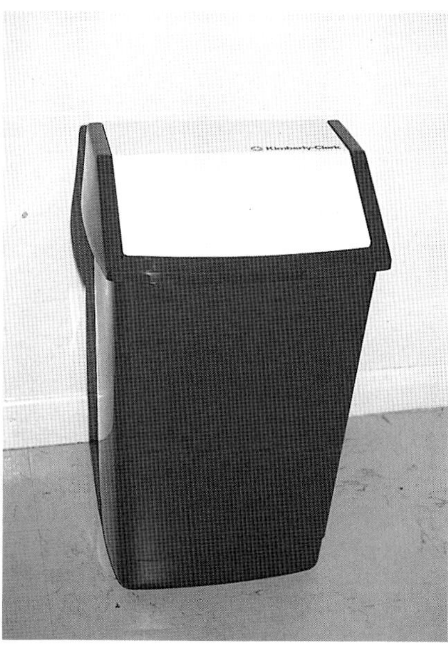

Fig. 3.2 A large waste-bin with disposable bin-liners is very useful (Kimberley-Clark).

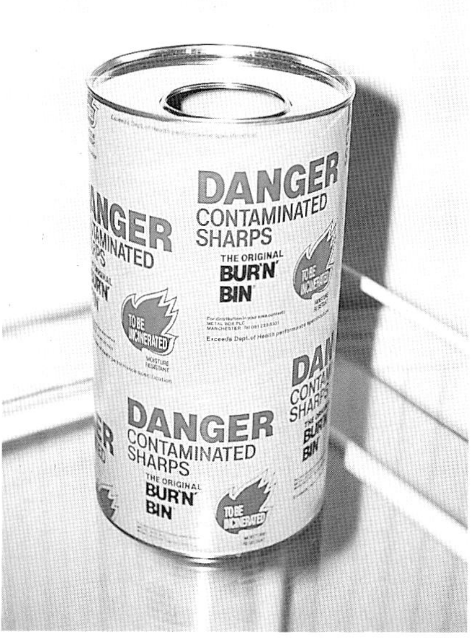

Fig. 3.3 A separate container is necessary for all needles, broken glass, and 'sharps'.

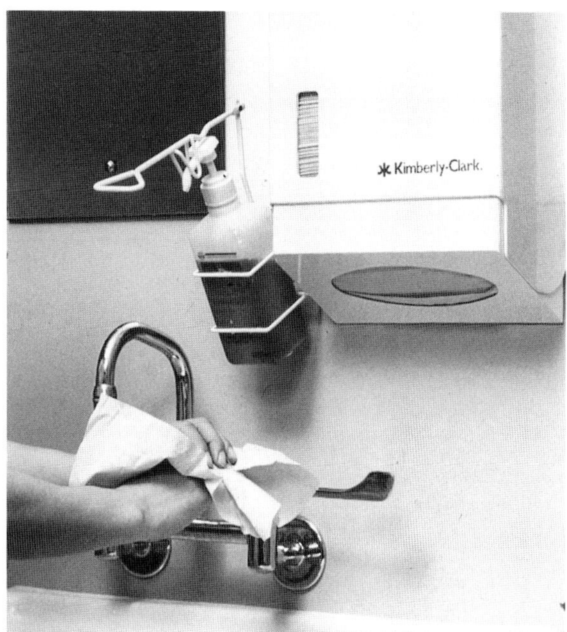

Fig. 3.4 Paper hand-towels: economical and hygienic (Kimberley-Clark).

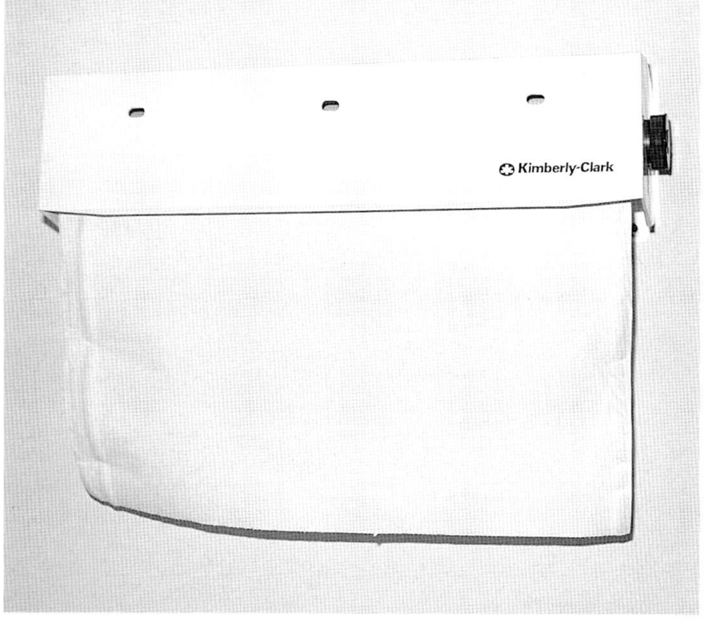

Fig. 3.5 The wider paper towelling is useful for couches and covering the operating theatre table (Kimberley-Clark).

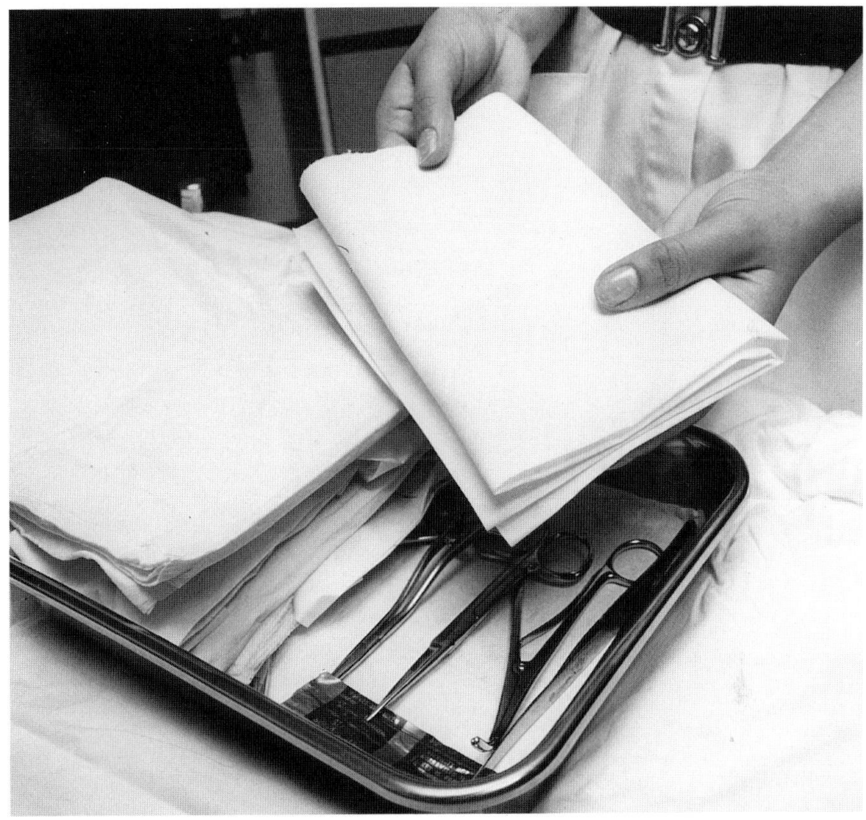

Fig. 3.6 Paper dressing-towels may also be included in CSSD instrument packs (Kimberley-Clark).

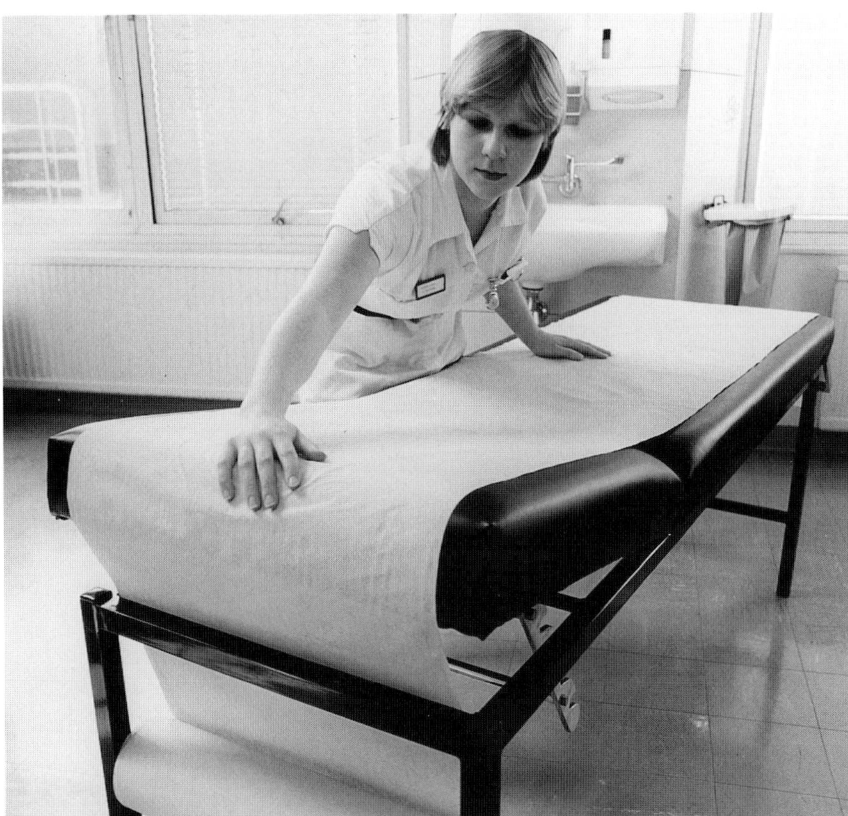

Fig. 3.7 Paper towelling being used to cover examination couch and operating area (Kimberley-Clark).

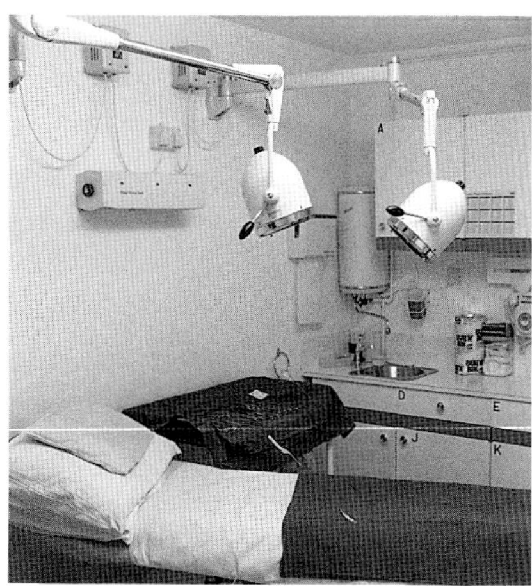

Fig. 3.8 Wall-mounted spotlights are ideal for most minor surgical procedures.

stands are made by the same firms. The large disposable sheets are excellent for placing on the operating theatre table underneath the patient, for protecting pillows, and for covering trolley shelves (Figs 3.4, 3.5, 3.6 and 3.7). Sufficient electric power sockets should be fitted, and a minimum of eight outlets provided.

Background illumination may be provided by fluorescent strip lighting which will complement natural light from windows. An extractor fan is not a luxury – there are many procedures such as opening perineal abscesses, sigmoidoscopy, and the use of electrocautery where a rapid change of air is desirable; because of this it is better to choose an extractor fan one or two sizes larger than recommended by the manufacturers. Finally, included amongst the fixtures and fittings is a small dangerous-drugs cupboard or drawer; this is recommended as some surgical procedures may require a premedication injection of such drugs as midazolam (Hypnovel) and fentanyl (Sublimaze).

3.2 THE OPERATING THEATRE TABLE

The most important item in any minor operating room is the table (Fig. 3.9) or couch for the patient. New operating theatre tables are expensive for the average practitioner, but by contacting local hospitals and clinics, a secondhand table may be found which will be more than adequate for minor surgery. The ability to raise and lower the patient, and, in particular, to be able to put the patient in the head-down position and elevate the lower limbs is a decided advantage over the fixed examination-couch type tables, and where possible it is worth waiting until a second-hand theatre table becomes available.

Having acquired the table, certain simple accessories such as an arm rest or lithotomy stirrups can be obtained and greatly increase the scope of the operations to be performed. Where space is restricted, a small Mayo-type tray which fixes to the side of the operating theatre table is a useful

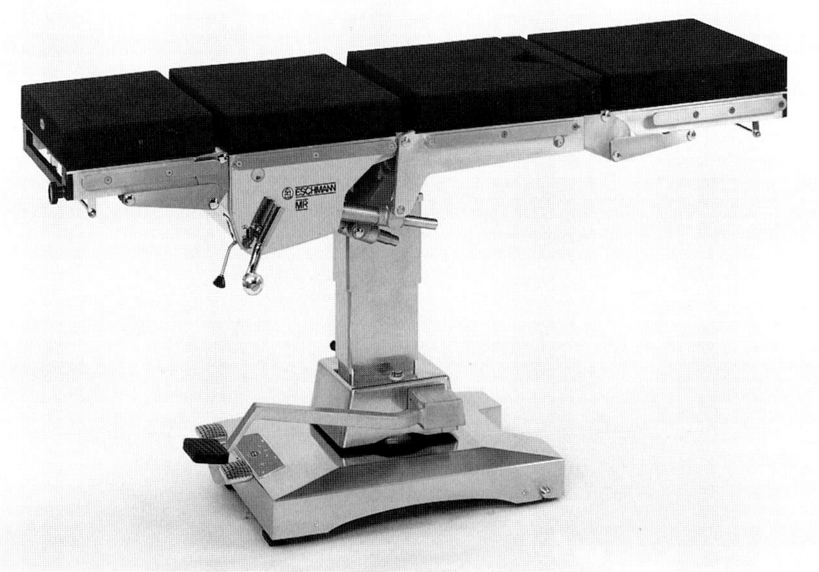

Fig. 3.9 Operating theatre table.

addition which can be recommended. One or two instrument trolleys should be purchased: preferably glass topped or stainless steel. Instruments for any operation may then be prepared in advance and the trolley brought to the patient for the operation. Again, new trolleys need not be felt to be essential as many very good second-hand ones can be found in most hospitals – perhaps needing slight repairs such as welding or repainting.

One operator's stool, adjustable in height, is needed; most minor operations can be readily performed with the patient lying down and the operator standing, but where any intricate surgery is being done, a comfortable stool for the surgeon makes the task easier.

As many minor operations are performed on the lower limbs, a chiropodist's chair for the patient would be a great help – as they are fairly bulky however, a large treatment room would be necessary.

3.3 ILLUMINATION

As previously mentioned, it is worth spending more on a good quality operating spotlight. For superficial minor surgical procedures, it is not necessary to install the large shadowless main operating theatre lights, but one or two good quality low-voltage spotlights are essential, preferably mounted permanently to the wall or ceiling (Figs 3.8 and 3.10). Most are now fitted with a plastic heat filter, tinted to give a more natural wavelength of light – many also have adjustable focus. Low-voltage (24 V) bulbs are preferred, especially the quartz halogen lamps, but each will need a special step-down transformer or rechargeable battery which needs to be fitted separately (Fig. 3.11).

In recent years, circular fluorescent lights surrounding a central 5 in. (12.7 cm) convex lens have been introduced, and these give excellent illumination coupled with magnification, particularly valuable for eye surgery and intricate hand surgery. There are several firms who make such lights, and each will provide lenses of different (or even combined) magnifications

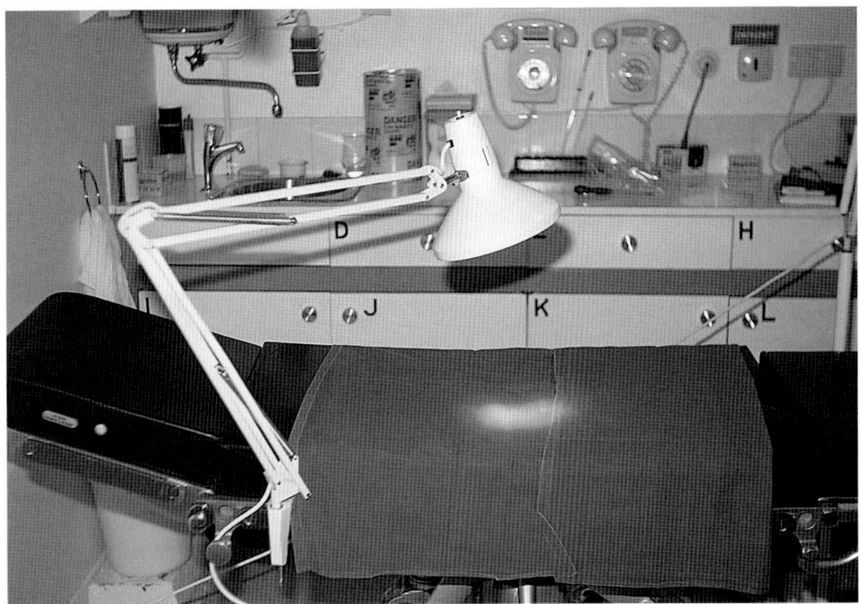

Fig. 3.10 Anglepoise-type spotlights are adequate where space is restricted, and give very good illumination (Ledu Lamps).

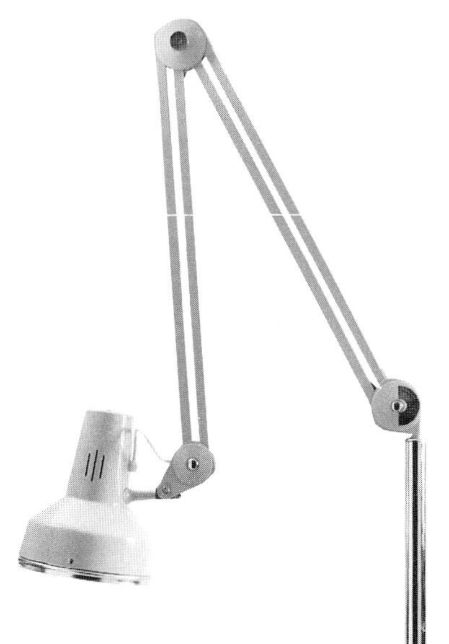

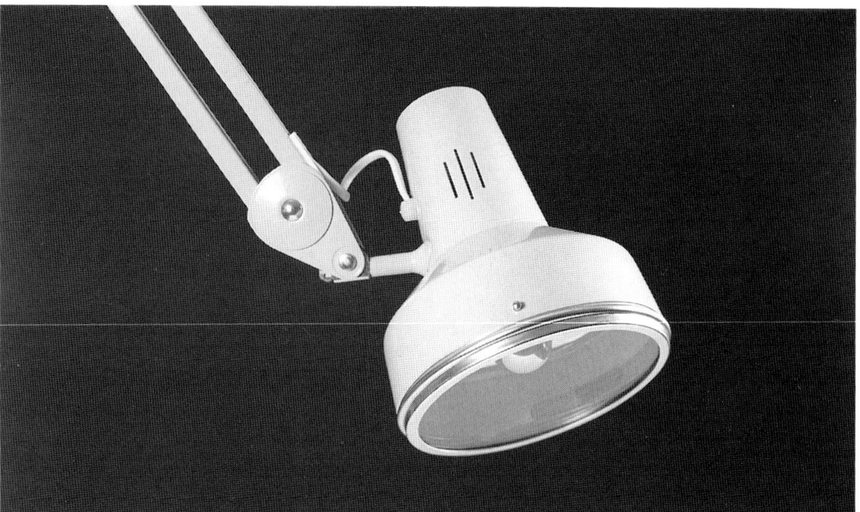

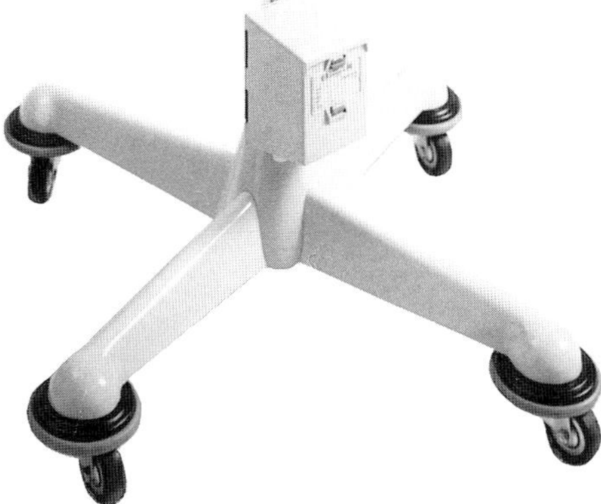

Fig. 3.11 A useful spotlight using low-voltage reflector bulb; may be wall or ceiling mounted or on castors.

depending on the needs of the operator (Fig. 3.12). These lights have the added advantages that no heat is generated, the light wavelength approximates to natural daylight, and they are light and manoeuvrable. Their only disadvantage is that they have to be interspersed between the patient and operator; and, where short focal length lenses are used, there is a risk of the operator's hands and instruments accidentally touching the under-surface of the unit.

Small head-mounted spotlights are favoured by some surgeons; the source of illumination may be a tungsten filament bulb or quartz halogen bulb mounted behind a convex lens, or a fibre-optic transmission system from a light source adjacent to the operator. Although giving good illumination, particularly inside cavities, they have the disadvantage that the operator is connected to batteries, transformer or light source and is not able to move about freely.

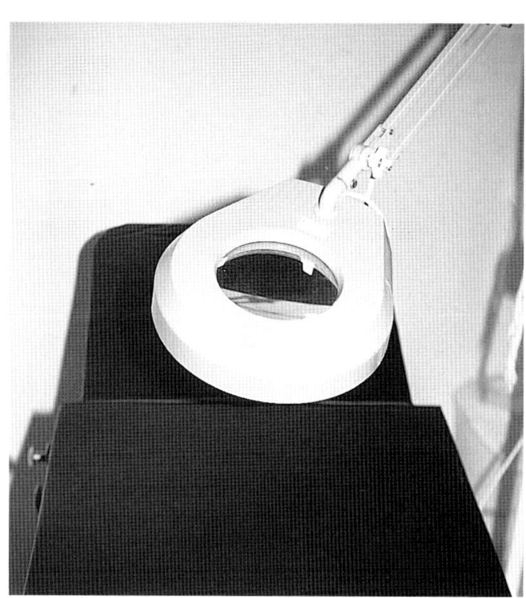

Fig. 3.12 Fluorescent circular magnifying light; extremely valuable for fine work e.g. eyes and removing splinters.

3.4 THE ELECTROCAUTERY

One of the most useful instruments for minor surgical procedures is the electrocautery: it consists essentially of a platinum wire which can be heated to red heat by means of an electric current (Figs 3.13, 3.14, 3.15 and 3.16) .

Application of the red hot wire to tissues will either cut them or seal any bleeding points by coagulation. It is thus ideal for removing small skin tags and papillomata, and for controlling the bleeding following curetting warts, granulomas, and similar lesions.

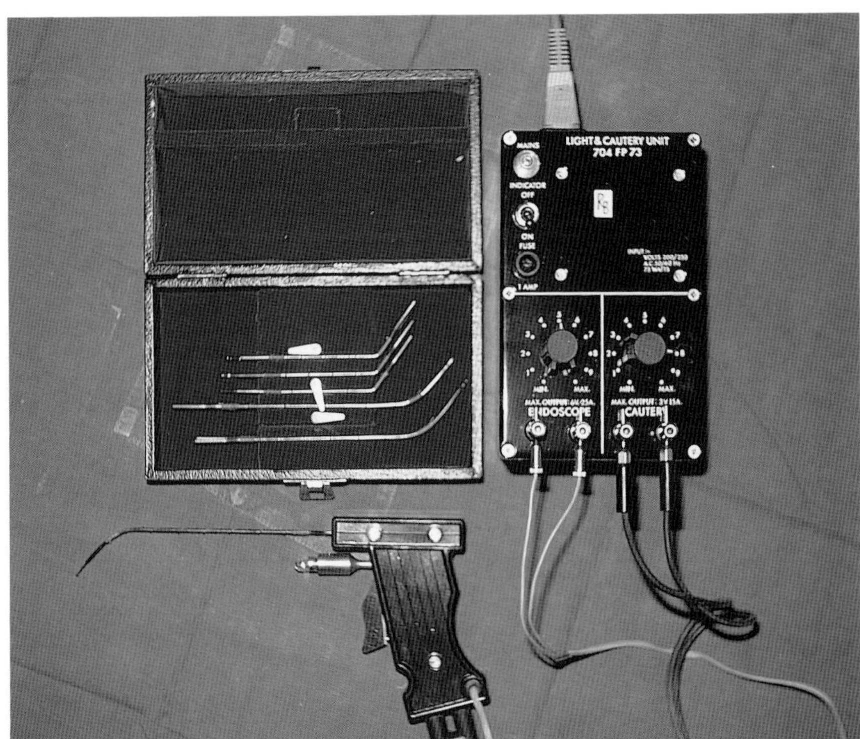

Fig. 3.13 Electrocautery transformer and selection of burners (Rimmer Bros Ltd).

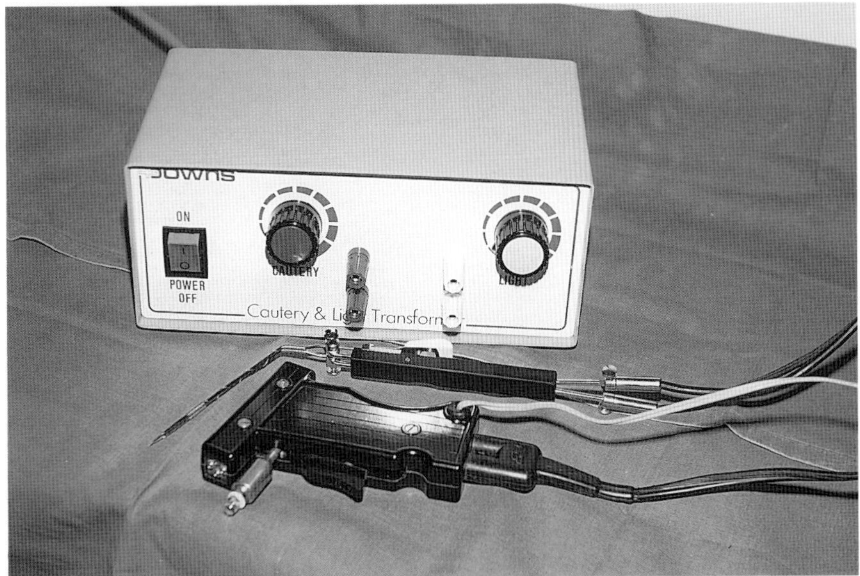

Fig. 3.14 Alternative electrocautery transformer with pistol-grip handle (Down Bros).

The earliest electrocauteries used a standard battery, and rheostat to control the temperature of the tip; subsequently with the change in domestic electricity supplies from direct current (DC) to alternating current (AC) it was possible to use step-down transformers and rheostats as

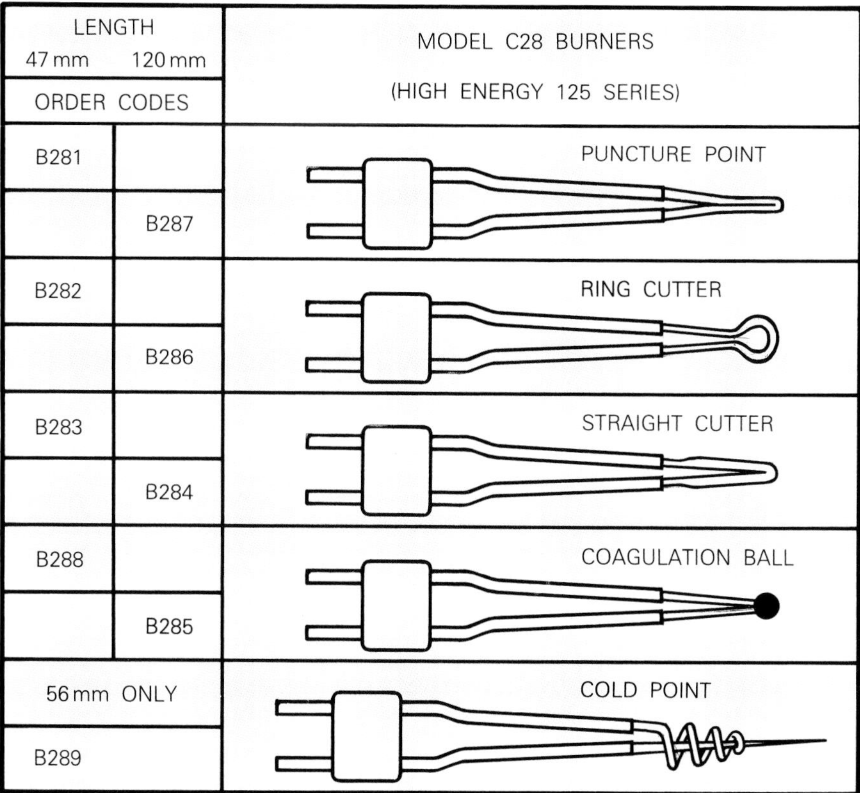

LENGTH 47 mm	120 mm	MODEL C28 BURNERS (HIGH ENERGY 125 SERIES)
ORDER CODES		
B281		PUNCTURE POINT
	B287	
B282		RING CUTTER
	B286	
B283		STRAIGHT CUTTER
	B284	
B288		COAGULATION BALL
	B285	
56 mm ONLY		COLD POINT
B289		

Fig. 3.15 A selection of the five most useful cautery burners. For most minor surgery work the short 47-mm length is the easiest to handle. The longer (120 mm) are useful for gynaecological use.

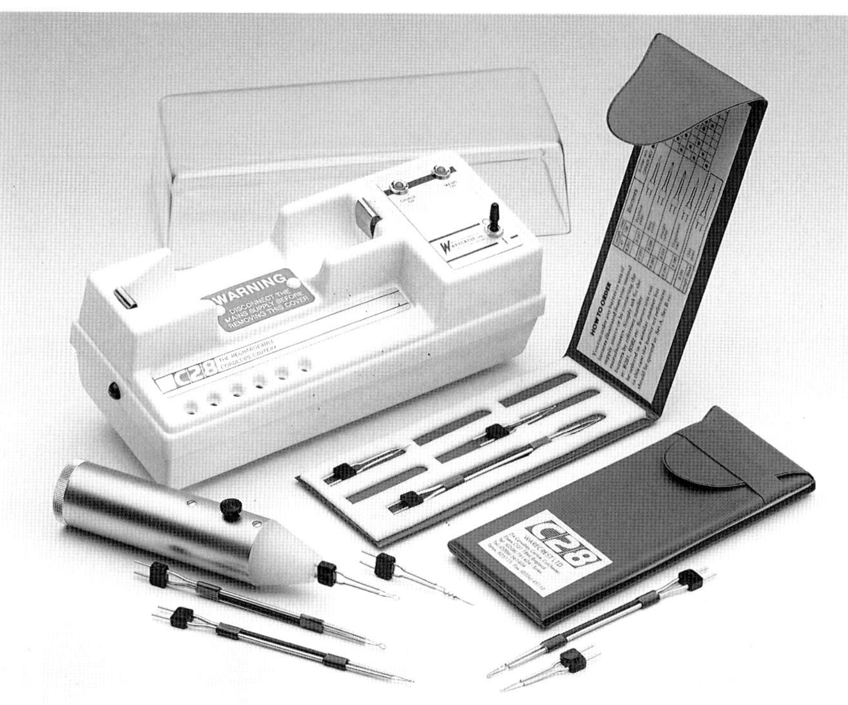

Fig. 3.16 The C28 rechargeable electrocautery: quick and simple to use (Warecrest Ltd).

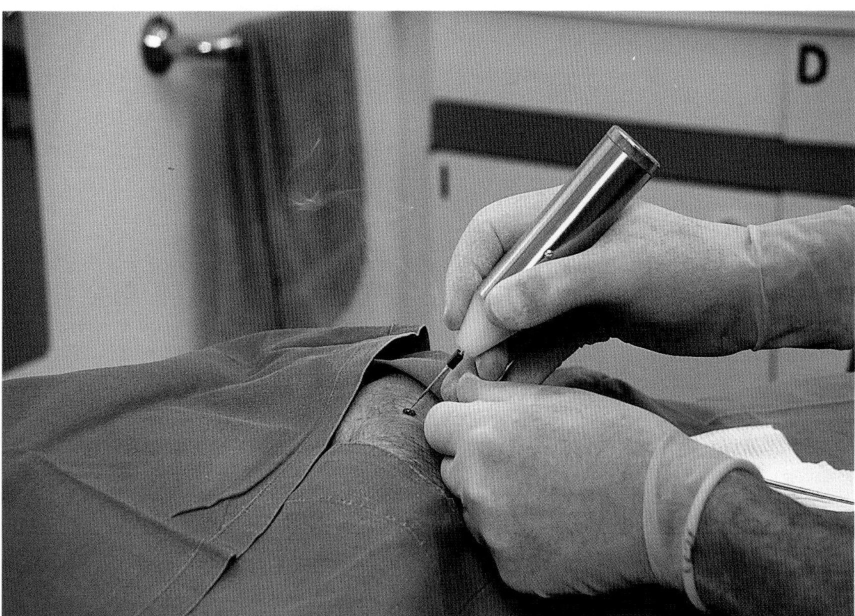

Fig. 3.17a The C28 cordless cautery in use (Warecrest Ltd).

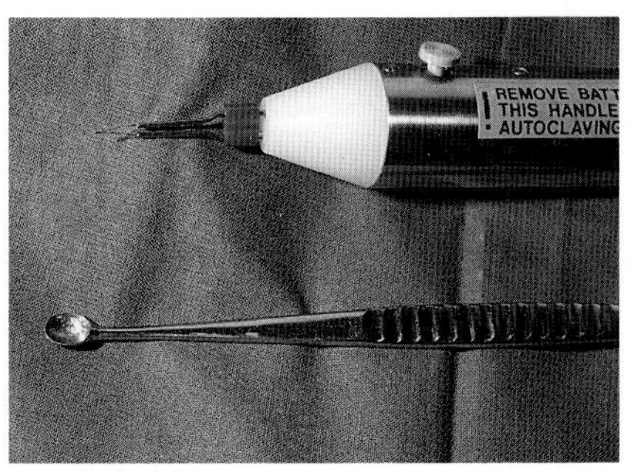

Fig. 3.17b Two of the most useful instruments for skin surgery: electrocautery and curette.

the source of current, with the great advantage that it avoided 'flat' batteries, provided the patient was within reach of a mains voltage socket.

More recently, with the introduction of nickel-cadmium rechargeable batteries with their ability to withstand high current drain without damage, several firms now produce portable rechargeable electrocauteries, with a variety of different burners (Fig. 3.17a, b).

One big advantage of the rechargeable cautery is the absence of long, trailing wires, and the fact that it can easily be carried between consulting rooms, or even to the patient's home for immediate use. The batteries may be kept on continuous low-current charge, and when fully charged will give one hundred or more burns before requiring recharging.

A variety of different shaped platinum burners is produced for different applications, some with a short and others with a long extension. In general the short burners give better control, and the most useful shapes are (Fig. 3.15):

1. Ball-ended burner – ideal for sealing some bleeding vessels and for destroying small superficial lesions.
2. Cutting electrodes (ring and straight) – suitable for dividing tissues. No force is needed – the heat of the tip does the cutting.
3. Small puncture electrode – suitable for releasing subungual haematomata, spider naevi, and dividing small papillomata.
4. 'Cold point' tip, consisting of a central firm needle-type electrode surrounded by a coil of platinum wire. Heat is transferred by conduction to the tip, which, as its name implies, does not reach such a high temperature as the platinum wire itself. The cold point burner is ideal for treating spider naevi and for releasing subungual haematomata.

All the burners will last many years with careful use, they do not corrode, and may be immediately sterilized merely by switching on the current and heating the tip to red heat for a few seconds.

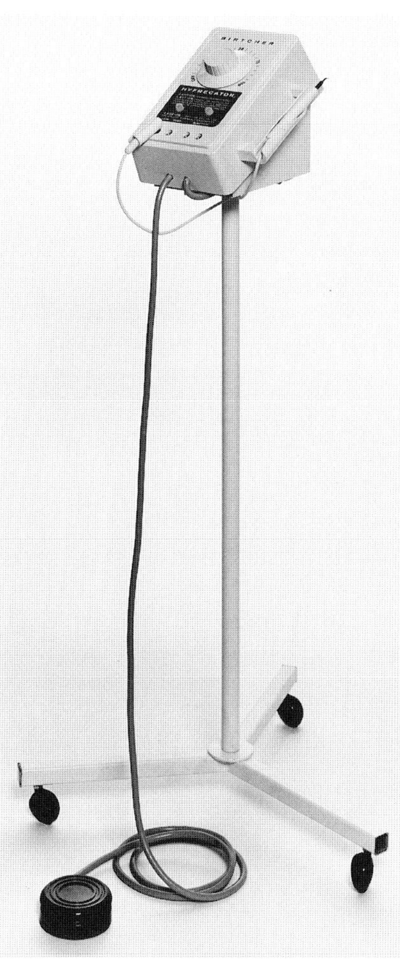

Fig. 3.18 The Birtcher Hyfrecator Model 733 on stand 708-1 (Birtcher Corporation, USA; Schuco International, London).

3.5 THE 'HYFRECATOR' OR UNIPOLAR DIATHERMY

Most surgeons will be familiar with the standard bipolar diathermy apparatus in use in most large operating theatres. In this, a very high-frequency current is passed through the patient's body and generates heat. By making one electrode relatively large and strapping it firmly to one limb, and by making the other electrode a pointed movable tip, sufficient heat is generated at the tip to coagulate or cut tissues. For major surgery such coagulating/cutting is standard practice, but the equipment is expensive, has to pass stringent tests for electrical safety, and is not really necessary or ideal for minor surgery.

One answer has been to produce the unipolar diathermy of 'Hyfrecator' (Fig. 3.18). This is a small, portable, instrument which by means of an adjustable spark gap or solid-state circuitry and transformer, produces a very high voltage and low current, sufficient to cause a spark to pass from the electrode tip to the patient without needing a second large pad electrode to complete the circuit. Three types of electrode are commonly used: the first is a fine wire electrode which may be inserted into the lesion to be destroyed. Passing a current through the tissues generates heat, which in turn coagulates the blood and cells; this 'desiccation' is particularly suitable for vascular haemangiomata. The second type of electrode is larger than the needle electrode, and is held a short distance away from the tissues; when the current is switched on, a stream of hot sparks passes between the patient and the electrode, and this is sufficient to destroy small areas of tissue. This technique is referred to as 'fulguration'. Thirdly, the Hyfrecator can be used for coagulation by using a double electrode which is connected to a lower voltage winding on the high-frequency transformer. By placing this double electrode on the surface to be treated and passing a slightly heavier current between the poles of the electrode, the underlying tissues are coagulated and destroyed.

The advantage of using the Hyfrecator is the absence of bleeding; its effect is very similar to that of the electrocautery, and the heat generated automatically sterilizes the area treated; a sterile dry dressing or no dressing at all is, therefore, all that is needed to promote healing. The disadvantage is that histological examination of the treated lesion is not usually possible due to the distortion of the cells from the heat; thus a preliminary biopsy needs to be done where the diagnosis is in doubt.

3.6 THE RADIO-SURGERY UNIT

Radio-surgery units (Fig. 3.19) use high-frequency electric currents (3.8 MHz) to both cut and coagulate tissues. There is much less tissue damage than with conventional electrocauteries and diathermy, and excellent cosmetic results can be obtained (Chapter 42). Cutting is by means of a fine-gauge needle or tungsten wire loop, and haemostasis by a ball-ended electrode. The instruments are small, portable and inexpensive. Where radio-surgery is used regularly, a Vapor-Vac smoke extraction unit is advisable as plumes of smoke are generated. Unlike the electrocautery, the electrode remains cold throughout the surgical procedure. No pressure is needed, and the surgeon needs to learn a completely new technique to use this equipment.

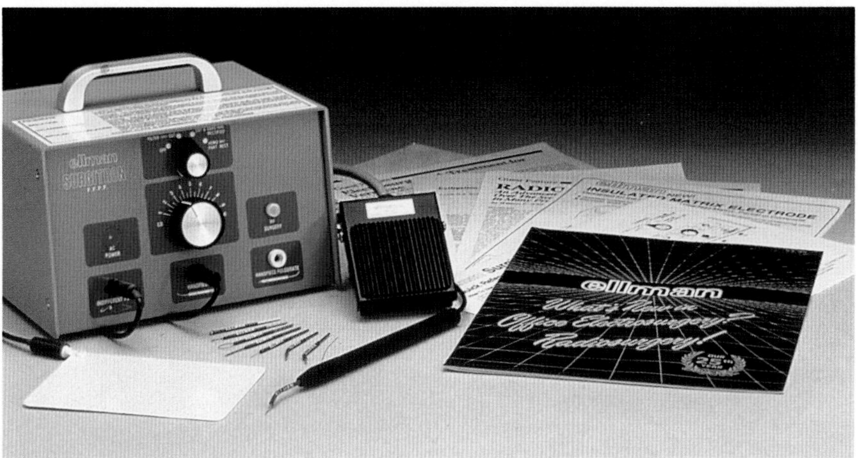

Fig. 3.19 The Ellman Surgitron FFPF radio-surgical instrument with footswitch assembly, Surgitron hand-piece, coated passive antenna and electrodes (Ellman International Inc. Hewlett, USA).

3.7 RESUSCITATION FACILITIES

Every doctor's surgery should possess some form of simple resuscitation equipment. Because patients suffering from a variety of diseases are constantly passing through the premises, sooner or later one will collapse with a myocardial infarction, major epileptic convulsion, cardiac arrest, simple haemorrhage or just a vasovagal 'faint'. Where any form of treatment is being offered, be it one hypodermic injection or minor surgical procedure, the practitioner must be prepared for the patient who will faint, or suffer an unexpected allergic reaction to the treatment. Should a patient 'collapse' on the premises the first prerequisite is a room or area sufficiently large to be able to allow the patient to lie on the floor with sufficient space around him or her for equipment, doctors, and assistants. The second requirement is the management of the unconscious patient – to maintain an airway and circulation, to prevent the inhalation of secretions or vomit, to establish a diagnosis, and render treatment.

Fortunately the majority of 'attacks' will be vasovagal, all of which will be expected to recover rapidly once the patient is lying flat, with or without elevation of the legs to assist venous return to the heart.

A clear resuscitation sheet, based on the first-aid manuals [3], supplemented with additional information for cardiac arrest and anaphylactic reactions should be on a wall in the treatment room for all staff to see.

Resuscitation equipment should comprise syringes and needles, a selection of drugs to be administered including diazepam, benzodiazepine antagonists (Anexate, flumazenil), morphine, adrenaline, lignocaine, atropine, verapamil, plasma expanders and hydrocortisone, together with intravenous cannulae, intravenous giving sets, bandages, and adhesive plasters. Simple disposable airways are valuable, and an Ambu type positive-pressure resuscitator is worth having. Where funds permit, and particularly where regular surgery sessions are undertaken, additional resuscitation equipment such as electric suction, ECG machines, oxygen giving sets, and cardiac defibrillators are a good idea even though the need for any of them hardly ever arises. In general practice it would be difficult to justify the purchase of such items as cardiac defibrillators, but it is the type of equipment often donated by charitable organizations or groups of patients, and

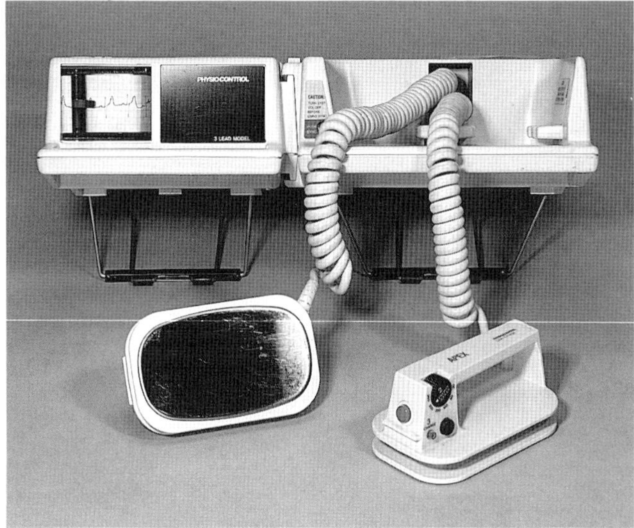

Fig. 3.20a Resuscitation equipment should always be available. This shows combined cardiac monitor and cardiac defibrillator (Physio Lifepak 5).

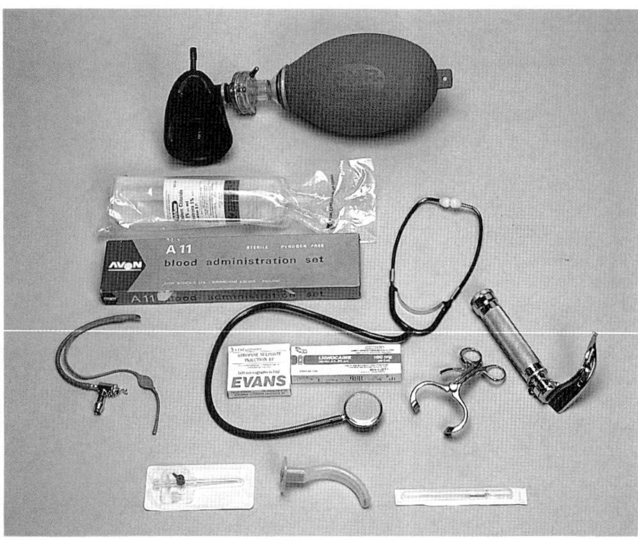

Fig. 3.20b Contents of simple resuscitation box. Main drugs, syringes, etc. kept separately.

Fig. 3.21 Portable resuscitation kits have the added advantage that they can be taken to the patient's home in addition to use at the surgery.

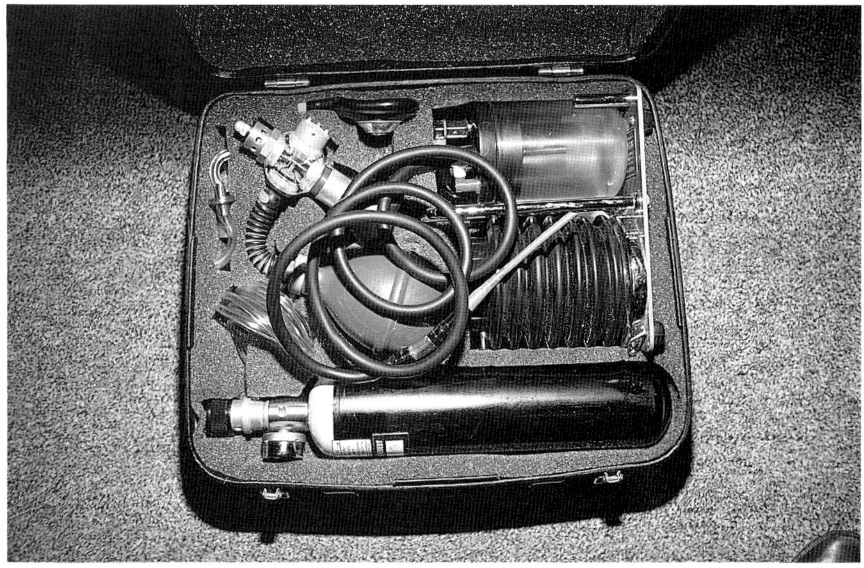

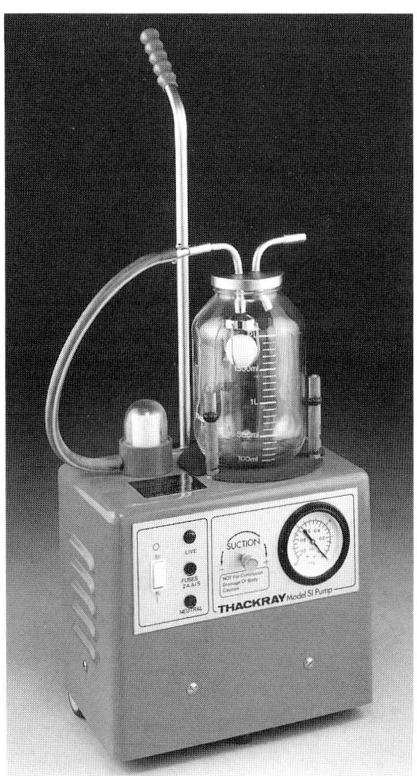

Fig. 3.22 Adequate suction equipment is valuable (Chas F. Thackray).

the possession of more sophisticated types of resuscitation equipment greatly adds to the practitioner's (and patient's!) peace of mind (Figs 3.20, 3.21 and 3.22).

3.8 STERILIZERS

Some means of sterilizing or disinfecting instruments and equipment should be included in the minor operating theatre. In recent years there has been a trend towards CSSD (Central Sterile Supplies Department) packs, where the instruments are cleaned, prepared and packed at a central sterilizing department, autoclaved in sealed paper envelopes, and delivered

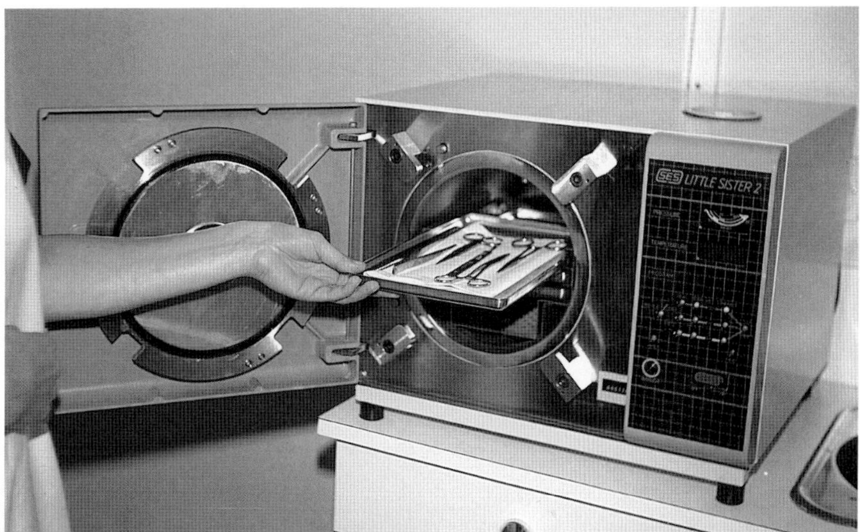

Fig. 3.23 Instruments being loaded into 'Little Sister Mk II' autoclave.

to the treatment room or surgery. Where such an arrangement can be made by the practitioner, this is ideal; every instrument is guaranteed to be sterile, together with all dressings, drapes, towels and gowns which are included in the pack. Where CSSD facilities do not exist, alternative methods can be employed.

Traditionally, the method of disinfecting instruments was by boiling in water for 5 min; bacterial spores and viruses may not be destroyed and thus the term sterilization should not strictly be employed. Most hot water disinfectors have a variable heat control indicator light and thermostat together with trays to hold instruments. Alternatively, a dry heat oven may be employed, heating the instruments to 160°C (320°F) for 1 hour; this is better than boiling, but has the disadvantage that plastics, paper drapes and dressings tend to be damaged. Where heat cannot be used for certain instruments such as fibre-optic cables, and endoscopes, soaking in a solution of glutaraldehyde is acceptable.

Perhaps the most efficient method of sterilizing instruments in a small treatment room is by using a small portable autoclave (Fig. 3.23). These utilize the same principle as the larger hospital equipment, viz. steam under pressure resulting in temperatures of 136°C (277°F) under a pressure of 30 lbf/in^2 (207 kN/m^2) for 2.5 min. This destroys all known organisms and can be used for most instruments. However, it has the disadvantage that instruments cannot be packed with dressings and drapes inside a sealed paper envelope as the smaller machines do not have a vacuum cycle to extract all the air.

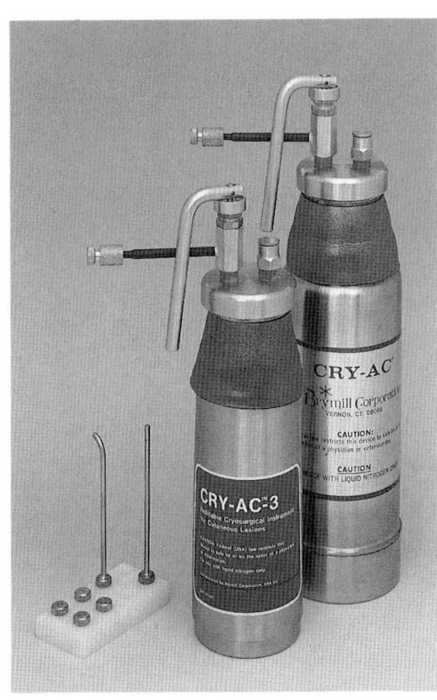

Fig. 3.24 Liquid nitrogen cryosurgical equipment: may be used either as cryoprobe or cryospray.

3.9 THE CRYOPROBE

In recent years there has been a renewed interest in cryotherapy where superficial lesions are destroyed by freezing. The common cryogens are carbon dioxide, nitrous oxide, and liquid nitrogen. The carbon dioxide and nitrous oxide equipment may be kept on the premises for immediate use. Liquid nitrogen, on the other hand, gives better results for many skin lesions, but some means of storage in a vacuum flask has to be arranged, and where this is not available, small quantities of liquid nitrogen need to be collected in advance. This has the slight disadvantage that patients need to be booked in advance for a 'session' (Fig. 3.24).

3.10 USE OF ENTONOX

An Entonox giving set is a very useful additional piece or equipment for any minor operating theatre. Originally designed for the relief of pain during labour, the equipment may be used for both adults and children in uncomfortable or painful procedures. Consciousness is not lost, the gas is self-administered, and recovery is rapid (Fig. 3.25).

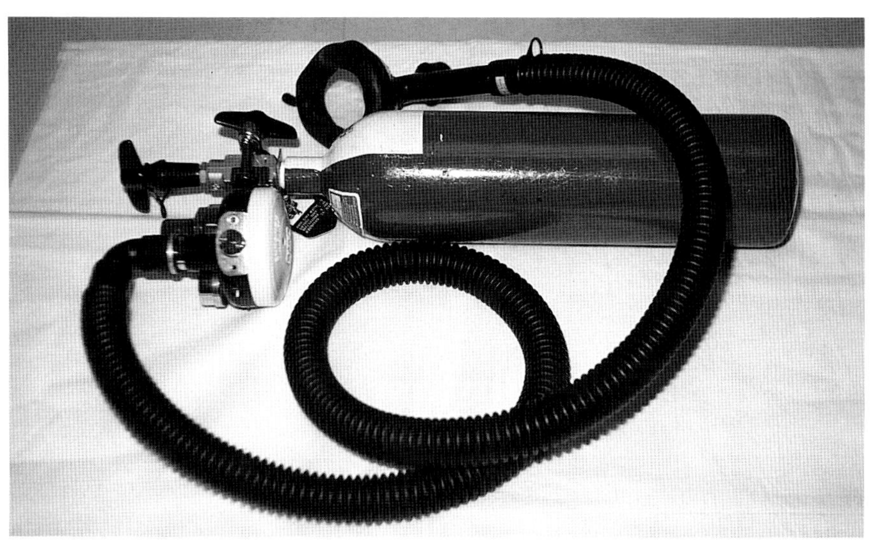

Fig. 3.25 Entonox (50:50 nitrous oxide : oxygen) is valuable for pain relief for procedures such as incision of abscesses, injections, and painful dressings.

3.11 DISINFECTANT DISPENSERS

Surgical scrub solutions are recommended for routine washing and hand-scrubbing prior to each operation; the two most commonly used agents being Hibiscrub (chlorhexidine gluconate 4% in detergent base) and Betadine surgical scrub (povidone-iodine 7.5% in detergent base). Each is supplied in a standard container which may be affixed to a wall-mounted dispenser, usually provided free of charge by the manufacturers.

3.12 SYRINGES AND NEEDLES

Standard 1 ml, 2 ml, 5 ml, 10 ml and 20 ml syringes with Luer fittings are needed for local anaesthetics, intravenous drugs, and for sclerotherapy of varicose veins. Three standard size Luer fitting needles are recommended 25 swg × 5/8 in. (0.5 mm × 16 mm), 23 swg × 1 in. (0.6 mm ×25 mm) and 21 swg × 1 1/2 in. (0.8 mm × 40 mm). In addition a standard dental syringe and 30 swg × 3/4 in. (0.3 mm × 19 mm) needle will be found to be invaluable for giving local anaesthetics in fingers and toes, and particularly for children. Dental cartridges of local anaesthetic can be quickly inserted in the syringe, and as nearly a painless injection as is possible can be made.

3.13 TOURNIQUETS

Where a bloodless operating field is required such as for ingrowing toe-nails, excision of ganglia, removal of foreign bodies, or exploration, a tourniquet is required. For fingers and toes, this need only be a length of rubber tubing, rubber strip, a wide rubber band, or even a surgical rubber glove with the tip cut off and rolled down the digit. However, for a whole limb, a proper orthopaedic tourniquet should be used (Fig. 3.26).

Fig. 3.26 Orthopaedic pneumatic tourniquet; this is better than a blood-pressure sphygmomanometer cuff if intravenous regional anaesthesia is undertaken.

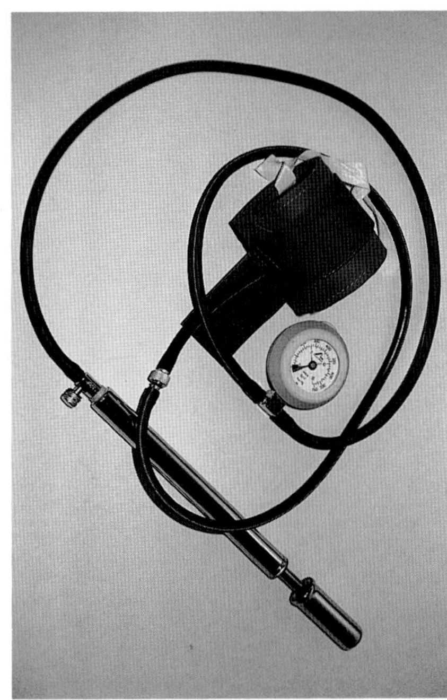

3.14 'SHARPS' CONTAINERS

Needles, broken glass ampoules and other 'sharps' need to be disposed of safely. They should be placed in a cardboard or plastic receptacle such as a 'burn-bin', which is subsequently incinerated (Fig. 3.3).

3.15 CLINICAL WASTE DISPOSAL

Blood-stained and contaminated dressings and paper drapes can be collected in plastic bin liners for eventual disposal by incineration (Fig. 3.2). Most local authorities provide special clinical waste disposal sacks and arrange for regular collection.

3.16 HOT-AIR HAND DRIERS

Unless the doctor uses separate sterile paper towels with each instrument pack, there is a possible risk of cross-infection and contamination from hand towels.

A simple method for drying hands after washing is to use an electric wall-mounted hot-air hand drier. A slight disadvantage is the noise, and a small risk of airborne droplet infection.

3.17 ALTERNATIVE LAYOUTS FOR MINOR OPERATING THEATRES

Where new premises are being designed, and where there are sufficient funds and space available, much improved minor operating facilities may be considered. There is much to commend dividing the total floor area into three separate areas, namely:

1. Administration and counselling
2. Utility and preparation
3. Treatment.

This division provides extra comfort for the patient, relatives and nurses, allows all the paperwork to be done away from the treatment area, allows more than one patient to be treated simultaneously, allows instruments and trolleys for the next case to be prepared outside the main treatment room area, and reduces risks of cross-infection (Fig. 3.27).

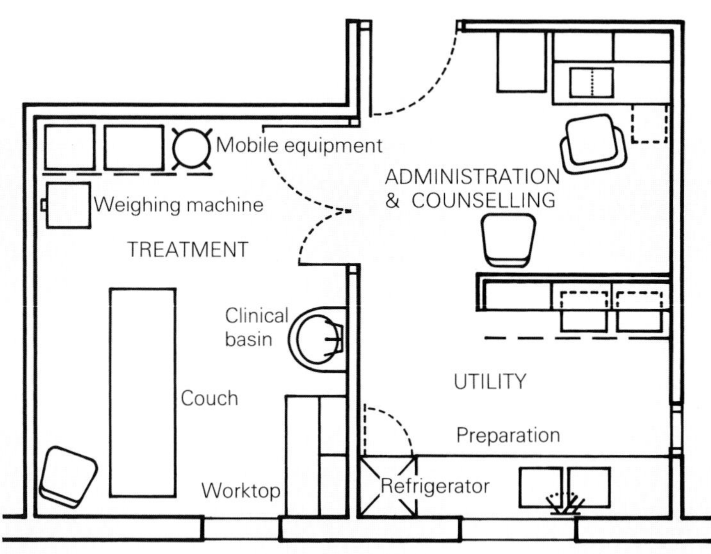

Fig. 3.27 Where space permits, improved minor surgery facilities may be offered by dividing the space into three separate areas as shown.

3.18 FIRST-AID BOX

It is often forgotten that, under the Health and Safety (First Aid) Regulations 1981, even doctors' surgeries need to have first-aid provisions. There should be a nominal appointed person to take charge of any accident, to ensure that it is reported and recorded, and a simple first-aid box installed in the building. It is not a good idea to rely on treatment room first-aid supplies.

The first-aid box should contain:

1. A guidance card on resuscitation
2. Individually wrapped sterile adhesive dressings
3. Triangular bandages
4. Medium-sized sterile wound dressings
5. Large sterile wound dressing
6. Safety pins
7. Sterile eye-pads and bandages.

First-aid boxes should not contain medications of any kind.

3.19 COMPARISON OF DIFFERENT INSTRUMENTS

There are now several instruments on the market which offer to treat skin lesions successfully – cryosurgery, electrocautery, hyfrecation and radiosurgery (plus laser for those who can afford it) – and it can be quite difficult for a practitioner to decide which instrument will be the best for his or her situation (Tables 3.1 and 3.2).

3.19.1 Cryosurgery

Liquid nitrogen will treat most superficial skin lesions including viral warts. Results are good, cryobiopsies can be obtained for histology, there is minimal scarring and most treatments are given without prior anaesthesia, although it can be quite painful and unacceptable to young children. More than one treatment may need to be given and supplies of liquid nitrogen need to be available easily. Maintenance costs are minimal and running costs are just the cost of the liquid nitrogen. It is very portable and may be taken to the patient's home.

Table 3.1 Comparison of cryotherapy, electrocautery, diathermy and radio-surgery and the different characteristics of each

Characteristic	*Cryosurgery*	*Cautery*	*Hyfrecator*	*Radio-surgery*	*Scalpel*
Cutting	No	Yes	No	Yes	Yes
Control of bleeding	No	Yes	Yes	Yes	No
Ability to obtain biopsies	Yes	Yes	No	Yes	Yes
Self-sterilizing	No	Yes	No	Yes	No
Production of sterilized cut	No	Yes	No	Yes	No
Healing time	Same	Same	Same	Same	Same
Production of scar tissue	No	Yes	Little	No	Yes
Ability to plane soft tissue	No	No	No	Yes	No
Portability	Yes	Yes	Yes	Yes	Yes
Initial costs	+++	++	+++	++++	+
Running costs	+	+	+	++	+
Need for local anaesthesia	No	Yes	Yes	Yes	Yes

Table 3.2 Comparison of cryotherapy, electrocautery, diathermy and radio-surgery in the treatment of different skin lesions

Uses	*Cryosurgery*	*Cautery*	*Hyfrecator*	*Radio-surgery*	*Scalpel*
Intradermal naevi	Yes	Yes	Yes	Yes	Yes
Spider veins	No	Yes	Yes	Yes	No
Viral warts	Yes	Yes	Yes	Yes	Rarely
Ingrowing toe-nails	Some	No	Some	Yes	Yes
Keratoses	Yes	Yes	Yes	Yes	Yes
Basal cell carcinoma	Yes	Yes	Yes	Yes	Yes
Skin tags	Some	Yes	Some	Yes	Yes
Kerato-acanthoma	Yes	Yes	Yes	Yes	Yes
Molluscum contagiosum	Yes	Yes	Yes	Yes	No
Pyogenic granuloma	Some	Yes	Yes	Yes	No
Seborrhoeic warts	Yes	Yes	Yes	Yes	Yes
Cervical erosions	Yes	Yes	Yes	Yes	No

Characteristic	Cryosurgery	Cautery	Hyfrecator	Radio-surgery	Scalpel
Cutting	No	Yes	No	Yes	Yes
Control of bleeding	No	Yes	Yes	Yes	No
Ability to obtain biopsies	Yes	Yes	No	Yes	Yes
Self-sterilising	No	Yes	No	Yes	No
Production of sterilised cut	No	Yes	No	Yes	No
Healing time	Same	Same	Same	Same	Same
Production of scar tissue	No	Yes	Little	No	Yes
Ability to plane soft tissue	No	No	No	Yes	No
Portability	Yes	Yes	Yes	Yes	Yes
Intial costs	***	**	***	****	*
Running costs	*	*	*	**	*
Need for local anaesthesia	No	Yes	Yes	Yes	Yes

Comparison of different instruments for treating skin lesions.

Characteristic	Cryosurgery	Cautery	Hyfrecator	Radio-surgery	Scalpel
USES					
Intradermal naevi	Yes	Yes	Yes	Yes	Yes
Spider veins	No	Yes	Yes	Yes	No
Viral warts	Yes	Yes	Yes	Yes	Rarely
Ingrowing toe-nails	Some	No	Some	Yes	Yes
Keratoses	Yes	Yes	Yes	Yes	Yes
Basal cell carcinoma	Yes	Yes	Yes	Yes	Yes
Skin tags	Some	Yes	Some	Yes	Yes
Kerato-acanthoma	Yes	Yes	Yes	Yes	Yes
Molluscum contagiosum	Yes	Yes	Yes	Yes	No
Pyogenic granuloma	Some	Yes	Yes	Yes	No
Seborrhoeic warts	Yes	Yes	Yes	Yes	Yes
Cervical erosions	Yes	Yes	Yes	Yes	No

Uses of different instruments for the treatment of skin lesions.

3.19.2 Electrocautery

The small, hand-held, cordless rechargeable cautery is an ideal instrument to start minor surgery. It can both cut and coagulate, is immediately available and can be used for the removal of most skin lesions, either alone or with a curette or scalpel. Local anaesthesia is necessary for many lesions. Maintenance costs are minimal and, with care, the burners last for years. Running costs are also minimal – the cost of electricity to recharge the batteries – and one single rechargeable cell needs replacing after several years of use. It produces thermal damage to delicate tissues with some degree of scarring. Histological specimens may be obtained in most cases. It is very portable and may be taken to the patient's home. Burners are self-sterilizing. One disadvantage is the smell of burning and the use of an extractor fan is advisable.

3.19.3 Hyfrecator

Another very useful instrument which is ideal for treating all superficial skin lesions, including keratoses, angioma, warts, molluscum, Bowen's and basal cell carcinomata. Local anaesthesia is necessary for all but the smallest lesions. Thermal damage occurs with consequent mild scarring. The electrodes are not self-sterilizing. It is excellent for vascular lesions and for haemostasis and epilation. The disadvantages include difficulty in obtaining specimens for histology and the smell of burning, so a good extractor fan or vacuum extractor unit is advisable. Maintenance and running costs are minimal, consisting only of the occasional replacement of flexible leads. It is portable and may be taken to the patient's home.

3.19.4 Radio-surgery

This combines both cutting and coagulation. There is minimal thermal damage to tissues and excellent cosmetic results are achieved with virtually no scarring. Lesions may be 'planed' down to skin level. There is minimal postoperative pain with rapid healing. Local anaesthesia is needed for most lesions. Specimens may be obtained for histology. Electrodes are self-sterilizing. Maintenance costs are minimal – mainly the cost of replacing wire electrodes and flexible cables. Running costs are also minimal – just the cost of electricity used. The smell of burning is more pronounced than with electrocautery or diathermy so a good extractor fan and vacuum extractor unit is necessary. It is semi-portable so may be taken to the patient's home.

4

Care of instruments and equipment

> *The instruments, and when and how they should be prepared, so that they may not impede the work, and that there may be no difficulty in taking hold of them, with the part of the body which operates. But if another gives them, he must be ready a little beforehand and do as you direct.*
>
> *Hippocrates, 460–377* BC

Like all mechanical and electronic equipment, surgical instruments require regular care and maintenance to retain their efficiency and prolong their useful life. Dirty, rusty forceps are not only a potential source of infection, but look unsightly, are difficult to use, and ultimately break prematurely.

4.1 CARE OF STAINLESS STEEL

Stainless steel is the material of choice for most surgical instruments; it combines a high resistance to corrosion and rust with an attractive finish. Even under ideal conditions the finest stainless steel instruments can become pitted and stained, so great care is needed with washing and cleaning, polishing, and lubrication. Rough handling or the use of abrasives can permanently mark stainless steel, so initially all instruments after use should be cleaned with a hard brush under running cool water. Very hot water will cause coagulation of blood and exudate and make subsequent cleaning harder.

If use of an ultrasonic cleaning bath using instrument detergents is available, this will be ideal and restore a high polish to most instruments (Fig. 4.1).

After washing, instruments should be carefully dried to avoid water remaining in any joint and causing corrosion. Lubrication using a water-soluble lubricant is strongly to be recommended and will greatly prolong the useful life of any instrument.

Saline solutions are a major cause of pitting, and instruments should never be soaked in them, nor should a saline solution be allowed to dry on an instrument.

Whenever cleaning or washing instruments, keep all ratchets unlocked and box joints open, and similarly avoid using wire wool or abrasives, iodine, bromine, aluminium chloride, or barium chloride. The same advice applies to surgical blades and needles, both of which may rust and corrode more easily than stainless steel instruments.

Serrated surfaces on artery forceps and needle holders can be effectively cleaned with a small brass wire brush obtainable from shoe shops.

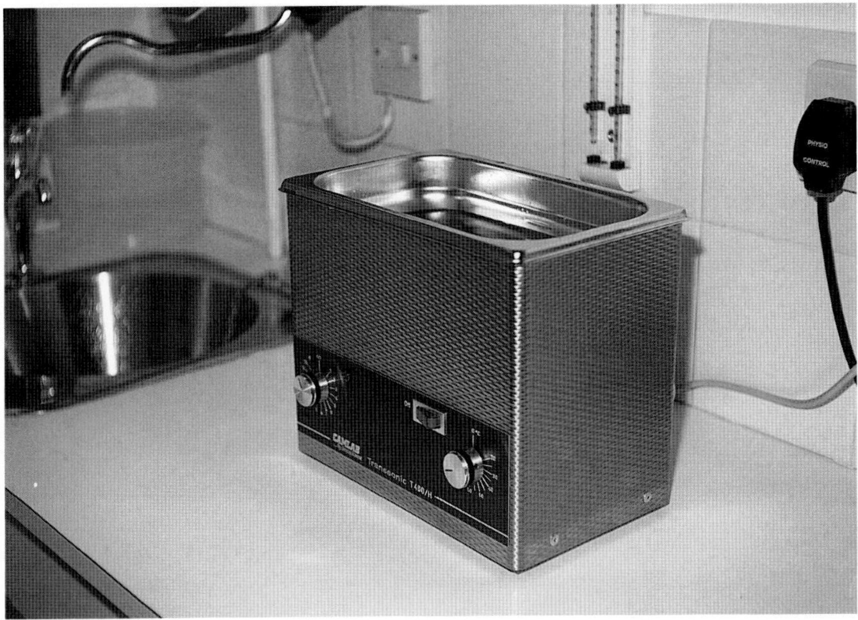

Fig. 4.1 An ultrasonic cleaning bath. This is an excellent method of keeping surgical instruments clean prior to sterilizing.

Plastic instruments or plastic parts of instruments are particularly vulnerable to corrosive agents, heat, rough handling and abrasive cleaners. They should be treated with great respect; generally, washing with warm soapy water with a soft cloth is sufficient. Sterilization may be by either soaking in antiseptic solutions or autoclaving at a lower temperature (115°C under 9 lbf/in^2 (62 kN/m^2) for 30 min) than is used for steel instruments. Cleaning and polishing should only be undertaken using recommended cleansers and polishers, as even ordinary domestic polishes can abrade perspex and similar plastics. Most plastics are best stored in a dry state rather than under prolonged soaking in antiseptic solutions.

4.2 ELECTRICAL SAFETY

It cannot be stressed enough that there should be the utmost regard for electrical safety at all times. Many modern instruments and pieces of equipment operate from mains voltage 110 or 240 V AC. All such instruments have to pass stringent safety tests during and after manufacture and can be assumed to be electrically safe on delivery. However, with use, cables become frayed, earth connections work loose or break, internal components move with vibration or accidental damage or unauthorized alteration to the circuitry or safety fuses occurs, resulting in potentially lethal voltages and currents reaching the patient. Obvious simple checks of plugs, fuses, and cables should be made regularly, and routine maintenance be performed by a qualified person at standard intervals as recommended by the manufacturer. Water and electricity do not mix (!) so it is imperative that all mains electrically operated instruments be kept dry. Low-voltage battery equipment is generally safe and may even be designed to work in damp or humid conditions. Earth connections and safety fuses should be regularly checked, making sure that the correct loading fuses are being used. Any frayed cables should be immediately replaced and any loose components such as switches and sockets dealt with. All equipment working from mains voltage should have a circuit breaker in the supply lines.

Cardiac defibrillators deliver a high voltage of several thousand volts, together with a relatively high current, making a lethal combination to the operator if any serious electrical fault should occur, it is thus even more imperative that servicing and maintenance of these instruments be entrusted to a qualified electrical engineer.

Electronic components comprising microchips and integrated circuits are generally very rugged and will withstand rough handling; they also operate at low voltages so are relatively safe, but they respond badly to high temperatures. Overheating should therefore be avoided and any ventilation apertures left uncovered; given these safeguards, they should give good service.

4.3 RECHARGEABLE BATTERY PACKS

Increasingly rechargeable nickel-cadmium batteries are being used for items of medical equipment. These are relatively expensive and have a limited life, although are electrically safe. Rechargeable batteries are capable of delivering a very high current on discharge, so should not be shorted, as this might result in fire. Another feature is that their life is extended by regular discharging and recharging. Thus, any piece of equipment containing rechargeable batteries should be regularly switched on, fully discharged and then fully recharged. As they can fail without warning, back-up batteries for essential pieces of equipment are a good idea.

5

Infection control

I tried the application of carbolic acid to the wound to prevent decomposition of the blood

Lord Joseph Lister, 1827–1912, letter dated May 27th 1866 to his father

Infection in general practitioner minor surgery is very rare: nevertheless, unless consistently high standards of preoperative, operative, and postoperative care are adopted, the incidence of infection and cross-infection will rise, producing anything from minor irritation to a major disaster.

Most cases of infection can be avoided by careful surgical technique, and meticulous attention to sterilization of instruments and dressings.

However, as well as the problems of common bacterial pathogens, doctors are now having to address themselves to the problems of methicillin-resistant *Staphylococcus aureus* (MRSA), viral agents such as hepatitis B, herpes and HIV infection, which may have very much more serious consequences.

Infection is also not always a one-way problem of patients infecting doctors or other patients: in a few instances an infected surgeon can infect the patient, or other colleagues. It is therefore important for all involved with minor surgery to be aware of the possible causative agents of infection, and to know how to avoid or treat them [4].

5.1 COMMON PATHOGENS

Bacterial pathogens include staphylococci and streptococci and are responsible for the majority of cases of cellulitis and abscesses seen on the skin. Most respond to appropriate antibiotics such as flucloxacillin.

Abscesses in the perineal area are frequently infected with anaerobic and mixed organisms: in these situations metronidazole or similar antibiotics may be necessary.

Where infection is suspected, a bacterial swab should be taken: this will often be helpful in ascertaining whether the infective agent was present before or after the surgical treatment, and will also guide the doctor to the most appropriate treatment.

Fungal infection of toe-nails and finger-nails may be easily recognized by sending nail clippings or even the complete nail for mycology. Such action may avoid the need for surgery and establish a definitive diagnosis.

Candida infections are generally not seen in minor surgery, and if so are readily treated with any of the antimycotic agents.

5.2 HEPATITIS VIRUSES

5.2.1 Hepatitis B (serum hepatitis)

This is one of the most infective viruses, causing serious illness. It may be transmitted from patient to patient by as little as 0.0001 ml of infected blood. The virus remains active for up to 6 months in dried blood, consequently instruments which have been poorly cleaned or disinfected may be responsible for infecting other patients, whilst poor surgical technique may result in the doctor becoming infected from the patient, or vice versa.

It has been estimated that there are possibly 200 million carriers of hepatitis in the world, representing up to 20% of the population in African, Pacific, and other tropical countries, and 0.5% of the population in northern Europe. Thus, statistically the doctor has a 1 in 200 chance of treating a hepatitis B carrier.

Worse still, if the doctor becomes accidentally infected with the hepatitis B virus, not only may the disease develop but the doctor may become a hepatitis B carrier and be a serious risk to patients.

For this reason, every doctor and nurse undertaking minor surgery should have a full course of hepatitis B vaccine, and a follow-up blood test to confirm immunity. It is probably good practice to be retested after five years to confirm continued protection.

5.2.2 Hepatitis C

Hepatitis C has recently been isolated as another blood-borne virus, capable of causing liver cirrhosis and liver failure. At the present time there is no vaccine available to protect against this organism.

5.3 HIV INFECTION

The acquired immune deficiency syndrome (AIDS) was first described in 1981 and the human immunodeficiency virus (HIV) was first identified in 1983. Also in 1983 the receptor cell for the virus was identified as the CD4 or T helper cell. Antibody tests were subsequently developed which revealed the HIV status of the individual. Subsequently in 1986 a second strain, HIV 2, was isolated.

Like hepatitis B the virus is present in blood and body fluids, but unlike hepatitis B is relatively easily destroyed outside the body, and is not as infectious as the hepatitis B virus.

Infection of the surgeon can occur from contamination from infected blood or body fluids, either through an open wound, from aerosol sprays, or from a puncture wound or needle-stick injury.

Following infection there is an asymptomatic period during which antibody to the virus is not yet present in the blood, and thus HIV tests will be negative. After approximately 6 months the infected individual may seroconvert, and the HIV antibody be detected. A high proportion will then progress to develop AIDS.

A common presenting feature in AIDS sufferers is Kaposi's sarcoma, with an incidence of between 25% and 50% . Biopsy of such lesions may be the first contact the doctor has with this disease as far as minor surgery is concerned.

Kaposi's sarcomas present as pink to purple blotches like a bruise or blood blister. They may be flat or raised. They are skin cancers arising from the endothelial cells such as those lining blood vessels.

Histologically, malignant transformation causes the endothelial cells to become stippled with spindle-shaped tumour cells; lymphatic obstruction may occur, but they do not metastasize, and remain multifocal, both on the skin and in the alimentary tract.

Despite the worry of surgeons about risks of infection, these remain small. Surgeons have been shown to contaminate themselves with blood in 8.7% cases, and sustain penetrating injuries in 1.7% cases, yet statistically the risk of seroconversion for a surgeon is one infection every 8 years in a high-risk area with a caseload of 15 000 patients per year, and as small as one infection every 80 years in a low-risk area. Thus the risk to the general practitioner minor surgeon is exceptionally low.

5.4 INFECTION CONTROL GUIDELINES

Obviously where the doctor suspects or knows that his patient may be HIV positive additional infection control protocols are carried out. This may not be entirely logical, and it is better to assume that every patient is potentially infectious, and to use the same standards of care and sterility throughout. In this way the unsuspected HIV-positive patient will not put either the doctor, his staff, or other patients at risk. As a general guide, therefore, the following procedures would seem to be reasonable.

1. For all patients wear latex/vinyl gloves and a plastic apron for all procedures in which exposure to blood and/or body fluids is anticipated.
2. Discard all sharps into a good-quality plastic sharps container. Never resheath needles after use. Do not break syringes, but discard syringe and needle in one piece. Where the needle needs to be removed, use a pair of forceps or needle-holding device. Incinerate the sharps container.
3. Specimens from patients infected with HIV or hepatitis should be placed in a sealed plastic bag and marked with warning tape.
4. Contaminated dressings and waste material should be placed in a yellow plastic bag for incineration via the local Environmental Health Department.
5. Any linen contaminated with blood or body fluids should be handled with gloves, and washed in a washing machine at the highest temperature setting.
6. For any spillage of blood or body fluids, wear an apron, and gently pour undiluted Milton or similar hypochlorite bleach over the spillage, cover with paper towels, leave for 30min and wipe up with disposable towels. Alternatively, sprinkle granular sodium dichloriso-cyanate (Na DCC), e.g. Presept granules, over spillage and wipe up with paper towels or a disposable cloth.
7. Cover any cuts or abrasions with a waterproof dressing.

5.5 PROCEDURES IN THE CASE OF ACCIDENTAL CONTAMINATION

Should the operator or assistant be accidentally contaminated, e.g. needle-stick injury, the site of entry should be immediately encouraged to bleed, should be thoroughly washed with warm, soapy water, and a sterile dressing applied.

An entry should be made in the Accident or Infection Book, with the date, circumstances, names of those present, name of the patient, nature of accident, and eventual outcome.

5.6 INFECTION BOOK

A separate Infection Book is a good idea: all cases of infection should be recorded, particularly the postoperative infection rate. Only by recording every case of infection can an accurate audit be made, and if the rate is unacceptable, steps taken to improve it.

6

Sterilizing and disinfecting instruments

In the course of the year 1864 I was much struck with an account of the remarkable effects produced by Carbolic Acid upon the sewage of the town of Carlisle, destroying the entozoa which usually infest cattle fed upon such pastures

Lord Joseph Lister, 1827–1912

Sterilization is the destruction of all living organisms. Contrary to popular belief an item may only be sterile or non-sterile – it cannot be nearly sterile. Disinfection, on the other hand, is the reduction of a population of pathogenic micro-organisms without achieving sterility. Not all bacterial spores are destroyed. There are five methods of sterilizing or disinfecting instruments in general practice:

1. Antiseptic solutions
2. Boiling
3. Hot air ovens
4. Autoclave
5. Use of CSSD facilities.

6.1 ANTISEPTIC SOLUTIONS

Traditionally 70% alcohol was the solution most widely used, subsequently with the addition of 0.5% chlorhexidine. This is widely used for emergency disinfection of surgical instruments requiring only 2 min immersion. Where instruments are left for longer periods or stored continuously, the addition of one tablet of sodium nitrite BPC 1 g will prevent rusting. As the tablet dissolves over several days, another is added.

The aldehydes are powerful disinfectors and sterilizers. A solution containing 2% glutaraldehyde will disinfect instruments if they are soaked for 10 min, and sterilize if left soaking for 10 hours. The disadvantages are that the solution needs to be fresh, and it can cause staining if left on the skin.

6.2 BOILING

This is still the most widely used method of disinfecting instruments in the world; it is simple, quick, and reasonably effective, but will not destroy certain bacterial spores and certain viruses. Normally, instruments are cleaned, and then boiled for 5 min (100°C or 212°F). It is obviously not suitable for dressings, drapes or paper (Fig. 6.1).

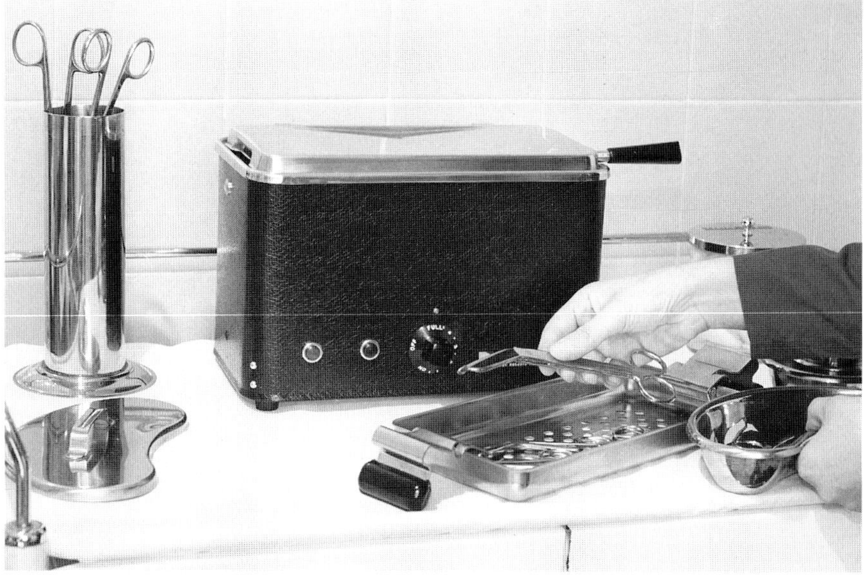

Fig. 6.1 Electric boiling water disinfector with thermostat and removable tray.

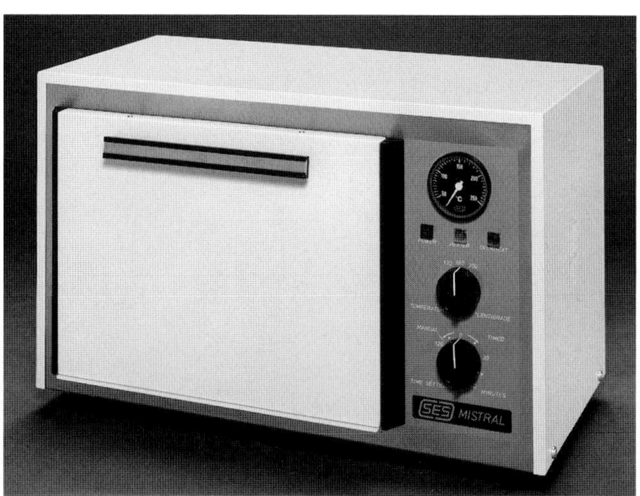

Fig. 6.2 Hot-air oven.

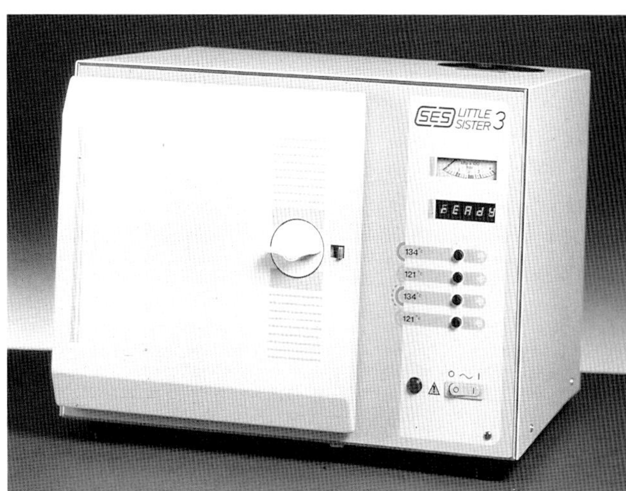

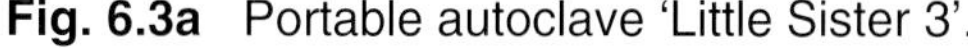

Fig. 6.3a Portable autoclave 'Little Sister 3'.

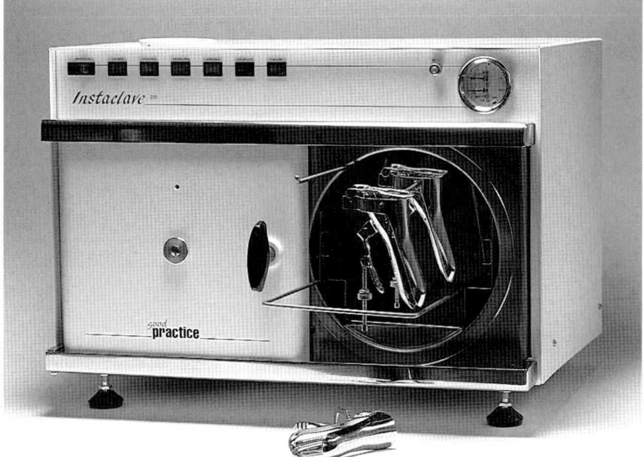

Fig. 6.3b Portable autoclave 'Instaclave' (Prospect Medical).

6.3 HOT-AIR OVENS

These are thermostatically controlled ovens, with an electric heating element, similar to a domestic electric oven. Instruments to be sterilized are heated to 160°C (320°F) for 1 hour. Sterilization is achieved, but it is not suitable for rubber, plastic or, to a lesser extent, paper items (Fig. 6.2).

6.4 AUTOCLAVES

Now considered to be the most efficient method of sterilizing instruments, packs and dressings, and suitable for most materials, an autoclave is basically a pressure cooker, and in fact, there is no reason why a domestic pressure cooker should not be used to sterilize instruments. The small autoclaves produced for the doctor's surgery offer a choice of temperatures, pressures and sterilizing times: typically a 'quick' cycle would heat the water to 134°C (273°F) for 3.5 min under a pressure of 30 lbf/in^2 (207 kN/m^2) whereas a slower cycle, more suitable for plastics, would heat the water to 115°C (239°F) under a pressure of 10 lbf/in^2 (69 kN/m^2). In practice, instruments are placed in the trays, the autoclave turned on, and left for the desired time. At the end of the cycle, the instruments are ready for use. The main disadvantage of the smaller autoclave is that instrument packs cannot be sterilized as there is not a vacuum cycle to extract air and dry the packs. However, most materials including rubber, plastics and metal can be readily sterilized, the only exception being sealed containers (Fig. 6.3a, b).

6.5 GUIDELINES FOR SELECTING STERILIZERS

In 1988 The British Medical Association Board of Science and Education reviewed the guidance issued by the Department of Health on sterilization and disinfection procedures in general practice [5].

To achieve sterilization using saturated steam (i.e. autoclaving) they recommended 2.2 bar pressure at 121°C for 15 min, or 134°C for 3 min.

Similarly, using dry heat, they recommended 160°C for 60 min holding time, or 180°C for 30 min.

It is important to re-emphasize that small portable autoclaves used in the general practitioner's surgery will only process unwrapped instruments for immediate use, and are not suitable for sterilizing instruments wrapped in any packaging, or for dressings and towels.

It is also important to note that sealed containers containing fluids should never be put in a portable autoclave because of the risk of explosion.

Features to look for in the selection of an autoclave in general practice are:

1. A preset automatic cycle
2. Safety interlocks which prevent opening during a sterilizing cycle
3. Thermocouple entry for testing
4. Visible instrumentation, giving temperature and pressure readings
5. Some means of monitoring the sterilizing cycle
6. Cycle/stage fault indicators

7. A cycle counter
8. Empty-chamber performance
9. Full-load performance
10. Water reservoir temperature
11. Safety cut outs
12. The ability to sterilize despite cycle interruption
13. Surface temperature
14. Electrical safety
15. Price.

All sterilizers should be commissioned before use, and regular maintenance carried out by a qualified engineer, recording the dates and results of tests in a hard-back book.

It would be a good idea for a doctor to seek written assurance from the supplier that their autoclave meets the recommendations and complies with the British Standards.

6.6 USE OF CSSD (CENTRAL STERILE SUPPLIES DEPARTMENT) FACILITIES

Most hospitals in Europe and North America now use large autoclaves for all routine instrument sterilization. As well as superheated water under pressure, the large machines have two vacuum cycles, a pre-vacuum pulsing stage which removes air from the load, ensuring efficient steam penetration, and a post-vacuum pulse stage which ensures a dry sterile load at the end of the cycle. Thus dressings, drapes, gowns, sheets and instrument packs can be sterilized and dried at the same time. In practice, instruments are prepacked in plastic or foil trays, together with any selected dressings and drapes, these are then enclosed in a paper envelope which is closed with a heat sensitive autoclave adhesive tape, and the whole enclosed in an outer paper envelope, similarly closed with the autoclave marking tape. This tape changes colour if the desired sterilizing conditions have been reached, and affords a visible proof of sterilization. This type of autoclave offers the best method of sterilization, and it is well worth the practitioner making arrangements, if at all possible, with a hospital Central Sterile Supplies Department. Not only will the GP's instruments and drapes be sterilized, but each will be cleaned and repacked in a sterile envelope ready for future use. Such packs may be stored at the surgery and used either on the premises or taken to the patient's home if needed for such conditions as draining malignant abdominal ascites or a minor operation on a housebound patient.

6.7 IMPROVISED METHODS OF STERILIZATION

There will be occasions when the doctor will not have access to CSSD facilities, hot-air ovens, or autoclaves, either as a result of location or failure of existing equipment. Under these circumstances it is possible to improvise techniques for sterilizing instruments as follows.

6.7.1 Hot-air oven

Instruments placed in a metal biscuit tin in a domestic oven and heated to 160°C for 1 hour or 180° for 0.5 hour will be adequately sterilized in the majority of cases.

6.7.2 Domestic pressure cooker

Satisfactory sterilization of instruments may be obtained using a domestic pressure cooker, which works on the same principle as an autoclave, i.e. superheated water under pressure. Indeed, one manufacturer of a domestic pressure cooker has produced an autoclave by simple modification (Fig. 6.4).

Generally 15 min at the highest pressure is adequate. For added reassurance, testing strips may be included with the instruments to indicate that sterilizing conditions have been met.

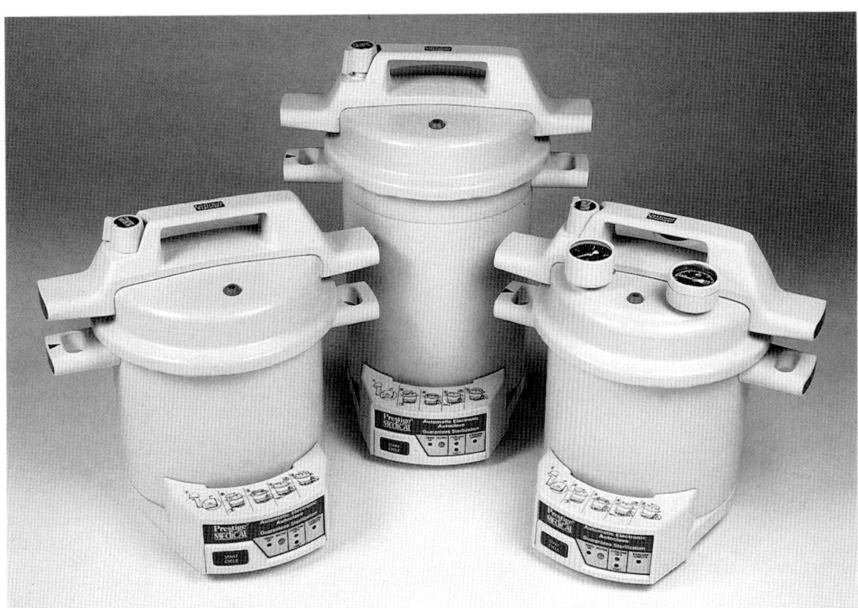

Fig. 6.4 'Prestige' autoclaves.

7

Assessment, preoperative preparation and skin preparation

One of the great advantages of general practitioner minor surgery is that the patient is frequently very well known to the doctor. The latter will therefore be fully aware of the patient's medical condition and what medication, if any, he or she is taking.

It is important to ascertain any relevant past problems with either local anaesthetics, dressings, plaster, or skin antiseptics, particularly any known sensitivities.

Of particular relevance is the patient's current medication, especially anticoagulant therapy, and drugs which could react with local anaesthetics such as the tricyclic antidepressants. Also of great importance is any condition which may jeopardize healing, such as a poor peripheral circulation, diabetes, scleroderma, polyarteritis, reduced immunity, or a tendency to produce keloid reactions.

At the initial assessment and consultation, a full explanation must be given to the patient of what to expect. It is still surprising to find patients who believe an operation will leave no scar! Obviously the type of scar, its length and situation needs to be discussed, and any possible complications which could arise. It is wise to record in the medical notes that this information has been given to the patient.

For many procedures skin preparation is probably not necessary; the removal of small skin tags with the electrocautery is certainly better done without applying any antiseptic solution to the skin – indeed if the electrocautery or diathermy is used shortly after applying an inflammable antiseptic such as alcohol or ether, serious burns could ensue. In any case, the temperature of the electrocautery wire is sufficiently high to sterilize the tissue during use. Similarly, operations on or near the eye are best performed without any prior disinfection of the skin or conjunctiva, and rarely does one see any infection.

For the majority of other minor operations some form of skin antiseptic is used; many commercially prepared solutions are available, containing either chlorhexidine 0.5% in isopropyl alcohol (Hibisol: ICI) or povidone-iodine 10% alcoholic solution (Betadine alcoholic solution: Napp). Coloured solutions have the added advantage that the operator can readily see where the antiseptic has been applied. As there are so many preparations available, the final choice depends on the preference of the individual doctor. Each antiseptic solution may either be painted on the skin using an absorbent swab, sprayed over the area from a pressurized applicator, or the affected part if small enough, such as a finger or toe, immersed in the solution.

Removal of hair by shaving is now rarely necessary – the majority of minor surgical procedures can be performed easily without; where sebaceous cysts occur on the head, and there is much hair, cutting away the minimum amount with stitch scissors or iris scissors is all that is necessary.

Although normal surgical practice is to apply skin antiseptics only before any operation, occasionally it helps to apply a second application after the skin has been closed, before a final sterile dry dressing is applied, to reduce any bacterial colonies secreted through the pores of the skin or which have contaminated the skin, either airborne or from the operator or assistant during the operation.

8

Anaesthesia

The powder benumbs the nerves of the tongue depriving it of feeling and taste

Albert Niemann, first description of cocaine, 1860

Modern anaesthetics have revolutionized surgical practice, and it should now be easily possible to perform any minor operation completely painlessly. It is worth taking time to fully anaesthetize the area and to have the confidence that it has been successful; to repeatedly ask a patient 'Can you feel this?' does nothing for their confidence; they will let the operator know if they can feel any pain!

Many different techniques are available, the most widely used being infiltration; some operations such as those on the eye may require two different methods such as surface anaesthesia of the conjunctiva and infiltration of the skin.

8.1 FREEZING

Most doctors have witnessed small abscesses being opened by freezing of the overlying skin with an ethyl chloride spray. Those doctors who have had such a procedure done to them will also say how ineffective it is, and how uncomfortable it is as the tissues thaw out. One suspects that most freezing was performed for the benefit of the operator and had a placebo effect at best for the patient! Ethyl chloride spray freezing was reserved mainly for incision of abscesses; if such abscesses were deeply situated it certainly would not offer much pain relief other than that achieved from the release of pus, and if very superficial probably was unnecessary as the overlying skin was now insensitive to pain. Thus as a method of anaesthesia it tends to have been superseded by other more effective agents (Fig. 8.1).

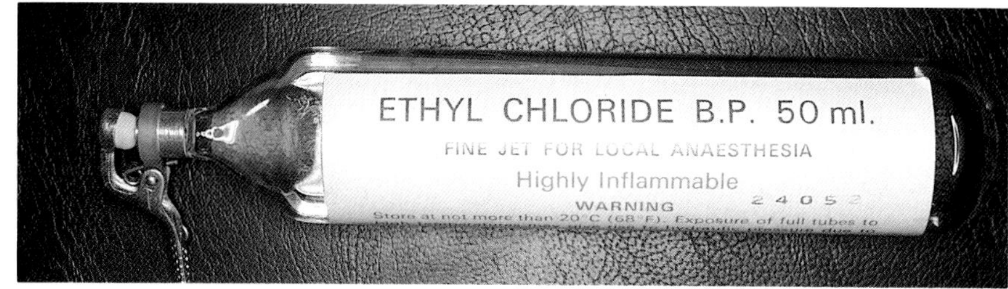

Fig. 8.1 Ethyl chloride spray; suitable for incision of certain abscesses, but not very effective for the majority of procedures requiring anaesthesia.

8.2 TOPICAL OR SURFACE ANAESTHESIA

Mucous membranes fortunately absorb local anaesthetics very rapidly, efficiently, and painlessly. Thus the cornea and conjunctiva can be readily anaesthetized with local anaesthetic drops, of which there are several varieties. Lignocaine (Xylocaine, UK; Octocaine, USA) is manufactured as a 4% eye-drops solution. Individual applications of oxybuprocaine hydrochloride 0.4% (Minims Benoxinate SNP 0.4%, UK) or amethocaine hydrochloride 0.5% (Minims Amethocaine SNP 0.5%, UK) are manufactured for once-only application. Onset of anaesthesia is rapid and lasts for up to 1 hour. The number of instillations is more important than the amount administered for each instillation to achieve anaesthesia.

Similarly the lining of the nose, buccal mucosa, larynx and pharynx, oesophagus, trachea, tympanic membrane, and urethra may all be anaesthetized using topical anaesthetic preparations.

Lignocaine aerosol spray (Xylocaine spray, UK; Octocaine spray, USA) is particularly useful for the nasal cavity, pharynx, and larynx, while lignocaine sterile gel (Xylocaine Gel 2%, UK; Octocaine gel 2%, USA) is extremely good for anaesthetizing the urethra.

As with all local anaesthetics, the maximum safe dose which can be given to any particular patient should be known and not exceeded; as doses for different anaesthetic agents differ, the doctor is advised to refer to the manufacturer's data sheet. Ask the patient if he or she is on any medication.

8.3 TOPICAL ANAESTHETIC CREAMS

In recent years, topical creams containing local anaesthetics have been introduced with the object of achieving anaesthesia of the skin. Absorption is poor under normal conditions, but by applying an occlusive dressing over the cream, and allowing 1 or 2 hours for the cream to be absorbed, satisfactory anaesthesia may be obtained for many superficial procedures.

Emla cream containing 25 mg lignocaine and 25 mg prilocaine per gram is manufactured in 5 g tubes, and is effective for anaesthesia of the skin prior to needle puncture or split-skin grafting. For needle puncture, 2 g are applied as a thick layer under occlusion for at least 60 min. For split-skin grafting or pinch grafting 2 g per 10 cm is applied as a thick layer under occlusion for at least 120 min.

Other uses include superficial anaesthesia prior to cauterizing molluscum contagiosum. However, the cream should not be applied to wounds, mucous membranes or to patients with atopic dermatitis.

Where time permits, its most useful application is in children prior to needle puncture, enabling infiltration anaesthesia to be accomplished painlessly.

8.4 INFILTRATION ANAESTHESIA

Most local anaesthetic agents can be given by injection and this method of infiltration is now widely used for producing anaesthesia, particularly for minor surgery. Certain points need to be borne in mind.

1. The finer the needle, the less the discomfort. If only small volumes of local anaesthetic are needed, a sterile 1 ml diabetic syringe and attached 30 swg needle is ideal (Fig. 8.2a). A small bleb of local

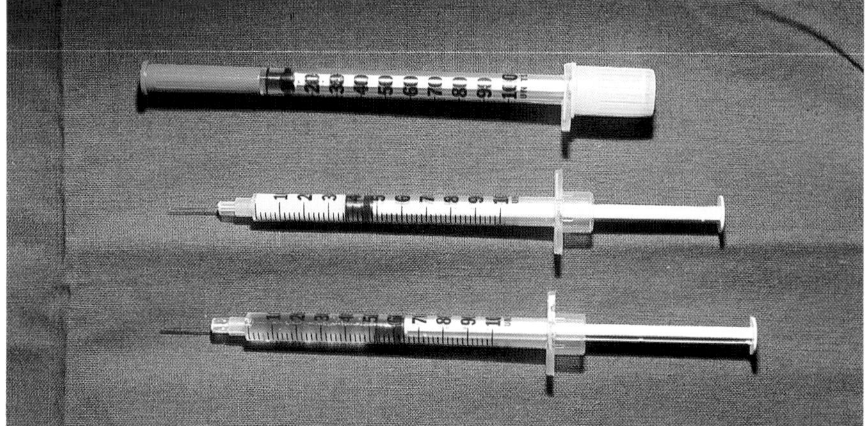

Fig. 8.2a For small volumes of local anaesthetic or steroids, sterile single-use diabetic syringes and needles are ideal. (**b**) Posterior tibial nerve block, excellent for producing anaesthesia of the sole of the foot.

(a)

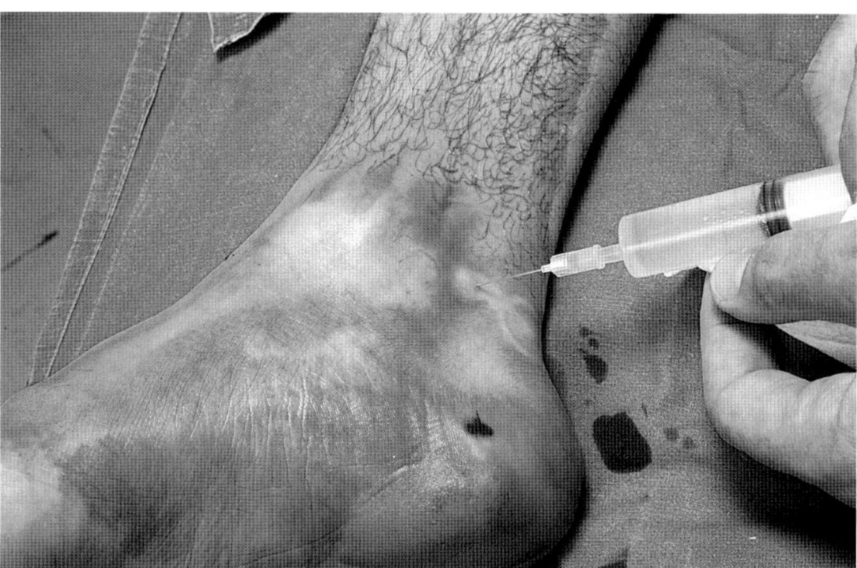

(b)

anaesthetic is raised in the skin initially before advancing the needle to deeper tissues.

2. Inject slowly as the needle advances, sudden injections of large volumes, even of local anaesthetic, cause pain.
3. If possible, ensure that the solution to be injected is at body temperature or at room temperature, injection of icy-cold solutions taken from a refrigerator causes discomfort.
4. Wait an adequate time for anaesthesia to develop; so often one sees a rapid injection of local anaesthetic followed immediately by a surgical procedure which can be felt by the patient, only to see full anaesthesia reached after the procedure is completed.
5. Use single-dose snap-open glass ampoules in preference to multidose vials; this reduces the risk of cross infection and reactions to the preservative.
6. Use only pre-packed sterilized disposable syringes and needles.
7. Do not open any sterilized pack until the moment of use.
8. Hands should be washed clean with Hibiscrub or similar agent and thoroughly dried – wet hands increase the risk of infection.

9. Do not touch the needle at all, and in particular, do not guide the needle with your finger.
10. Advise the patient that neither of you should talk or cough while the needle is exposed to the air and during the injection; droplet infection can occur otherwise, and for this reason it is still good practice to wear a mask, particularly if aspirating or injecting a joint.
11. Where intra-articular injections are to be given, it is still a good idea to swab the skin with an antiseptic such as povidone-iodine in spirit or a similar preparation. For other superficial injections it is probably not necessary to use any skin antiseptic.
12. Do not exceed the manufacturer's recommended dose of local anaesthetic.
13. Beware of using local anaesthetics with added adrenaline and never, never use these for fingers, toes, tip of the nose, ear, or penis in case prolonged vasoconstriction results in ischaemia and gangrene.
14. In a vascular area, occasionally withdraw the plunger of the syringe to check that the needle is not inside a vein. Probably some 'reactions' and 'allergic responses' to local anaesthetics have been due to inadvertent intravenous injection of the anaesthetic with or without added adrenaline.
15. Remember that adrenaline can interreact with certain drugs such as antidepressants: ask patients if they are taking any medication.
16. Caution should be observed in patients with epilepsy.
17. Weaker solutions of local anaesthetics cause less discomfort during administration.
18. In the presence of infection, e.g. infected ingrowing toe-nail, greater volumes of local anaesthetic are needed due to increased vascularity.

8.5 MECHANISM OF ACTION OF LOCAL ANAESTHETICS

Chemically the three most widely used local anaesthetics, lignocaine, bupivacaine and prilocaine, are classified as amides. They are metabolized in the liver. Clearance rate is fastest with prilocaine, followed by lignocaine and slowest with bupivacaine.

Prilocaine and bupivacaine are vasodilators, whilst lignocaine appears to cause no effect on blood vessels.

It is interesting to speculate how local anaesthetic agents work: their speed of action suggests that they may prevent depolarization and thus non-conduction. Sensory fibres are blocked faster than motor fibres, and their action is slower in inflamed tissues and mucous membranes.

8.6 WHICH LOCAL ANAESTHETIC?

Several well-known local anaesthetic agents are manufactured, and each gives very adequate anaesthesia. Different surveys have shown slight variations in toxicity between different local anaesthetics, but the three most widely used agents are currently lignocaine (Xylocaine, UK; Octocaine, USA) bupivacaine (Marcain, UK; Marcain, USA) and prilocaine (Citanest, UK; Xylonest, USA). Where small volumes are being used, there is little to choose between the three local anaesthetics; where intravenous injections are used, prilocaine appears to be the drug of choice at present.

Each of the above anaesthetics is also manufactured with added adrenaline as an option; this has the effect of causing localized vasoconstriction and thus prolonging the action of the anaesthetic drug. However, as previously emphasized, any of the preparations with adrenaline should be treated with great respect and should never be used for digital anaesthesia – the constriction of digital arteries could result in gangrene of fingers or toes. This also applies to the tip of the nose, tip of the ear, or penis. For this reason, as an added safeguard, all local anaesthetics containing adrenaline should be kept separately from the plain injections, and should be clearly marked.

8.7 MAXIMUM DOSE OF LOCAL ANAESTHETICS

As a guide, the maximum safe dose of each of the three local anaesthetics is shown below for an average adult of 70 kg.

Lignocaine 200 mg
Bupivacaine 140 mg
Prilocaine 400 mg.

This represents, respectively, 20 ml of 1% lignocaine (or 40 ml of 0.5% lignocaine), 28 ml of 0.5% bupivacaine (or 56 ml of 0.25% bupivacaine), and 40 ml of 1% prilocaine (or 80 ml of 0.5% prilocaine). Dosages should be correspondingly less in the elderly, debilitated, and young, and basically it should be remembered that the correct dose is the smallest dose required to produce the desired anaesthesia.

8.8 TOXICITY OF LOCAL ANAESTHETICS

The three local anaesthetic agents, lignocaine, prilocaine and bupivacaine are remarkably free from side-effects, and in over 15 000 personally administered injections I have not seen a serious reaction. Occasionally one sees the vasovagal reaction or faint, but even these are rare if the patient is lying flat.

Nevertheless, toxic reactions have been reported, and the doctor should be aware of what might be expected. Two types of reaction can occur – either stimulation or depression of the cerebral cortex and medulla respectively.

Where there is stimulation the patient may feel apprehensive, dizzy, complain of blurred vision, nausea, tremor, convulsions, and respiratory arrest.

In depression of the brain, respiratory arrest, cardiovascular collapse, and cardiac arrest may occur, often with little warning.

Toxic reactions are most likely to be seen if the technique of intravenous regional anaesthesia (Bier block) is used and there is a failure of both pneumatic cuffs, allowing a bolus of local anaesthetic agent into the circulation. Prilocaine can cause methaemaglobinaemia.

8.9 NERVE BLOCKS

Any nerve in the body can be 'blocked' by infiltrating local anaesthetic around it – the only caution is to ensure that the local anaesthetic is not injected into the nerve itself, which could result in permanent damage to the nerve. It is, therefore, important, if the patient complains of pain in the distribution of the nerve during injection, that the needle be withdrawn and the injection tried again in a different site.

One of the most useful nerve blocks is the posterior tibial nerve block. As a method of producing anaesthesia of the sole of the foot it is ideal, as in this area the skin is particularly thick, and injections through the horny layer cause intense pain, and largely defeat any object of painless surgery!

The posterior tibial nerve is a branch of the sciatic nerve; it passes down the back of the calf in company with the posterior tibial vessels to the interval between the heel and the medial malleolus where it ends under the cover of the flexor retinaculum by dividing into the medial and lateral plantar nerves, which between them supply the sole of the foot. The posterior tibial nerve may be blocked as it passes behind the medial malleolus, before it divides.

8.10 TECHNIQUE OF POSTERIOR TIBIAL NERVE BLOCK

A point is chosen exactly midway between the medial malleolus and Achilles tendon at the level of the ankle, and the overlying skin painted with povidone-iodine alcoholic solution (Betadine) or similar antiseptic.

A sterile syringe with 25 swg needle is used to draw in 5 ml of 1% lignocaine with added adrenaline 1:200 000. A small weal of local anaesthetic is raised at the point between the medial malleolus and Achilles tendon, and then the syringe is directed at 45° in a horizontal plane, aiming the needle at the underlying bone. When this is reached, the needle is withdrawn 2 mm and the plunger gently withdrawn to check that the needle is not inside a vein. Then 2–5 ml local anaesthetic solution is injected around the posterior tibial nerve and the needle is withdrawn (Fig. 8.2b).

Anaesthesia of the sole of the foot gradually develops over the ensuing 10 minutes and will last for up to 2 hours. As the overlying skin at the ankle is so much softer than the horny layers on the sole of the foot, an injection may be given painlessly at this site. The method is particularly useful for suturing lacerations on the sole of the foot or for the treatment of verrucae or other intradermal lesions.

One word of caution – proprioception depends on sensory impulses received from the soles of the feet; therefore it is inadvisable to perform a posterior tibial nerve block on both feet simultaneously otherwise the patient may fall over and be unable to maintain his or her balance.

8.11 ULNAR NERVE BLOCK

The sensory distribution of the ulnar nerve in the hand is shown in Fig. 8.3. As can be seen, only the little finger can be totally anaesthetized.

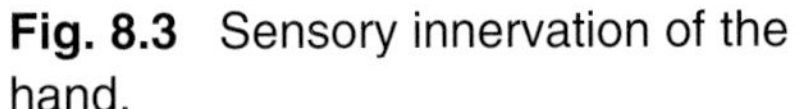

Fig. 8.3 Sensory innervation of the hand.

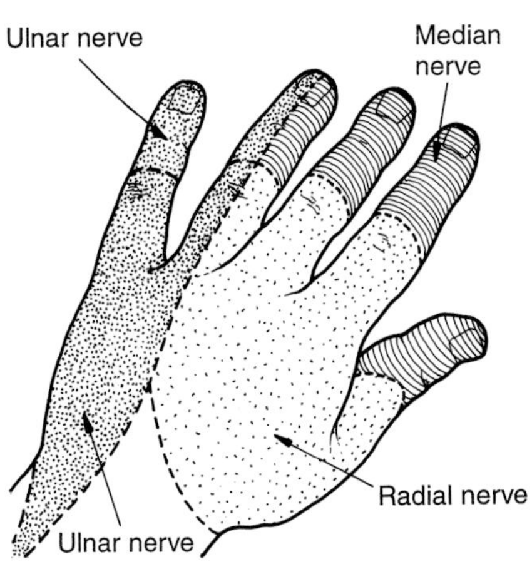

8.11.1 Technique

The ulnar nerve at the wrist lies lateral to the tendon of the flexor carpi ulnaris, which runs down the ulnar border of the arm and is inserted into the pisiform bone. The nerve can usually be palpated as it passes lateral to this tendon proximal to the pisiform bone.

Using 1% lignocaine, a small weal is raised in the overlying skin, and the needle inserted perpendicularly, lateral to the tendon over the nerve (Fig. 8.4). As the needle penetrates the deep fascia it may touch the nerve, causing paraesthesia.

Five millilitres of 1% lignocaine is now injected.

The dorsal sensory branch of the ulnar nerve frequently arises proximal to this point, so in order to block this as well, a further 5 ml of 1% lignocaine is injected subcutaneously from the medial side of the level of the ulnar styloid, extending under the skin to the middle of the back of the wrist (Fig. 8.5).

As with other nerve blocks, sufficient time should be allowed for the local anaesthetic to be absorbed by the nerve. It is also important not to inject the anaesthetic directly into the nerve; should the patient complain of pain, the needle should be either withdrawn or repositioned and the injection reattempted.

8.12 RADIAL NERVE BLOCK

The radial nerve supplies the sensation at the back of the lateral part of the hand as shown in Fig. 8.3. It accompanies the radial artery in the forearm, and then separates about 7 cm above the wrist, passing deep to the tendon of brachioradialis muscle, subsequently dividing into digital branches.

To block the radial nerve, it is useful to identify the 'anatomical snuff box' by fully abducting the thumb, revealing a depression over the base of the first metacarpal. This space is bounded anteriorly by the tendons of

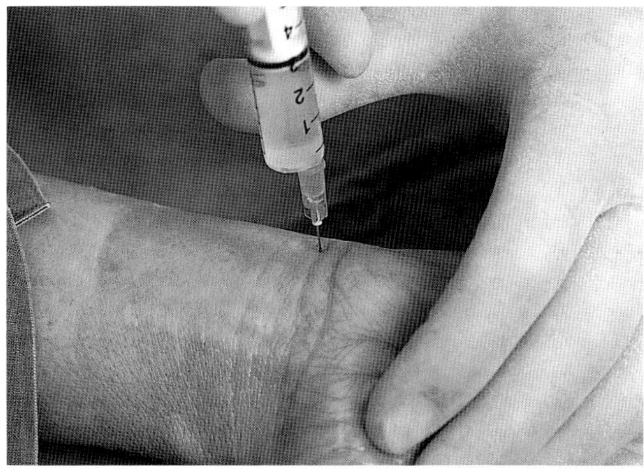

Fig. 8.4 Ulnar nerve block (see text).

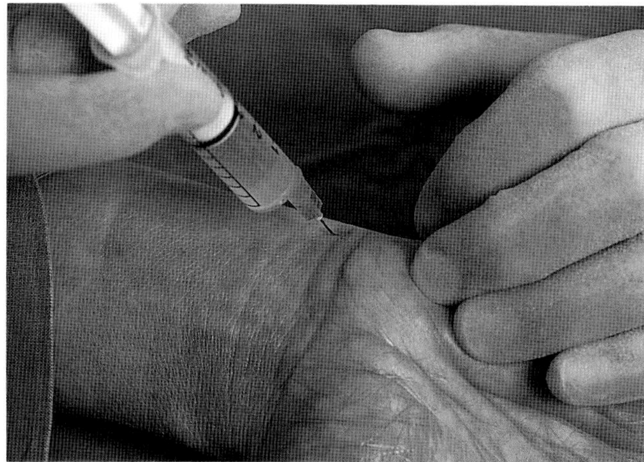

Fig. 8.5 Ulnar nerve block (see text).

abductor pollicis longus and extensor pollicis brevis together, and posteriorly by the tendon of extensor pollicis longus.

8.12.1 Technique

Five millilitres of 1% lignocaine is used. A small weal is raised in the overlying skin and 3 ml injected subcutaneously in the anatomical snuff box (Fig. 8.6). Two millilitres are then injected subcutaneously over the lower end of the radius.

Sufficient time (10 minutes or more) is allowed for the anaesthetic to work.

8.13 MEDIAN NERVE BLOCK

The sensory distribution of the median nerve is shown in Fig. 8.3, where it can be seen to supply the palmar surface of the hand including half the thumb, palmar surface of the 1st and 2nd fingers, and half the palmar surface of the 3rd finger (ring finger).

At the wrist, the median nerve lies between the flexor carpi radialis tendon laterally and the flexor digitorum sublimis and palmaris longus tendon medially.

8.13.1 Technique

The needle is inserted just lateral to the palmaris longus tendon, a weal raised in the overlying skin, and 5 ml of 1% lignocaine injected around the nerve (Fig. 8.7).

Allow sufficient time for the local anaesthetic to be absorbed (10–15 minutes). As with other nerve blocks it is important not to inject directly into the nerve; if pain is experienced by the patient, withdraw and change the site of injection.

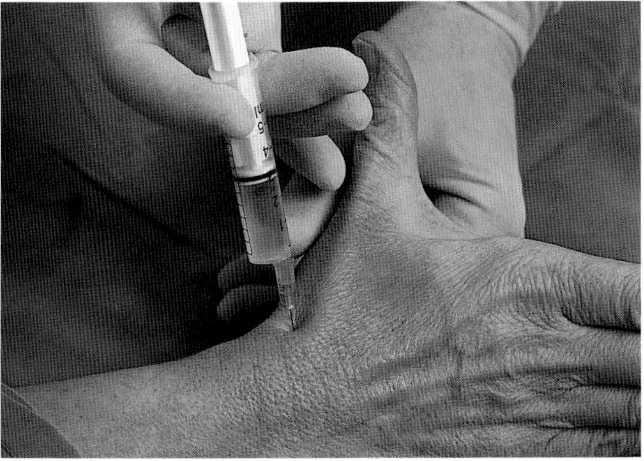

Fig. 8.6 Radial nerve block demonstrating injection site in 'anatomical snuff-box'.

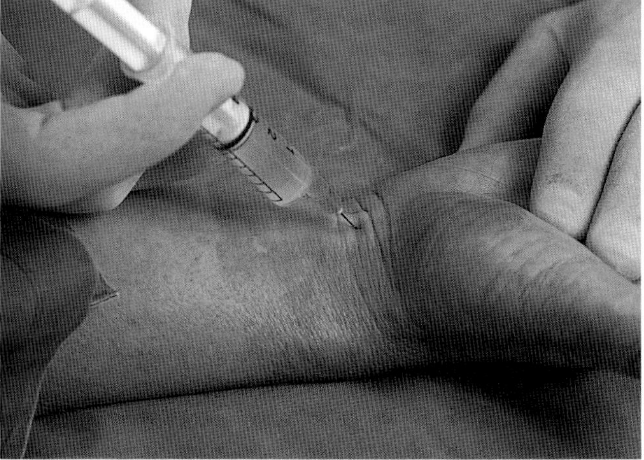

Fig. 8.7 Median nerve block. Injection site is identical to that for injection of the carpal tunnel.

8.14 DIGITAL NERVE BLOCKS

This technique is used to anaesthetize fingers or toes. With the exception of the thumb and large toe, each digit is supplied with plantar or palmar and dorsal digital nerves on each side, all of which will need to be blocked to achieve anaesthesia. The thumb and big toe have additional digital nerve branches, and these also need to be blocked for complete anaesthesia.

8.14.1 Contraindications for digital nerve block

1. Adrenaline must never be used with the local anaesthetic as vasoconstriction, ischaemia, and possible gangrene can occur.
2. Any condition where there is reduced peripheral circulation, e.g. diabetes, Raynaud's disease, scleroderma, and polyarteritis.
3. Infection. Only consider local infiltration if it can be given at least one phalanx distance away from any infected area.

8.14.2 Technique

Plain lignocaine without added adrenaline is used. After cleaning the skin, a weal is raised over the dorsum of the base of the proximal phalanx.

The needle is now advanced, injecting as it proceeds, distributing local anaesthetic under the skin in the direction of the digital nerves. It is now nearly withdrawn, and the same procedure followed on the other side.

In the case of the thumb and big toe, a 'ring block' is usually necessary, whereby the digit is encircled with a ring of local anaesthetic.

At this stage it is usual to apply a tourniquet around the base of the digit; this helps to distribute the local anaesthetic around the digital nerves, and helps to prolong the action of the drug.

Where there is infection, cellulitis, or suppuration, it is frequently found to be difficult to anaesthetize adequately a digit. In such situations it is necessary to use larger amounts of local anaesthetic and to allow longer for anaesthesia to develop.

8.15 LOCAL INFILTRATION AND BLOODLESS FIELD

Where the doctor requires a bloodless field and anaesthesia in a limb, a safer alternative to a Bier's block is to infiltrate the area with local anaesthesia and then apply an orthopaedic tourniquet and Esmarch bandage. This is particularly effective for decompression of the carpal tunnel and release of trigger finger, and exploration for foreign bodies.

8.15.1 Technique for producing anaesthesia and bloodless field in the arm

The following items are required:

1. Orthopaedic tourniquet
2. 3 in. Esmarch bandage
3. Syringe and needles
4. 1% Lignocaine

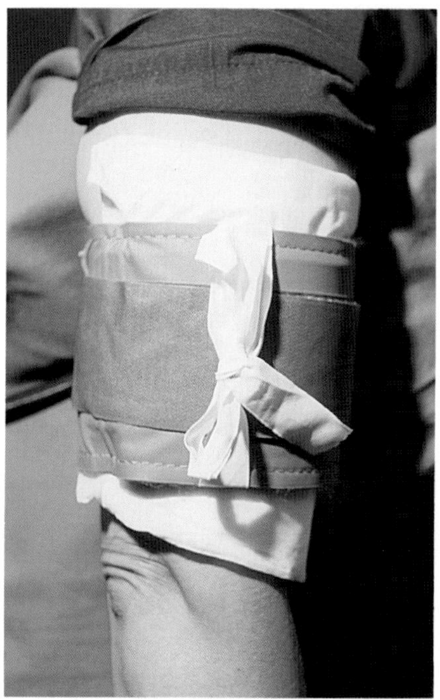

Fig. 8.8 Orthopaedic tourniquet applied to the upper arm over a layer of cotton-wool.

The orthopaedic tourniquet is applied to the upper arm over a layer of cotton-wool (Fig. 8.8). The site of the operation is then anaesthetized using local infiltration of 1% lignocaine. Povidone-iodine in spirit is applied to the operation site and covered with a sterile pad. The 3 in. Esmarch bandage is then applied to the elevated limb, starting at the extremity and working proximally as far as the orthopaedic tourniquet (Fig. 8.9). At this stage the tourniquet is inflated to above arterial pressure and the Esmarch bandage released.

The operation site is now anaesthetized and bloodless.

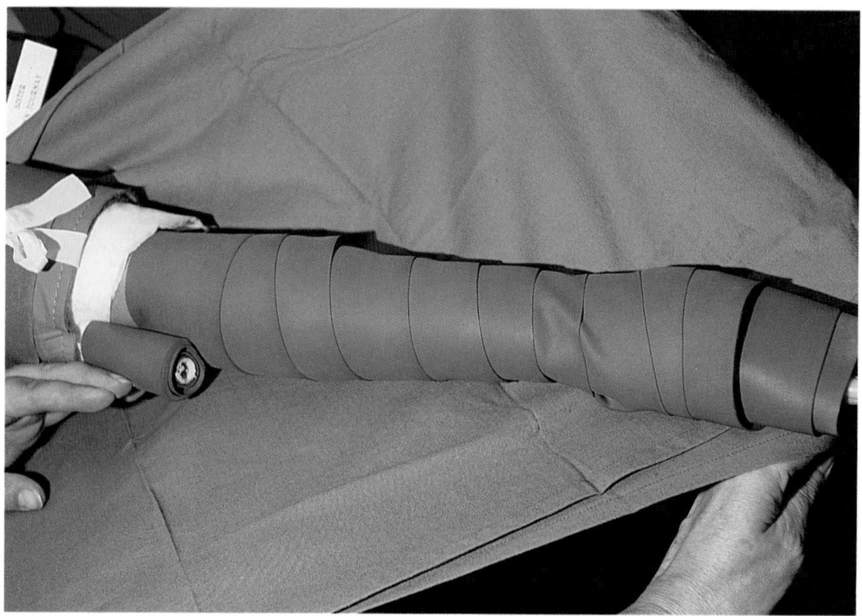

Fig. 8.9 Esmarch bandage applied to the elevated limb.

Caution

Because the application of a tourniquet above arterial pressure can cause discomfort or even pain, it is quite helpful to give the patient an intravenous premedication injection of midazolam and fentanyl prior to applying the tourniquet. For a fit, healthy, young adult the average doses are 4 mg midazolam and 100 μg fentanyl; these doses should be reduced proportionately in the young, elderly or frail.

8.16 AMNALGESIA

In this technique the awareness of painful stimuli is reduced and the patient, although appearing to be fully conversant with what is happening, has no recollection of it afterwards. This is achieved very simply by an intravenous injection of midazolam with or without an added analgesic such as fentanyl. For the average fit, healthy adult, midazolam 2–6 mg is usually sufficient, with the dosage correspondingly reduced for younger patients and the elderly. This technique is particularly valuable for the patient with malignant ascites who requires paracentesis and who will doze throughout the procedure, and have no recollection of it afterwards.

If given at the surgery, it is wise to allow the patient to rest for 1 hour afterwards and under no circumstances should they drive a car for the next 12 hours.

The sedative effects of benzodiazepines can now be reversed with intravenous Flumazenil.

8.17 ENTONOX INHALATION

A mixture of equal parts of oxygen and nitrous oxide is manufactured as Entonox (British Oxygen; Nitronox, USA) and is widely used for obstetric analgesia. The apparatus is patient controlled and exceptionally safe. The giving set attaches to a cylinder of Entonox and the patient can breathe directly via a low-pressure actuating valve in the set (Fig. 8.10). It is a most valuable piece of equipment in the minor operating theatre.

Twenty breaths of the gas will enable the doctor to remove splinters from under finger-nails, incise superficial abscesses, change painful dressings, and carry out painful procedures. It may also be used to reduce the

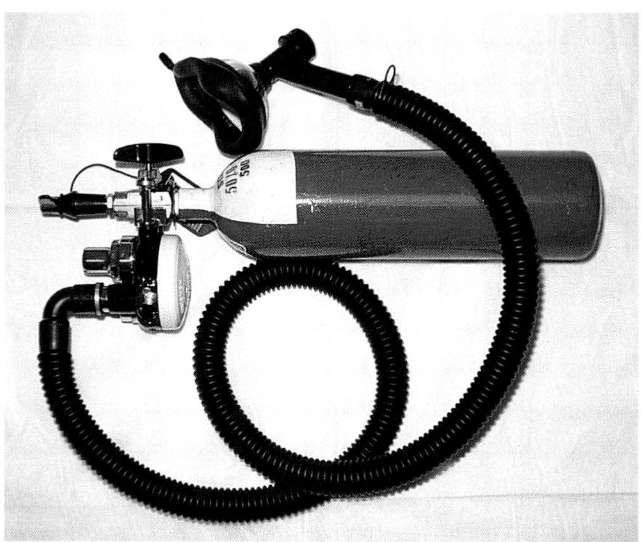

Fig. 8.10 Entonox giving set.

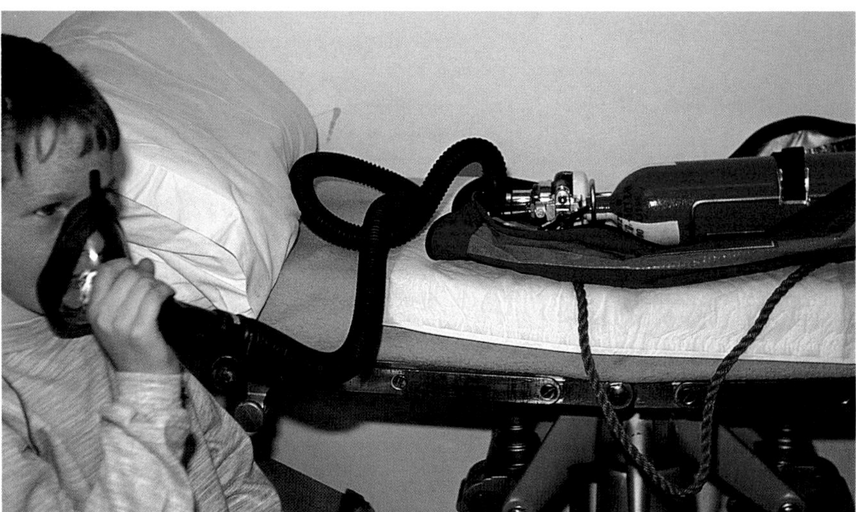

Fig. 8.11 Young patient using Entonox prior to removal of a splinter from under a finger-nail.

pain of giving a local anaesthetic injection, particularly in the sole of the foot, a technique appreciated by children and the nervous.

Furthermore, as recovery is so rapid the patient may leave the surgery as soon as the treatment is completed and no restrictions need be imposed regarding driving or cycling home. Even quite young children can be encouraged to use the Entonox 'mask' (Fig. 8.11).

8.18 GENERAL ANAESTHESIA

Few GPs now give general anaesthetics outside hospital premises. This contrasts with 50 years ago when chloroform, ether, nitrous oxide and pentothal were all widely used in the patient's home and doctor's surgery. Where a practice has facilities to give general anaesthetics, a doctor with a special interest in anaesthetics, and full recovery and resuscitation equipment, there is no reason why some of the minor operations mentioned should not be done under a general anaesthetic, particularly short-acting intravenous anaesthetics for such conditions as opening abscesses or the removal of toe-nails. On the whole, however, the doctor will find that all the minor operations described in this book can be very adequately and safely performed under local anaesthesia.

8.19 LOCAL ANAESTHETIC TECHNIQUE IN GENERAL PRACTICE

A frequent cause for discomfort to the patient is the allowance of insufficient time for the local anaesthetic to work, this applies particularly to infiltration anaesthesia and nerve blocks.

It can usually be avoided by giving the local anaesthetic before scrubbing up, using a sterile, no-touch technique, as follows:

1. The area to be anaesthetized is painted with povidone-iodine in spirit (Betadine alcoholic solution).
2. Without donning sterile gloves, but using a no-touch technique, local anaesthetic is drawn into a syringe.
3. The needle is changed for the finest gauge consistent with the operation.
4. Without touching the exact point of entry of the needle with the fingers, the local anaesthetic is injected.
5. The doctor may now scrub up while the assistant repaints the skin with povidone-iodine in spirit and applies any drapes.
6. By the time the doctor has scrubbed up, assembled all instruments and sutures, and applied any additional sterile drapes, the operation site should be fully anaesthetized.

9

Surgical techniques

And whosoever comes suffering from sores, with wounded limbs, or with wasted bodies, he (Aesculepius) delivers them, different ones from different pains, tending some with kindly incantations, giving some soothing potions, while he set some on their feet again with the knife.

Pindar, Pythian Ode III

One aim of each operation will be to achieve as neat a scar as possible. Many patients will expect to end up with no scar at all, and it is perhaps wise to warn them at the first consultation that it is physically not possible to achieve such a result. However, by observing a few simple rules it is possible to obtain a nearly invisible scar in most cases.

Skin is a living tissue, and must be treated gently and with respect. Good healing will only occur if the cut edges are held in exact position, and under no tension. Tissues should be cut with a sharp scalpel rather than scissors, which have a shearing action.

Dissection should be likewise with a sharp scalpel rather than gauze.

Haemostasis should be achieved carefully, although in most minor surgical procedures this is not a major problem.

Sutures should be the finest, consistent with the ability to hold the wound together, and should be removed at the earliest opportunity (Fig. 9.1).

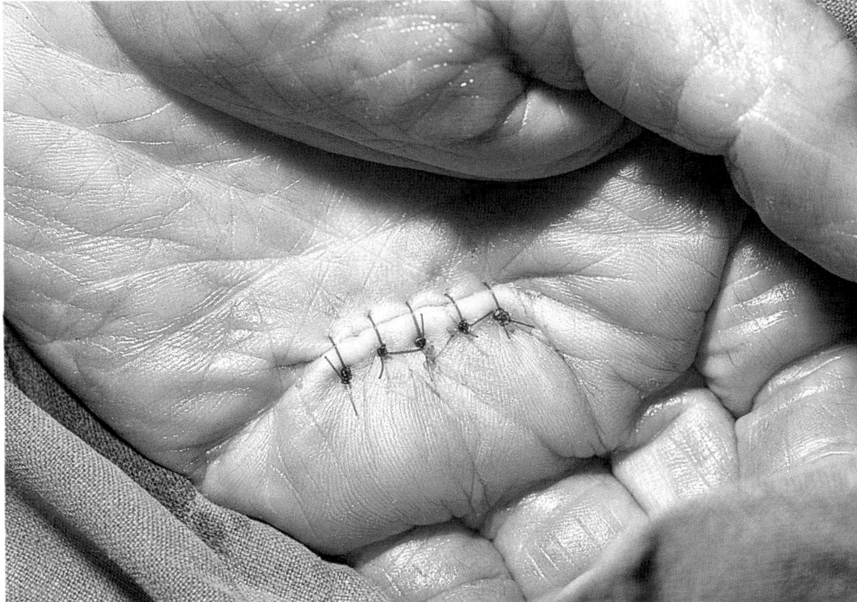

Fig. 9.1 Use the finest gauge sutures, closely spaced together, preferably in the line of a skin crease, to obtain the neatest scar.

Subcutaneous absorbable sutures should be placed as deep as possible, and be as few as possible, and the knots tied in the deeper plane.

Absorbable sutures should, in general, not be used for the skin where a good cosmetic result is required.

Many fine, closely positioned sutures are preferable to a few widely spaced stitches. Tissues should be handled as little as possible, and particularly not with any crushing forceps. Single skin hooks should be used to hold or retract skin flaps.

The surgeon who inserts the sutures should be the person who removes them, or at least supervises their removal. Only by personally examining each wound postoperatively can improvements in technique be achieved.

9.1 HAEMOSTASIS

Bleeding may occur from fine capillaries or visible blood vessels, either arteries or veins.

9.1.1 Fine capillaries

When any tissue is cut there is fine capillary oozing. Most of this will stop spontaneously; some will be reduced if adrenaline is included with the local anaesthetic, but in the remainder firm pressure is all that is required. However, pressure needs to be applied for a realistic time – up to 3 min in some cases – and this needs to be timed using a clock or timer.

Unusual capillary bleeding may occur where there are coagulation defects or abnormal capillaries, e.g. the patient may be taking anticoagulant therapy, there may be a blood dyscrasia, or more rarely vitamin C deficiency or thrombocytopenia.

9.1.2 Visible blood vessels

Bleeding from visible blood vessels is usually more brisk than from capillaries, and often the exact source of bleeding cannot immediately be seen. In this case the application of firm pressure with a swab for 1–3 min whilst spasm of the vessel is occurring will often be all that is required.

If on carefully removing the swab a bleeding source can be identified it should be picked off with a pair of fine artery forceps. As little surrounding tissue as possible should be included in the jaws of the forceps.

Having grasped the blood vessel, it must then be secured by tying a fine absorbable suture around it. As the first part of the knot is tied, the forceps are gradually released, at the same time tightening the knot; the forceps are then removed.

If the blood vessel can be seen, and has not been divided, it may be secured by tying two ligatures around it and then dividing between them.

9.2 TISSUE HEALING

For good healing to occur each surface must be cleanly cut, have a good blood supply and be in good apposition. Where a surgical incision has been made the above conditions can usually be met: where, however, there is a contused traumatic wound, accurate apposition of clean healthy tissues may not be possible, and in this situation it is necessary to trim the traumatized edges with a scalpel. Similarly, any foreign bodies should be carefully removed prior to closure.

In a connective tissue injury, the blood filling the cavity forms a fibrin clot, this becomes replaced by granulation tissue, which then becomes replaced by fibroblast proliferation. Eventually collagen fibrils form, fibrous tissue develops, the scar becomes avascular, pale, and predominantly collagen. This gradually shrinks over the ensuing months and years.

Occasionally the healing process 'overshoots' producing a hypertrophic or keloid scar. This process is not fully understood, but it is known to happen more frequently in pigmented skin, and in certain sites of the body, notably over the front of the sternum and shoulder, and in patients of Afro-Caribbean origin.

9.3 SURGICAL TECHNIQUE USING PIGS' TROTTERS

Whilst most doctors will have had more than adequate training in surgical techniques, nevertheless different procedures may be tried using pigs' trotters, obtainable from any butchers or supermarket. The skin texture is very similar to human skin, and incisions, suturing techniques, electrocautery, cryotherapy, and various alternative methods of skin closure may be practiced (Fig. 9.2). Furthermore, pigs' trotters also provide an ideal medium for teaching suturing techniques to practice nurses and trainees.

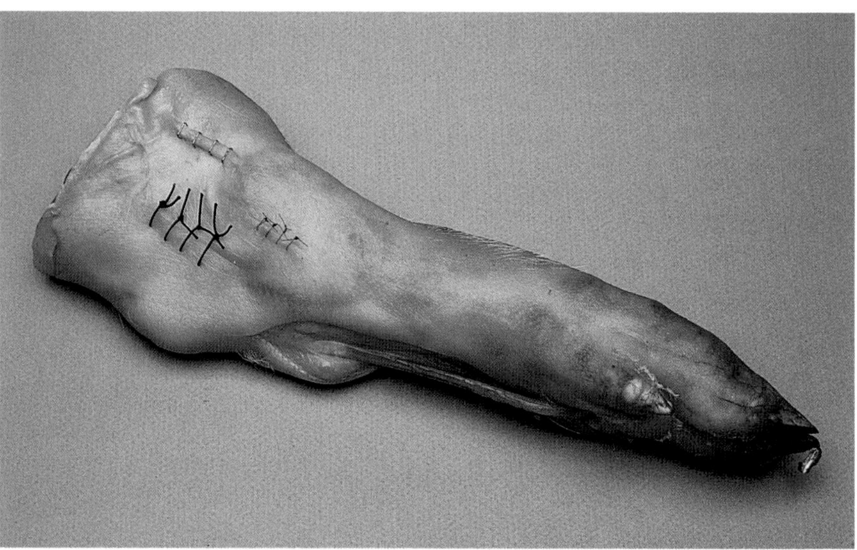

Fig. 9.2 Pigs' trotters may be used to practise suture technique and other minor surgical procedures.

9.4 SURGICAL TECHNIQUE USING SKIN SIMULATORS

Skin simulators designed to simulate conditions met in minor surgery without the use of biological material are now available. They are remarkably realistic, and models of sebaceous cysts, lipoma, peri-anal haematoma, as well as skin are all available from Limbs and Things Ltd, Bristol (Figs 9.3–9.10). Skin simulators are also available from Ethicon, Edinburgh.

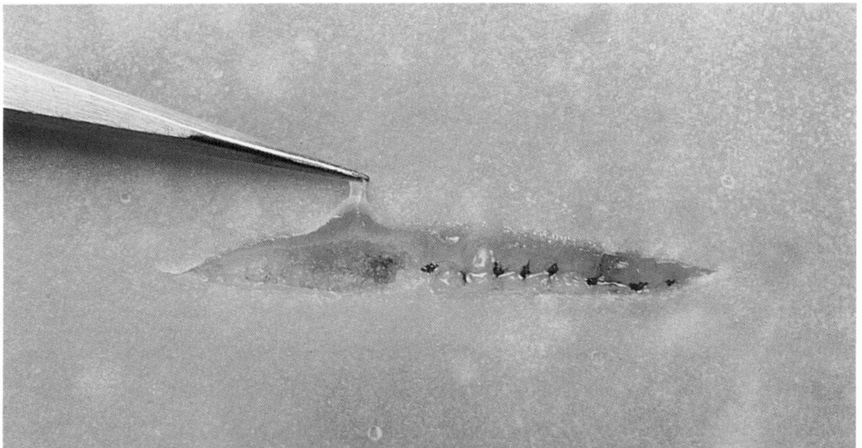

Fig. 9.3 Model of skin with three layers – epidermis, dermis and subdermis – for practising suturing, undercutting and knot tying (Limbs & Things Ltd, Bristol, UK).

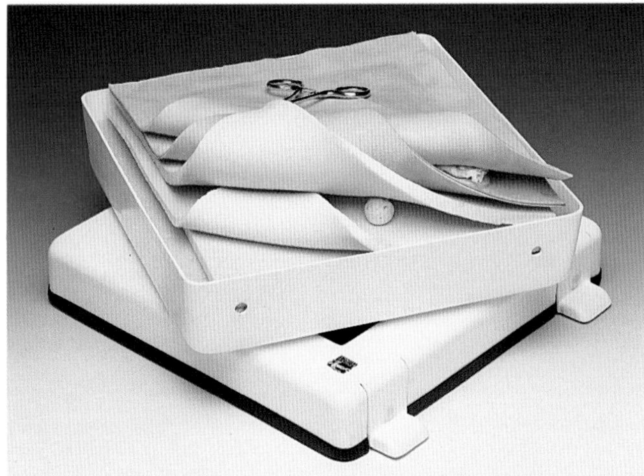

Fig. 9.4a Model with several layers representing different tissue planes in which a series of lumps and bumps can be inserted (Limbs & Things Ltd, Bristol, UK).

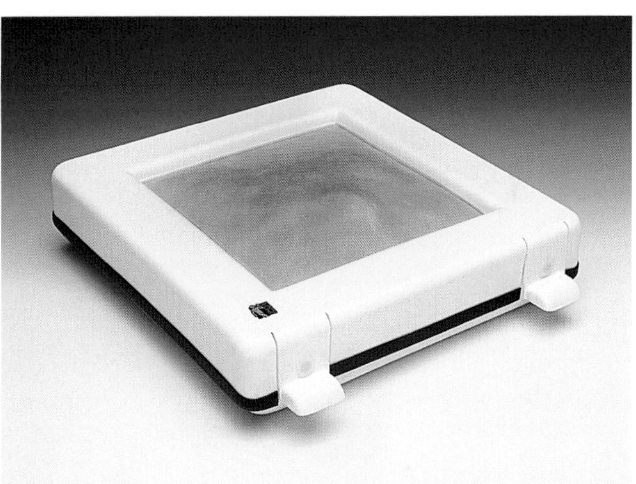

Fig. 9.4b Model with 'lump' situated between layers, simulating a cyst (Limbs & Things Ltd, Bristol, UK).

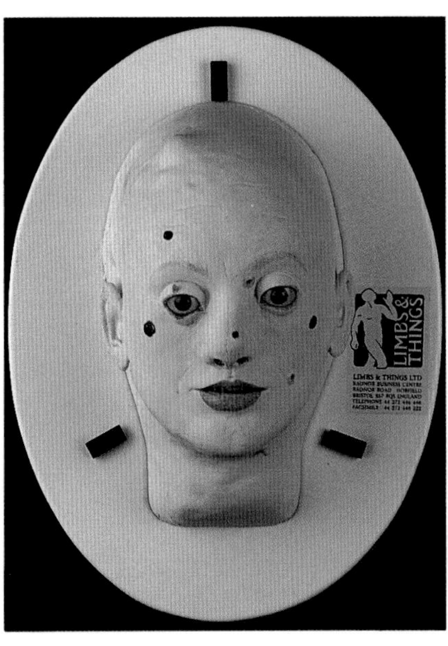

Fig. 9.5a A model face with a variety of different lesions including sebaceous cyst, meibomian cyst, mucous cyst, skin tags, crusty warts, basal cell carcinoma, keratoacanthoma and malignant melanoma (Limbs & Things Ltd, Bristol, UK).

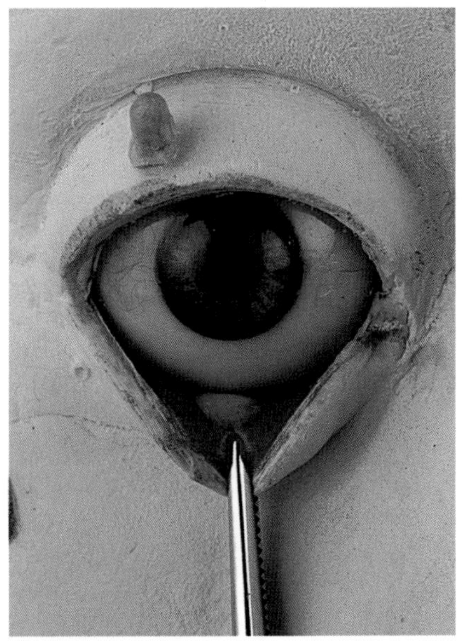

Fig. 9.5b A realistic meibomian cyst in the lower eye-lid (Limbs & Things Ltd, Bristol, UK).

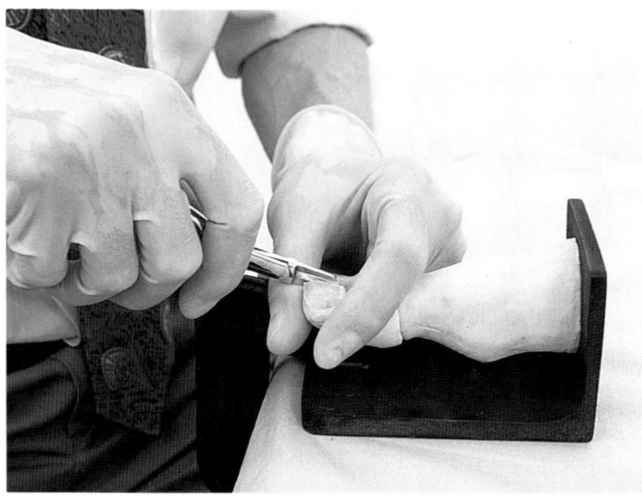

Fig. 9.6a Model to mimic an inflamed ingrowing toe-nail. Detachable toe ends can be inserted into the 'foot' (Limbs & Things Ltd, Bristol, UK).

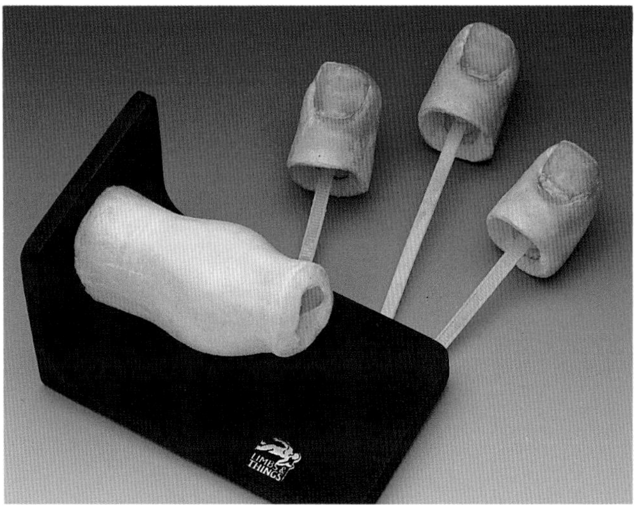

Fig. 9.6b A selection of 'toe ends' and the 'master toe' (Limbs & Things Ltd, Bristol, UK).

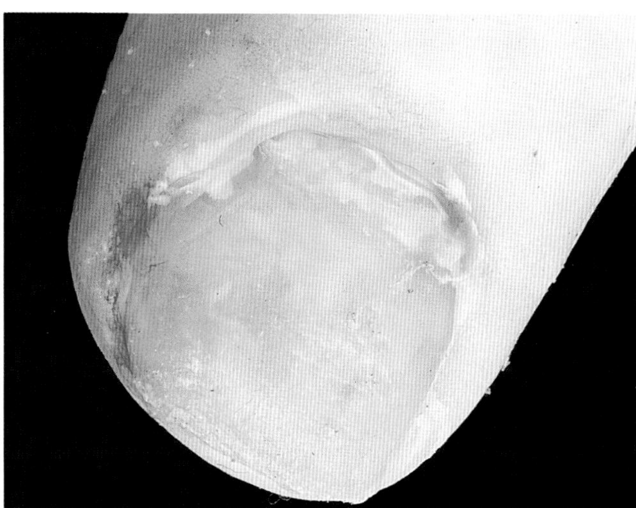

Fig. 9.6c A remarkably realistic inflamed ingrowing toe-nail (Limbs & Things Ltd, Bristol, UK).

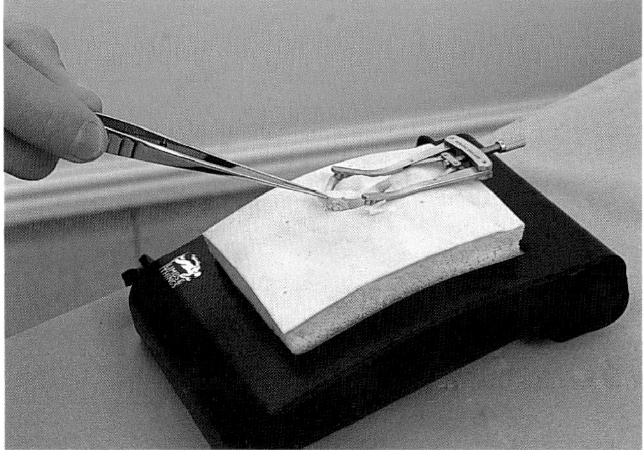

Fig. 9.7 A lipoma being dissected out (Limbs & Things Ltd, Bristol, UK).

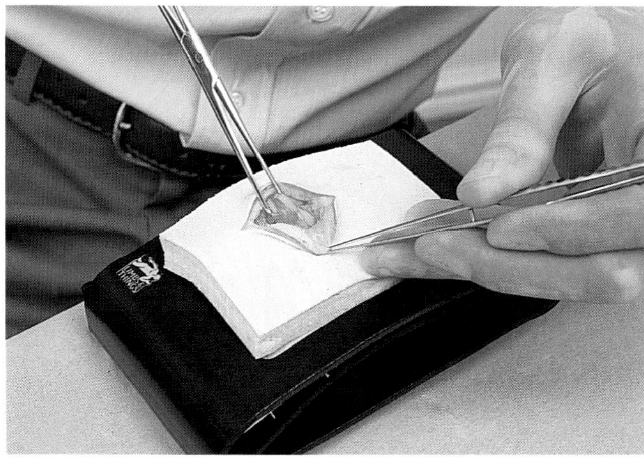

Fig. 9.8 A sebaceous cyst containing realistically unpleasant smelling material in the centre. Beware of puncturing it! (Limbs & Things Ltd, Bristol, UK).

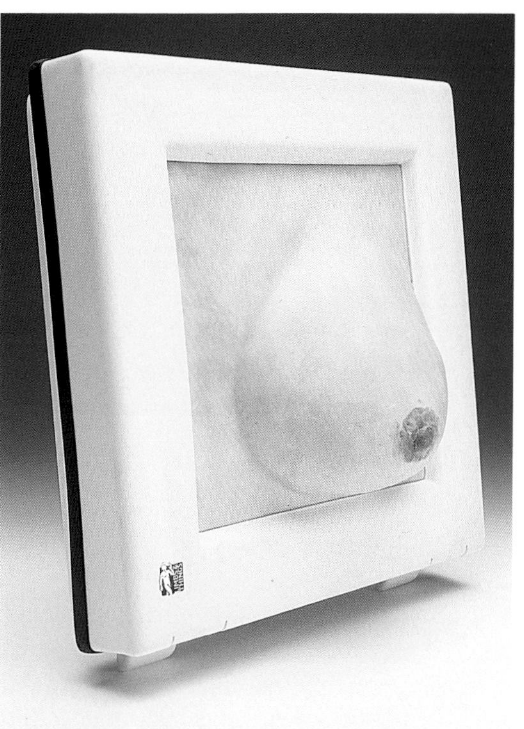

Fig. 9.9 A model of the breast containing a simulated fibroadenoma, carcinoma and benign cyst (Limbs & Things Ltd, Bristol, UK).

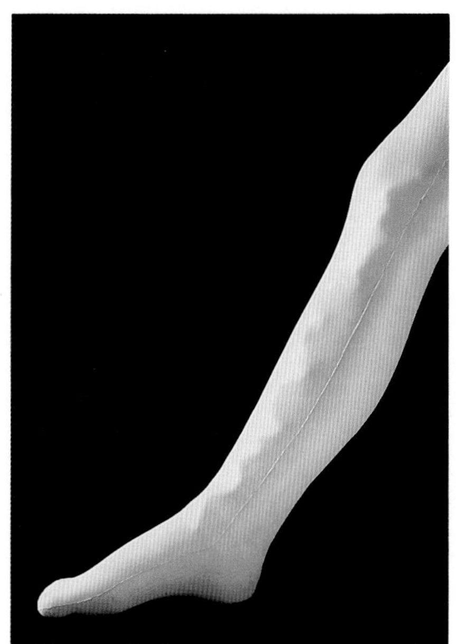

Fig. 9.10a A highly convincing leg with varicose veins containing 'blood' and veins which collapse when the limb is elevated (Limbs & Things Ltd, Bristol, UK).

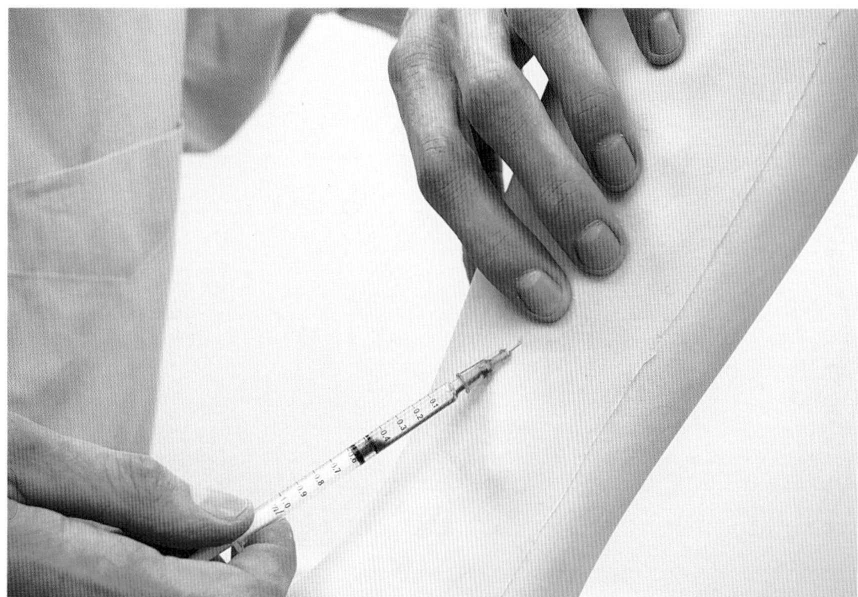

Fig. 9.10b Practising sclerotherapy (Limbs & Things Ltd, Bristol, UK).

10

Incisions

There are three ways of opening an abscess so as to give outlet to the matter: by caustic, by incision, or by the introduction of feton. The first is more agreeable to timid patients who are afraid of the pain of incision
Encyclopaedia Britannica, 1797

Patients judge their surgeons by the end result which can be seen, viz. the operation scar. With a little forethought and variation in technique, almost invisible scars can be produced, depending on the knowledge of certain lines on the body, first described by Langer [6] in 1861. Until that time operative incisions were made where they would be most effective to excise the pathological lesion with little regard to the resultant scar. Textbook of plastic surgery then reproduced pictures of Langer's lines designed to give optimum healing and the neatest scars [7, 8, 9] and it was not until 1950 that some doubt was cast on this atlas of lines for incision by Smith [10]

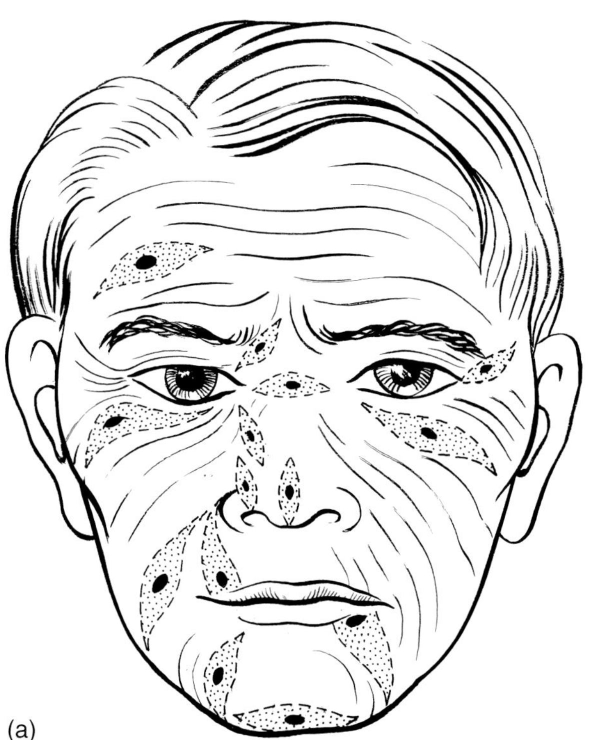

(a)

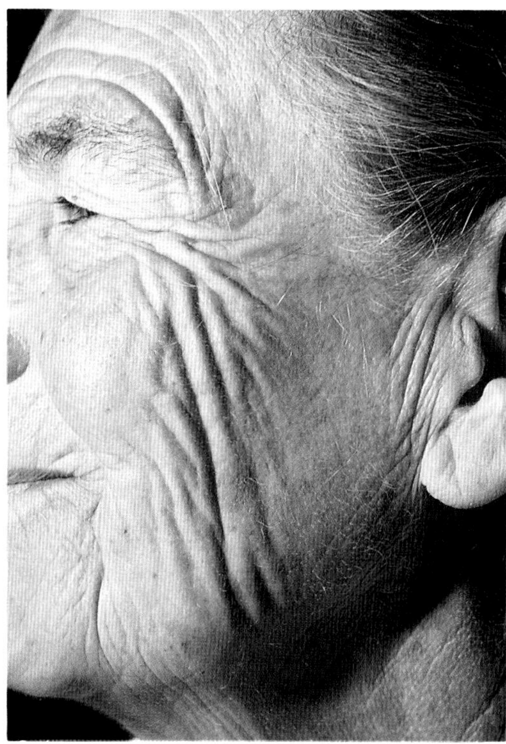

(b)

Fig. 10.1a Wrinkle lines and optimal sites for incisions on the face. (**b**) Incisions made in the line of skin creases will give the neatest scars.

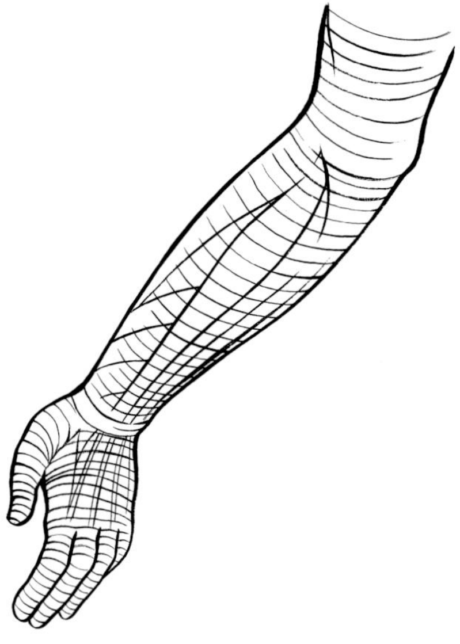

Fig. 10.2 Langer lines for the forearm, and sites for incisions, across underlying muscles.

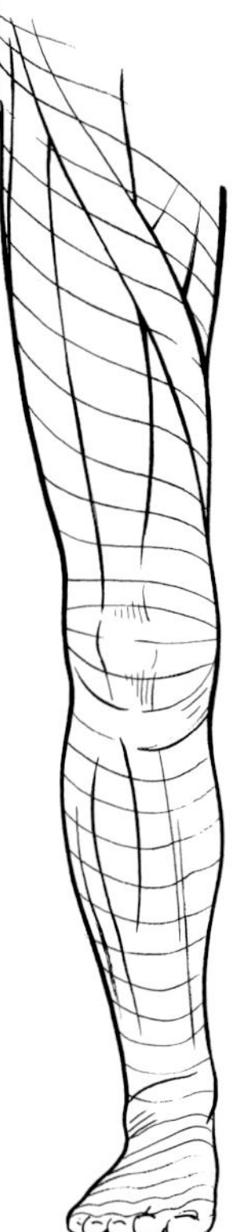

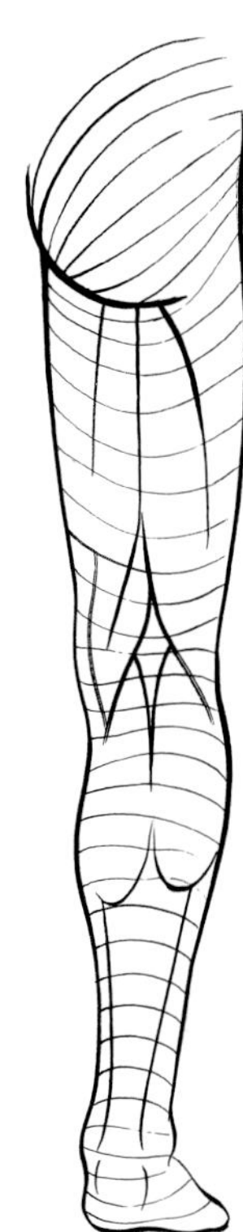

Fig. 10.3 Langer lines for the lower limb, crossing the direction of the underlying muscles.

Fig. 10.4 Langer lines for upper limb.

and subsequently in 1951 by Kraissl [11] who compared the traditional Langer lines with wrinkle lines or skin creases. Most wrinkle lines run perpendicular to the action of underlying muscles, and it is common experience that incisions made in these wrinkle lines give the neatest scars with minimum disruption of function. Thus, in planning the elective incision the following points should be borne in mind:

1. Look for natural creases and if possible follow these lines (Figs 10.1–10.4).
2. Where there is an underlying joint the incision should be placed transversely across it to prevent loss of function.
3. To demonstrate some wrinkles, gently compress the relaxed skin in different directions to ascertain the line, or ask the patient to contract the underlying muscles.
4. In many parts of the body, traditional Langer lines are at variance with natural wrinkle lines; in these situations it is better to use the skin creases.

One of the most important aspects in achieving a neat scar is the avoidance of tension; this may mean careful undercutting to approximate the skin edges, and the placing of many fine sutures rather than widely placed interrupted sutures of inappropriately thick suture material. Tension may also be minimized by subcutaneous absorbable sutures, and externally by the use of Steri-strips in addition to sutures.

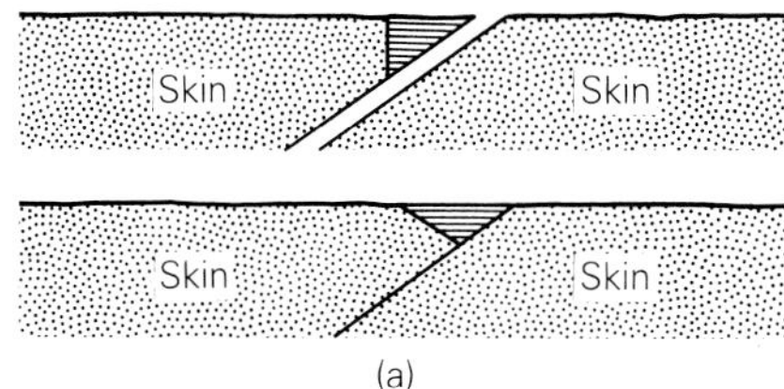

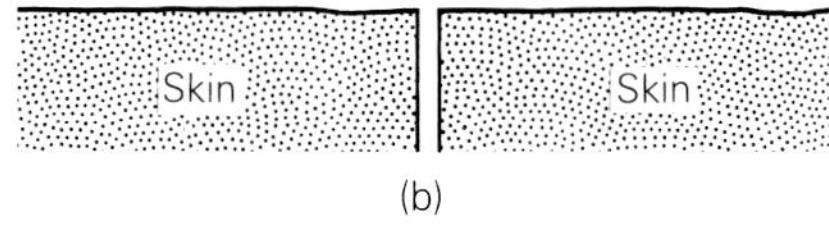

Fig. 10.5 Technique of skin incision. (**a**) Incorrect: oblique incision, resulting in broad scar; (**b**) correct: vertical incision giving linear scar. (Redrawn from B.A. Maurice, *Surgery for General Practitioners*, by permission of Oxford University Press.)

Infection is a potent cause of unsightly scars – often as a result of an infected subcutaneous haematoma. The latter can be minimized by careful attention to haemostasis at the time of the operation, the obliteration of any dead spaces, and, where appropriate, the insertion of a small drain for 48 hours postoperatively.

10.1 TECHNIQUE OF SKIN INCISION

Whichever scalpel blade is used, one paramount principle must be adhered to – the incision through the skin must be at right-angles and never slanted or oblique (Fig. 10.5). Secondly, the scalpel blade should cut completely through the epidermis and dermis in one stroke if at all possible. Thirdly, try to estimate the length of the scar at the outset: a neater scar will result if the original scar is not lengthened: too short a scar will necessitate undue traction on the skin edges and unnecessarily traumatize the tissues. Fourthly, keep the skin under tension while making the incision (Fig. 10.6). This is necessary otherwise the skin will tend to ruck up ahead of the scalpel. Tension is most easily applied using thumb and forefinger as shown.

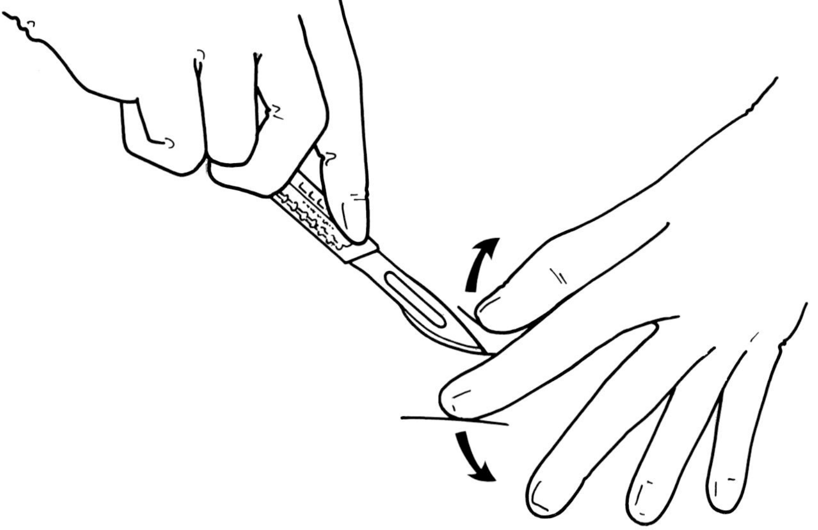

Fig. 10.6 Technique of skin incision keeping the skin under tension with finger and thumb. (Redrawn from B.A. Maurice, *Surgery for General Practitioners*, by permission of Oxford University Press.)

10.2 DEEPER DISSECTION

Scalpel dissection and radiowave surgery produce the least tissue trauma. Curved McIndoe scissors have the advantage that they may be used for both blunt and sharp dissection, whilst curved mosquito forceps can be used for blunt dissection by inserting the closed forceps in the wound and opening the blades. Blunt dissection will often reveal underlying vessels and nerves.

At the earliest opportunity, retractors should be inserted in the wound to improve the operator's view. These may be self-retaining, single skin-hooks, or combined 'cat's paw' retractors, held by an assistant.

A single suture placed in the dermis is a simple effective means of applying traction.

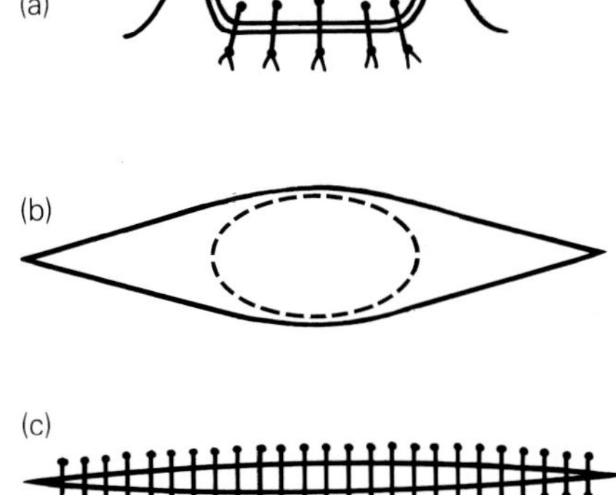

Fig. 10.7 Development of 'dog-ear'. (**a**) Tension on stitches of circular excision causes dog ear at each end. (**b**) Ellipse lengthened so tension is evened out over full length of incision. (**c**) Scar longer but cosmetically better. No dog ears. (Redrawn from B.A. Maurice, *Surgery for General Practitioners*, by permission of Oxford University Press.)

Cutaneous nerves should be divided with a scalpel if they cannot be preserved. This may produce anaesthesia in the distal part of the incision, but with careful closure a high proportion will recover.

10.3 EXCISION

Much of minor surgery entails the excision of a skin lesion, be it a small intradermal naevus or a basal cell carcinoma. This will, of necessity, leave a skin defect to dose, and whether an unsightly scar or a near invisible scar ensues will depend on how the excision is planned and how the gap is closed.

If a disc of skin is removed and the edges pulled together, there is a risk that the centre will have an impaired blood supply and fail to heal, and also a risk of producing a 'dog-ear' at each end of the scar (Fig. 10.7a). However, if instead of a disc an elongated ellipse is removed and the edges undermined, the skin will come together more easily, and there will be no dog-ears (Fig. 10.7b).

Next, the direction of the final scar needs to be calculated. This will need to lie along a skin crease or Langer's lines to give the neatest scar. Joining the points of the ellipse will give the line of the final scar (Fig. 10.7c, 10.9, 10.10).

As a skin incision heals from side to side, a longer incision with no tension will heal better than a shorter one under tension.

10.4 TECHNIQUE FOR REMOVAL OF A 'DOG-EAR'

If despite careful planning of the excision, a dog-ear is produced at the end of the scar, it may be eradicated as follows:

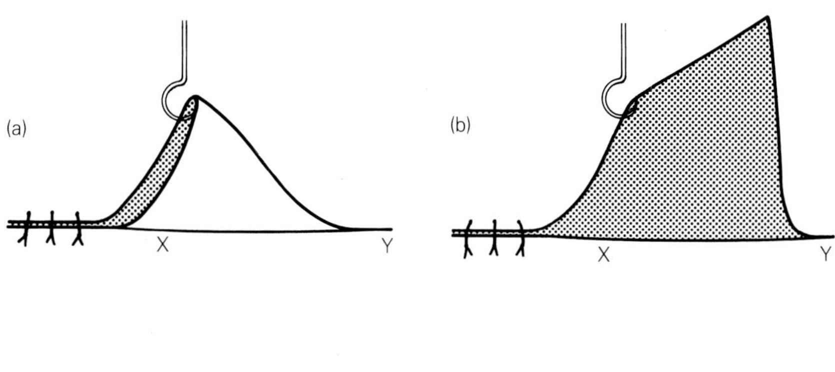

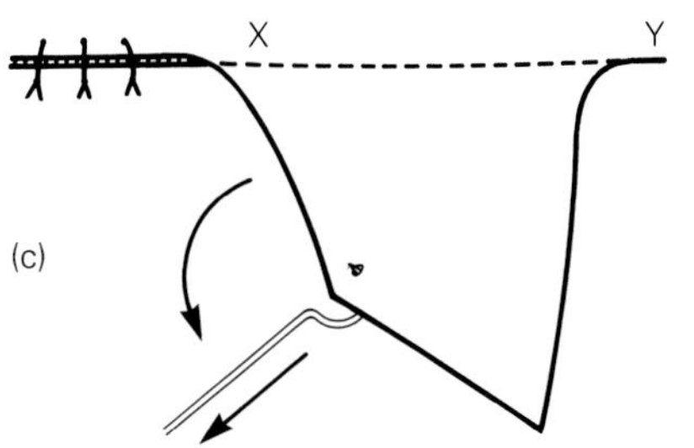

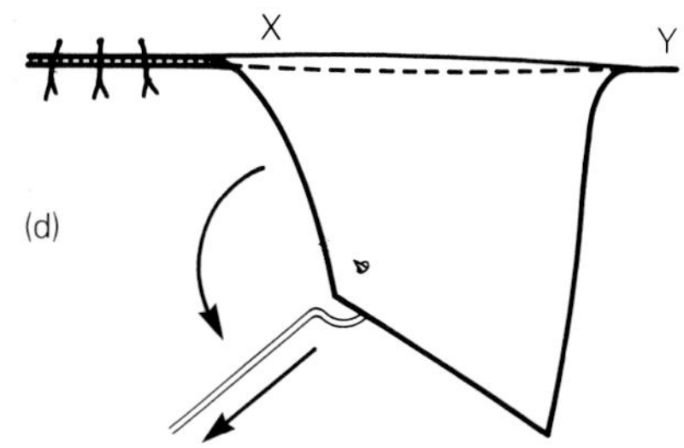

Fig. 10.8 Removal of 'dog-ear'. (**a**) 'Dog-ear' held up with skin hook. Incision at right-angles to skin, X–Y. (**b**) 'Dog-ear' after first cut held up. Undersurface of skin; skin hook in same place. (**c**) Flap now lying flat. Underlying skin incision line; skin hook in same place. (**d**) Flap excised. Along X–Y. (Redrawn from B.A. Maurice, *Surgery for General Practitioners*, by permission of Oxford University Press.)

1. The centre of the incision is sutured as far as possible.
2. The remaining dog-ear is lifted up with a single skin hook.
3. The base is cut with a scalpel as shown in Fig. 10.8, at right-angles to the skin.
4. The flap of skin is now pulled over the same line cut on the opposite side (see Fig. 10.8a, b, c, d).

The excess dog-ear is excised, and the wound sutured.

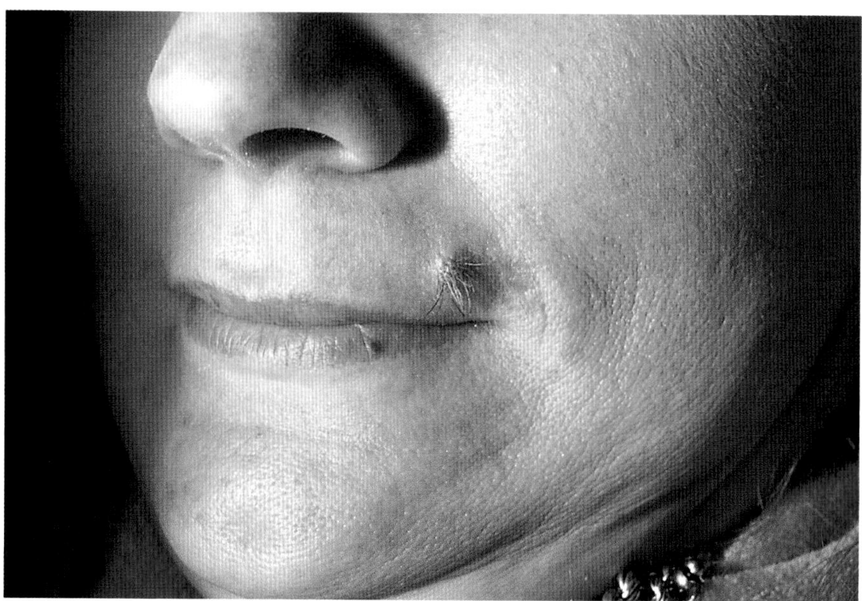

Fig. 10.9 Pigmented hairy intradermal melanocytic naevus on face.

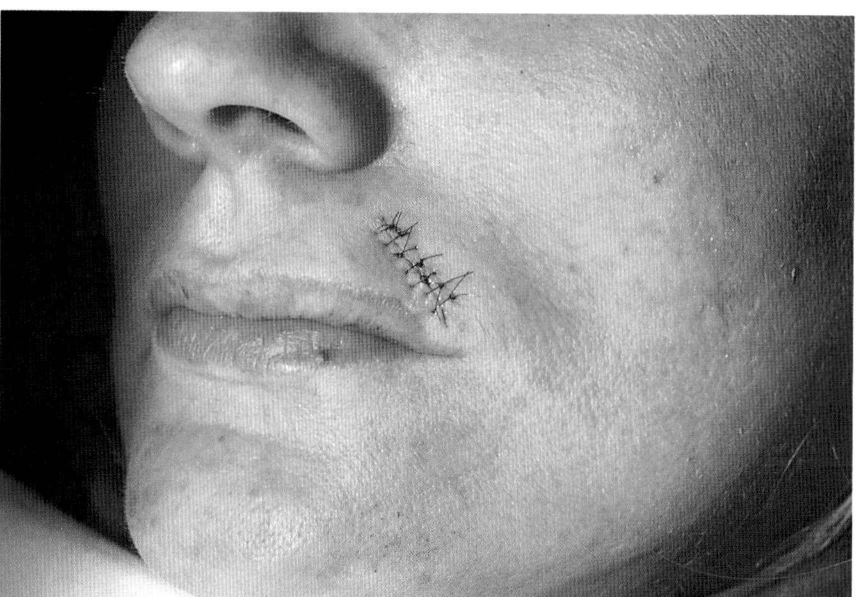

Fig. 10.10 Excision by ellipse with final scar lying along a skin crease. Multiple 6/0 monofilament Prolene sutures which were removed after 4 days.

11

Skin closure

Sutures are best made of soft thread, not too hard twisted that it may sit easier on the tissues, nor are too few nor too many of either of them to be put in

Aulus Cornelius Celsus, 25 BC–AD 50

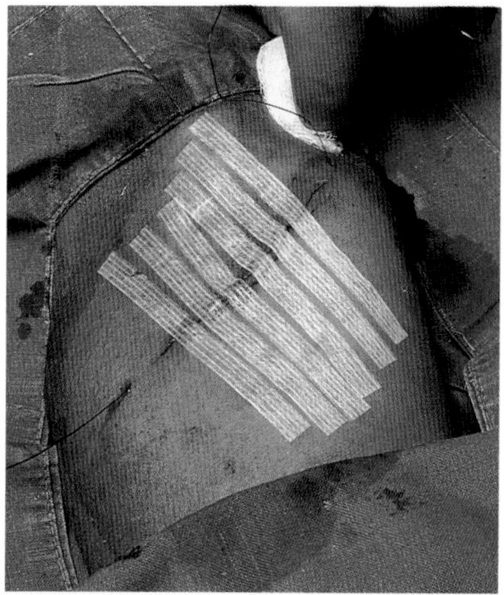

Fig. 11.1 Steri-strips may be used both to close a wound and also to give additional support for sutures (3M).

Following any operation, if skin edges are closely approximated without tension, healing will generally occur in ten days. Traditionally surgeons have used interrupted sutures to hold the skin edges together, but stitches are not always necessary nor desirable and many alternative methods have been used in an attempt to give as neat a scar as possible.

The simplest method of skin closure is self-adhesive tape; where tension can be avoided, excellent results are obtained and it is particularly suitable for small superficial lacerations on the face and fingers. Ordinary, non-stretch, self-adhesive plaster tape can be used, but better results are obtained with purpose made sterile strips (Steri-strips 3M) which can be readily applied and which have good tensile strength (Figs 11.1 and 11.2).

It is important if using sterile strips that good adhesion is obtained; thus the skin must be thoroughly dry, and if in an area where increased perspiration occurs, extra adhesion may be obtained by first painting the skin with tinct. benz. co. or collodion prior to applying the Steri-strips. Additional external support can be given by careful bandaging, and if the original wound is clean, may be left undisturbed for up to ten days. Most lacerations on fingers and toes can be satisfactorily closed using Steri-strips supplemented with tubular cotton stockinette bandage. It is important that

A

B

C

D

E

Fig. 11.2 Skin closure strips are ideal for small wounds and for giving additional support during healing.
Size A 3 mm × 75 mm
Size B 6 mm × 50 mm
Size C 6 mm × 75 mm
Size D 6 mm × 100 mm
Size E 12 mm × 100 mm.

Fig. 11.3 Simple method of closing a small laceration of the scalp by knotting a few strands of hair on either side of the wound.

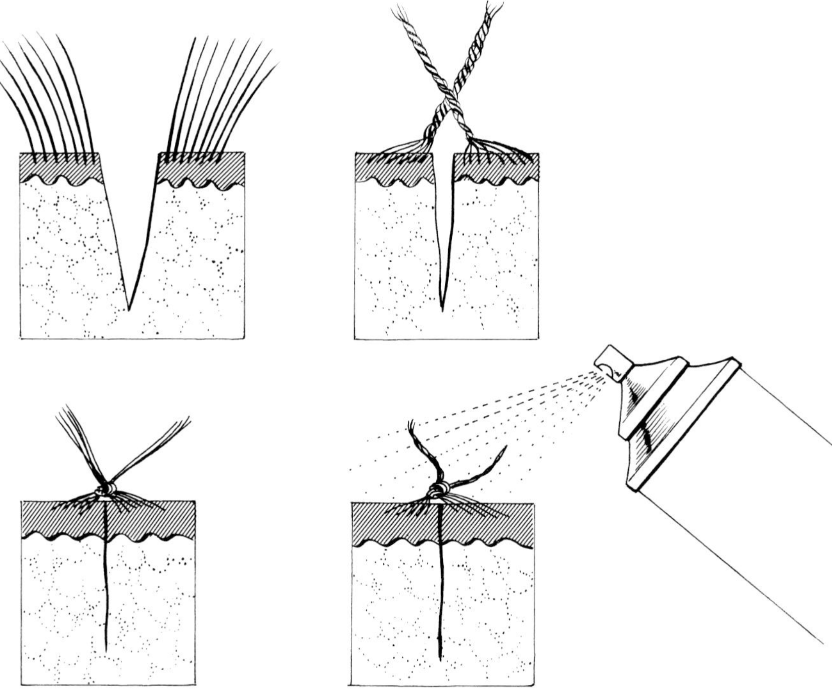

Fig. 11.4 Another simple method of suturing a wound using a hypodermic needle and some nylon fishing line.

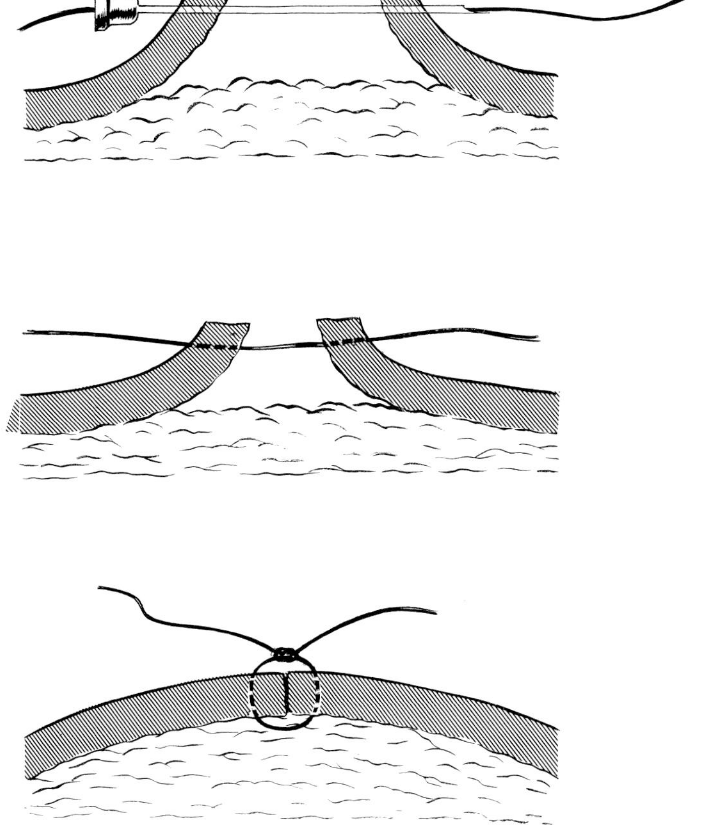

the strip does not completely encircle the digit in case oedema occurs and the Steri-strip then acts as a tourniquet with ensuing ischaemia or necrosis. In very young children sutures may be preferable to sterile strip closure in case the child inadvertently pulls off the dressing and strips before healing has occurred.

Faced with a small laceration on the scalp satisfactory skin closure may often be achieved merely by twisting a few strands of hair on either side of the wound and knotting them together over the laceration (Fig. 11.3). Spraying the knot with Nobecutane spray, tinct. benz. co. or collodion will prevent the knot slipping, and the knot may then be cut free after ten days when healing has occurred. Another 'first-aid' method of skin closure in the absence of suitable suture materials uses hypodermic needles and nylon fishing line! The needles may be inserted through the skin edges from one side to another, the nylon thread passed through the lumen of the needle which is then withdrawn over the thread, leaving the nylon ready to be tied. Very satisfactory skin closure may be achieved using this simple procedure (Fig. 11.4).

11.1 SUTURES

The doctor looking through a catalogue of surgical sutures will find a bewildering array of materials in all sizes, colours, absorbability, needle sizes etc. Basically the majority of surgical sutures will be either absorbable or non-absorbable. Absorbable sutures as their name implies slowly dissolve as the tissues heal, and therefore do not need to be removed; non-absorbable sutures do not dissolve, and need to be removed. The different sutures are described in the following sections.

11.1.1 Interrupted, plain

This is the commonest method of suturing. The needle is inserted through the skin, across the subcutaneous part of the wound, through the skin on the opposite side, and then knotted, bringing the edges together. As most suture materials have a tendency to slip, a reef knot with one additional throw (surgeon's knot) is used.

11.1.2 Interrupted (mattress)

Where skin edges may not approximate accurately due to laxity of the tissues or any other reason, good apposition may be achieved by including the skin edges in the suture (vertical mattress). Interrupted sutures give a neat scar but are occasionally quite difficult to remove.

11.1.3 Subcuticular sutures

These are becoming increasingly popular and will give an extremely neat scar providing the skin is not under tension (Fig. 11.5a, b). A straight needle is preferable, although cutting curved needles can be used. The needle is inserted through the skin about 1–2 cm away from, but in line with, the incision. It is passed under the skin to emerge in the subcuticular

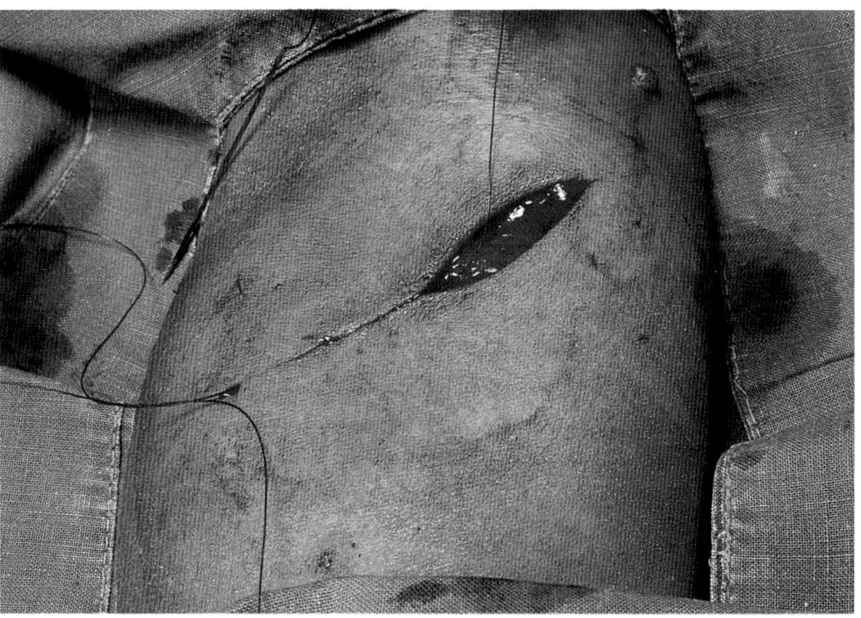

Fig. 11.5a A subcuticular stitch gives a neat scar and takes less time to insert than interrupted sutures.

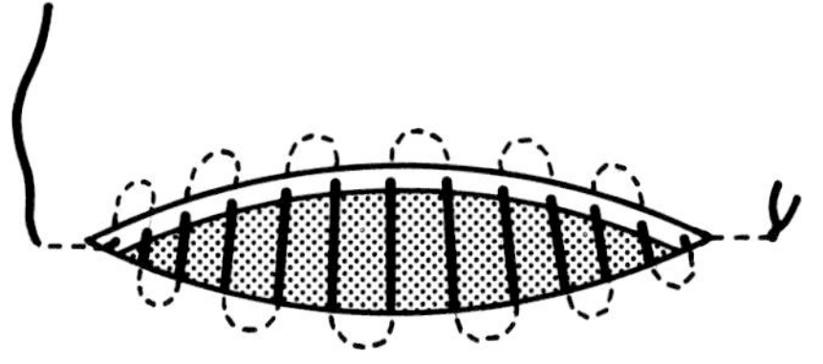

Fig. 11.5b Subcuticular stitch. (Redrawn from B.A. Maurice, *Surgery for General Practitioners*, by permission of Oxford University Press.)

layer on one side of the wound; it is then passed backwards and forwards across the wound, eventually emerging beyond the other end of the incision corresponding to where the suture commenced. By applying traction to both ends of the suture, the skin edges are approximated neatly, and the part of the suture remaining visible is fixed to the skin either with tape, dressings or a single 'button'. Removal is effected by cutting one end flush with the skin, and firmly pulling the other.

11.1.4 Continuous and blanket stitch

These tend to be used for longer scars, and are generally seldom used for minor surgical incisions. As their name implies, a continuous stitch extends from one end of the wound to the other; it is quick to insert, difficult to achieve even tension and even spacing of the stitch, not easy to remove, has an increased risk of infection during removal, and does not allow the removal of individual sutures should fluid collect under the scar and require drainage.

11.2 SUTURE MATERIALS

Every doctor has a personal selection of preferred suture materials; listed in the following sections are the various types available.

11.2.1 Plain catgut

This is made from purified ribbons of animal intestines, which are spun into a strand, electronically gauged, and then polished. It is absorbed by body enzymes; originally it was very popular, but has tended to be superseded by synthetic absorbable sutures in recent years.

11.2.2 Chromic catgut

This is made from ribbons of animal intestines, spun into a strand, exactly as plain catgut, but treated so that the strength of the suture is maintained for a considerably longer time than plain catgut. It is still used in obstetrics, and for approximating subcutaneous tissues, but is being superseded by synthetic materials.

11.2.3 Braided silk (Mersilk)

The raw silk is treated and de-gummed prior to braiding, resulting in a compact braid which ties easily; it used to be extremely popular but has now been superseded by monofilament nylon and Prolene sutures.

11.2.4 Monofilament polyamide 6 and 66 (Ethilon)

These are synthetic, monofilament sutures, whose smooth surface does not appear to support bacterial growth. They can be difficult to knot, but are useful for subcuticular sutures.

11.2.5 Monofilament polypropylene (Prolene)

The advantage of polypropylene is that it is supple, ties securely and handles well. As with other monofilament synthetic sutures, knots need to be square ties with additional throws, and in addition, damage from forceps and needle holders should be avoided to prevent fracture of the material. It is extremely smooth and suitable for subcuticular stitches. It is now one of the most popular materials for skin sutures.

11.2.6 Polyglycolic acid synthetic absorbable sutures (Dexon)

These sutures, introduced in recent years, are extremely popular, they appear to cause virtually no tissue reaction as they dissolve, compared with considerable histological tissue reaction with catgut. Their rate of absorption is considerably slower than even chromic catgut, and may take several weeks. It is an ideal suture material for all subcutaneous skin closures.

11.2.7 Coated polyglactin 910 (Vicryl)

Coated Vicryl is a multifilament synthetic absorbable suture, manufactured as a copolymer of glycolide and lactide. Individual filaments are braided together and then treated with an absorbable coating. This coating allows smooth passage of the suture through the skin, and also makes the tying of knots easy.

Absorption is by hydrolysis and appears to cause only minimal tissue reaction.

It is now one of the most popular and widely used sutures for subcutaneous use, with tensile strength lasting at least 28–40 days.

All suture materials are now graded by metric gauge, which indicates the actual diameter of the suture in tenths of a millimetre, and this gauging has now been adopted by both European and United States Pharmacopoeia, replacing the former system of 0 gauges thus:

USP/BP	Metric
7/0	0.5
6/0	0.7
5/0	1.0
4/0	1.5
3/0	2.0
2/0	3.0
0	3.5

11.2.8 Polybutester (Novafil)

This is a monofilament suture which is easier to handle and knot than some earlier monofilament sutures.

A selection of the most widely used suture materials is now included in the Drug Tariff and doctors in the UK can now prescribe these for use on their National Health Service patients. For minor surgical procedures, the following 'short-list' will provide a basic treatment set.

1. Sterile monofilament polyamide 6 Ethilon 1.5 metric gauge (formerly 410) Ref. W 319. Ideal for most skin closures.
2. Sterile braided silk metric 1 (formerly 5/0) Mersilk Ref. W 535. Useful for suturing the scalp but gradually being superseded by monofilament Prolene sutures.
3. Sterile coated Vicryl (undyed) 1.5 metric (formerly 4/0) (polyglactin 910) Ref. W 9951.
   Ideal absorbable suture for subcutaneous closure. Good tensile strength for 4 weeks.

11.3 SKIN CLOSURE STRIPS

These are used as an alternative to sutures or to supplement sutures to give additional support. Certain sites such as fingers are better closed with sterile skin closure strips rather than suturing, if possible. When used on digits, care must be taken not to encircle the finger or toe completely with the strip, as a tourniquet effect may result.

Improvised skin closure strips may be made from Sellotape, micropore tape, or adhesive zinc oxide plaster.

If applied carefully between sutures at the time of skin closure, they may be left undisturbed when the sutures are removed, thus giving extra strength and support to the wound.

11.4 SKIN CLOSURE CLIPS

These are generally not used for minor surgical procedures, although some surgeons favour their use; the disadvantages are that they require a special instrument to remove them and they can be uncomfortable for the patient, but on the other hand they can give extremely good skin closure and a very neat scar. Most manufacturers now produce sterile disposable packs of clips (Ethicon Proximate disposable skin stapler) (Figs 11.6 and 11.7).

Fig. 11.6 Wound closure using the Proximate skin stapler.

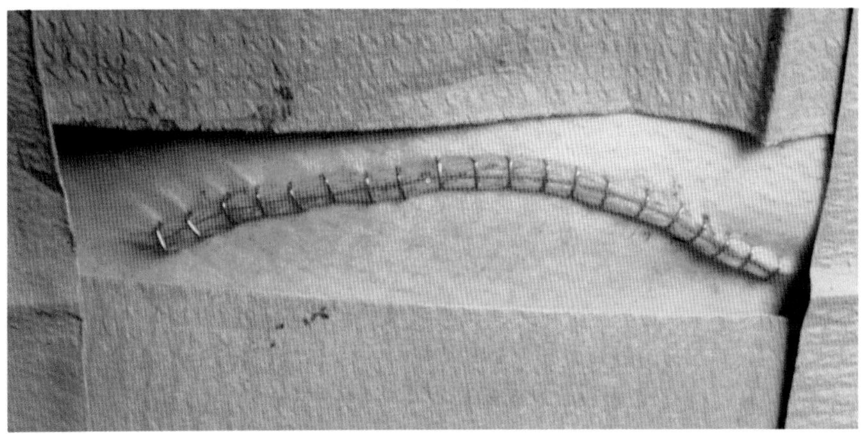

Fig. 11.7 Use of Proximate stapler.

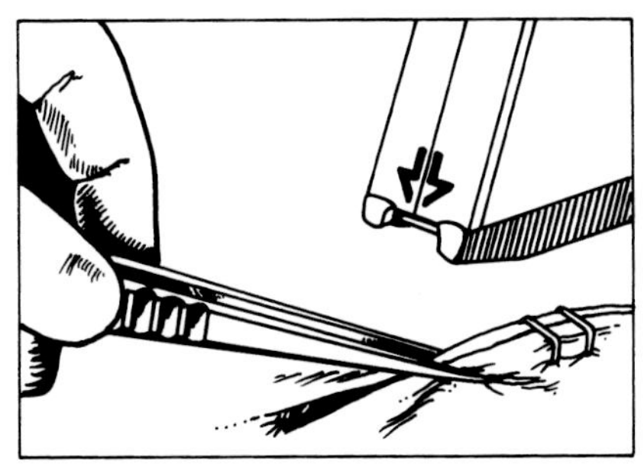

1. Evert and approximate skin edges as desired. Several techniques are suggested: (**a**) With one tissue forceps, bring skin edges together until edges evert.

11.5 DRAINS

Although widely used for operations on the neck, breast, thorax and pelvis, drains are generally not necessary when performing minor surgical procedures. Where good haemostasis has been achieved, and any dead space closed, haematoma formation is unlikely. If drainage is thought necessary, a small piece of rubber or plastic tubing may be inserted under the sutures and removed after 48 hours.

11.6 STITCHCRAFT AND KNOTS

Practice at tying knots is essential; knots may be formed using two hands as with tying shoe-laces, with one hand, or using instruments.

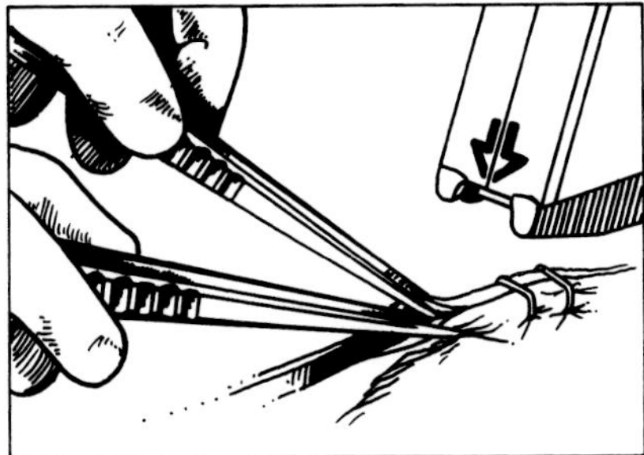

(**b**) With two tissue forceps, pick up each wound edge individually and approximate the edges.
(**c**) Apply tension to either end of the incision, such that the tissue edges begin to approximate themselves. One forceps can be used to ensure that the edges are everted.

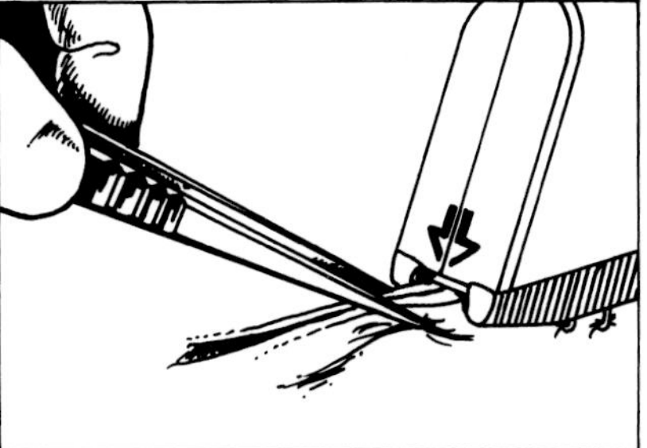

2. Position the instrument very lightly over the everted skin edges, aligning the instrument arrow with the incision. Pressing down on the instrument too heavily may make staple removal difficult.

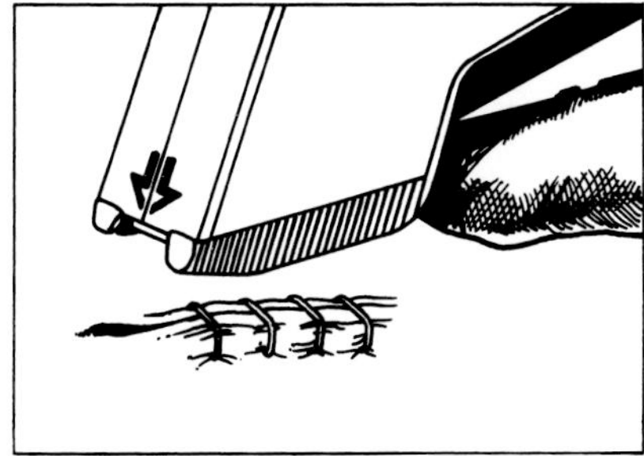

3. With one firm action squeeze the trigger until the trigger motion is halted. Release the trigger and back the instrument off the staple; the anvil easily slides out from under the staple.

11.6.1 One-hand tie

The one-hand tie may be practised using a piece of string to tie up a parcel; the instrument tie is most easily practised using surplus sutures and pigs' trotters.

In all techniques, the ends of the sutures should be kept taut at all times to avoid slippage (Fig. 11.8).

However, correct tightening of the knot is important to avoid eversion of the skin edges and to promote good healing (Fig. 11.9).

Where an assistant is available, the use of two single skin-hooks, one at each end of the incision, helps to align the edges and makes accurate approximation easier (Fig. 11.10).

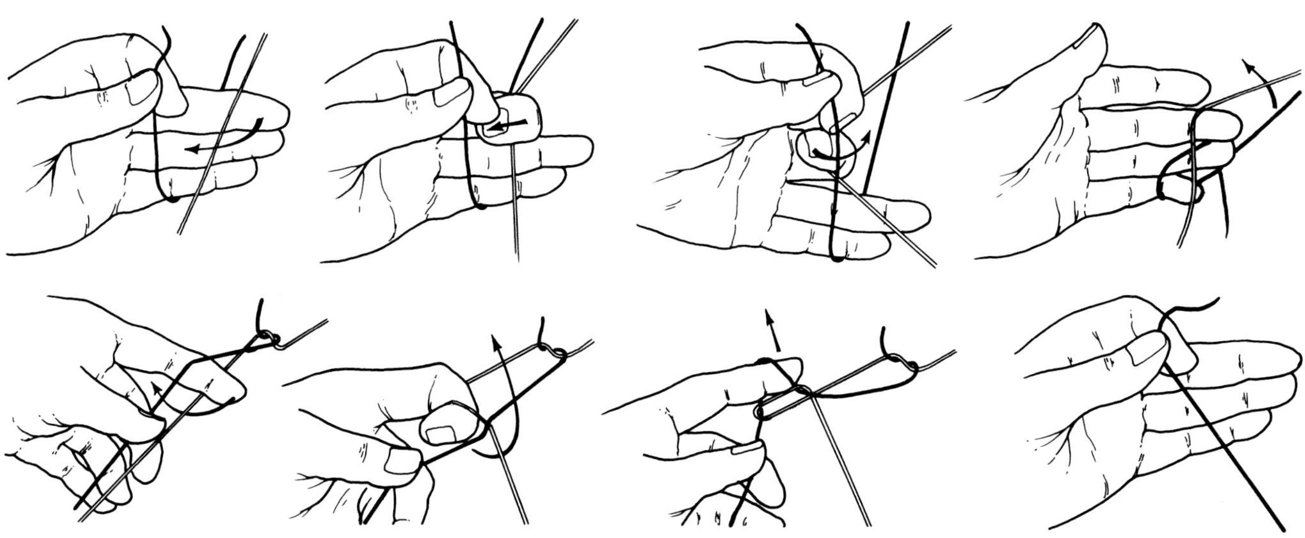

Fig 11.8 One-hand tie.

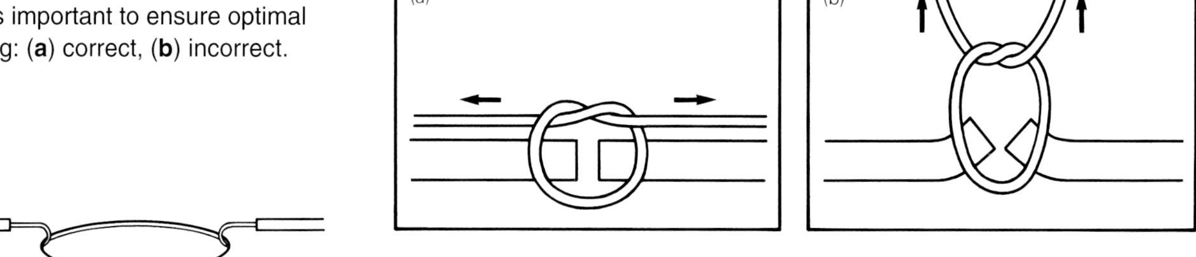

Fig. 11.9 Correct tightening of the knot is important to ensure optimal healing: (**a**) correct, (**b**) incorrect.

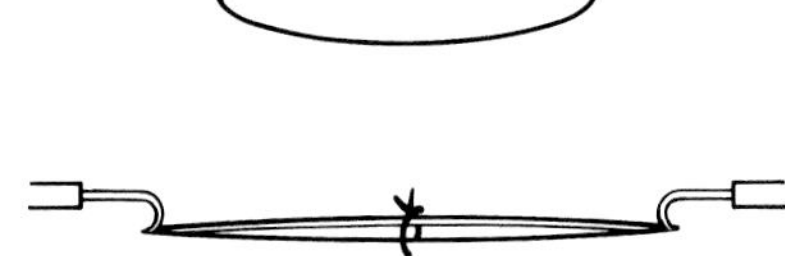

Fig. 11.10 Placing a skin hook in each end of the incision helps to align the edges prior to suturing. (Redrawn from B.A. Maurice, *Surgery for General Practitioners*, by permission of Oxford University Press.)

11.6.2 Instrument ties

Instrument ties are more suitable for minor surgery, using less suture material.

Having passed the suture through both ends of the wound, a short end is left protruding. Holding the needle end of the suture in the left hand, the suture is looped around the end of the needle holder once or twice depending on the type of knot. Still with the loops around the end of the needle holder, the short protruding end is grasped with the tips of the

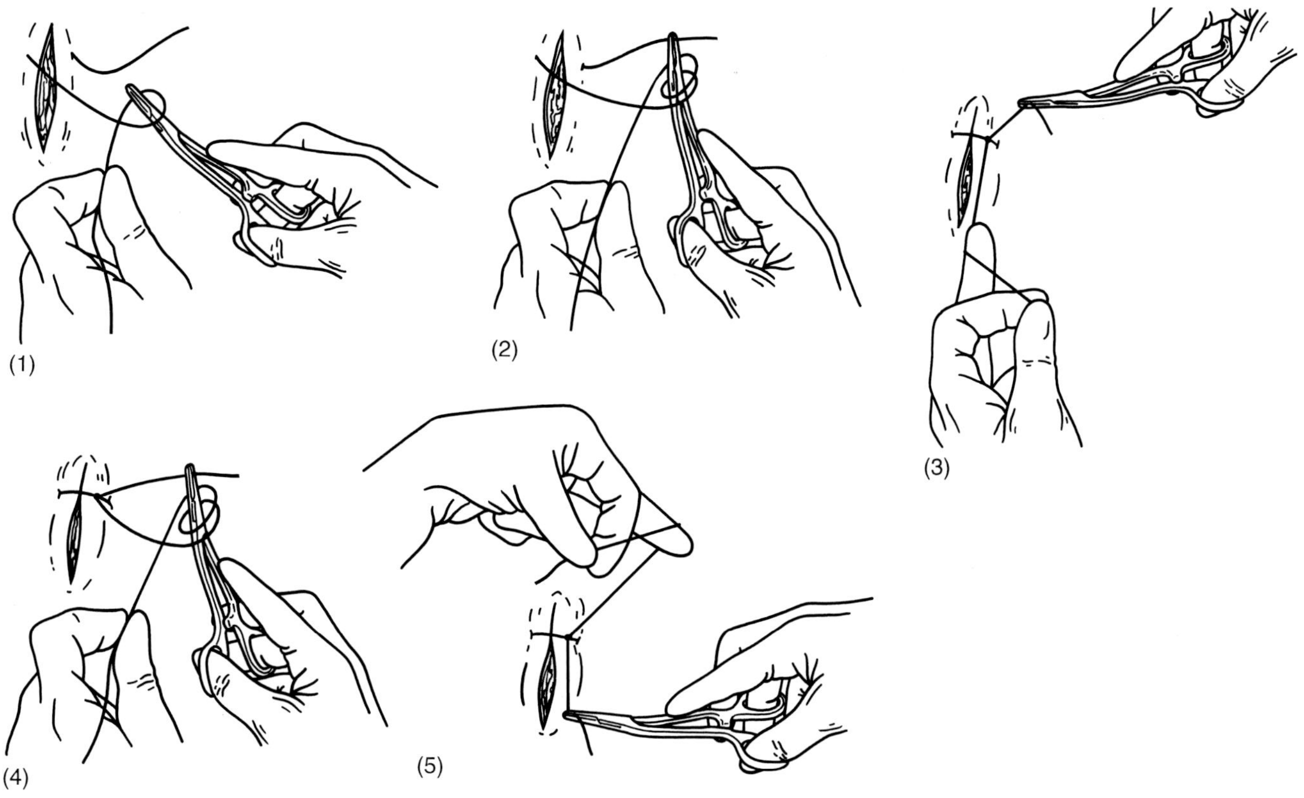

Fig. 11.11 Instrument tie, five stages. (From B.A. Maurice, *Surgery for General Practitioners,* by permission of Oxford University Press.)

needle holders and pulled back through the loops. By pulling both the end of the suture and the needle holder in opposite directions, the first throw of the knot is tied. The process is then repeated, but on the second throw the suture is looped round the needle-holder in the opposite direction (Fig. 11.11).

11.6.3 Three types of knot are used (Fig. 11.12)

1. Reef knot
2. Surgeon's knot
3. Nylon knot

For most situations a surgeon's knot comprising two throws followed by one throw as a reef knot is most suitable. Having tied the first throw, it may be 'locked' by pulling the knot to one edge of the wound. This allows the second throw to be formed without the first throw slipping.

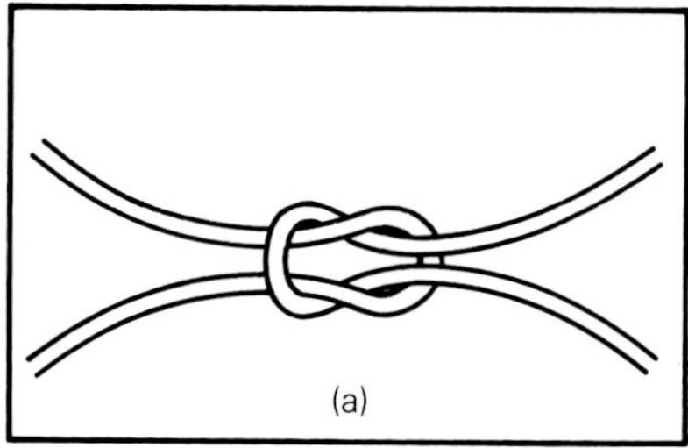

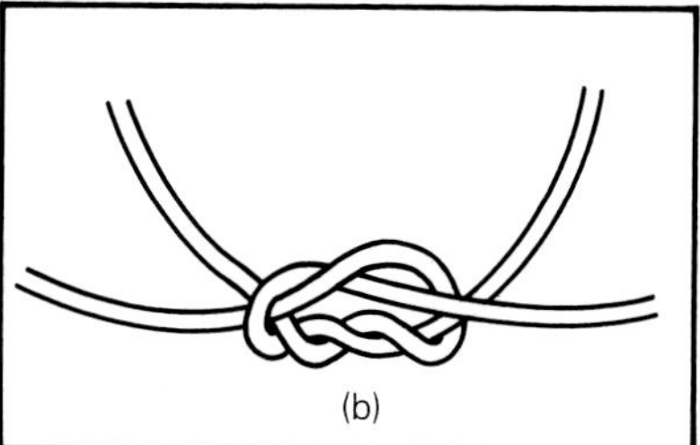

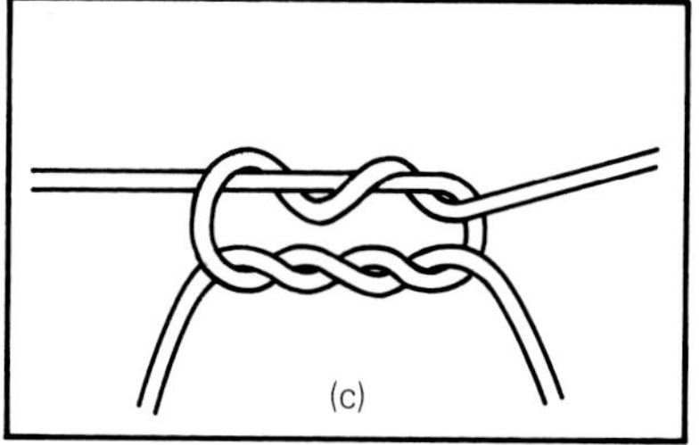

Fig. 11.12 Different types of knots used in suturing: (**a**) reef knot, (**b**) surgeon's knot, (**c**) nylon knot.

Generally, when cutting sutures inside a wound the ends should be cut as short as possible. Outside the wound, sufficient length should be left to make removal easy.

Where very fine, smooth sutures have been used, e.g. on the face, and there is a risk of the suture slipping, the wound may be painted with tinct. benz. co. or sprayed with Nobecutane, which will not only form a transparent dressing but will 'glue' the knots together.

Although this method is popular with the person inserting the sutures, it is not always popular with the person removing them!

11.6.4 Types of sutures

For minor surgery the three most frequently used sutures are:

1. Simple interrupted
2. Vertical mattress interrupted
3. Subcuticular or intradermal continuous (see Fig. 11.5).

11.6.5 Simple interrupted sutures

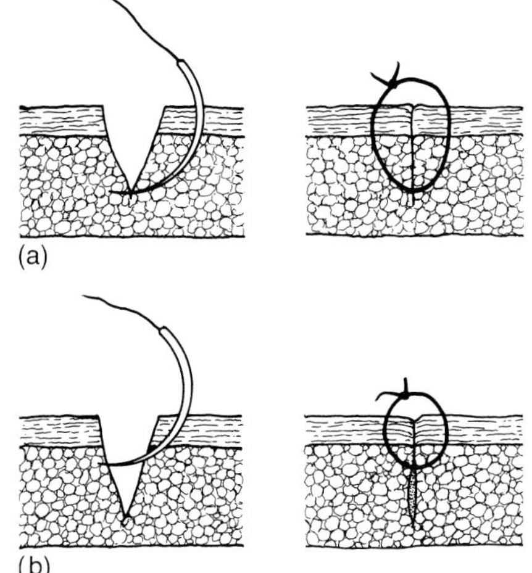

Fig. 11.13 Simple interrupted sutures: (**a**) correct, (**b**) incorrect

To achieve the neatest results the following principles need to be adhered to:

1. The needle should be pushed through the skin at right-angles.
2. The exit tract should likewise be at right-angles to the skin.
3. The distance of the entry site from the edge of the wound should be equal to the depth of skin through which the suture is passing (Figs 11.13 and 11.14).
4. Where deep tissues need to be sutured, a subcutaneous suture of an absorbable material, e.g. 1.5 coated Vicryl, will reduce tension on the skin edges and give a neater scar (Fig. 11.15).
5. Practise on pigs' trotters!

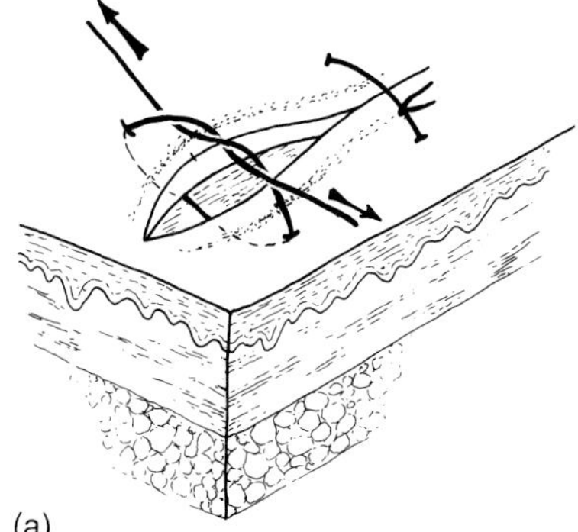

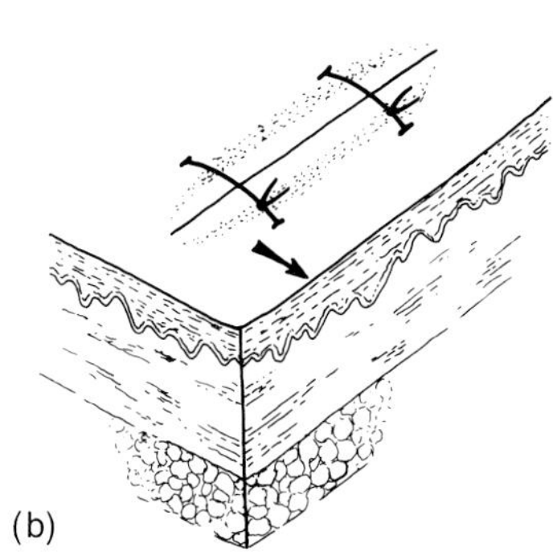

Fig. 11.14 Simple suture. (**a**) The suture is laid evenly across the wound; (**b**) positioning the knot to one side.

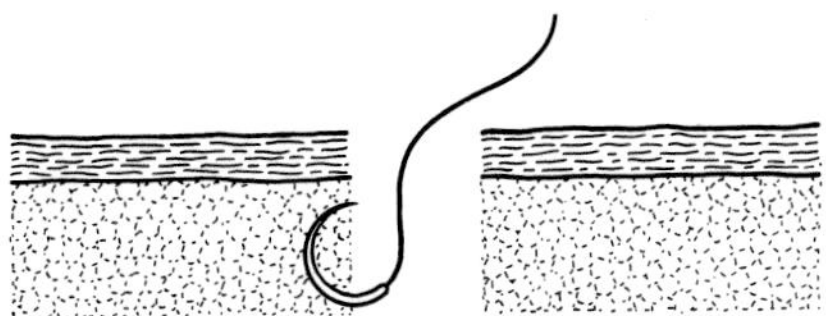

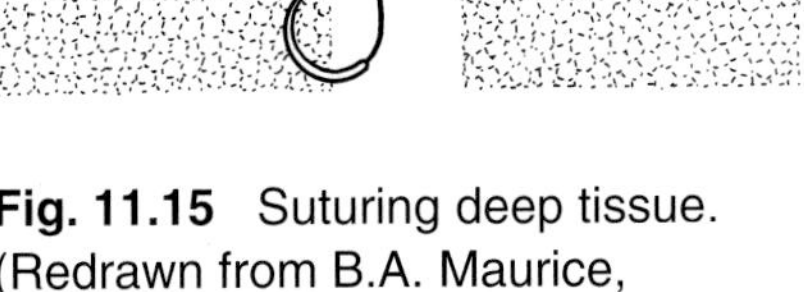

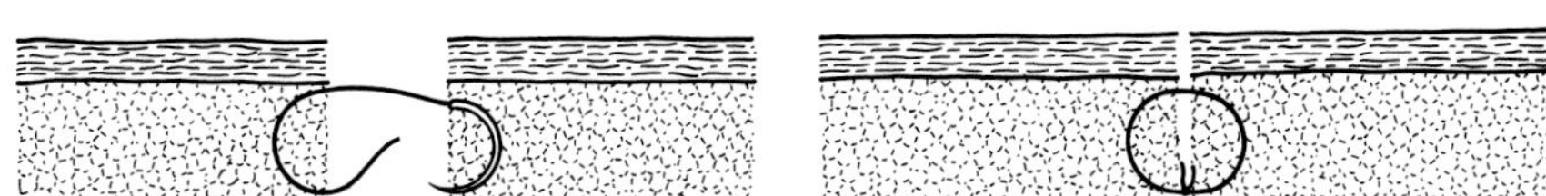

Fig. 11.15 Suturing deep tissue. (Redrawn from B.A. Maurice, *Surgery for General Practitioners*, by permission of Oxford University Press.)

11.6.6 Vertical mattress interrupted suture

This is a very useful stitch when the tissues are lax and the edges tend to invert. It apposes the skin layers accurately, but should not be used if the skin circulation is poor. Tension can be less to take account of any post-operative oedema.

The following principles should be followed:

1. The needle tract should be at right-angles to the skin.
2. It is a slightly deeper stitch which can incorporate the subcutaneous layer.
3. The entry site is judged to be the same distance from the entry site to the point where it comes out of the deep tissue.
4. The inner part of the stitch should be made 2 mm from the skin edge and come out half-way through the thickness of skin (Fig. 11.16a,b).
5. Practise on pigs' trotters or skin simulators.

11.6.7 Subcuticular or intradermal continuous sutures

Where the edges of the wound can be brought together easily without tension, and where the risk of subcutaneous haematoma formation is slight, a subcuticular or intradermal continuous suture gives the neatest scar.

Monofilament nylon, Ethilon, or Prolene are used. The stitch starts outside the wound at the end of the incision and passes backwards and

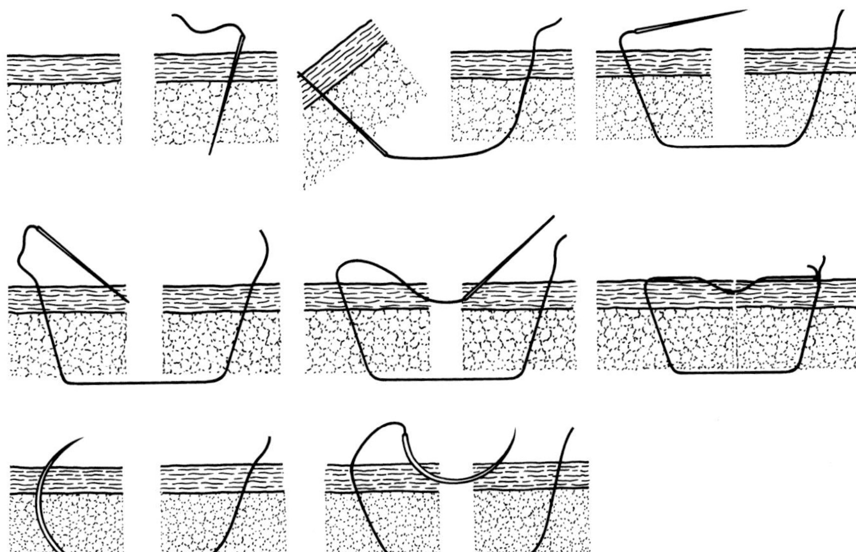

Fig. 11.16a Vertical mattress suture: stages using straight needle. (Redrawn from B.A. Maurice, *Surgery for General Practitioners*, by permission of Oxford University Press.)

Fig. 11.16b Vertical mattress suture using curved needle. (Redrawn from B.A. Maurice, *Surgery for General Practitioners*, by permission of Oxford University Press.)

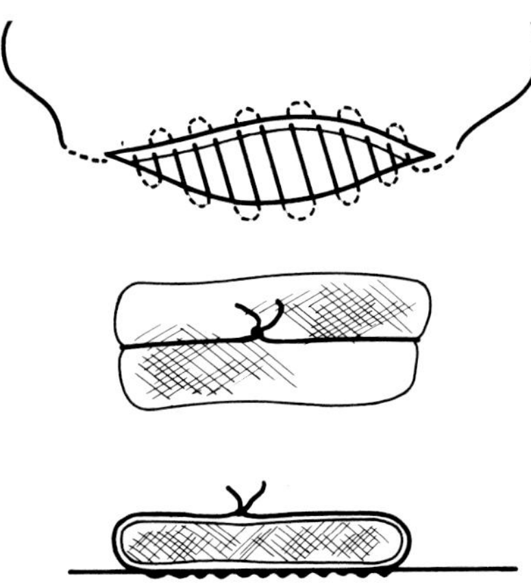

Fig. 11.17 Subcuticular suture and method of securing ends by tying over a small gauze swab.

forwards under the surface of the skin, emerging outside the end of the wound at the opposite end.

This leaves two ends which need to be secured. One method is to use 'buttons' or split 'lead' shot, but a simpler method is to tie the ends over a gauze swab and then tape the swab to the skin (Fig. 11.17).

To remove this suture, one end is divided flush with the skin, and traction is applied at the opposite end.

11.7 THE USE OF TISSUE ADHESIVE

Following anecdotal reports of accidental adhesion of skin using 'super glue', manufacturers have now produced a medical tissue adhesive. It is made as a sterile solution of n-butyl-2 cyanoacrylate monomer sealed in single-dose plastic vials. To help to identify the thickness of adhesive applied, a blue dye is added (Fig. 11.18).

Histoacryl (enbucrilate) blue is especially suitable for the closure of minor skin wounds without suturing, and also for sealing sutured skin wounds. When applied to the skin, it rapidly polymerizes into a firm adhesive bond in the presence of anions, especially hydroxyl ions, i.e. when contact is made with water or tissue moisture.

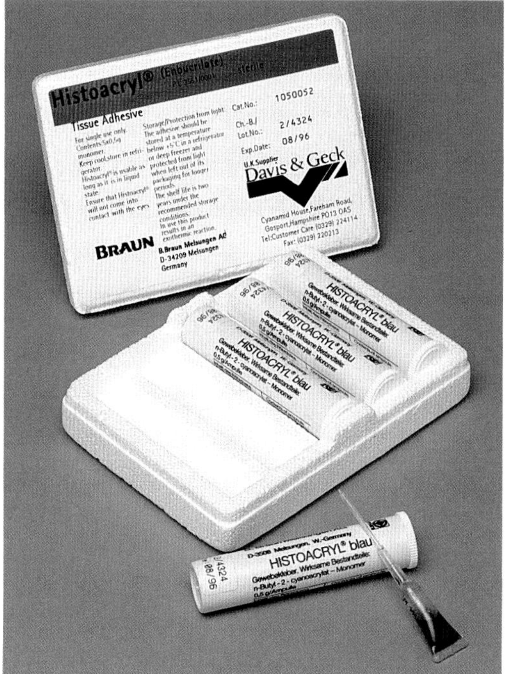

Fig. 11.18 Histoacryl blue tissue adhesive. Ideal for small lacerations in children.
(Kindly provided by Davis and Geck, Hampshire, UK.)

11.7.1 Technique

It is important to clean, dry, and check whether the edges of the wound will approximate without tension. Histoacryl blue may then be applied as spots or evenly along the length of the wound and the edges held together accurately for 1 min.

The correct method of closure of a skin laceration using tissue adhesive is shown in Figs 11.19 to 11.30.

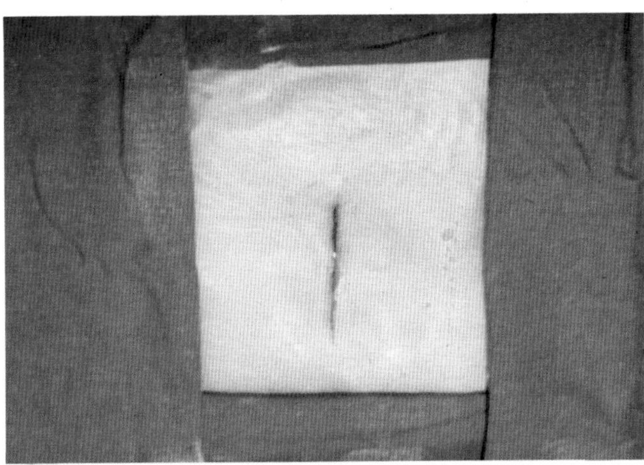

Fig. 11.19 Typical wound suitable for tissue adhesive. (Kindly provided by Davis and Geck, Hampshire, UK.)

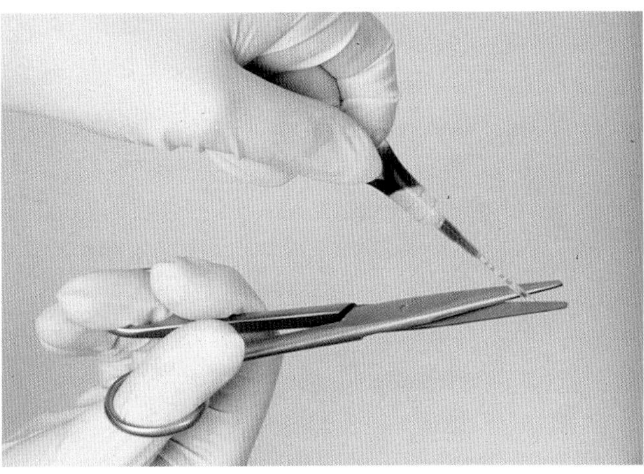

Fig. 11.20 Cutting off the tip of the nozzle – always hold upright and point away from the patient.
(Kindly provided by Davis and Geck, Hampshire, UK.)

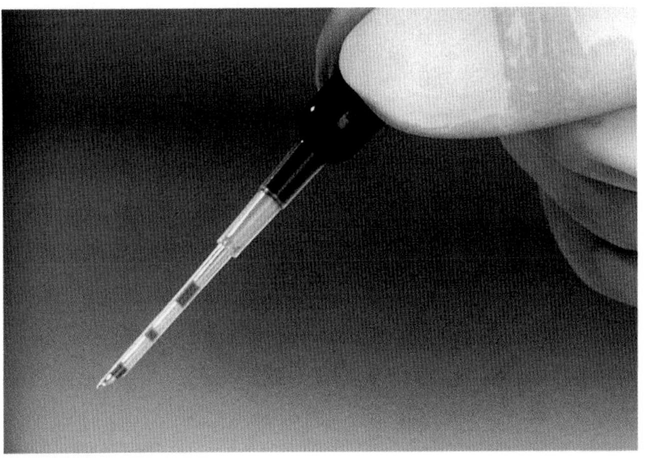

Fig. 11.21 Squeeze adhesive to the tip of the nozzle, away from the patient, to check flow.
(Kindly provided by Davis and Geck, Hampshire, UK.)

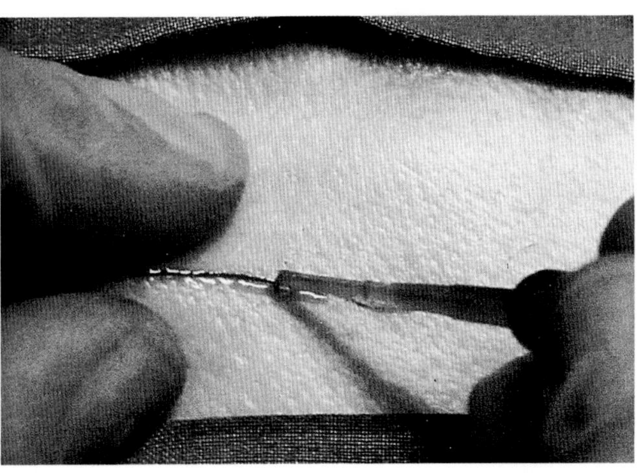

Fig. 11.22 Apply adhesive to the surface of the apposed wound edges – **not** into the wound.
(Kindly provided by Davis and Geck, Hampshire, UK.)

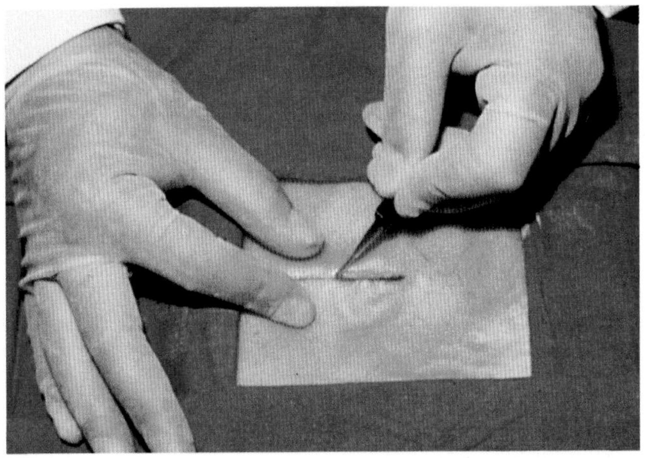

Fig. 11.23 Appose wound edges with fingers **before** applying adhesive.
(Kindly provided by Davis and Geck, Hampshire, UK.)

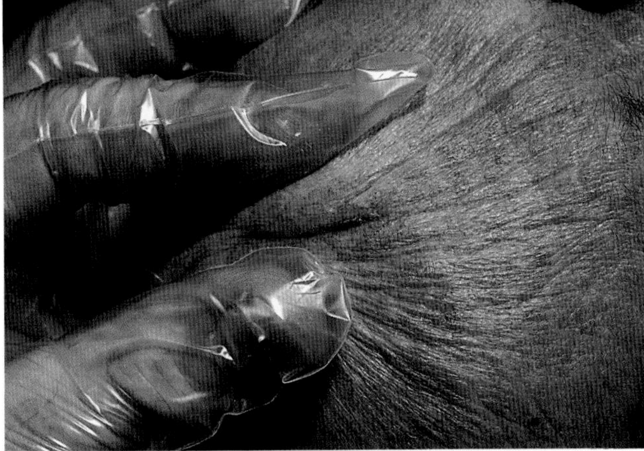

Fig. 11.24 Closing wound on scalp with finger pressure
(Kindly provided by Davis and Geck, Hampshire, UK.)

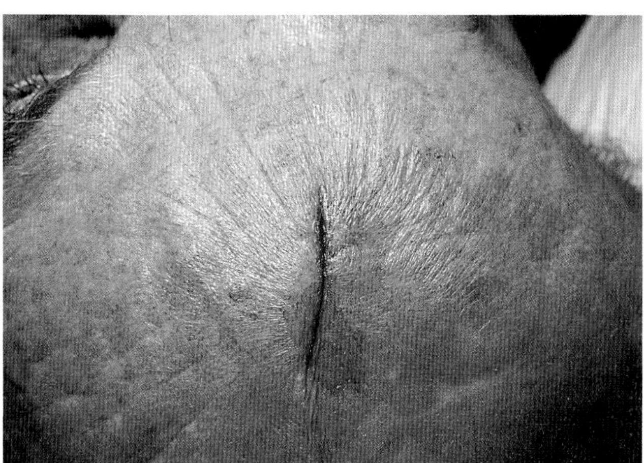

Fig. 11.25 Same wound immediately after closure with tissue adhesive.

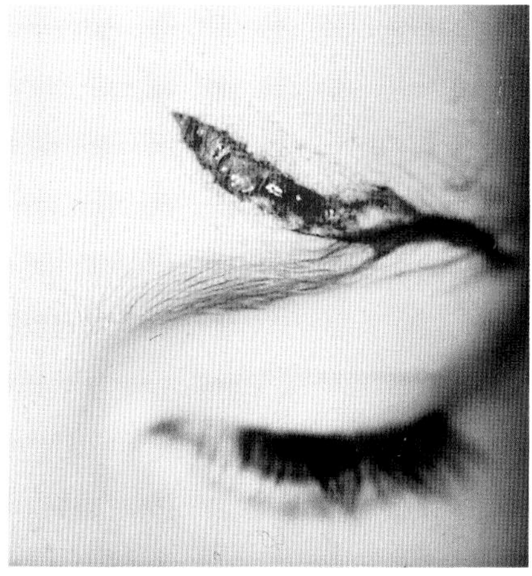

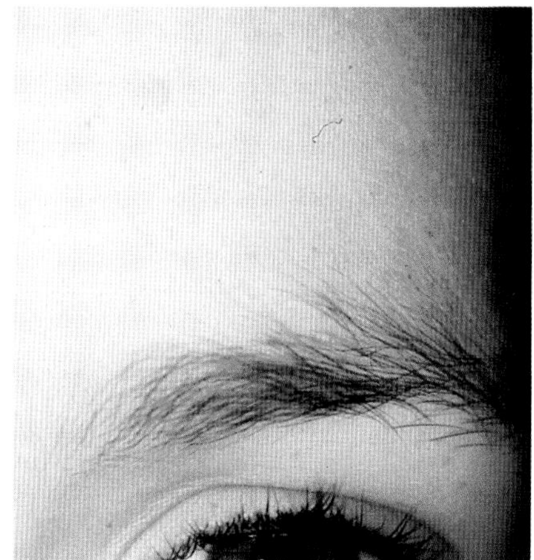

Fig. 11.26 Five-year-old child with laceration above eye-brow (photograph taken by Dr David Watson at Lewisham Hospital).

Fig. 11.27 Same patient, 6 months later (photograph taken by Dr David Watson at Lewisham Hospital).

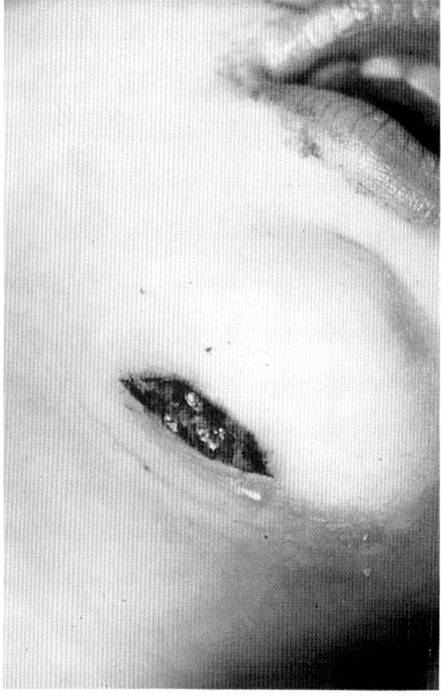

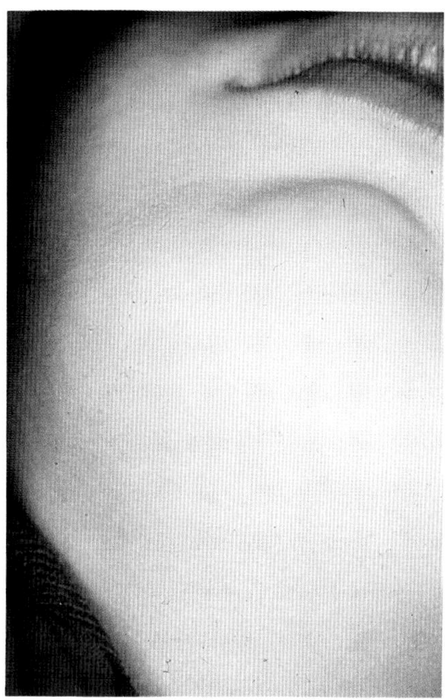

Fig. 11.28 Four-year-old child with laceration beneath chin (photograph taken by Dr David Watson at Lewisham Hospital).

Fig. 11.29 Same patient 3 months later (photograph taken by Dr David Watson at Lewisham Hospital).

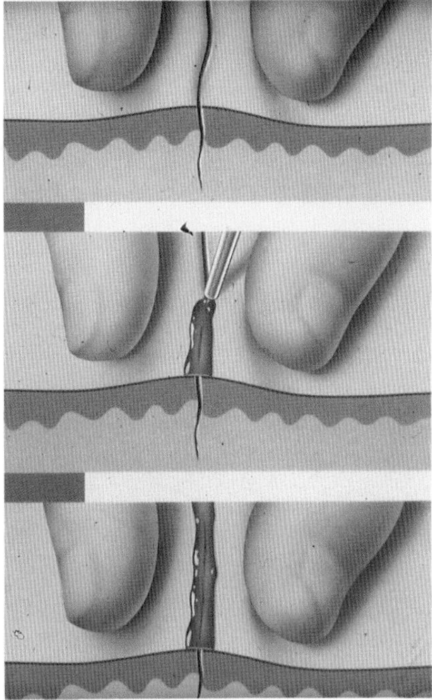

Fig. 11.30 Diagram to show application of adhesive to surface of closed wound and not between the wound edges.
(Kindly provided by Davis and Geck, Hampshire, UK.)

Caution

It is vital to approximate the edges accurately before applying the adhesive, as polymerization time is only 20 seconds and mistakes cannot be corrected! It should also be noted that heat is produced during polymerization; thus the thinnest layer possible should be applied to avoid thermal damage to the skin.

Further, Histoacryl should not be applied to blood vessels in case intravascular thrombosis occurs; care should also be taken to avoid contact with the cornea or conjunctiva.

Instruments, clothes, swabs, gloves or fingers which come into contact with Histoacryl will adhere to it, so extreme care needs to be taken. Instruments accidentally contaminated with the glue may be cleaned with dimethyl formamide or acetone.

It is recommended that the glue be kept in a refrigerator or freezer and protected from the light. It has a shelf life of 2 years.

Because no local anaesthetic is necessary, it is an ideal method of skin closure for small wounds in young children. Also as no sutures need to be removed, follow-up visits are virtually eliminated.

12

Suturing lacerations

If thou examinest a man having a wound in his ear, cutting through the flesh, the injury being in the lower part of the ear, and confined to the flesh, thou shouldst draw it together for him with stitching behind the hollow of his ear.

Edwin Smith, Surgical Papyrus, 3000–2500 BC

One of the first skills to be acquired by medical students in their clinical training is the suturing of wounds; in the emergency department they meet a variety of injuries and lacerations, and on the maternity wards they learn how to repair perineal tears and episiotomies. House-surgeons assist at many surgical procedures and are often responsible for suturing the wound at the end of the operation. Thus all doctors by the time they qualify are able to suture the majority of wounds likely to be encountered in any minor surgical operation. If it is considered necessary to suture a wound, the following general principles should be borne in mind:

1. Healing will occur more readily if the skin edges are accurately and carefully apposed to each other.
2. There should be minimum or no tension on the skin edges if at all possible. This may be achieved by careful undercutting of the skin prior to suturing.
3. The skin edges should be slightly everted; this is done by applying slight traction to the skin edge and including slightly more of the dermal layer than skin in the stitch.
4. Many fine sutures, equally placed close together are preferable to larger sutures spaced further apart.
5. Any 'dead space' should be closed either with subcutaneous absorbable sutures, or by including this layer in the skin stitches.
6. All stitches should only remain in place as long as they are needed to give support. Thus stitches on the face may be removed as early as 48 hours to 5 days, whereas those on the abdominal wall and foot should remain for 10 days or more.
7. All wounds should be as clean as possible.
8. There should be the minimum of handling and tissue trauma from forceps.
9. Additional support may be given by the use of sterile adhesive strips which can remain in place after the stitches have been removed.
10. Practice at different suturing techniques is most easily acquired using pigs' trotters.

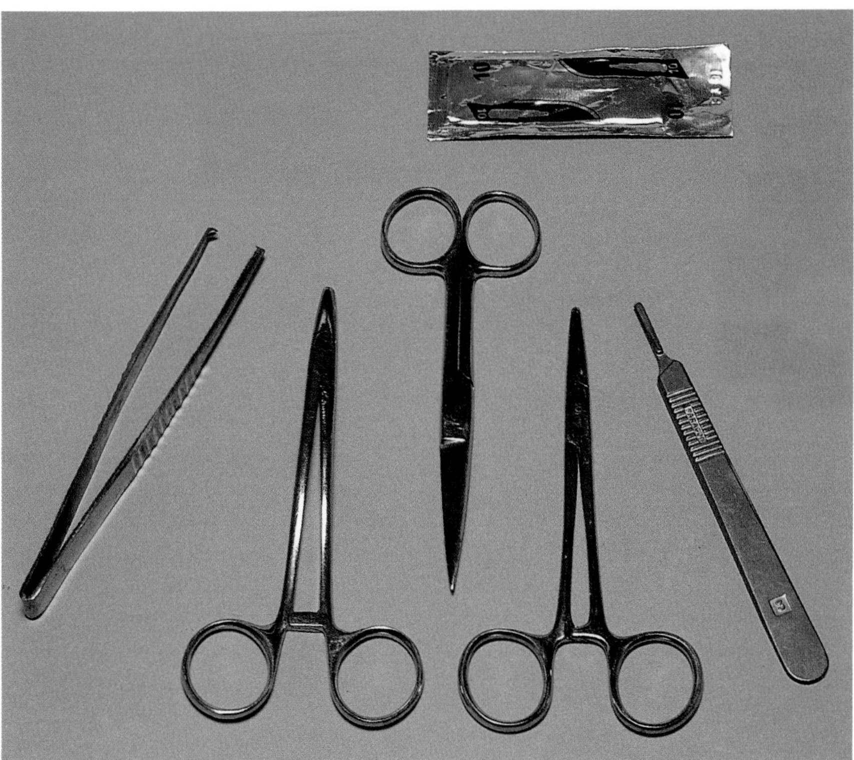

Fig. 12.1 Basic instrument set suitable for most suturing.

12.1 INSTRUMENTS REQUIRED

The following 'basic set' is recommended for routine suturing and many simple surgical procedures (Fig. 12.1).

Kilner needle holder 5¼in. (13.3 cm)
Scalpel handle size 3
Scalpel blades 10 and 15
Pair standard stitch scissors (sharp/sharp) 5 in. (12.7 cm)
Pair toothed dissecting forceps 5 in. (12.7 cm).

Suture material – this is individual preference, but the finer the suture the better, consistent with giving adequate support.

W 319 Ethilon monofilament nylon 1.5 on curved, reverse-cutting needle.
W 507 Ethilon monofilament nylon 0.7 on slim blade curved cutting needle.
W 539 Ethicon Prolene 1.5 on slim blade curved cutting needle.

Syringes and needles and local anaesthesia – the 2 ml syringe is sufficient for small lacerations, 10 ml or even 20 ml for larger. The finest gauge needles should be selected, and a dental syringe with a screw-on 30 swg (0.3 mm) needle is ideal for children.

12.2 TECHNIQUE FOR SUTURING LACERATIONS

The patient should be lying comfortably on a couch or operating theatre table, this is preferable to the patient sitting or standing as the most unexpected patients faint during a simple suturing procedure; it is also more comfortable for both the patient and doctor. Good illumination is essential, and the wound should first be carefully inspected to determine the extent and nature of the injury, and to ascertain whether any other injury to underlying structures has occurred. Having excluded other injuries, the area should be anaesthetized. This is most conveniently done by infiltration as described in Chapter 8 using first a dental syringe and 30 swg (0.3 mm) needle, changing to a longer needle and larger syringe if necessary, always remembering the maximum dose of anaesthetic which may be given to this particular patient (take care with the very young and very old).

After allowing a few minutes for anaesthesia to develop, the area may be again inspected, carefully palpated, cleaned thoroughly, and any hairs clipped away from the immediate operative field.

At this stage the doctor will need to decide whether deep tissues will require suturing as well as skin, and if so, catgut, Dexon or preferably coated Vicryl sutures should be inserted. As a general guide, the less deep sutures that are inserted, the better, compatible with achieving haemostasis and closing any 'dead' spaces.

Any bleeding points may be dealt with by electrocautery, ligature, clipping, or just firm pressure for a few minutes. Next an attempt should be made to bring the edges of the wound together to see if undue tension will be created. If this is likely, the skin should be widely undercut to help approximate the edges. Any ragged edges should be carefully trimmed, and dead tissue excised.

Using the toothed dissecting forceps to hold the skin edges, interrupted sutures are inserted, tying the knots on the same side and avoiding any tension, taking into account the fact that tissues may swell during the first 2 days following injury.

If an assistant is available, two Gillies skin hooks can be used, one at either end of the wound, applying traction, which aligns the wound nicely, and makes insertion of sutures easier (see Fig. 11.10). A dry dressing may now be applied, with or without a covering of Nobecutane spray on the skin.

Deep, dirty, penetrating wounds should be cleaned as thoroughly as possible, and the patient given prophylactic antibiotics and a reinforcing tetanus immunization if not up-to-date. Dirty contaminated grazes can be scrubbed using chlorhexidine in detergent (Hibiscrub) after first anaesthetizing the area with infiltration anaesthetic.

12.3 TECHNIQUE FOR CLOSURE WITH 'GLUE'

Where the edges of the wound can be brought together easily, it may be appropriate to consider one of the cyanoacrylate glues. After drying the edges with absorbent gauze, the glue is applied using a glass rod. The edges are then held firmly together for 2 minutes. Care must be taken not to stick the operator's fingers to the patient's skin!

Normally no anaesthetic is needed, and no further follow-up required.

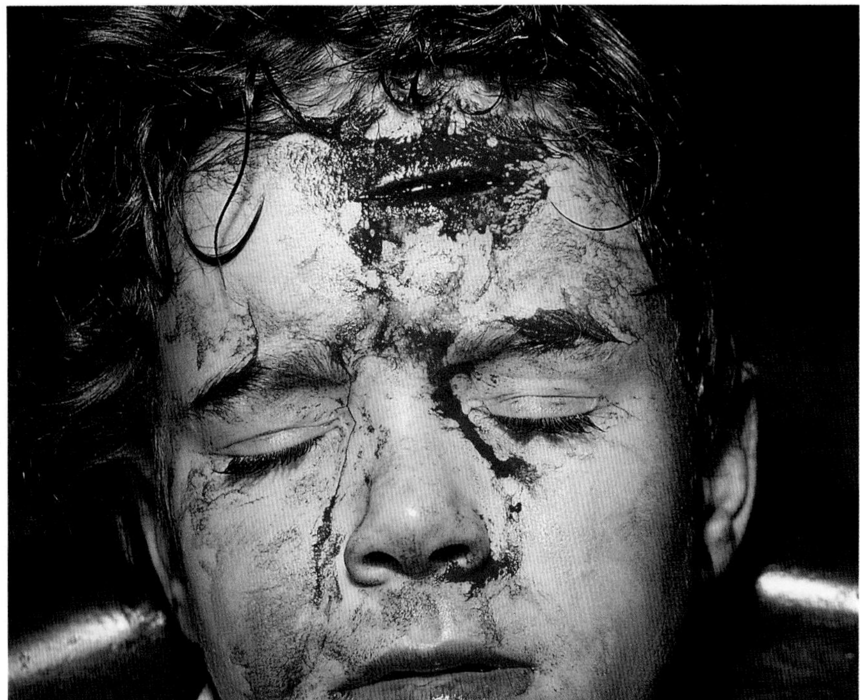

Fig. 12.2 A common injury.

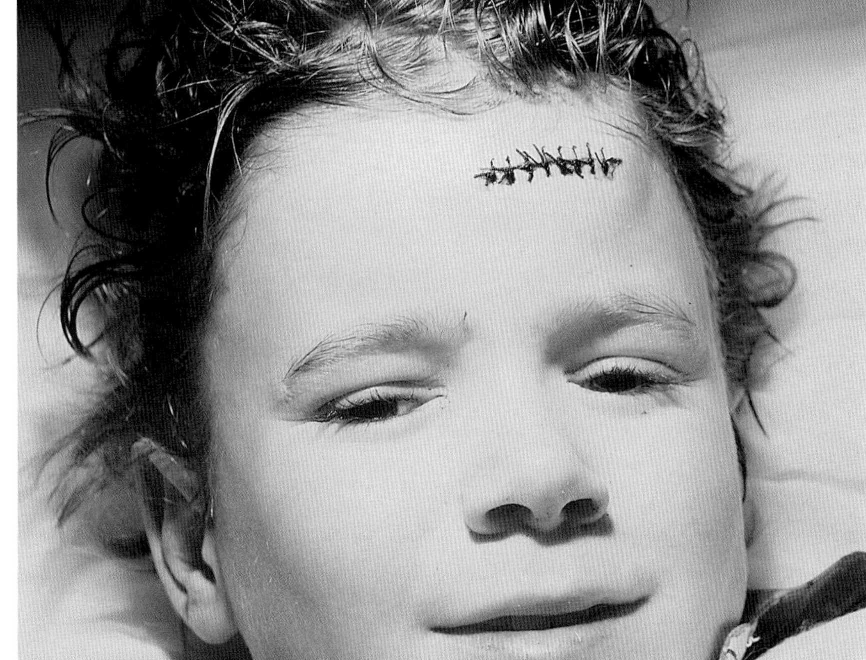

Fig. 12.3 'No hard feelings!'

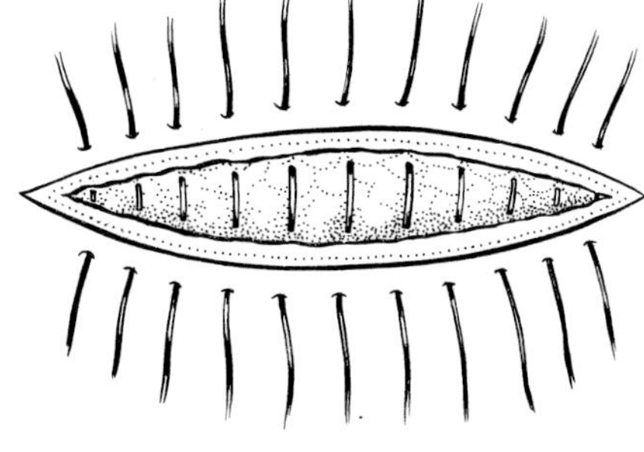

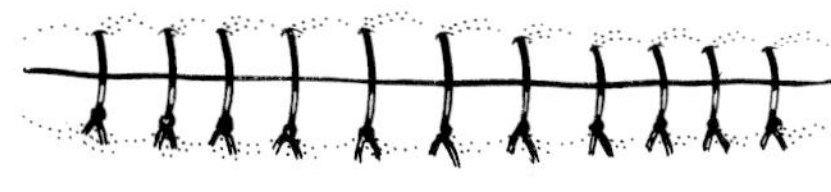

Fig. 12.4 Skin closure with interrupted sutures.

12.4 CHOICE OF SKIN CLOSURE

Mention has already been made about alternative closures to sutures, these should always be borne in mind when faced with a laceration. It may be more appropriate to use a subcuticular stitch, sterile self-adhesive strips, or clips, or just a firm dressing.

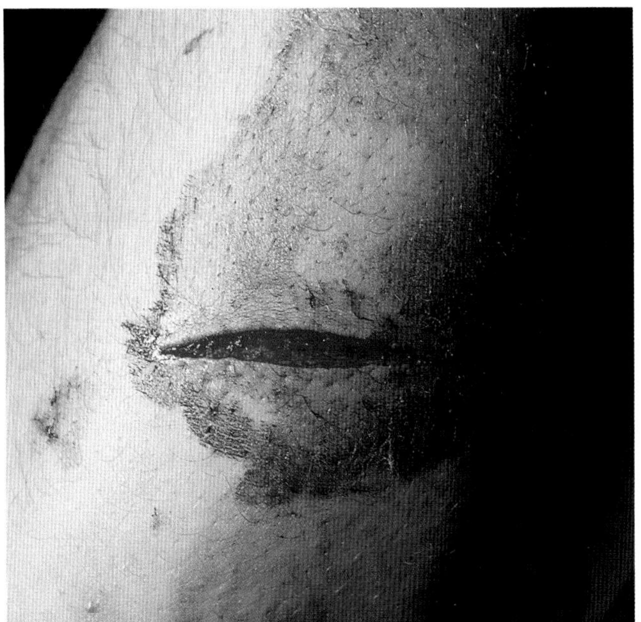

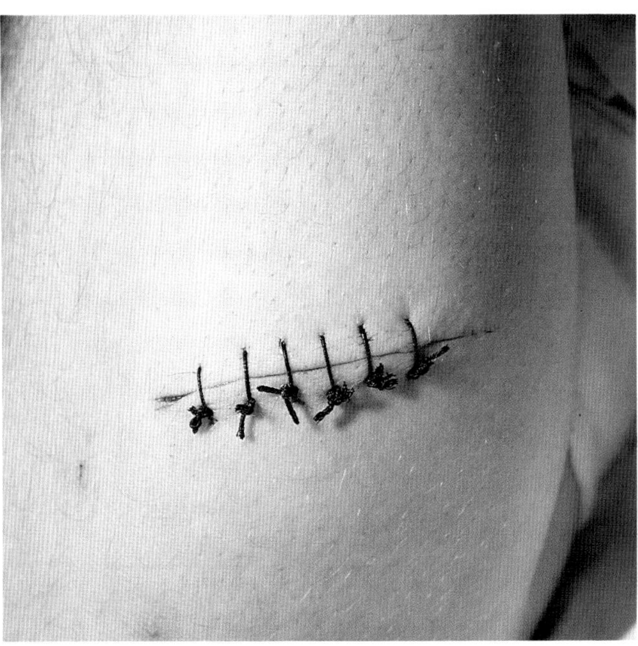

Fig. 12.5a, b A laceration from a sharp knife is easily closed using interrupted non-absorbable sutures, preferably monofilament Prolene

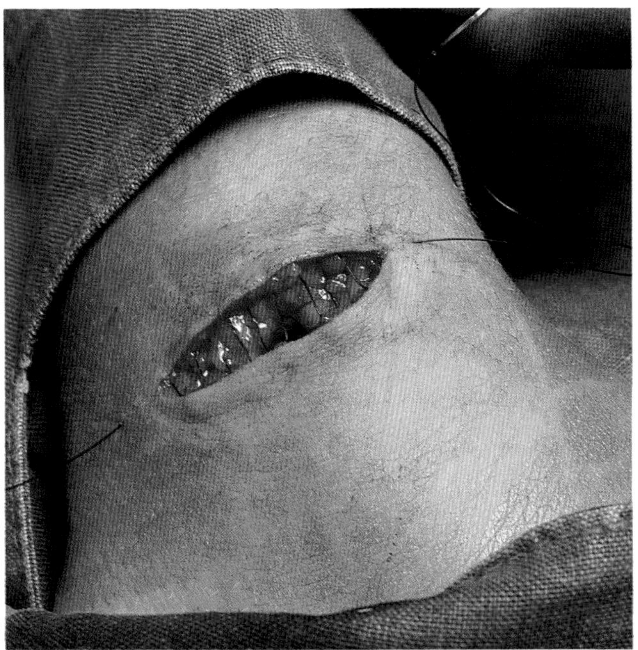

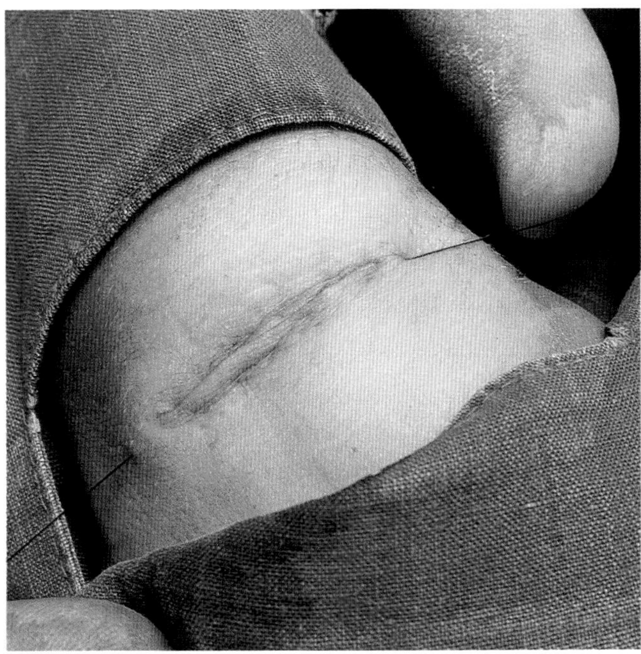

Fig. 12.6a, b Where the edges of the wound can be approximated without tension, and the site splinted afterwards, a subcuticular suture may give a neater scar.

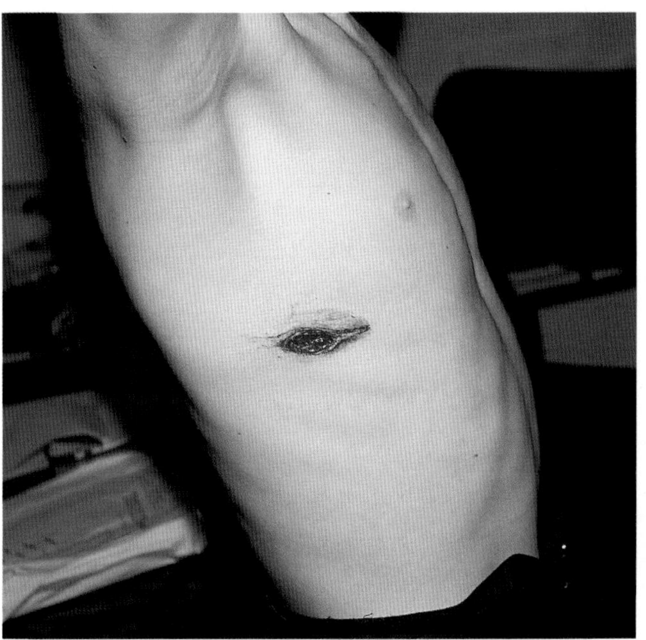

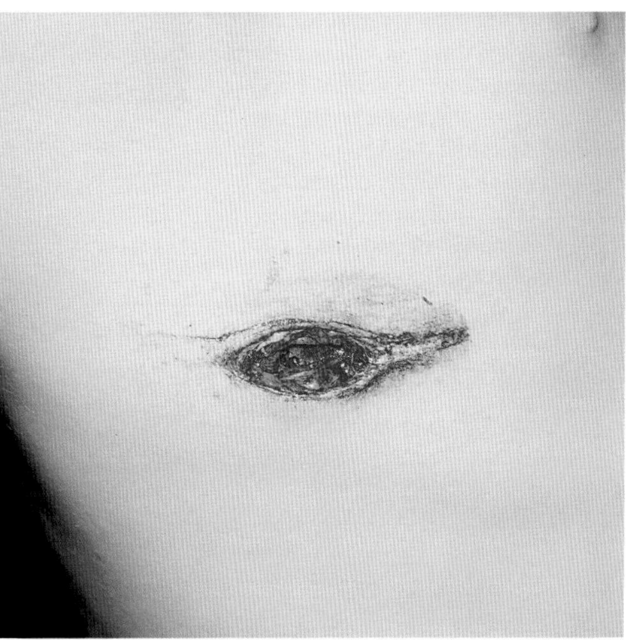

Fig. 12.7a, b Beware of wounds which may extend deeper than appears at first sight.

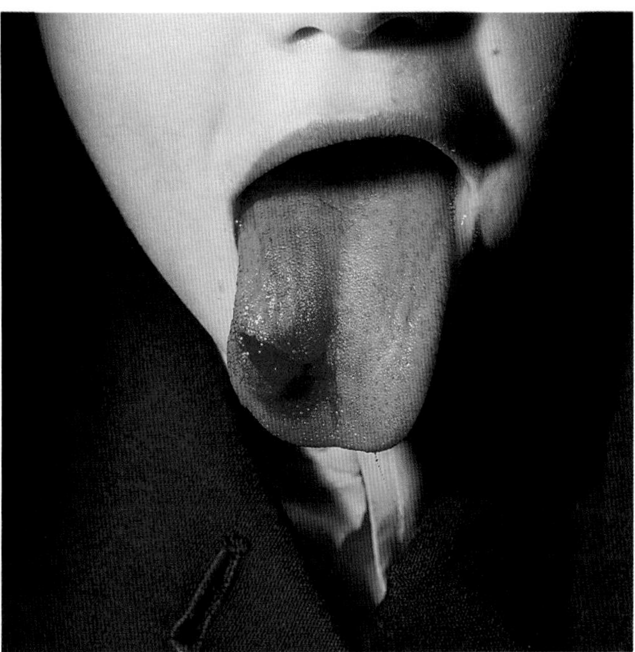

Fig. 12.8 Small lacerations on the tongue often heal without any attention. Deeper cuts require suturing, using an absorbable material.

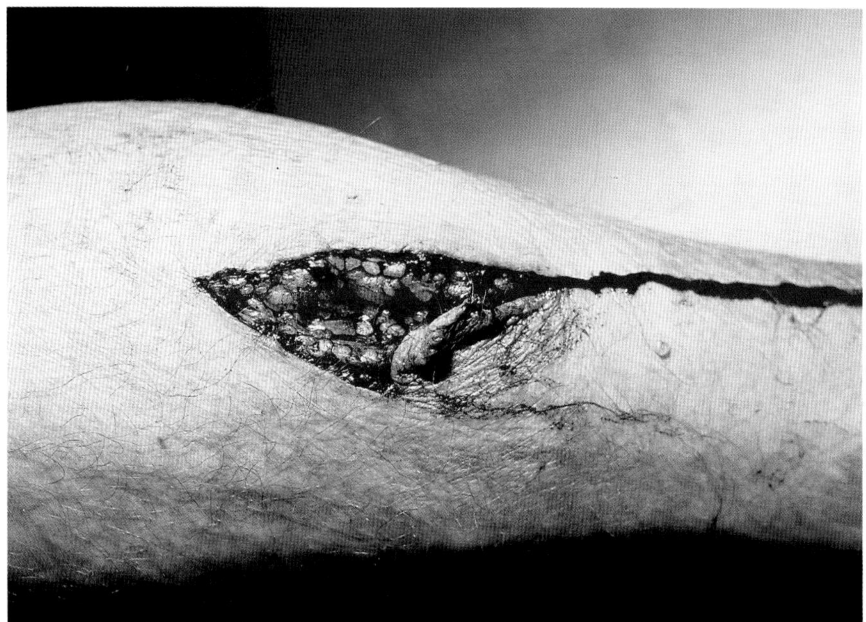

Fig. 12.9 Lacerations over the anterior surface of the tibia, particularly in elderly women, are difficult to heal. Any tension in the wound must be avoided. In the above wound the skin flap should be carefully stretched back to its original position and Steri-strips, a sterile pad and a firm compression bandage applied. This can give better healing than the use of sutures.

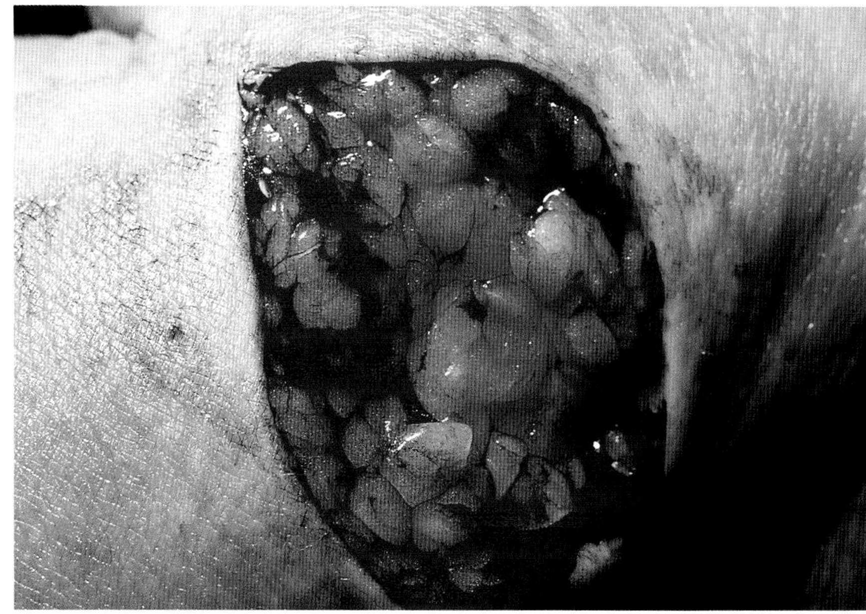

Fig. 12.10 Before excising any lesion decide whether the edges can be brought together without undue tension. This wound will need undercutting, subcutaneous supporting sutures and many fine sutures, supported with large self-adhesive skin closure strips, kept on for several weeks after the sutures have been removed.

13

Dressings

Now, after thou hast stitched it, thou shouldst bind it with fresh meat the first day. Thou shouldst treat it afterwards with grease and honey every day until he recovers

Edwin Smith, Surgical Papyrus, 3000–2500 BC

It has been suggested that dressings on surgical wounds are unnecessary, that they merely prevent the doctor and patient observing what is happening underneath, and this is certainly true on many occasions. Every doctor will have observed how well incisions heal on the scalp and face, where no dressings are used.

13.1 REASONS FOR USING DRESSINGS

Where dressings are used, they probably help in four ways:

1. Absorption of any secretions
2. Protection from contamination
3. Additional support during the healing phase
4. Limitation of excessive movements during healing.

13.1.1 Absorption of secretions

Any wound which is discharging or oozing will be helped by the application of an absorbent sterile, dry dressing, which must be changed frequently.

13.1.2 Protection from contamination

If a surgical operation has been performed under sterile conditions, and primary skin closure is expected, a sterile dry dressing firmly applied at the end of the operation should be left undisturbed until the sutures are removed. Peeping under the dressing 'to see how it is healing' is to be condemned: this only increases the chances of cross-infection. Only if there is a definite indication such as unexpected pain, swelling, fever, or signs of infection should the original dressing be disturbed – in every other case leave well alone!

13.1.3 Additional support

Sutures alone may not give adequate support to a healing wound, and in this case a dressing firmly bandaged in place will give additional external support, reduce tension on the stitches, and promote healing.

13.1.4 Limitation of movement

Wounds on the limbs may be subjected to excessive forces during healing, for example transverse wounds near the knee joint may tend to pull apart during walking and kneeling, by applying a thick layer of bandage, limitation of movements of the joint will be achieved, and promote healing. Similarly on the hand or fingers where sterile strips may have been used in preference to sutures, but by themselves are not strong enough to withstand full movements, supportive bandaging will supplement the Steri-strips and avoid the need for suturing.

13.2 TYPES OF DRESSING

13.2.1 Non-adherent dressings

Where there is considerable discharge either from an ulcer, burns, blisters, or sinuses, ordinary dry dressings may become adherent and difficult to remove. In such cases non-adherent dressings may be used, such as Melolin X-A, Johnsons N.A. dressing, Vaseline-impregnated gauze or similar preparations.

13.2.2 Antibacterial dressings

These consist of *tulle gras* dressings impregnated with antibacterial substances. They are of limited use and carry the risk of causing skin sensitization. In certain situations such as ingrowing toe-nail operations where there is known to be heavy infection, the routine use of such dressings appears to accelerate healing, e.g. Inadine (povidone-iodine).

13.2.3 Acrylic resin aerosol dressings (Nobecutane)

These consist of acrylic resin dissolved in a mixture of acetate esters in aerosol containers. By spraying on the skin from a distance of 20 cm a protective film is produced. This is useful on sites where conventional dressings would be difficult to keep in place e.g. the scalp; in other sites it may be used instead of a dry gauze dressing, particularly after sutures have been removed.

13.2.4 Cotton conforming bandages (Kling, Crinx, Easifix and Kurlex)

These lightweight bandages are so designed that they will bandage irregular surfaces and maintain even tension. They are cheap, efficient, and widely used.

13.2.5 Elastic bandages

Where firm external elastic support is required, for example on the legs to control varicose veins, elastic web bandages are ideal. Wounds and ulcers on the lower leg tend to heal more slowly, the more so when oedema is present. The early application of firm elastic bandages reduces oedema and accelerates healing. They are frequently used in the treatment of varicose veins and varicose ulceration.

13.2.6 Elasticated net stockinette (Netelast)

This elastic tubular dressing is designed to hold dressings in place in sites such as the axilla, breast, perineum, buttock, and scalp; it is manufactured in different widths, and with ingenuity all parts of the body can be covered. It has the advantage of being extremely comfortable but does not give much compression.

13.2.7 Elasticated tubular stockinette (Tubigrip)

For additional elastic support, elasticated tubular stockinette is used; particularly for wounds on arms and legs. As with the elastic net stockinette it is manufactured in various sizes to suit most parts of the body. It is used to give compression for sclerotherapy for varicose veins.

13.2.8 Cotton surgical tubular stockinette (Tubegauz)

This is a non-elastic, cotton stockinette, which is ideal for bandaging fingers and toes. It is manufactured in various widths, and is applied with a special tubular applicator using a twisting action to increase compression if required (Fig. 13.1a, b).

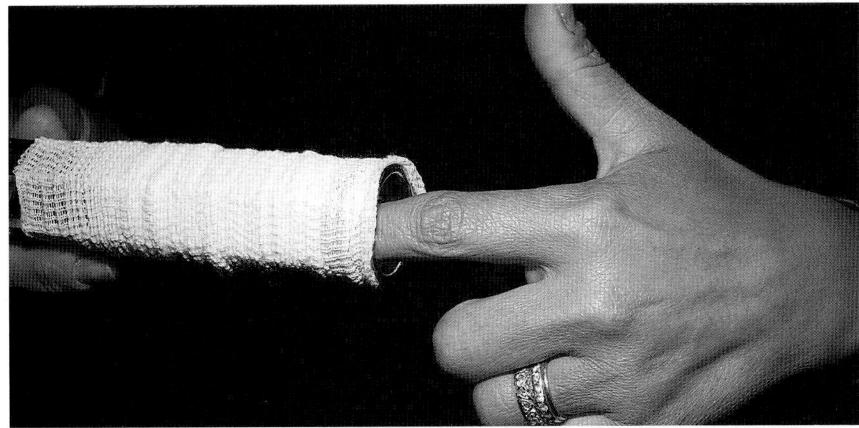

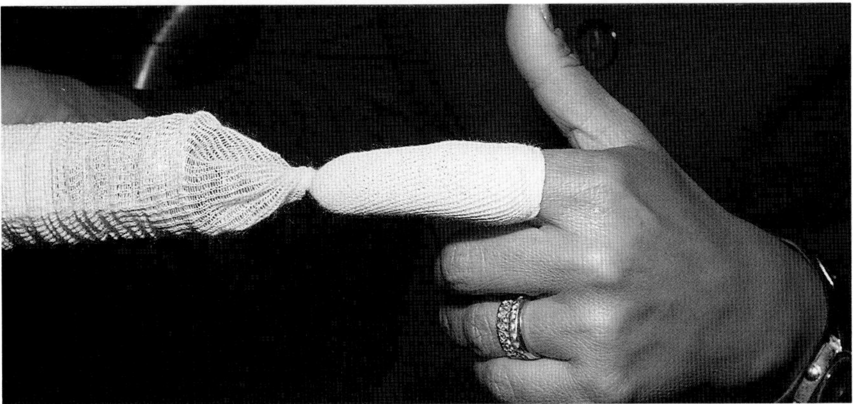

Fig. 13.1a, b Application of cotton tubular stockinette bandage to finger: ideal for gentle compression. Multiple layers will give additional splintage to the digit, thus often making suturing unnecessary.

14

Suture removal

> *If thou examinest a man having a wound in his lip, piercing through to the inside of his mouth, thou shouldst examine his wound as far as the column of the nose: thou shouldst draw together that wound with stitching*
>
> *Edwin Smith, Surgical Papyrus, 3000–2500* BC

The shorter the time sutures are *in situ*, the neater the scar. However, if they are removed too soon, there is a risk of the wound gaping; consequently a compromise has to be reached, and the optimum time will vary in different sites on the body. Thus the majority of sutures are removed on the tenth postoperative day, but on the face it is preferable to remove them very much earlier, and on the foot it might be advisable to leave them a day or two longer. It is also possible to remove alternate sutures one or two days before the remainder, and this improves the appearance of the final scar. Where it is desirable to remove sutures early, but the practitioner feels the wound may not be firmly adherent, additional external support may be given using sterile self-adhesive strips.

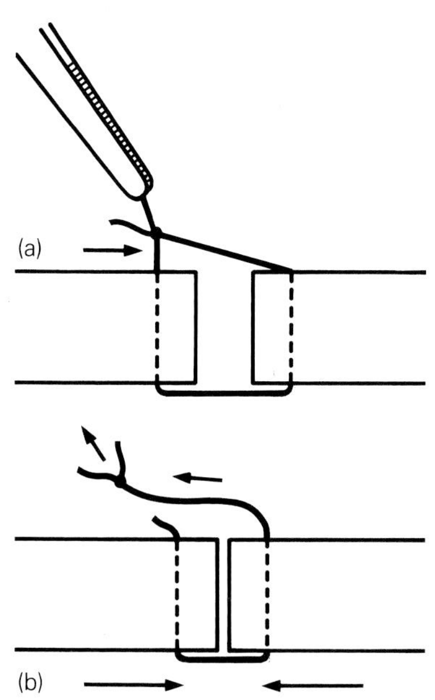

Fig. 14.1 Removal of stitches. (**a**) Cut under knot; (**b**) as the stitch is pulled out, the edges are drawn together.
(Redrawn from B.A. Maurice, *Surgery for General Practitioners*, by permission of Oxford University Press.)

14.1 TECHNIQUE OF SUTURE AND CLIP REMOVAL

Unfortunately, a wound which has healed well may be contaminated by poor suture removal technique resulting in stitch abscesses and an infected scar. Where possible the sterile dressings applied at the time of the operation should be left undisturbed until the sutures are to be removed. A sterile dressing pack should be used, and a no-touch technique employed, using sterile instruments. The doctor or nurse should either wear a mask or not talk during the actual procedure to reduce droplet cross-infection.

Fine sutures are best removed using a pair of iris scissors and dissecting forceps; most other sutures may be removed using either standard pointed stitch scissors or prepacked disposable stitch cutters and forceps. To minimize any risks of contamination, the knot should be picked up with forceps and one side of the suture cut flush with the skin; it may then be removed by carefully pulling on the knot (Fig. 14.1).

14.1.1 Subcuticular stitch removal

One end of the subcuticular stitch is cut flush with the skin, while the other end is grasped with artery forceps and traction applied. Additional support may be given by the application of sterile self-adhesive strips, which can be applied either at the time of the original operation or at the time of suture removal.

14.1.2 Removal of skin clips

Skin clips require a small pair of clip removers: these bend the clip open and cause minimum trauma to the skin. The blade is inserted under the clip and by applying pressure with the second blade, the clip opens (Fig. 14.2).

Skin stapling can result in minimal scarring (Fig. 14.3).

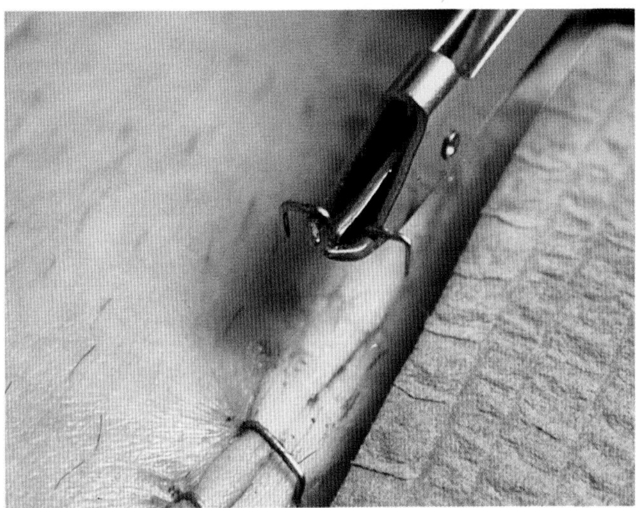

Fig. 14.2 The Proximate skin staple remover in use.

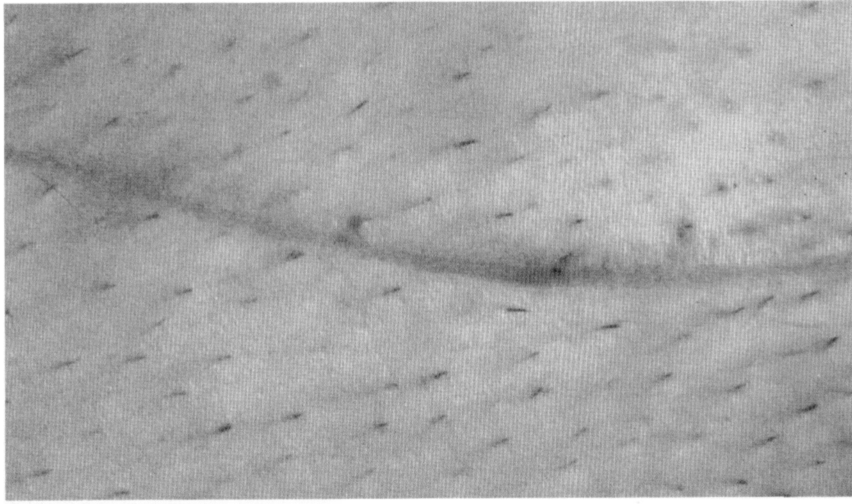

Fig. 14.3 Typical scar following skin stapling.

15

Chemical cauterization

Warts ... They may be removed also by the knife and the parts from whence they are cut afterwards touched with lunar caustic (silver nitrate) to prevent them from returning. But when this method is practised the operator ought to be certain that he has removed the wart entirely, for where part has been left, the most formidable symptoms have sometimes ensued

Encyclopaedia Britannica, 1797

The application of caustic chemicals to the tissues can be used to advantage to treat certain lesions; they are cheap, easily obtainable, effective and quick to apply and no special instruments are required. The two disadvantages of using chemicals are difficulty in controlling the exact area treated and the fact that only superficial lesions can be treated. Nevertheless, three substances are used commonly in medical practice, silver nitrate, liquefied phenol and monochloroacetic acid.

15.1 SILVER NITRATE

This has been used for centuries and is well known to most doctors; when applied to moist tissues, it causes them to turn white due to the formation of silver chloride; this then gradually turns black when exposed to light. Unless both patient and operator are particularly careful, accidental touching of the skin with the silver nitrate will result in stubborn, unsightly, black stains which are extremely difficult to remove. Similarly if left on plastic work-surfaces in the surgery, silver nitrate will cause permanent black staining.

It is produced as a solid pointed stick which may be fixed in a holder, or more recently, individual wooden applicators with a small, hard bead at the tip containing 75% silver nitrate. These are disposable, avoid any risks of cross-infection, and are easier and cleaner to handle. Finally, silver nitrate is made as a solution of any desired strength for topical application.

15.1.1 Granulations

These respond well to the application of silver nitrate, often being cured with just one application. Following separation of the umbilical cord in the newborn infant, occasionally messy granulations occur; one or two applications of silver nitrate and a dry dressing are all that is required.

15.1.2 Vaginal vault granulations

Vaginal vault granulations following hysterectomy are easily treated with topical silver nitrate, rarely needing more than two applications.

15.1.3 Small granuloma pyogenicum

If curette and electrocautery is not available or appropriate, the application of silver nitrate may result in a cure.

15.1.4 Epistaxis

Repeated nose-bleeds in children and young adults frequently occur from the small leash of blood vessels in 'Little's area' which are readily visible. The application of silver nitrate directly to this area often results in cure; it is slightly uncomfortable at the time of application and causes reflex watering of the eyes, but is usually acceptable to children (Chapter 32).

15.1.5 Cervical erosions

Many cervical erosions are asymptomatic and need no treatment; where the patient is experiencing an increased discharge or has symptoms of pain suggesting infection or cervicitis, cauterization of the cervix with silver nitrate may be tried. Using the applicator, the whole of the erosion, including the external cervical os is treated with silver nitrate; the area so treated becoming white. The patient is warned to expect an increased, watery vaginal discharge for 1 or 2 weeks while healing is occurring. Some doctors like the patient to use an antiseptic vaginal cream twice daily during this healing phase.

15.1.6 Ingrowing toe-nails

A silver nitrate caustic applicator has been traditionally used for ingrowing toe-nails for years; it is suitable for the treatment of any granulations which occur, but the black staining is a disadvantage, and alternative methods may be more appropriate (Chapter 30).

15.1.7 Chronic sinus or fistula

Long-standing suppuration and discharge through a skin sinus or fistula may result in the formation of fleshy polypi and/or heaped-up granulations. Both may be helped by the application of silver nitrate, often on more than one occasion. Where possible, the underlying cause of the fistula or sinus should be treated.

15.1.8 Chronic conjunctivitis

A weak aqueous solution of silver nitrate may be used to treat patients with chronic inflammation of the eyelids – the so-called 'silvering of the eyelids'. Benoxinate drops are instilled prior to the application of 1% silver nitrate, which is then washed out with normal saline.

15.2 PHENOL (CARBOLIC ACID)

Phenol crystals or pure liquefied phenol containing 80–90% w/w in water may be used for cauterization, while weaker solutions may be used for injection into hydrocele cavities (Chapter 22) or for the injection of haemorrhoids (Chapter 36). In each case the treatment relies on the irritant effect of the phenol on the tissues. Used as a 5% solution in glycerin, phenol may also be used for intrathecal and superficial nerve blocks.

The main use of liquefied phenol in general practitioner minor surgery is for ingrowing toe-nails, where it is used to cauterize and destroy the nail matrix (Chapter 30). In this situation, its threefold action of cauterization, destruction of nerve endings and sterilization makes it an ideal agent.

15.2.1 Granulations

The application of liquefied phenol is often an effective treatment for granulation tissue – more than one treatment may be necessary, and a delayed 'phenol reaction' may be seen on the 8th–10th day with increased inflammation and discharge.

15.2.2 Molluscum contagiosum

This condition is caused by a virus infection, and is typified by small, pearly, hard papules with an umbilicated centre. It may be treated with liquefied phenol by dipping a sharpened wooden applicator in phenol and then piercing each individual papule, transferring a minute quantity of phenol inside each spot.

15.2.3 Chronic paronychia

Following loss of the nail 'quick' and subsequent infection, often with yeasts, chronic paronychiae may be treated with phenol applied directly with a small wooden applicator sharpened in the shape of a chisel, dipped in phenol. This treatment may be supplemented with topical and occasional systemic antimycotics.

15.2.4 Ear-lobe cysts

Small infected cysts, particularly those occurring in the lobes of the ears may be treated effectively by incision, evacuation of any contents, and the application of pure liquefied phenol on a small wooden applicator and cotton wool.

15.2.5 Hydrocele and epididymal cysts (Chapter 22)

Aspiration alone rarely cures either of these conditions, but aspiration followed by the injection of 2.5% aqueous phenol results in 90–100% cure; the treatment needs to be repeated more than once.

15.2.6 Injection of haemorrhoids

Despite many alternative and more sophisticated treatments for haemorrhoids, 5% oily phenol still remains the treatment of choice for many doctors for their patients with haemorrhoids. The injection is given submucosally in doses of 0.5–5 ml (Chapter 36).

15.3 MONOCHLOROACETIC ACID

This is a simple, effective treatment for small warts, xanthelasmata, and superficial skin lesions.

15.3.1 Warts

Monochloroacetic acid may be 'pricked' into a wart using a pointed wooden applicator. The concentrated 'saturated' solution should be used. It will be noticed that initially the acid is rapidly absorbed by the wart. More is applied and 'pricked in' until no more is absorbed. Any surplus acid is mopped off the wart which is then left exposed to the air and kept dry. Healing occurs in 8–14 days; and the treatment may be repeated if necessary (Chapter 27).

15.3.2 Xanthelasma (Xanthoma)

This is a deposit of excess lipids in the skin; commonly found on the medial side of upper and lower eye-lids. Biochemical abnormalities are often not demonstrated and if treatment is requested they may be removed by surgery, electrocautery, cryotherapy, radio-surgery or the very careful application of monochloroacetic acid on a small wooden applicator.

15.3.3 Superficial skin lesions

Small naevi, plane warts, superficial keratoses etc. may all be treated by the careful application of monochloroacetic acid as an alternative to radio-surgery, electrocautery, diathermy or cryotherapy.

16

The electrocautery

> *Put an assortment of olivary cauteries on the fire, large and small, and blow on them until they are well heated. Take one, large or small, apply the cautery to the artery itself after having quickly removed the finger, and keep it there until bleeding is arrested*
>
> *Albucasis,* AD *936*

From the earliest times, physicians have used instruments heated to red-heat and applied to wounds to control haemorrhage and destroy diseased tissues. The use of an electric current instead of a fire to heat the instrument, enabled much greater control of the cauterization to be achieved, and in practice today most electrocauteries comprise a handle incorporating a switch, and a platinum wire electrode which can be heated to red-heat by the passage of an electric current through it.

Early instruments used a dry battery and rheostat to control the current, and, therefore, the temperature of the wire. These were not entirely satisfactory as the current drain was considerable and the batteries soon became exhausted, often in the middle of a surgical procedure.

With the advent of domestic electricity supplies, lead-acid accumulators were used which could be recharged at a convenient time and were still portable enough to be taken to a patient's home or doctor's treatment room. Furthermore they could withstand heavy current drain for several hours. As most domestic electricity supplies were direct current, transformers could not be used, and the only means of producing a low voltage and high current necessary for an electrocautery was by means of a heavy-duty variable resistance or rheostat, a method which was wasteful of electricity and not particularly safe for the patient.

The invention of the step-down transformer whereby the domestic electricity supply of 110 V (or subsequently 240 V) alternating current, could be transformed to any chosen voltage now enabled equipment previously run from batteries to be used on domestic supplies, with no worry about unexpected battery failure. In addition, the low-voltage winding of the transformer could be isolated completely from the primary, high-voltage winding, thus ensuring complete electrical safety for the patient and doctor.

Modern cautery transformers still employ this same principle, incorporating a rheostat to vary the output current (Figs 16.1 and 16.2). Unlike many electronic components the electrocautery works equally well on direct current or alternating current; thus there is no necessity to rectify the alternating output from the transformer.

More recently nickel-cadmium rechargeable batteries have been introduced; they have the ability to withstand a heavy current drain, are light in

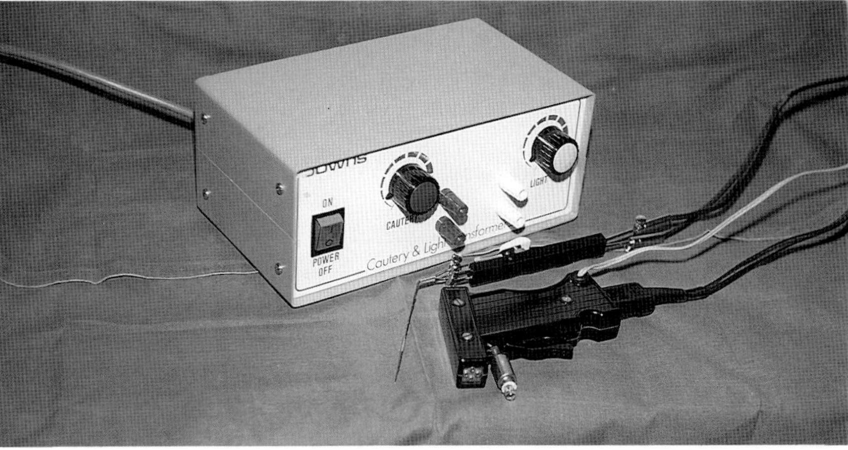

Fig. 16.1 A cautery-light transformer with pistol grip and Mark Hovell handles (Down Bros, Mitcham, Surrey).

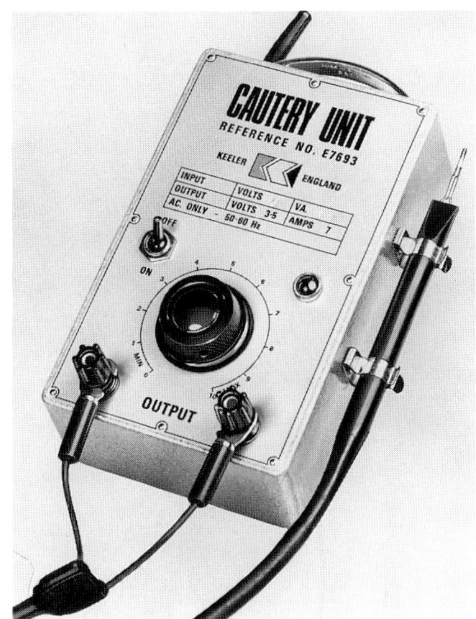

Fig. 16.2 A cautery designed for ophthalmic use but very suitable for minor surgical procedures (Keeler Instruments Ltd, London).

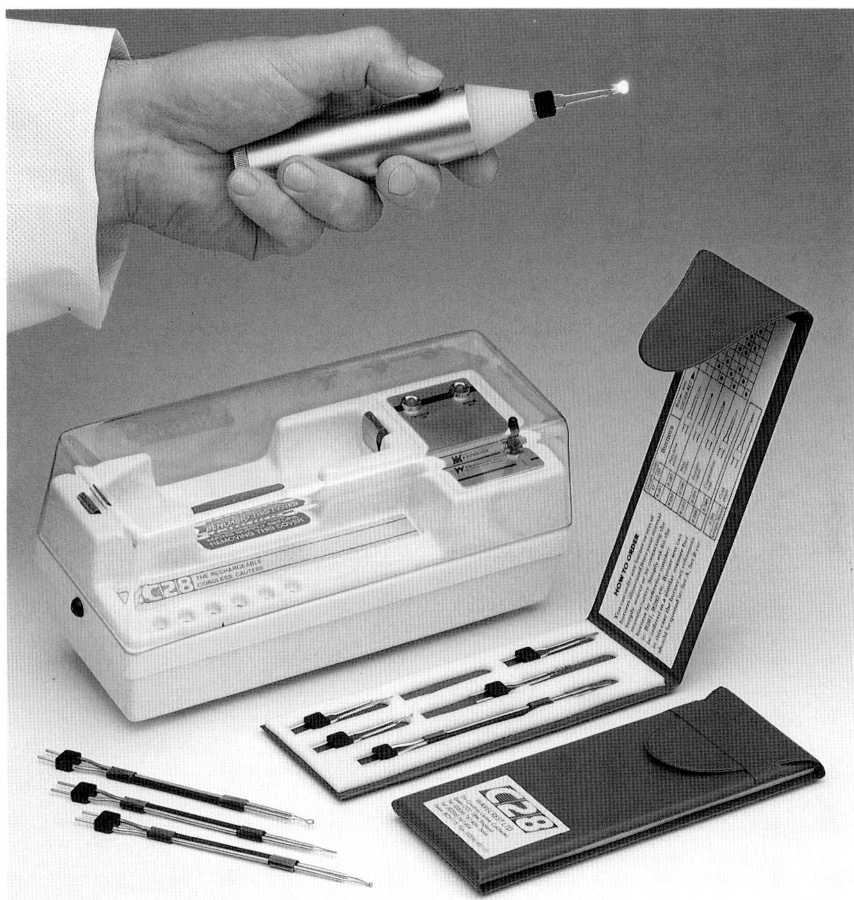

Fig. 16.3 Model C28 cordless rechargeable battery cautery. Quick and simple to use (Warecrest Ltd).

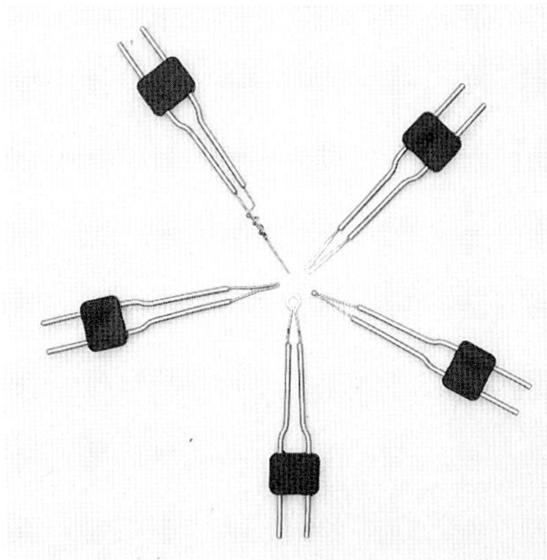

Fig. 16.4 Five cautery burners for use with C28 rechargeable cordless electrocautery.

weight, and a completely portable instrument can be produced with no attached wires (Fig. 16.3 and 16.4). However, unless regularly recharged, the batteries can fail suddenly, more so than conventional dry cells, so some form of stand-by is desirable. Also, after several hundred recharges, the batteries lose their ability to retain a charge, and need to be replaced.

Finally, small, lightweight, disposable cauteries have been introduced, incorporating dry-cell, non-rechargeable batteries. These are extremely light, very portable, and most useful for fine cauterization (Fig. 16.5).

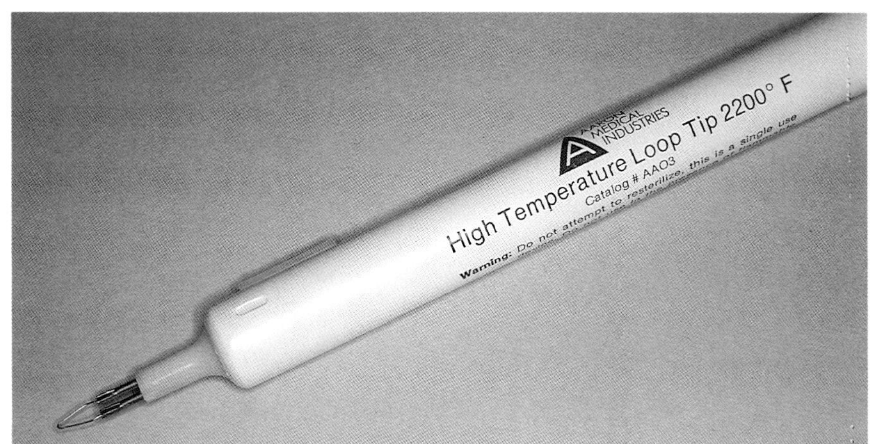

Fig. 16.5 Disposable electrocautery (Aaron Medical Industries, USA, Cardiokinetics Ltd, UK).

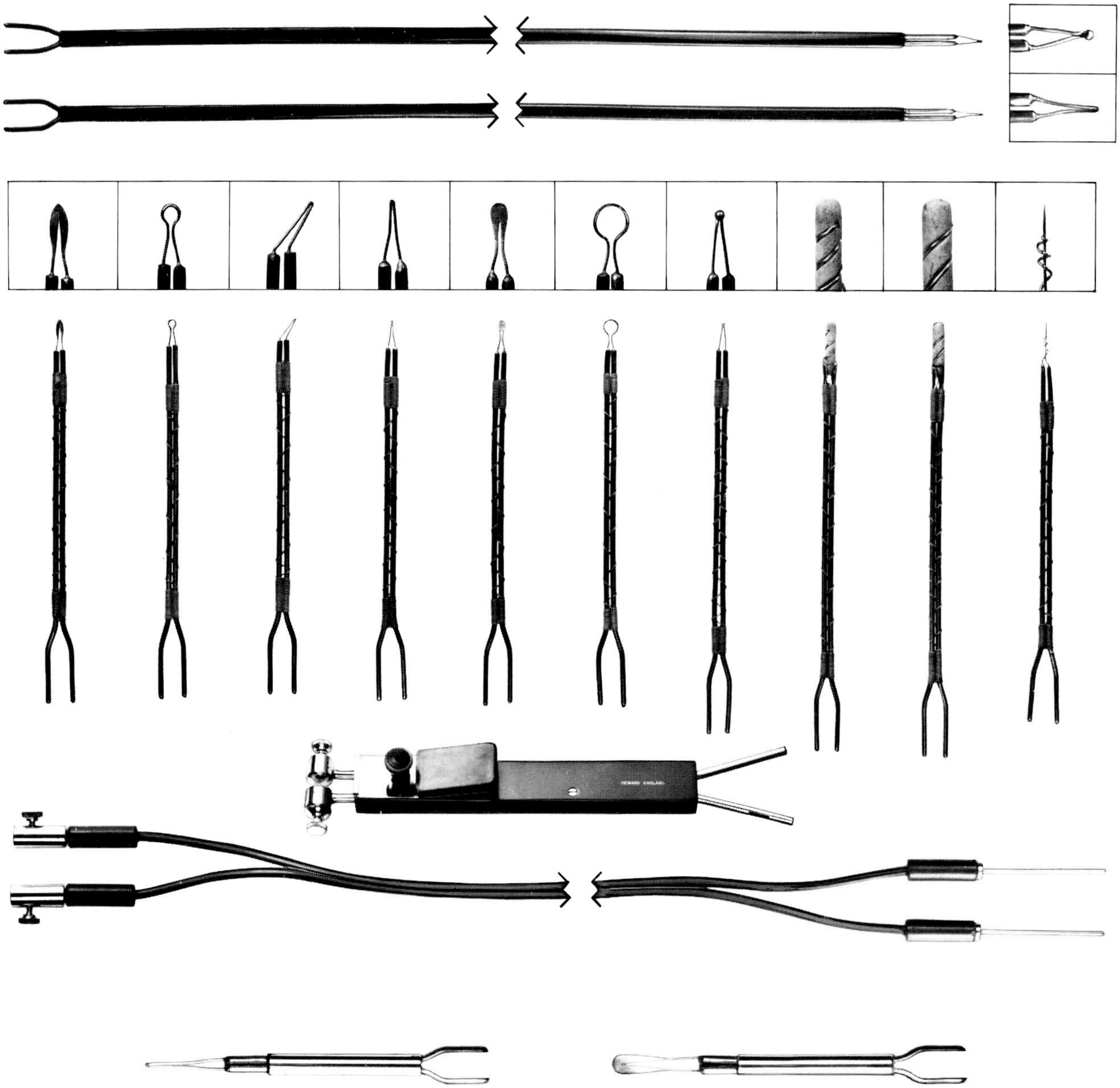

Fig. 16.6 A selection of cautery burners, together with Mark Hovell's cautery handle (Seward Medical).

The doctor purchasing an electrocautery will be faced with a bewildering array of different burners, handles, and transformers (Fig. 16.6). For the majority of minor surgery, a portable rechargeable cautery will give the best results. There are no trailing wires, the instrument may be taken between consulting rooms and also to the patient's home, and the risk of inadvertently putting too high a voltage across the burner is eliminated.

Burners come in two lengths, long and short. For the majority of cases the short burner is easier to handle and gives better control. The longer burners are mainly for use in cauterizing the cervix through a vaginal speculum.

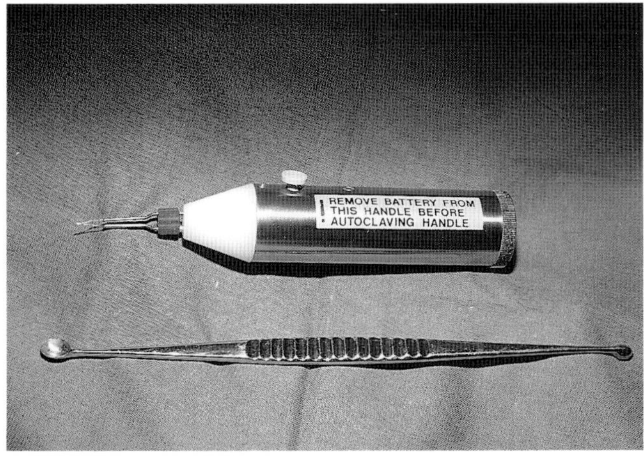

Fig. 16.7 C28 rechargeable cautery with Volkmann double-ended sharp-spoon curette: two of the most useful instruments for skin surgery.

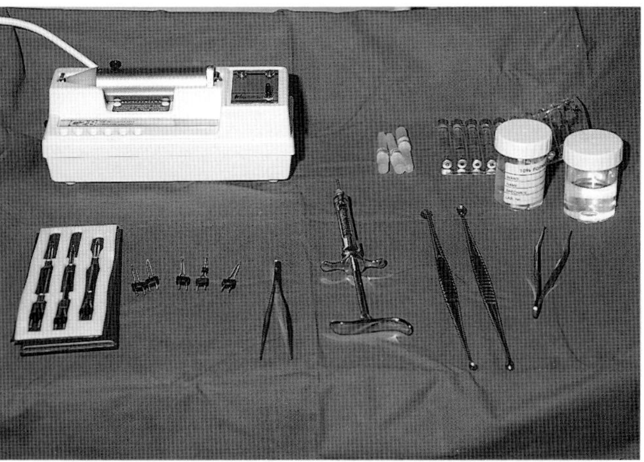

Fig. 16.8 Rechargeable cautery and holder, curettes, dental syringe, and local anaesthetic plus fine-toothed dissecting forceps, selection of cautery burners, and histology pots.

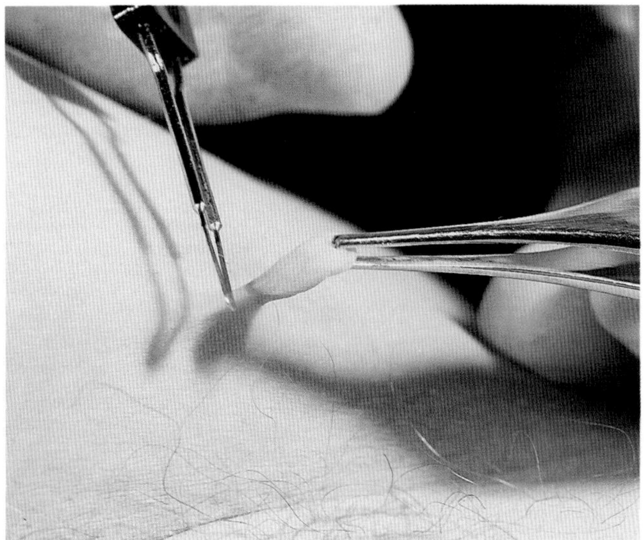

Fig. 16.9 Small skin tag being removed with cutting burner. Small lesions need no local anaesthetic.

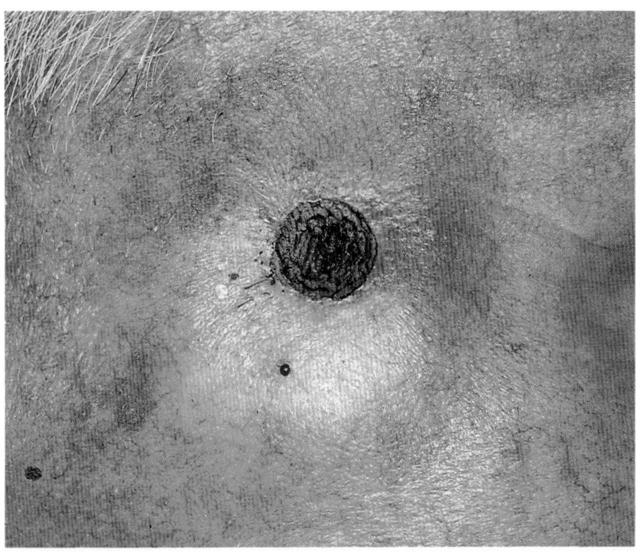

Fig. 16.10 Appearance of the base of a lesion removed with the curette, and cauterized using the ball-ended platinum burner.

A few basic instruments plus an electrocautery will enable a doctor to perform much simple skin surgery (Figs 16.7 and 16.8).

Of the many different shaped burners, the following will be found to be most useful:

1. Cutting electrode. This may be used for dividing skin tags and papillomata as well as removing some intradermal naevi (Figs 16.4 and 16.9).
2. Ball-ended coagulating electrode. This is one of the most useful burners for sealing small bleeding points: although more expensive than the other burners, it will be found to be the most frequently used (Figs 16.4 and 16.10).
3. 'Cold-point' burner. Instead of the heat being produced directly by the platinum wire as in other burners, the 'cold-point' has a central needle-like electrode, around which is wound a heating element. Heat is transferred by conduction to the tip. It is ideal for releasing subungual haematomata, and especially for treating spider naevi, where the needle tip is pressed against the feeding arteriole and effectively seals it (Figs 16.11 and 16.12).
4. Simple Λ-shaped burner. This is useful for a variety of lesions and can be used to both cut and coagulate (Figs 16.13, 16.14, 16.15 and 16.16).

16.1 USES OF THE ELECTROCAUTERY

16.1.1 Haemostasis

Small bleeding vessels can be readily sealed by the application of the electrocautery burner. The operator will soon discover the optimum temperature of the wire; generally a dull cherry-red is about right. If not hot enough, the wire will adhere to the tissues – if too hot, it will burn through bleeding vessels without sealing them; an adjustment on the rheostat is all that is required.

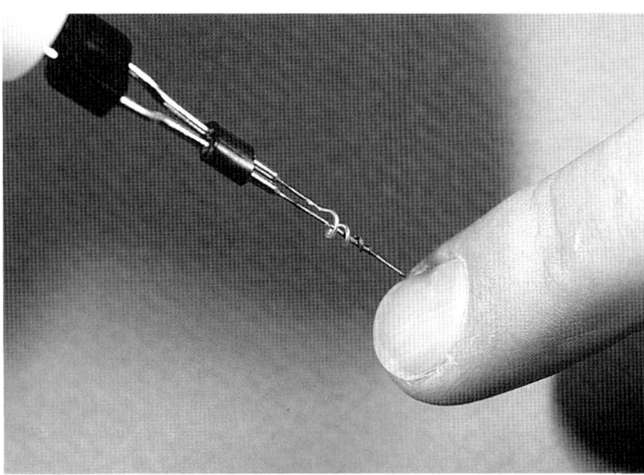

Fig. 16.11 The 'cold-point' cautery burner; ideal for subungual haematoma and spider naevi.

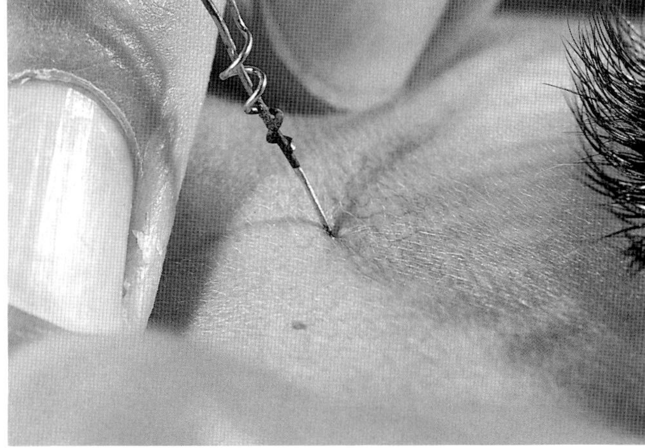

Fig. 16.12 The 'cold-point' burner being used to treat a spider naevus.

16.1.2 Skin tags (Chapter 26)

These may be picked up with fine-toothed forceps and divided easily with the electrocautery. No pressure is required, a repeated small movement of the red-hot wire will neatly separate the lesion from the base, with no bleeding.

16.1.3 Subungual haematoma (Chapter 42)

Resting the electrocautery tip against the nail and switching on the current results in a small painless hole in the nail with immediate release of blood. The 'cold-point' electrode gives the neatest result.

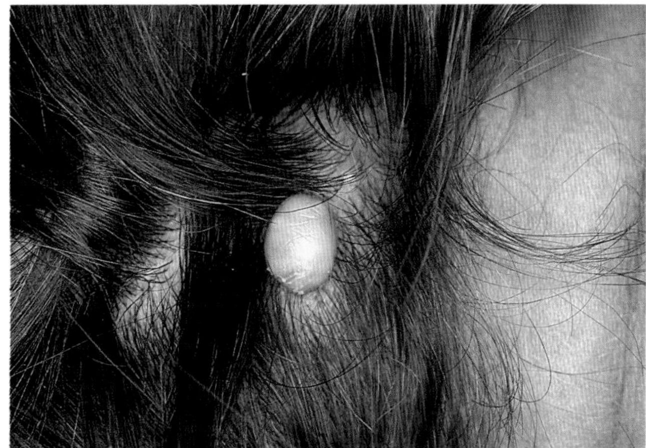

Fig. 16.13 Papilloma on scalp. Base is infiltrated with local anaesthetic.

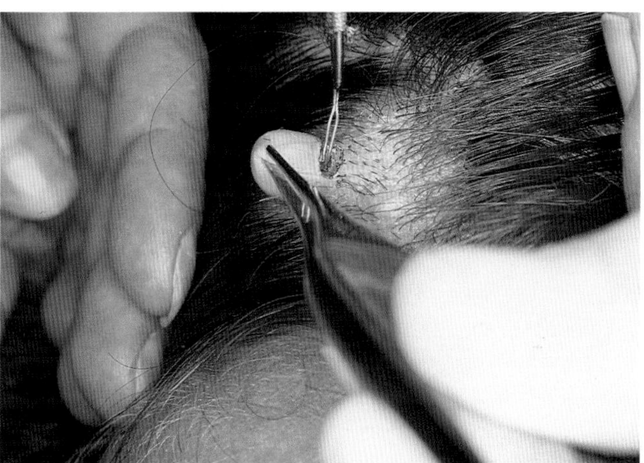

Fig. 16.14 The papilloma is picked up with forceps and separated with the electrocautery.

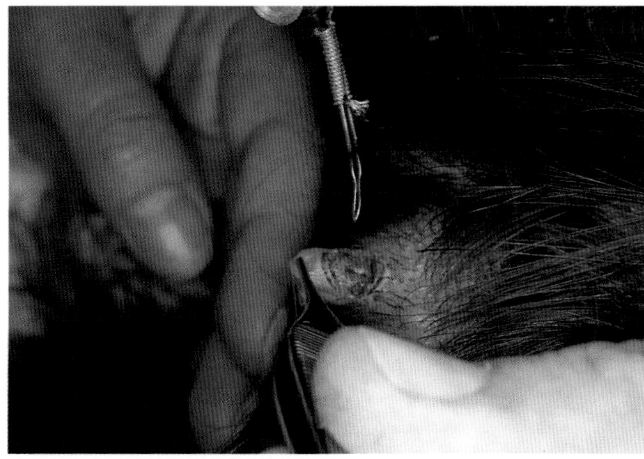

Fig. 16.15 Papilloma nearly separated from its base; notice absence of bleeding.

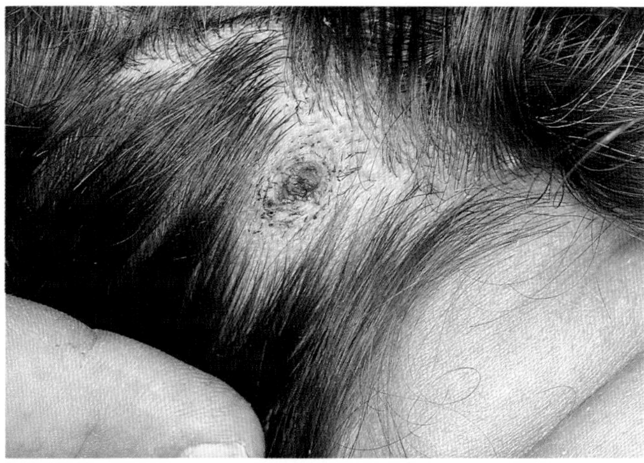

Fig. 16.16 The end-result immediately after removing papilloma. No dressing required.

16.1.4 Accessory digits (Chapter 42)

Where there is no underlying bony connection, accessory digits may be easily separated at birth using the electrocautery alone.

16.1.5 Basal cell carcinoma (Chapter 25)

Many small basal cell tumours of the skin may be curetted and the bases extensively cauterized with the electrocautery, with very good results.

16.1.6 Cauterization of the cervix (Chapter 38)

Cervical erosions are easily treated with the electrocautery; generally no anaesthetic is necessary and the results are good.

16.1.7 Condylomata (Chapter 38)

Individual condylomata may be destroyed using the electrocautery, small lesions will not require anaesthesia, larger ones can be infiltrated prior to treatment.

16.1.8 Entropion (Chapter 31)

Spot burns with the cautery help to produce fibrosis in the skin/muscle operation for entropion.

16.1.9 Epistaxis (Chapter 32)

Mild epistaxes are best treated with silver nitrate cauterization, but stubborn epistaxes may be treated with electrocautery to Little's area after preliminary topical anaesthesia. Beware of perforating the nasal septum.

16.1.10 Granuloma pyogenicum (Chapter 25)

These vascular lesions are ideally treated with curette and electrocautery.

16.1.11 Haemangioma of the lip (Chapter 45)

After infiltrating with local anaesthetic, a haemangioma on the lip can be treated very effectively by inserting the electrocautery into the centre of the lesion.

16.1.12 Intradermal lesions (Chapter 25)

Small intradermal lesions may be destroyed by the application of the electrocautery alone; larger lesions may be curetted followed by electrocautery to the base.

16.1.13 Keratoacanthoma (Chapter 25)

Curette followed by cauterization of the base is a simple and effective method of treating this rapidly growing tumour.

16.1.14 Molluscum contagiosum (Chapter 25)

Small lesions are better destroyed with phenol or iodine pricked into each spot, but equally good results may be obtained using the cautery.

16.1.15 Solar keratoses (Chapter 25)

Most solar keratoses may be removed with a sharp curette and the base cauterized using an electrocautery.

16.1.16 Spider naevi (Chapter 25)

If the central vessel of a spider naevus is touched with the electrocautery, rapid cure results.

16.1.17 Squamous celled carcinoma (Chapter 25)

Small squamous celled tumours may be curetted, followed by liberal cauterization of the base.

16.1.18 Warts and verrucae (Chapter 27)

Almost all warts and verrucae can be removed with a sharp-spoon curette, cauterizing the base afterwards.

16.1.19 Xanthomata (Chapter 45)

Used with care, the electrocautery may be a suitable treatment for small xanthelasmata.

16.2 COMPARISON BETWEEN INSTRUMENTS

16.2.1 Mains-operated cauteries

The design of mains-operated electrocauteries has changed little over the last 50 years. Basically they consist of a mains transformer with a lead to a switched handle. Mains-operated instruments have the advantage that higher currents and therefore higher temperatures may be obtained. This can be useful if a large lesion is being removed. A second advantage is that the instrument is always immediately ready for use and does not need prior recharging.

The main disadvantage of mains-operated electrocauteries is the trailing wires to the handle and burner, which makes a completely sterile technique difficult unless the connecting wires and handles are sterilized each time they are used. They are also not as portable as the disposable or rechargeable cauteries.

Because the current and voltage may be increased by using the rheostat, although higher temperatures may be achieved, there is also the risk of overheating and destroying the burners accidentally.

16.2.2 Rechargeable cauteries

The advantages of rechargeable cauteries are:

1. The absence of any trailing wires.
2. Greater portability, enabling the doctor to take it easily between consulting rooms, and even to the patient's home.
3. May be used where there is no electricity supply.
4. No risk of accidentally destroying the burners by overheating.
5. The handle may be enclosed in a sterile plastic sheath if a sterile operating field is required.

The disadvantages of rechargeable cauteries are:

1. The battery may fail without warning. This may generally be prevented by adequately charging prior to use.
2. The heat at the tip is less easily controllable than with a rheostat, and may be insufficient to deal with large, vascular lesions.

16.2.3 Disposable cauteries

The advantages of disposable cauteries are:

1. Cheaper to buy at the outset but more expensive in the long run;
2. No trailing wires;
3. Very portable.

The disadvantages are similar to those of the rechargeable cauteries, i.e.:

1. Battery may fail without much warning;
2. Insufficient heat may be generated for large vascular lesions;
3. The burners are generally more fragile and there is less choice of burner.

16.3 HAZARDS WITH INFLAMMABLE ANTISEPTICS

Spirit-based skin antiseptics or any other inflammable skin application should never be used with the electrocautery or diathermy because of the risk of burns to the patient.

In fact, it is unnecessary to use any antiseptic as the heat of the platinum burner is self-sterilizing.

17

The unipolar diathermy

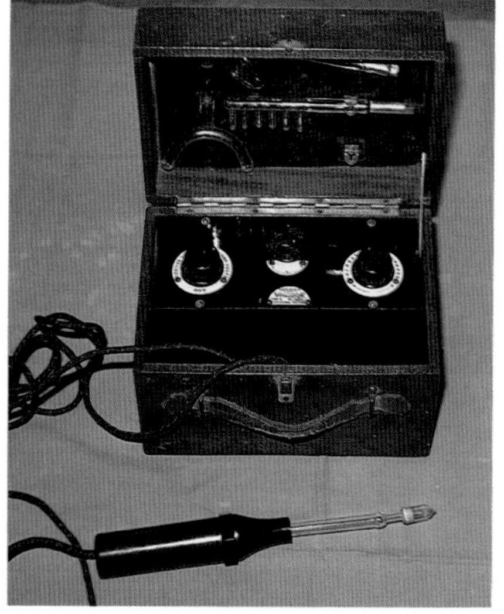

Fig. 17.1 A domestic 'high-frequency machine' which belonged to the author's grandfather; 1910 approx. This produced similar currents to the modern Hyfrecator.

An ailment I will treat ... with the fire-drill
Edwin Smith, Surgical Papyrus, 3000–2500 BC

High-frequency electric currents have been used for minor surgical procedures for 200 years. Early machines used rotating mica discs to generate static electricity which was stored in large Leyden jar condensers, connected to a spark gap and electrodes which were applied to the patient [12]. By the beginning of the 20th century, portable machines were in production (Fig. 17.1) which used batteries or domestic electricity supplies; the spark gap was still utilized and is still used in some machines today, being superseded by solid-state electronic circuitry (Fig. 17.2a, b).

The bipolar diathermy machine is a standard item of equipment in almost every operating theatre in the world. A low current at very high frequency and high voltage is passed through the patient. Two electrodes are needed to complete the circuit – one is large in area and is usually strapped to the patient's thigh, the other is usually connected to diathermy forceps or an electrode. If this latter electrode is placed in contact with the patient, a current sufficient to heat the tissues is generated. By varying the waveform and intensity of the current, tissues may be coagulated or cut.

The unipolar diathermy utilizes a similar principle – it generates a very high voltage, at very high frequency but relatively low current, but unlike the biopolar diathermy does not require a large second electrode to be connected to the patient. This makes it more suitable for use in minor surgery where large currents are not needed. A high-frequency current

Fig. 17.2a, b The Birtcher Hyfrecator Plus 7-797.

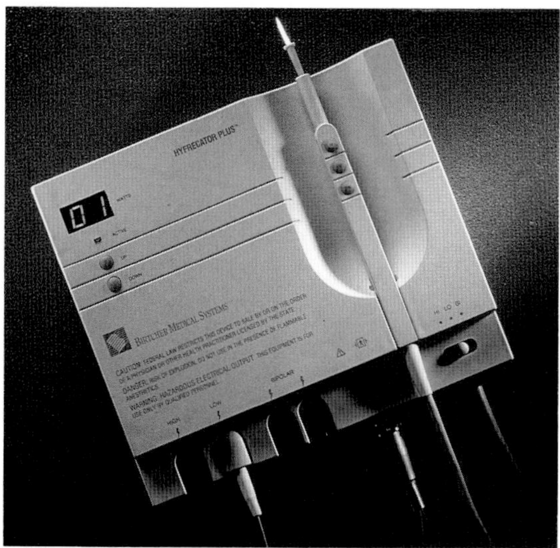

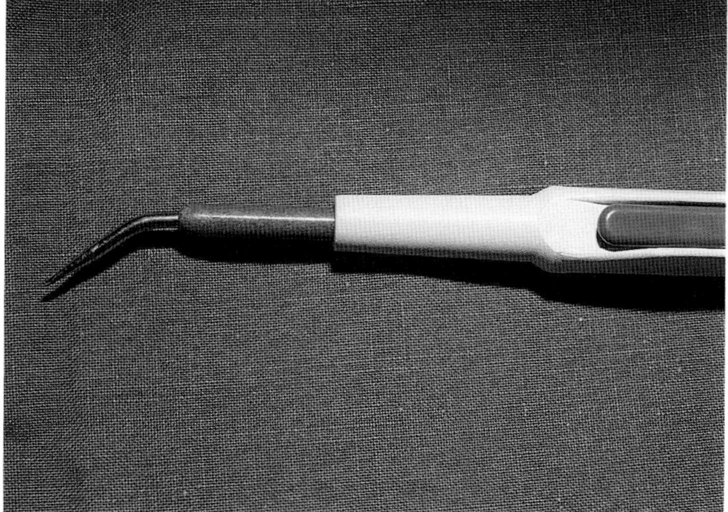

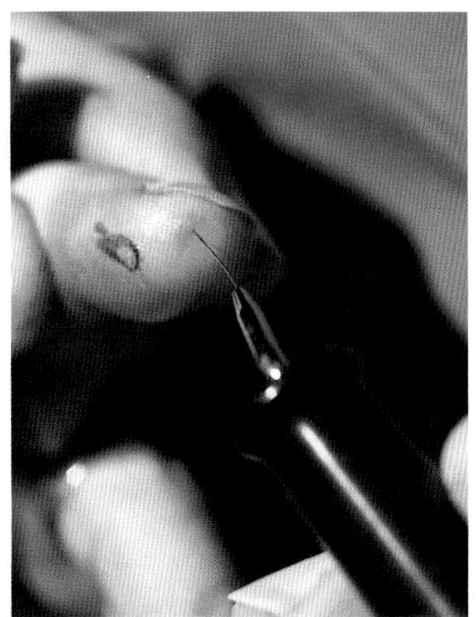

Fig. 17.3 The needle electrode of the unipolar diathermy being used to treat a wart on the finger-tip.

may be used in one of three ways, viz: desiccation, fulguration and coagulation.

In desication the electrode is inserted into the lesion to be treated to the depth at which the tissue is to be destroyed. The heat generated in the electrode dries out, and thus destroys the tissue which separates in a few days (Figs 17.3 and 17.4).

Fulguration is achieved by holding the electrode just above the surface to be treated and drawing a stream of sparks from the electrode to the point of treatment. The tissues are charred and destroyed, being rejected in a few days (Fig. 17.5).

In coagulation a bipolar electrode is used which is connected to a separate winding on the transformer. It is placed on the surface to be treated and an electric current flows between the two poles of the electrode, generating heat and thus destroying the tissues (Fig. 17.6). Similarly, bipolar forceps may be used to coagulate small bleeding vessels (Fig. 17.7).

As individual machines vary, the doctor who has not used a Hyfrecator before can experiment using a piece of raw meat held in the hand, and applying different electrodes – desiccation, fulguration and coagulation.

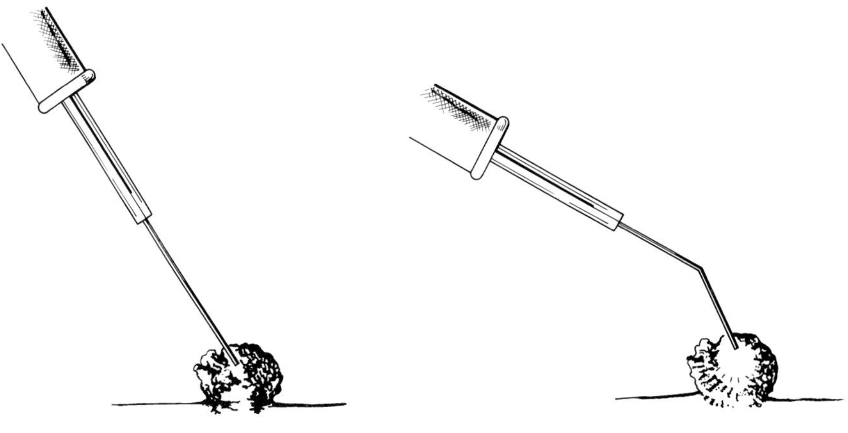

Fig. 17.4 Desiccation of a wart by inserting a needle electrode into the lesion and passing a current through it. This generates heat within the wart and destroys it.

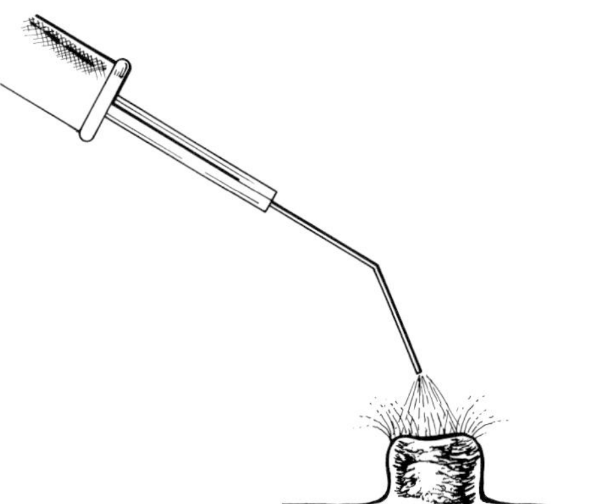

Fig. 17.5 Fulguration of a wart by holding the electrode just above the lesion and allowing a stream of sparks to pass from the electrode to the wart, thus generating heat and destroying it.

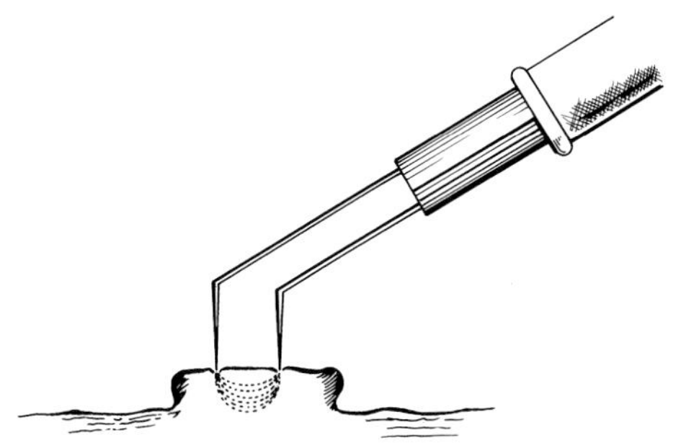

Fig. 17.6 Coagulation using a bipolar electrode pressed against the skin. Tissue destruction is confined to the area between the electrodes.

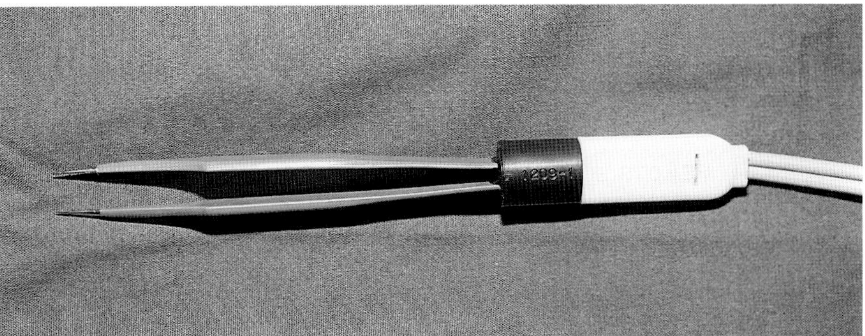

Fig. 17.7 Bipolar forceps for coagulating bleeding vessels: used with Hyfrecator or diathermy.

The depth and extent of treatment can then be assessed by cutting through the meat and examining the lesions produced.

Small cutaneous lesions and those affecting the cervix, vagina and bowel can be treated without the need for a local anaesthetic. For the majority of other lesions, however, it is more comfortable to infiltrate with local anaesthetic prior to treatment.

17.1 ADVANTAGES OF HIGH-FREQUENCY CURRENTS

1. Quick, effective destruction of lesions with no blood loss.
2. Accuracy – most lesions can be destroyed with minimal damage to adjacent tissues.
3. The treated area is left sterile.
4. Good cosmetic results with little postoperative pain.
5. Excellent for vascular lesions.

17.2 DISADVANTAGES OF HIGH-FREQUENCY CURRENTS

As with the electrocautery the lesion is destroyed and cannot be examined histologically, except by taking a preliminary biopsy.

17.3 SOME APPLICATIONS OF HIGH-FREQUENCY TREATMENT

17.3.1 Warts

Infiltrate the base of the wart with local anaesthetic and desiccate it with a fine needle electrode inserted to base of wart.

17.3.2 Verrucae

The technique is similar to that for warts.

17.3.3 Haemangiomata

As with warts use a method of desiccation. Haemangiomata may require more than one treatment, depending on their size.

17.3.4 Large haemangiomata

Infiltrate the base with local anaesthetic and then use bipolar coagulation. Treatment may need to be repeated.

17.3.5 Spider naevus

Local anaesthesia is not used. The needle electrode should be inserted into the main blood vessel usually in the centre.

17.3.6 Xanthelasma

The treatment is light fulguration with or without local anaesthesia.

17.3.7 Solar keratosis

Infiltrate with local anaesthetic; then curette followed by fulguration to the base.

17.3.8 Cervical erosions

These may be treated with fulguration without local anaesthesia.

17.3.9 Papillomata

Small papillomata may be desiccated or fulgurized without anaesthesia. Larger lesions should have the base anaesthetized first.

17.3.10 Naevi

Large naevi may be better excised, but small naevi can be easily destroyed by desiccation. If pigmented, the area desiccated should include a narrow area of healthy adjacent skin.

As can be seen, almost any skin lesion can be effectively treated with a high-frequency current; as the tissue immediately following treatment is sterile, healing may be promoted by the application of a sterile dry dressing, and advising the patient to keep the area dry until healing is complete.

18

Cryotherapy

Thou shalt make for him cool applications of ice and salt for drawing out the inflammation from the mouth of the wound

Edwin Smith, Surgical Papyrus, 3000–2500 BC

The first recorded use of cold for medical treatment was in the Edwin Smith Surgical Papyrus (3000 BC). Hippocrates describes the use of snow and ice for relieving pain and arresting haemorrhage (400 BC) but it is only in the last 100 years that freezing as a recognized treatment has achieved popularity.

Liquid air, liquid oxygen, and carbon dioxide snow were used at the beginning of the 20th century [13, 14, 15], and in 1950 liquid nitrogen was used successfully to treat a variety of skin lesions [16, 17, 18, 19, 20]. More recently, nitrous oxide has been used as a cryogen, utilizing the Joule Thompson effect to cool a probe applied to the lesion.

The boiling points of gases found in the atmosphere are shown in Table 18.1. As can be seen, nitrogen has the most advantages in that it is freely available (78% of the air in the atmosphere is nitrogen), is often a waste product in industry, is not inflammable, is chemically inert and has the fourth lowest freezing point. Because of these features, liquid nitrogen is now the cryogen of choice in medicine.

Gas	% in atmosphere	Boiling point
Nitrogen	78.1	– 196
Oxygen	20.9	– 183
Argon	0.93	– 186
Carbon dioxide	0.30	– 79
Neon	0.018	– 246
Helium	0.005	– 269
Freon 12	—	– 30
Nitrous oxide	—	– 89

18.1 MECHANISM OF ACTION

If human tissue is cooled to –25°C partial destruction occurs, and if cooled to –50°C total destruction takes place. Modern needle thermocouples now enable accurate observation of the effects of freezing and the relationship between probe temperature and depth of tissue destruction.

The result of freezing is the formation of ice crystals in the intracellular and extracellular fluids, resulting in cell dehydration, shrinkage, abnormal concentrates of electrolytes within the cells, thermal 'shock' and denaturation of lipid–protein complexes, and cell death.

It is found in practice that better results are obtained with a quick freeze and a slow thaw cycle, and it also seems better to give the lesion a second freeze immediately after the first freeze has thawed. This double freeze–thaw cycle is common to all freezing agents, whether spray or probe.

Following cryosurgery, a blister may develop, which dries to a scab in about 1 week and eventually separates. Occasionally a blood-filled blister results which, although looking alarming, heals quickly.

During the healing phase, which is usually surprisingly free from pain, depigmentation may occur in the treated skin and a narrow area

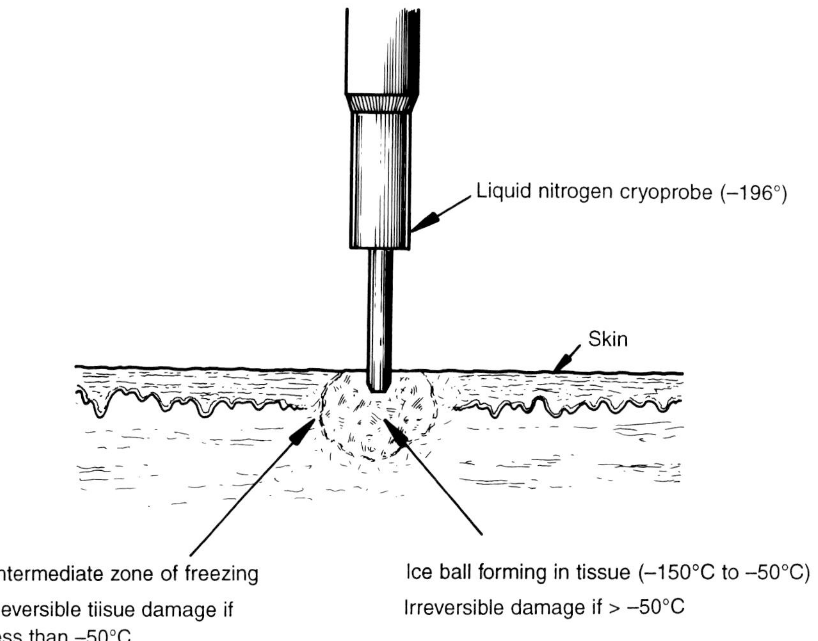

Fig. 18.1 Cross-section of lesion treated by freezing.

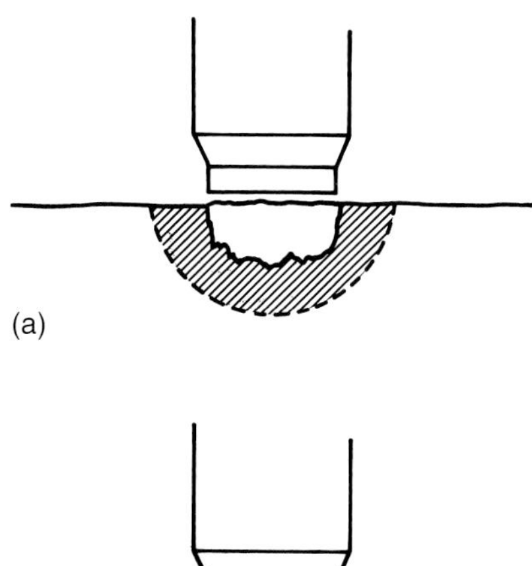

Fig. 18.2 (**a**) Hemisphere of ice must extend beyond the lesion in order to include whole volume. (**b**) Insufficient area of freezing leaves base of lesion still active.

Tissue temperature	Percentage survival
0 - –10°C	100%
–11- –20°C	67%
–21 - –30°C	38%
–31 - –40°C	14%
–41 - –50°C	3%
–51 - –60°C	0%

surrounding it: this should be explained to the patient, particularly if they are dark-skinned. Normally the pigment returns after several months.

Most lesions do not require additional local anaesthesia, although freezing of lesions on the digits may cause pain, and this may preclude its use in young children.

It is still possible to infiltrate the base of a lesion with local anaesthetic prior to freezing if the doctor judges that the procedure may give unacceptable discomfort to the patient, but the effects of freezing in this case may not be quite as predictable.

Whichever method of freezing is employed, the object is to produce a subcutaneous hemisphere of ice, in which is included the lesion to be destroyed (Fig. 18.1). Thus, the circumference of ice needs to extend beyond the edge of the lesion (Fig. 18.2).

A good way of demonstrating this is to practise on a pig's trotter, freezing an imaginary lesion and then bisecting the skin with a scalpel to observe the depth of frozen tissue. Tissue destruction is directly proportional to the degree of freezing as shown in Table 18.2.

18.2 INDICATIONS FOR CRYOSURGERY

Most superficial skin lesions may be treated with cryosurgery, with the exception of melanoma and certain intradermal naevi. Shallow lesions such as solar keratoses and seborrhoeic warts are ideal for treatment, and will respond to any of the different freezing agents.

The most widely used application for cryosurgery is in the treatment of warts, common warts, verrucae, and genital warts. In this situation, in addition to tissue destruction it is thought that the release of the wart virus into surrounding tissue may stimulate the immune mechanism and thus accelerate the clearance of warts in other areas of the body as well. Liquid nitrogen is probably the freezing agent of choice, as carbon dioxide and nitrous oxide rarely produce sufficient depth of cell destruction.

With experience, the doctor may also consider treating small basal cell carcinomata, small squamous cell carcinomata, and keratoacanthomata. These will require liquid nitrogen, an adequate freeze and meticulous follow-up, and confirmation of diagnosis by means of a cryobiopsy. Occasionally other factors such as the age of the patient may determine the size and site of the lesion to be treated (Fig. 18.24).

Pigmented lesions, and particularly melanomata are not suitable for cryosurgery.

Certain vascular lesions and haemorrhoids have been treated with cryosurgery; although successful, the postoperative phase is often prolonged, with blood-stained discharges, and is generally less well accepted by the patient.

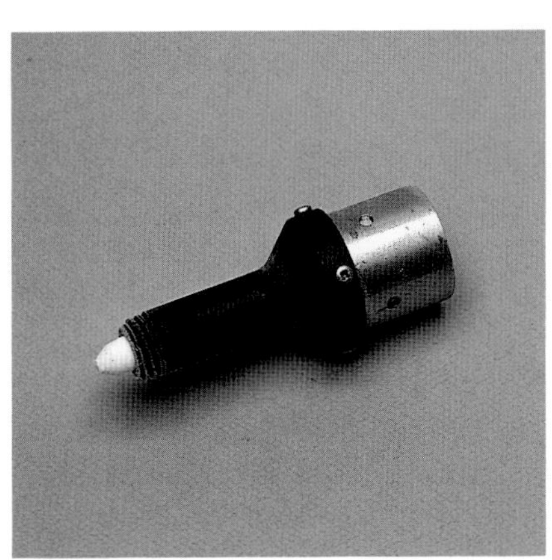

Fig. 18.3 A carbon dioxide pencil which can be made from a J-size CO_2 cylinder.

18.3 CRYOSURGICAL EQUIPMENT

Three main freezing agents are commonly employed for cryosurgery: carbon dioxide snow, nitrous oxide and liquid nitrogen.

18.3.1 Carbon dioxide snow

This is produced from a cylinder of compressed gas, and employs the Joule–Thompson effect whereby cooling occurs on expansion of the gas within a confined chamber. The snow is then compacted into a pencil applicator (Fig. 18.3), which is pressed against the lesion. Temperatures of –78.5°C are achieved. Carbon dioxide snow may also be mixed with acetone to produce a freezing sludge for treating larger areas of skin.

It is the least effective freezing agent, but is simple, cheap, readily available, and suitable for treating superficial lesions such as solar keratoses and seborrhoeic warts.

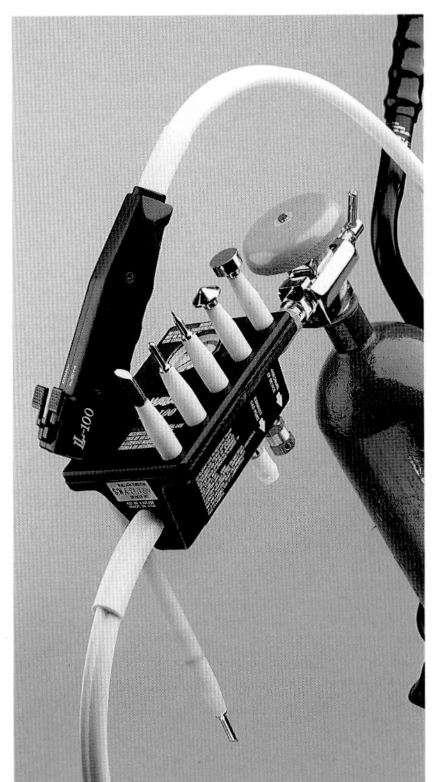

Fig. 18.4 The Wallach LL50X nitrous oxide cryosurgical instrument with selection of probes and 'instant thaw' trigger (Prospect Medical Ltd).

18.3.2 Nitrous oxide

Nitrous oxide is supplied under a pressure of 800 lb/in^2 in cylinders. A nitrous oxide cryoprobe consists of a reducing valve which attaches to the cylinder, and a length of connecting tube to a handle on which is screwed a cryoprobe (Fig. 18.4). A control tap on the handle causes cold nitrous oxide to reach the probe tip, resulting in freezing, or stops the flow of nitrous oxide, which builds up pressure and consequently warms, resulting in thawing.

This freezing–thawing facility is a great advantage and enables the probe to be disconnected easily from the skin after treatment.

Nitrous oxide cannot be sprayed on the skin, so only a probe can be used with this method of cryosurgery. In general practice, nitrous oxide has the advantage that it is always immediately available for use, unlike liquid nitrogen, which may have to be collected from an outside source.

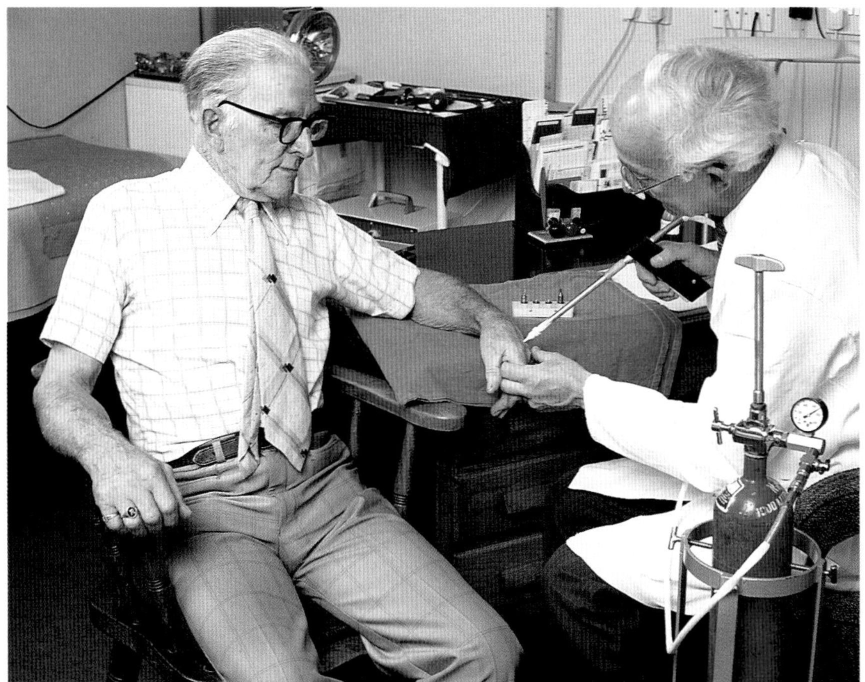

Fig. 18.5 The nitrous oxide cryoprobe in the surgery; treatment is quick and effective.

Fig. 18.6 The nitrous oxide cryoprobe applied to solar keratosis, back of hand.

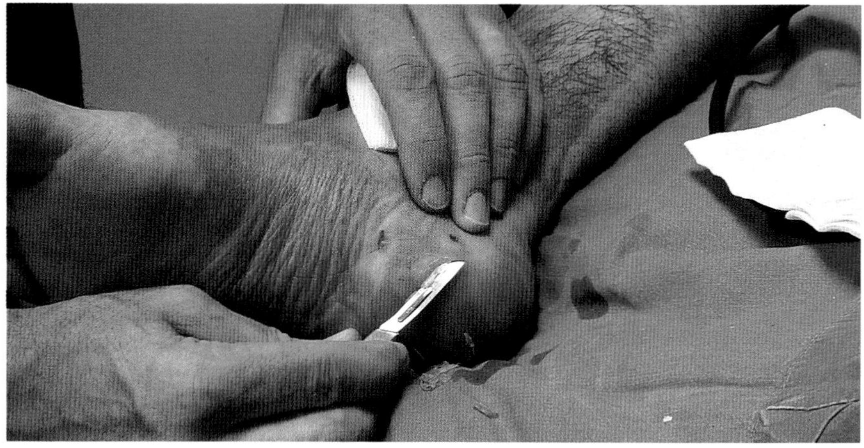

Fig. 18.7 Hard skin overlying a wart or verruca should be pared down with a scalpel prior to freezing.

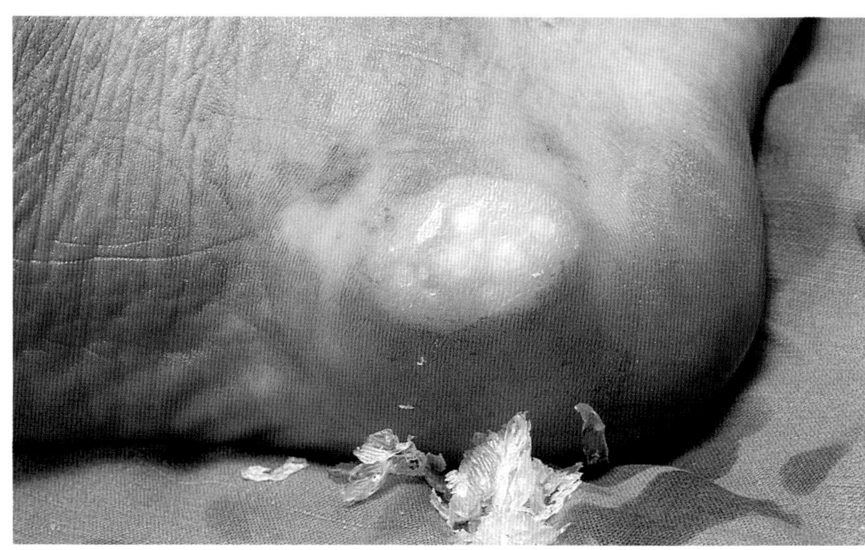

Fig. 18.8 Hard skin pared away, exposing verrucae.

Technique of using the nitrous oxide cryoprobe

Different size and shaped cryoprobes are available: the one approximating most closely to the lesion to be treated is chosen and fitted to the handle (Figs 18.5 and 18.6).

Any hard skin overlying the lesion (e.g. wart) is pared down with a scalpel (Figs 18.7 and 18.8), and a small quantity of water-soluble jelly (e.g. K-Y jelly) is applied either to the skin or to the probe, which is then pressed against the lesion and freezing commenced (Fig. 18.9).

Within a short time, ice forms at the probe tip, and causes the probe to adhere to the lesion. At this stage, by applying slight traction to the probe, the skin may be lifted away from underlying structures and thus reduce the likelihood of damage (Figs 18.10 and 18.11). Freezing is continued until a rim of ice 1–2 mm around the outer edge of the lesion is seen.

By switching off the nitrous oxide and pressing the 'thaw' switch, the probe tip warms up and detaches itself from the skin. The frozen area is now allowed to thaw, the probe reapplied, and a second freeze given, followed by a second thaw.

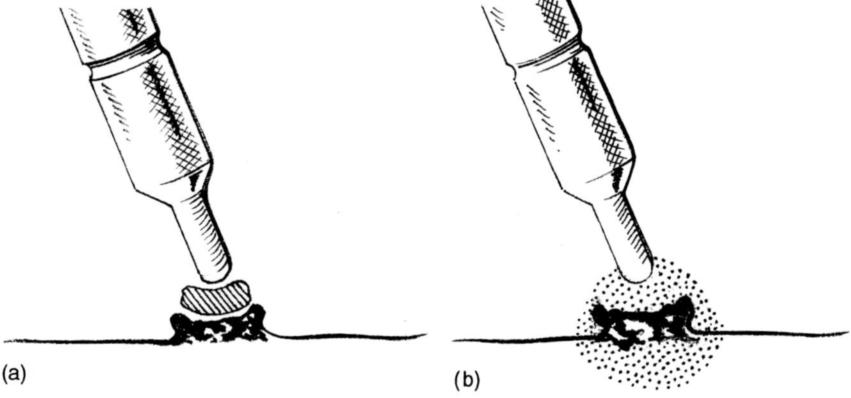

Fig. 18.9 Using a cryoprobe, a small quantity of water-soluble jelly (e.g. K-Y) is applied to the lesion and the probe pressed against it: freezing then causes the probe to adhere to the skin.

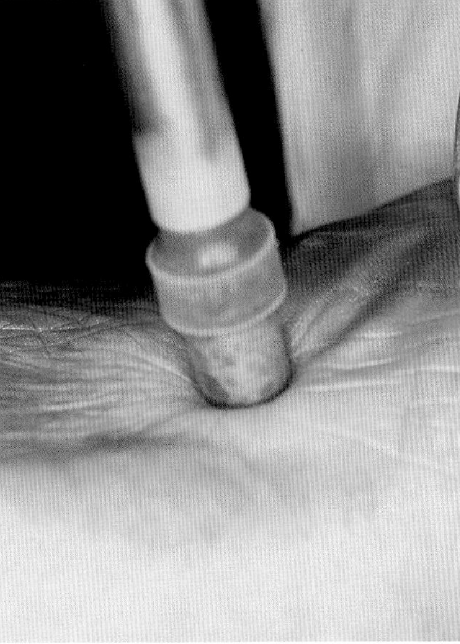

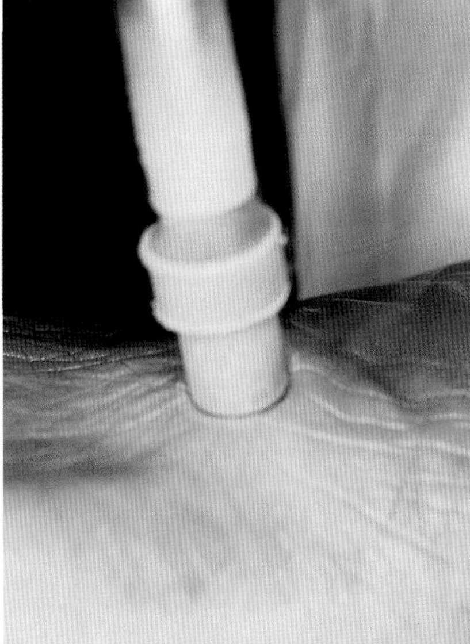

Fig. 18.10 The cryoprobe is applied to the lesion, which has been smeared with water-soluble jelly to help adhesion.

Fig. 18.11 Once the probe is adherent to the skin, it may be gently withdrawn as shown.

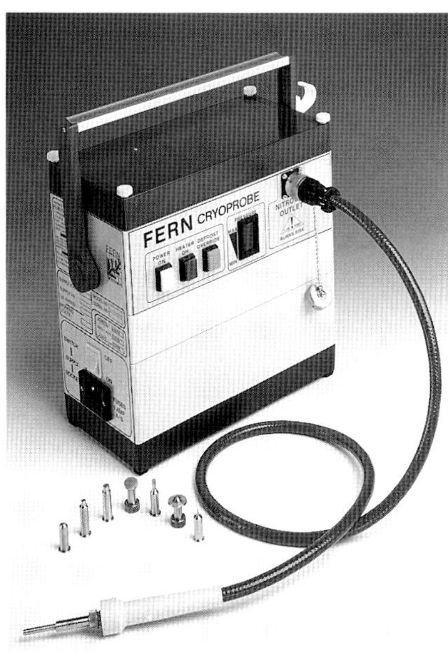

Fig. 18.12 The Fern cryoprobe: this utilizes liquid nitrogen, and has a thawing facility. A spray attachment is also available (Medinox International Ltd).

The patient is warned to expect some throbbing or discomfort over the next few hours: no dressing is necessary, but if a marked inflammatory reaction is expected, for example a large area frozen in an area of thin skin, it may be reduced by an application of a potent fluorinated steroid cream (e.g. Dermovate) under a dressing on completion of freezing.

There is a risk of cross-infection using the same cryoprobe: although this seems to be minimal, nevertheless it should be borne in mind when treating several patients, and the probes either autoclaved or wiped with a suitable antiseptic solution.

18.3.3 Liquid nitrogen

Liquid nitrogen is now the most widely used freezing agent, and in recent years a variety of liquid nitrogen cryosurgery instruments has been introduced (Figs 18.12, 18.13a, b and 18.14).

Liquid nitrogen itself is a waste product from industry and is relatively cheap. It boils at 196°C and needs to be kept in a Thermos-type container; even then it is continually evaporating and gradually reverts to nitrogen gas.

Where a doctor or practice considers using liquid nitrogen, a decision needs to be made either to collect small quantities from a nearby source at regular intervals, or to invest in a large Dewar-type flask which will store up to 3 months' supply of liquid nitrogen at one filling, and from which small quantities may be drawn off when needed.

The disadvantage of collecting quantities from an outside source is that patients need to be called back a second time and a special clinic arranged at which all may be treated at one session.

Fig. 18.13a The Cryo-jet (liquid nitrogen) with spray attachment (Cryomedical Instruments Ltd). (**b**) The Wallach liquid nitrogen ultra-freeze CY-6500 (Prospect Medical Ltd).

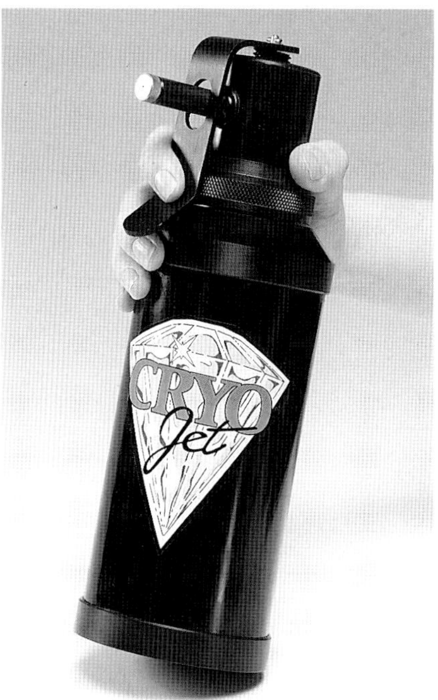

(a)

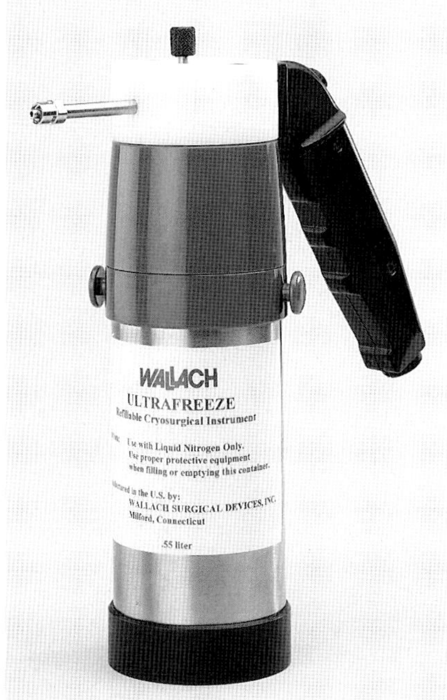

(b)

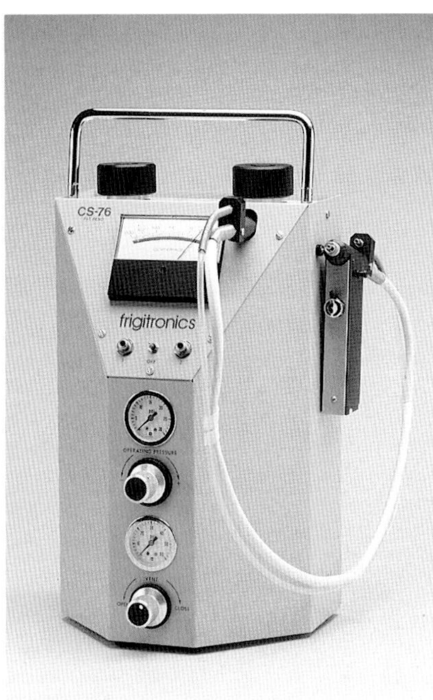

Fig. 18.14 The CS-76 liquid nitrogen cryosurgical unit, which is self-pressurizing, portable, and non-electric. It may be used with spray needles and closed-end probes (Frigitronics Ltd, Downs Surgical plc).

18.3.4 Methods of using liquid nitrogen

Four techniques of freezing using liquid nitrogen are available:

1. Cryospray
2. Cryoprobe
3. Individual probe
4. Cotton-wool swab applicator.

18.3.5 Cryospray

Most instruments designed for cryospray consist of a double-insulated Thermos-type flask, with screw-on lid and pressure safety valve, with a finger-operated on/off valve which delivers liquid nitrogen under moderate pressure to a spray-tip with a variable diameter hole. Liquid nitrogen is then sprayed as a fine jet on the lesion to be treated, with the nozzle held about 1 cm away from the lesion (Figs 18.15–18.19).

As with other cryotherapy techniques, best results are obtained with two freeze–thaw cycles. Furthermore, evidence suggests better results are also obtained with a relatively quick freeze and a relatively slow thaw.

Having given two freezes, the patient is warned to expect some discomfort, and if a marked inflammatory reaction is expected, a potent fluorinated steroid cream is applied under a dressing.

Cryospray treatment is remarkably simple to apply but has inherent dangers, the main one being the risk of damage to underlying structures such as digital nerves and tendons. It is not a treatment to be undertaken lightly or delegated to an untrained assistant.

18.3.6 Cryoprobe

As with nitrous oxide, cryoprobe attachments are available to screw to the liquid nitrogen outlet in place of the spray applicator. They consist of hollow metal probes of different diameters through which the liquid

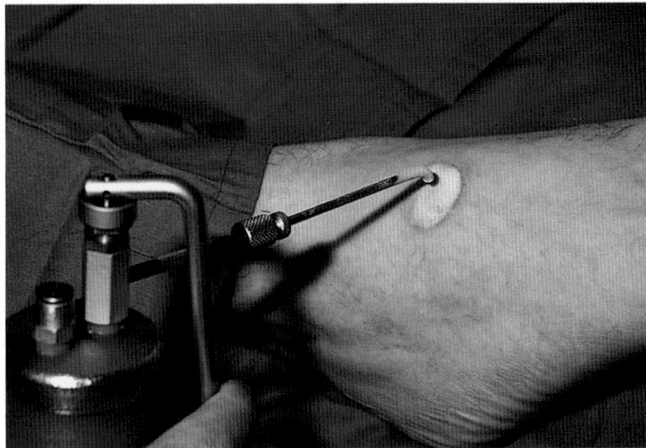

Fig. 18.15 Liquid nitrogen cryospray. The spray nozzle is held about 1 cm away from the lesion.

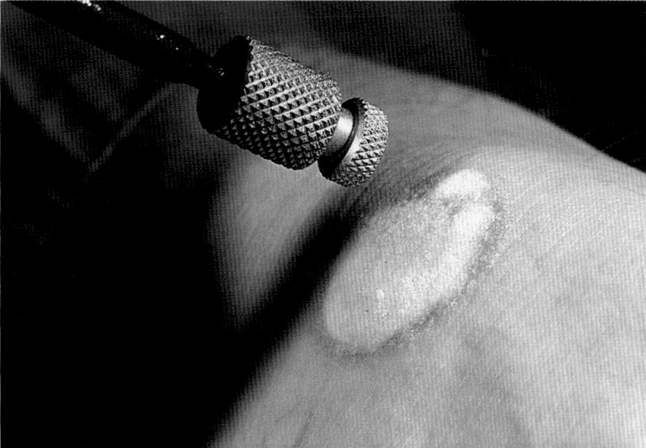

Fig. 18.16 Freezing occurring over the surface of the lesion. Two freeze-thaw cycles are recommended.

nitrogen is passed (Fig. 18.20). Here it evaporates, cools the tip of the probe to −196°C, and the nitrogen gas is then led away through a flexible exhaust tube attached to the side of the probe.

18.3.7 Technique for liquid nitrogen cryoprobe

This is similar in some respects to that used with nitrous oxide.

The probe nearest in size to the lesion is chosen. Any hard skin overlying the lesion (e.g. wart) is pared down, and a small quantity of water-soluble jelly (e.g. K-Y) is applied either to the lesion or to the tip of the probe, which is then pressed against the lesion and freezing commenced.

As soon as a rim of ice is seen forming at the tip of the probe, gentle traction is applied to the probe, thus pulling the skin away from underlying structures and reducing the risk of damage.

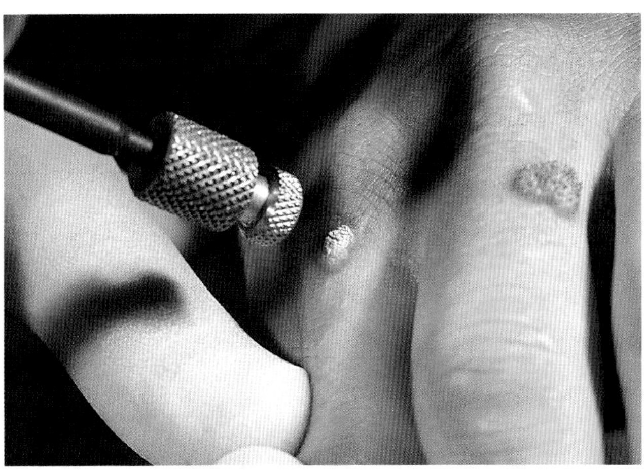

Fig. 18.17 Small warts are easily treated with a fine-aperture cryospray nozzle.

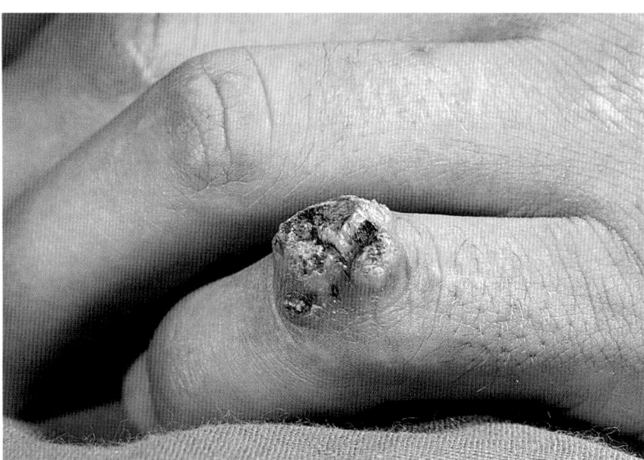

Fig. 18.18 Large solitary wart over 5th interphalangeal joint.

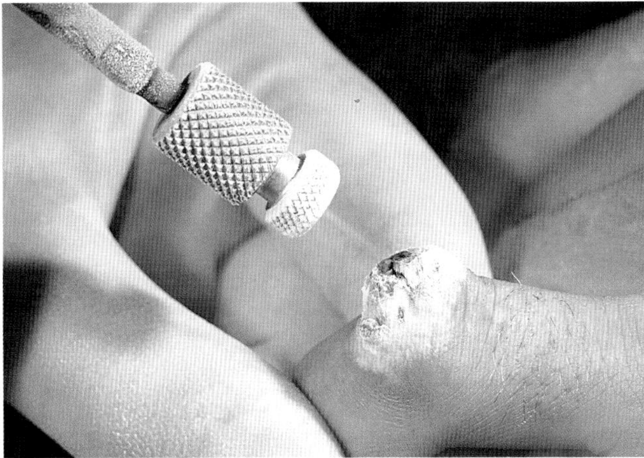

Fig. 18.19 Treatment of large wart with liquid nitrogen cryospray. Caution is needed to avoid damage to underlying structures, in this case extensor tendons and joint.

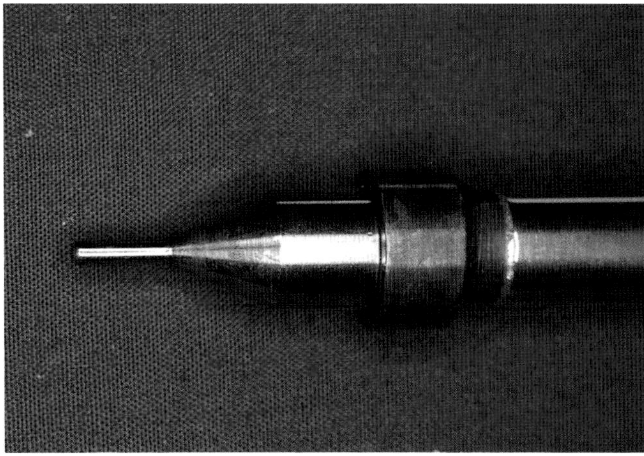

Fig. 18.20 Cryoprobe for use with liquid nitrogen.

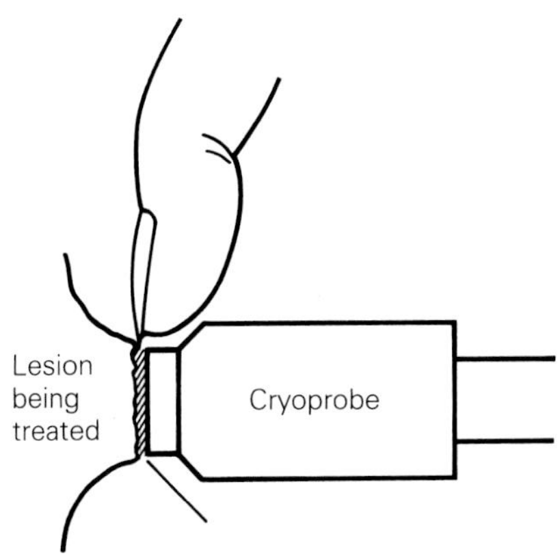

Fig. 18.21 Method of separating cryoprobe from lesion using finger-nail to snap off line of adherence.

Freezing is continued until a rim of ice 1–2 mm wide is seen surrounding the lesion. At this stage, freezing is discontinued, and with the majority of liquid nitrogen cryoprobes it will be necessary to separate the probe from the skin using pressure with the finger-nail in order to snap off the probe from the lesion (Fig. 18.21).

Where the doctor treats large numbers of patients with liquid nitrogen, it is worth investing in one of the machines which has a built-in heating cable to thaw the probe-end and also to keep the transfer tube supple (Fig. 18.12).

As with the nitrous oxide cryoprobe, two freeze–thaw cycles are recommended for best results; the possibility of cross-infection can be prevented by sterilizing the probe tip between patients.

18.3.8 Individual probe

A simple, cheap, metal probe can be used successfully for cryotherapy using the same method as is used for cotton-wool applicators (Fig. 18.22).

Liquid nitrogen is poured into an insulated polystyrene cup, and the metal probe dipped in until boiling stops, indicating that the probe is at –196°C.

It is removed, the tip wiped clean with a dry swab, and applied to the skin lesion, which has been pared down if necessary and covered with a thin film of water-soluble jelly (Fig. 18.23). The mass of the metal probe is such that quick freezing occurs, followed by a slow thaw, and separation occurs without difficulty as the probe warms up.

All the advantages of a cryoprobe accrue, without the need to purchase expensive equipment.

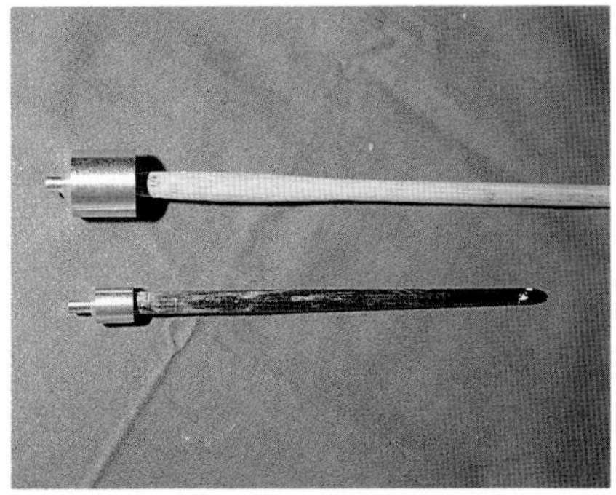

Fig 18.22 Simple, inexpensive probes for use with liquid nitrogen: made from aluminium or copper.

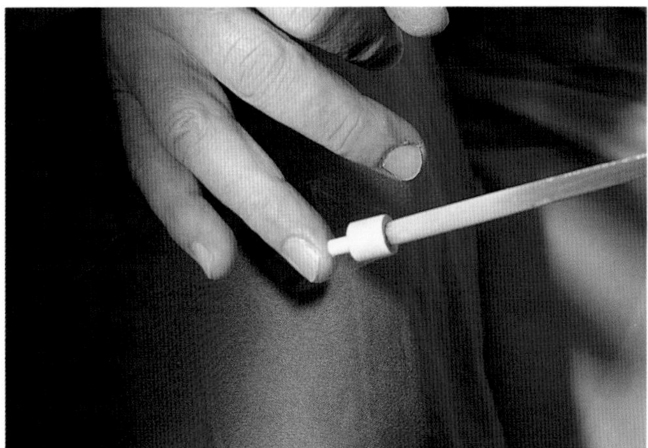

Fig. 18.23 Individual probe being used to treat digital wart.

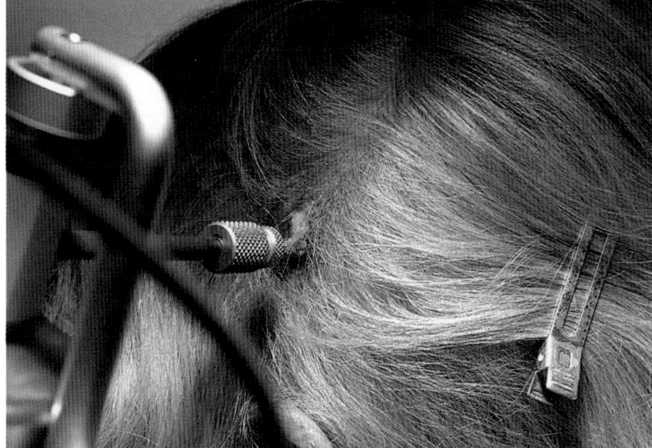

Fig. 18.24 Liquid nitrogen cryospray used to treat basal cell carcinoma on scalp of patient aged 98. Complete healing in 10 weeks.

18.3.9 Cotton-wool applicator

One of the earliest methods of applying liquid nitrogen was by means of a cotton-wool swab, dipped in liquid nitrogen and pressed against the lesion. Treatment is quick, simple, cheap and effective. Swabs should not be re-inserted in the liquid nitrogen as it has been shown that the human wart virus can remain alive in liquid nitrogen and there is the risk of cross-infection. Cotton-wool swabs are not as precise or as effective as the purpose-designed cryoprobe (Fig. 18.25).

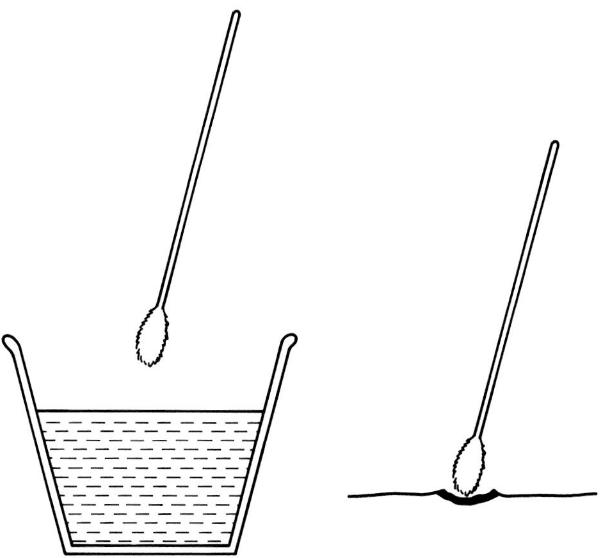

Fig. 18.25 Cotton-wool swab dipped in liquid nitrogen and applied to lesion.

18.3.10 Use of auriscope speculum for accurate freezing

Small cutaneous lesions may be frozen very precisely by choosing an appropriately sized auriscope speculum, placing it over the lesion, and spraying liquid nitrogen into the open end (Fig. 18.26).

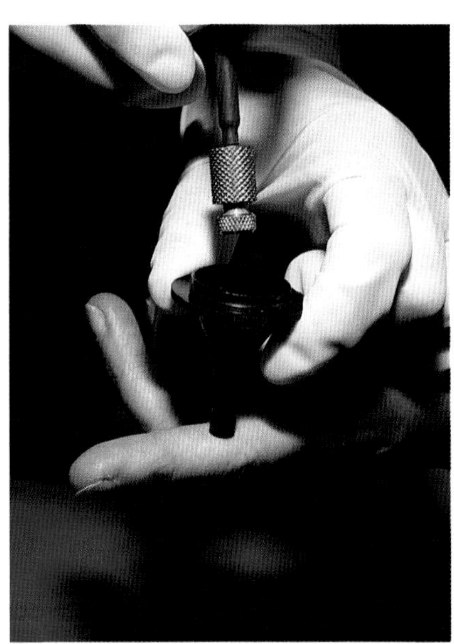

(a)

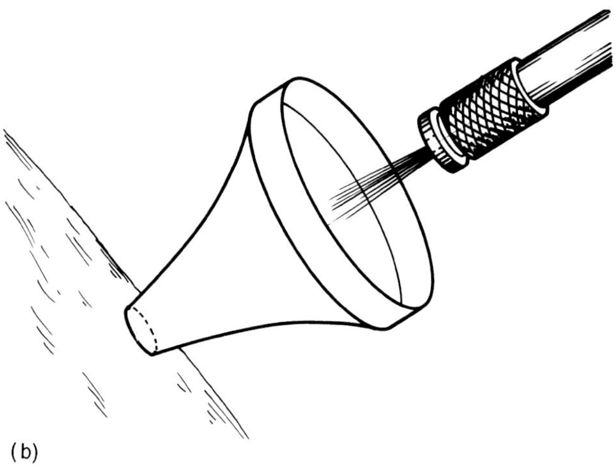

(b)

Fig. 18.26a, b Precise freezing may be obtained using an auriscope speculum.

18.3.11 Use of adhesive putty

This is normally used for sticking posters to walls, but can be used in cryotherapy for treating irregularly shaped lesions, particularly if near the eye, ear or mouth. The edge of the lesion is first identified using a marker pen and the putty is applied around it. When the spray is applied, the putty freezes to the skin and protects it. A narrow margin under the edge of the putty will also be frozen.

18.4 CONTRAINDICATIONS AND DANGERS OF CRYOSURGERY

18.4.1 Contraindications

Because cryosurgery is now so widely used, it is sometimes forgotten that there may be conditions where freezing may be contraindicated.

The doctor or nurse should consider the following as possible reasons for not using freezing agents on the skin:

1. Any known intolerance to cold;
2. Raynaud's disease;
3. Cold urticaria;
4. Cryoglobulinaemia;
5. Pyoderma gangrenosa;
6. Auto-immune diseases;
7. Agammaglobulinaemia;
8. Poorly controlled diabetes mellitus;
9. Dark skin where hypopigmentation following treatment would be unacceptable.

18.4.2 Dangers of cryosurgery

Because cryosurgery looks so easy, it is often forgotten that liquid nitrogen causes tissue death. Thus underlying structures may be irreparably damaged, e.g. cutaneous nerves and tendons [21]. It is therefore vital to be aware of the exact anatomy, and avoid damage to underlying structures.

Beware of warts on the sides of fingers!

Secondly, when transporting liquid nitrogen ensure that it is in a proper flask with a safety release valve for gas. A domestic vacuum flask is not the most suitable container and if it is used, under no circumstances should the lid be screwed down, otherwise it will explode because of the build-up of pressure.

Similarly, when transferring liquid nitrogen from one container to another, wear goggles and use protective gloves if at all possible. Splashes of liquid nitrogen on the hand, fortunately, do not generally cause burns.

Thirdly, when carrying a full flask of liquid nitrogen ensure that it remains upright and does not tip over. This applies particularly when transporting a container in a motor vehicle, and ensure adequate ventilation when transporting by car, preferably placing the container in the boot.

18.5 CRYOBIOPSY

One major advantage of cryotherapy is the ability to take a cryobiopsy to establish a diagnosis. This is done while the tissues are frozen, either with a punch biopsy forceps or curette (Figs 18.27 and 18.28). A small piece of alginate dressing is placed in the wound to check bleeding as thawing occurs, covered by a dry, sterile dressing. Unlike cauterization with heat, freezing does not damage the histology of the cells; the cryobiopsy may therefore be placed directly in 10% formol-saline and sent for routine histology exactly as any other specimen (Figs 18.29, 18.30 and 18.31).

Freezing also produces thrombosis in the microcirculation after 24 hours, so that provided the diameter of the vessels involved is small enough, many vascular lesions can be treated. Intradermal haemangiomata, particularly on the face, may be given repeated short freezes every 6 weeks, which will result in a gradual regression and total cure.

Following treatment of any lesion, the area should be kept as dry as possible and if necessary covered with a dry, sterile dressing.

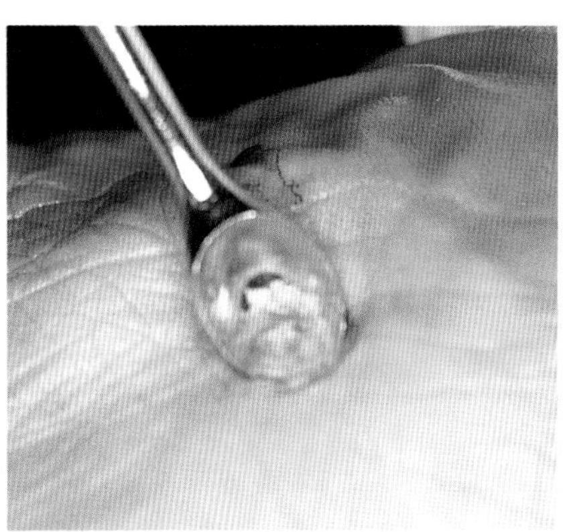

Fig. 18.27 A cryobiopsy may easily be taken with a sharp-spoon curette.

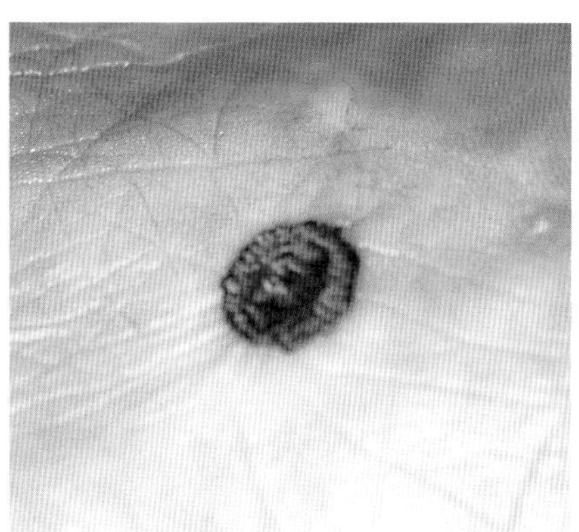

Fig. 18.28 If necessary the base may be cauterized with the electro-cautery as well.

18.6 SUCCESS RATES FOR CURING LESIONS

The success rates for curing various lesions are shown in Table 18.3.

Table 18.3 Success rates for various lesions

Lesion	*Cure rate*
Viral warts (hands)	75% if treated at 2–3 week intervals
Verrucae	60% if treated at 2–3 week intervals
Molluscum contagiosum	Similar to hand warts
Actinic keratoses	Nearly 100%
Seborrhoeic warts	Nearly 100%
Dermatofibroma	85% when treated at 2–3 week intervals
Tattoos	50% for small tattoos but high morbidity
Ingrowing toe-nails	50–60%
Labial mucoid cysts	85%
Synovial cysts	60%

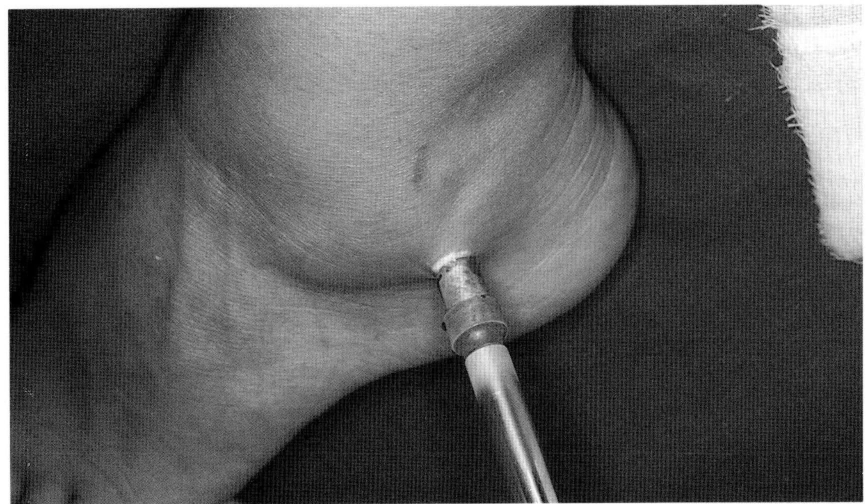

Fig. 18.29 The cryoprobe applied to a wart on the foot.

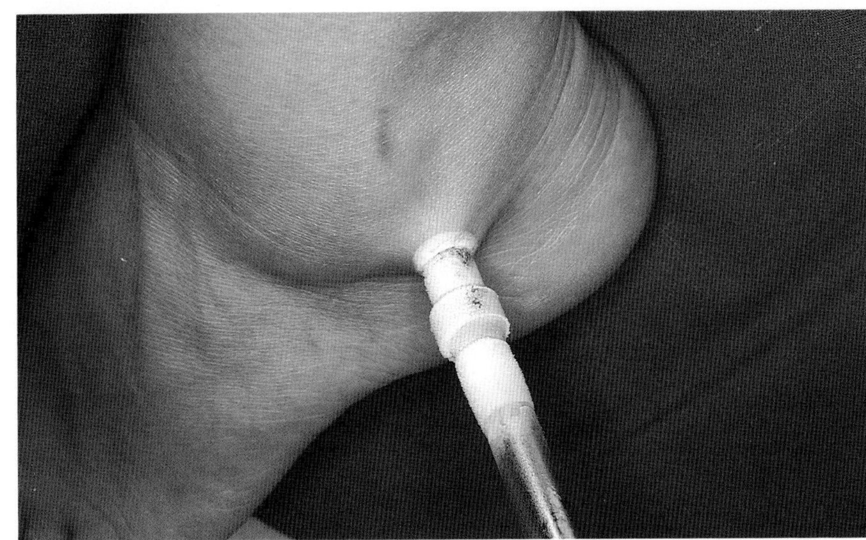

Fig. 18.30 Once the probe is adherent to the wart, gentle traction may be applied.

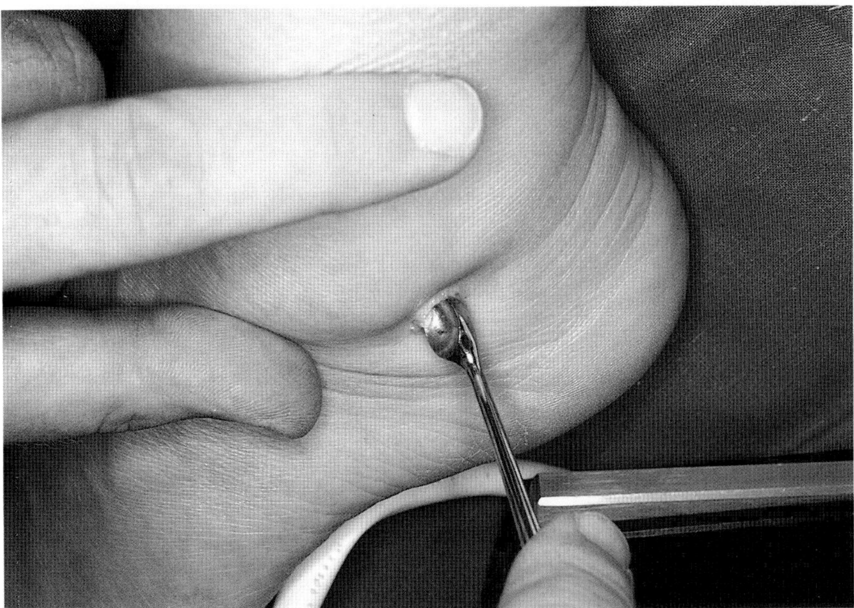

Fig. 18.31 A cryobiopsy may easily be performed, or the wart removed completely using a sharp-spoon curette.

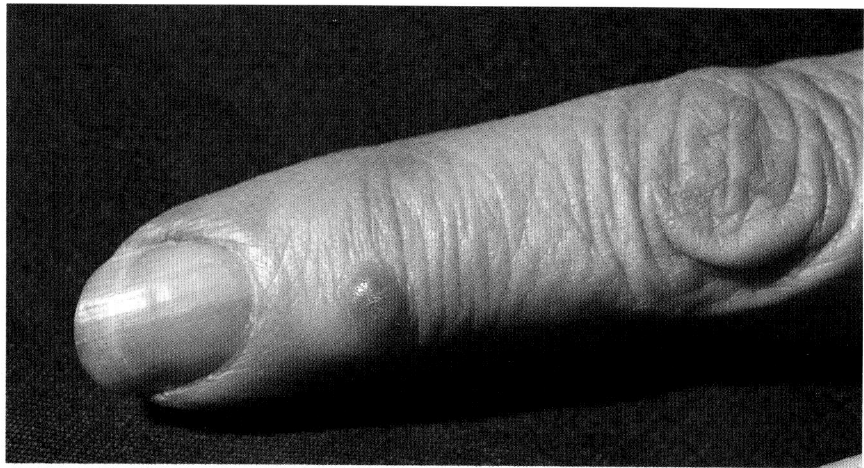

Fig. 18.32 Small ganglion over distal interphalangeal joint often disperses after cryotherapy.

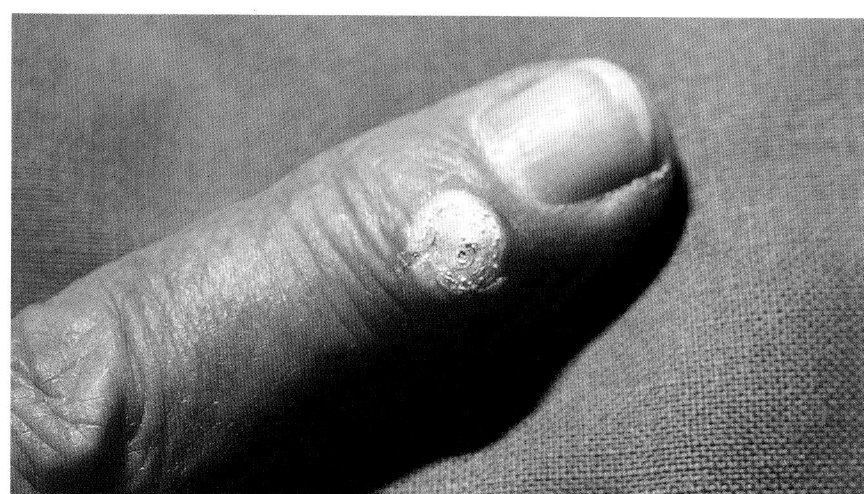

Fig. 18.33 Ganglion frozen with liquid nitrogen. Care needs to be taken to avoid damaging underlying structures.

Fig. 18.34 Information leaflet given to each patient receiving cryotherapy.

Postoperative instructions following liquid nitrogen treatment

1. Liquid nitrogen destroys tissues by freezing to –196°C. This results in ice forming inside the cells, and as this thaws, it causes cell death.
2. Immediately following treatment, apart from a slight discomfort, it will look as if nothing has happened to the skin.
3. Gradually, over the next few days, swelling, reddening, and sometimes blistering will occur.
4. Following this stage, healing occurs, which is usually remarkably pain-free, and leaves only a very slight scar, or none at all.
5. In dark skins, there is usually an area of depigmentation following cryotherapy; this normally recovers over the next year.
6. Reaction to liquid nitrogen is very variable; in some patients quite alarming looking blistering can occur, together with swelling of the surrounding tissues. Despite this, satisfactory healing still occurs.
7. Keep the treated area dry for 6 days if at all possible; it does not need any dressing unless blistering has occurred, in which case a simple non-stick dressing may be applied.
8. It is important to check with your doctor whether you need to be seen again, as more than one session is occasionally needed to cure some lesions.
9. If you have any queries, please do not hesitate to contact the surgery.

19

Histology

Although many skin lesions have characteristic or virtually diagnostic clinical appearances, histological examination of excised lesions is essential in ensuring a precise pathological diagnosis.

As a general guide, therefore, it is advisable to send all specimens for routine histological examination. Even quite innocent-looking skin lesions can occasionally turn out to be early neoplasms. The doctor is then in difficulties if he has thrown away the original specimen and a further lesion appears at the site of the first excision. Another advantage of sending all specimens for routine histology is to increase the doctor's diagnostic acumen. Only by comparing the histological report with the original clinical diagnosis can the accuracy of the latter be improved.

One point which is often overlooked is the importance of giving the histopathologist all relevant information about the specimen in order to obtain an accurate diagnosis.

In many cases precise diagnosis involves interpretation of the histological changes seen in a tissue section in the light of the clinical circumstances; for example, squamous cell carcinoma and keratoacanthoma both look alike histologically, but can be more readily differentiated if the history about the length of time the lesion has been present is given on the request form.

Most pathologists would like the following minimum clinical information with every specimen:

Name
Address
Age
Sex
History, including duration
Site of lesion
Size of lesion
Method of removal (e.g. excision, biopsy or curettage)
Clinical diagnosis.

19.1 HISTOLOGICAL APPEARANCES OF COMMON LESIONS (Figs 19.1–19.16)

For a more comprehensive account of histology, the reader is referred to one of the many histopathology textbooks. However, it is helpful to have a little knowledge of the histological appearances of the commonly encountered skin lesions seen in minor surgery, and the following have been chosen as being representative. They have been grouped into epidermal lesions of increasing severity, followed by dermal lesions.

1. Normal skin
2. Sebaceous cysts (pilar, tricholemmal, and epidermoid)
3. Viral wart
4. Molluscum contagiosum
5. Melanocytic naevus (junctional naevus stage)
6. Melanocytic naevus (compound naevus stage)
7. Melanocytic naevus (intradermal naevus stage)
8. Seborrhoeic wart (basal cell papilloma)
9. Keratoacanthoma
10. Basal cell carcinoma (rodent ulcer)
11. Squamous cell carcinoma
12. Malignant melanoma
13. Keloid scar
14. Haemangioma
15. Blue naevus (benign dermal melanocytoma)
16. Histiocytoma.

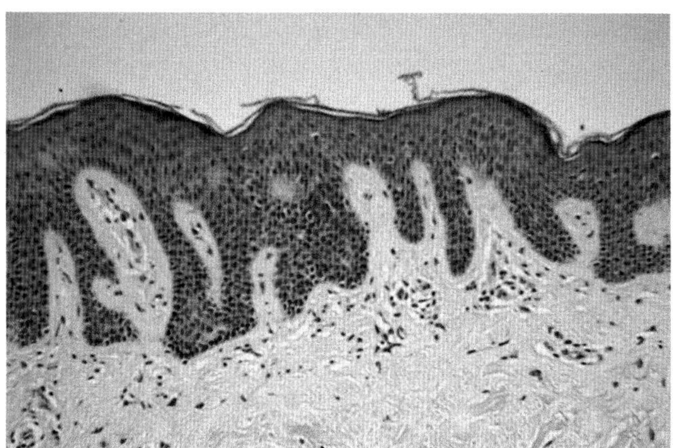

Fig. 19.1a Histological appearance of normal skin showing the keratinizing stratified squamous epithelium of the epidermis overlying the connective tissue structure of the dermis. (Scattered pale-staining melanocytes are present in the basal layer of the epidermis.)

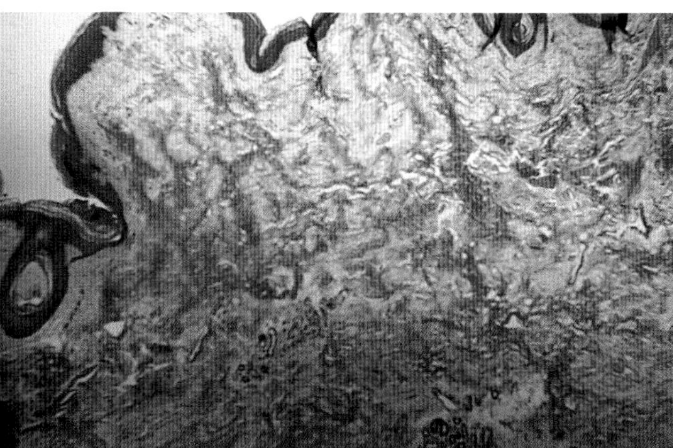

Fig. 19.1b Section of normal skin including sweat glands in lower dermis.

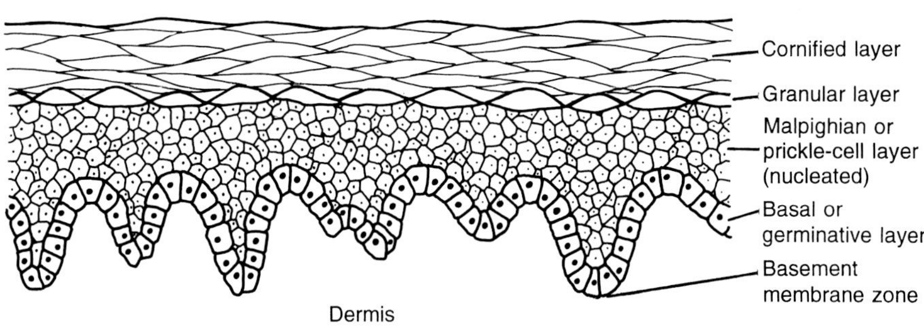

Fig. 19.1c Diagrammatic appearance of normal skin histology.

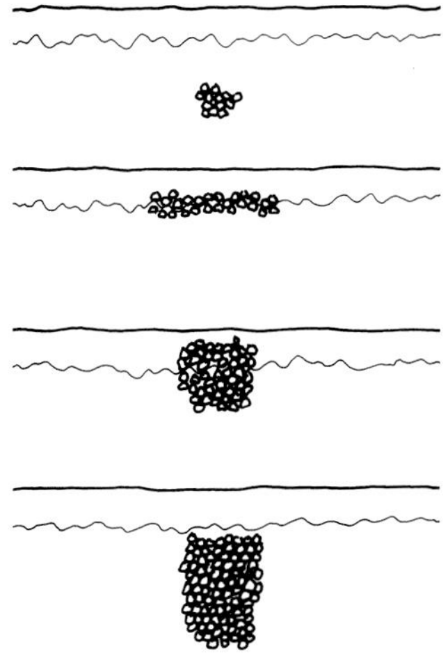

Fig. 19.1d Evolution of naevi showing histology.

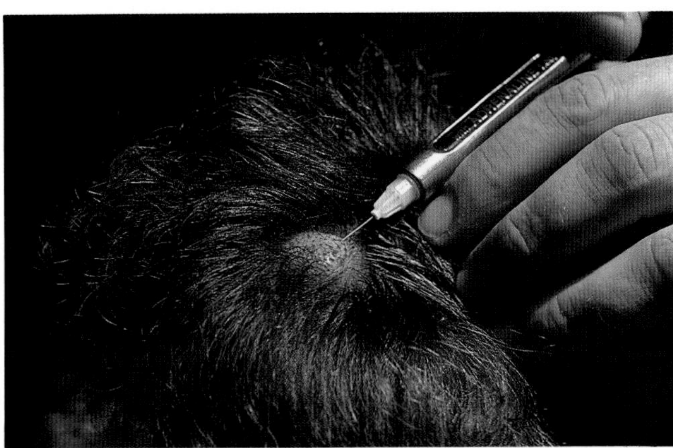

Fig. 19.2a Sebaceous cyst (pilar cyst). Common, benign, they may grow to very large size. Note central punctum.

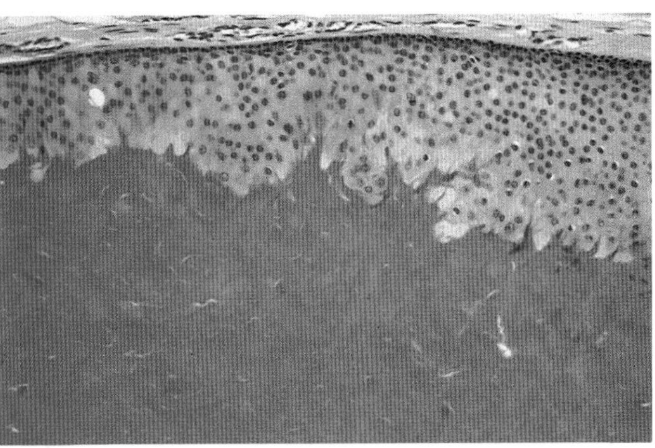

Fig. 19.2b Pilar cyst. Histological appearance. Note cyst lining corresponds to hair follicle outer sheath with no granular layer. Amorphous eosinophilic content.

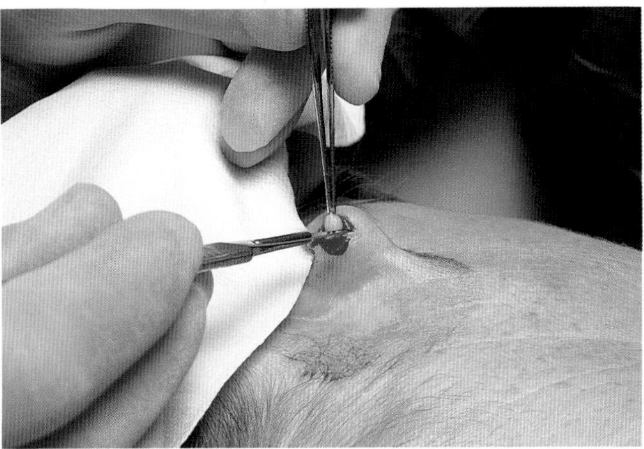

Fig. 19.2c Epidermoid or inclusion cyst being removed from ear-lobe.

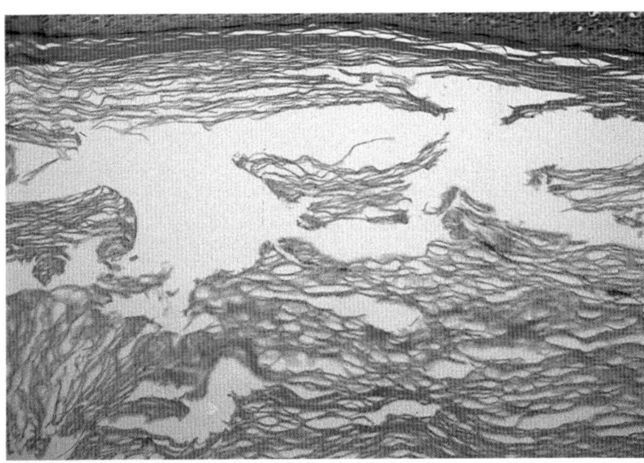

Fig. 19.2d Epidermoid cyst. Note cyst lining corresponds to the epidermis including the granular layer. The content is keratin.

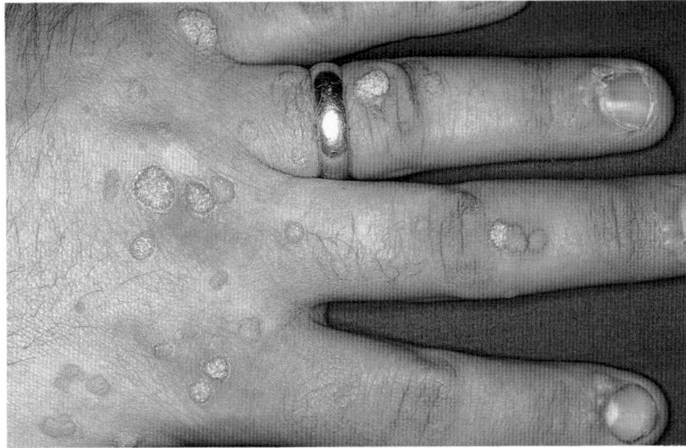

Fig. 19.3a Viral wart (verruca vulgaris). Usually multiple, raised, hyperkeratotic, and commonly found on the hands and feet.

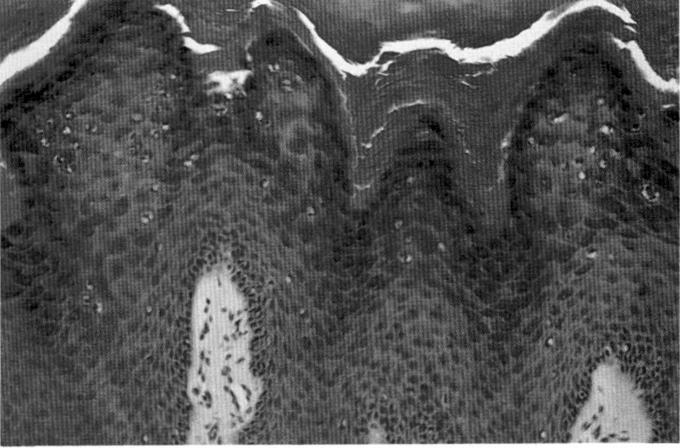

Fig. 19.3b Viral wart – histology. Note papillomatous structure with surface hyperkeratosis, acanthosis, and cytoplasmic vacuolation in scattered cells in the upper Malpighian and granular layers, indicating viral aetiology.

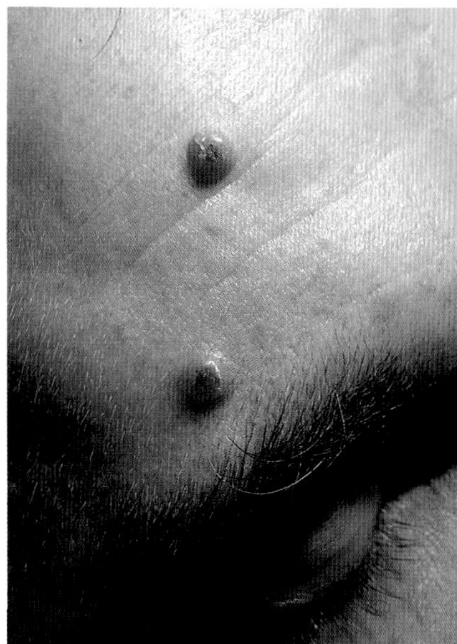

Fig. 19.4a Molluscum contagiosum. Multiple, umbilicated lesions commonly found in children under five. Solitary, large lesions seen in adults, similar in appearance to warts.

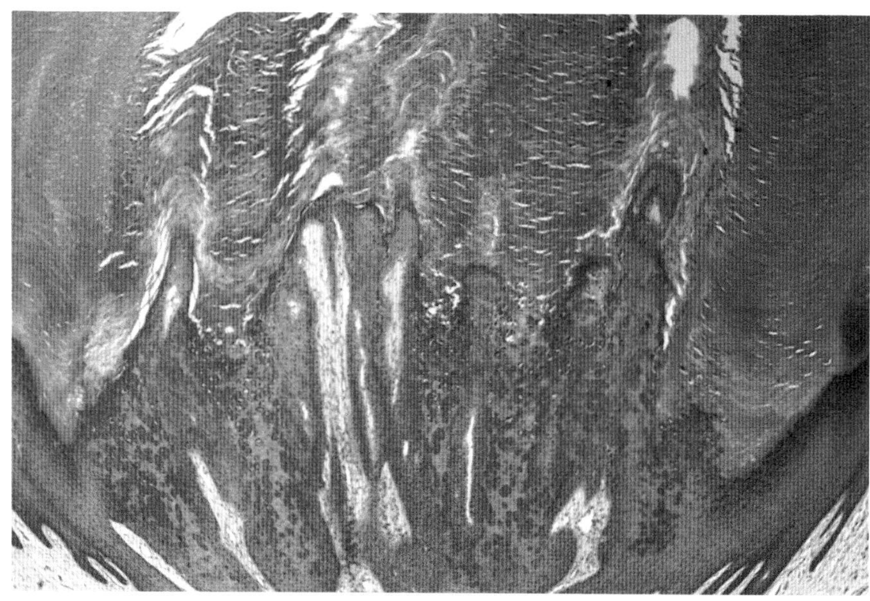

Fig. 19.4b Molluscum contagiosum – histological appearance. Note surface parakeratosis and acanthotic epidermis with numerous molluscum bodies, granular eosinophilic cytoplasmic masses in the cells of the Malpighian, granular, and horny layers.

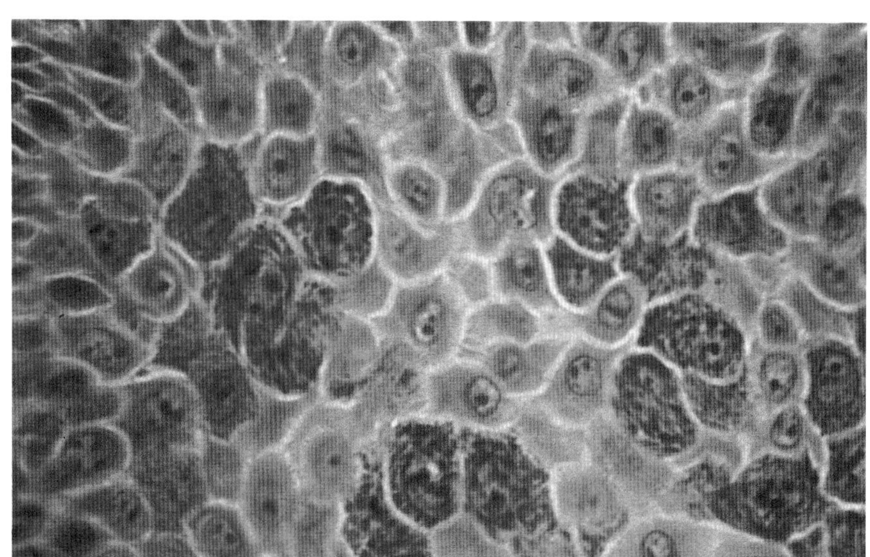

Fig. 19.4c Molluscum contagiosum – higher magnification of epidermal cells distended by intracytoplasmic, eosinophilic, virus-containing molluscum bodies.

Sebaceous cysts are rarely of 'sebaceous gland' origin. They are usually either pilar (tricholemmal) or epidermoid (implantation) cysts.

19.1.1 Evolution of the naevus (Fig. 19.1d)

Melanoblasts migrate in fetal life from the neural crest to the junction between the dermis and epidermis. An arrest of this migration in the dermis may form a 'blue naevus'.

In childhood, junctional activity is usual and the naevus is termed a **junctional** naevus.

In early adulthood, melanocytes may also migrate into the dermis as well as the dermo-epidermal junction to form nests and columns of cells. This is now a **compound** naevus.

In late adulthood through to old age all the activity is now in the dermis. Schwann cells may appear with the melanocytes and there may be less pigmentation as the naevus matures. This is now an **intradermal** naevus.

19.1.2 Benign melanocytic naevus

The common pigmented mole or naevus, also known as a benign melanocytic naevus, progresses through three evolutionary stages before ultimate involution.

Commonly arising in adolescence, the earliest stage is that of junctional naevus, followed by compound and intradermal naevus stages.

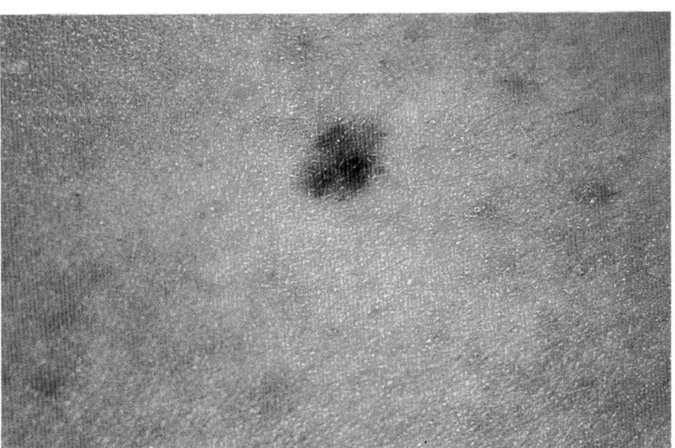

Fig. 19.5a Benign melanocytic naevus. Dark discrete lesion with smooth edges and even colour. Junctional naevus stage.

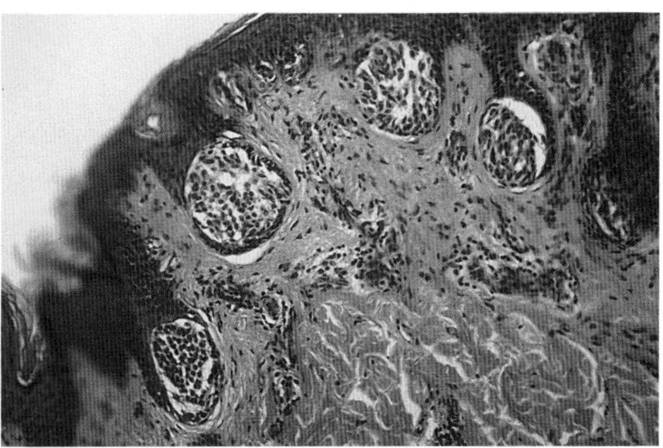

Fig. 19.5b Benign melanocytic naevus (junctional naevus stage). Histological appearance: note nests of proliferating melanocytes in the basal layer of the epidermis at the epidermodermal junction. No dermal involvement.

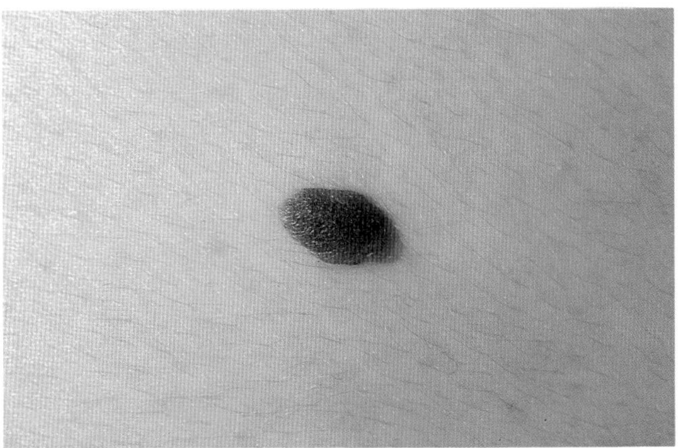

Fig. 19.6a Benign melanocytic naevus (compound naevus stage).

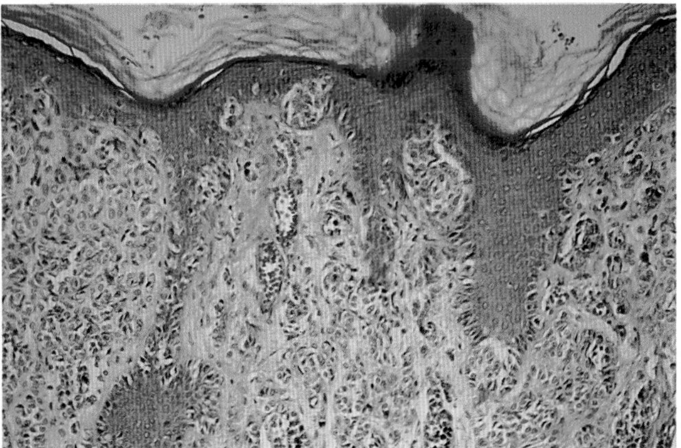

Fig. 19.6b Benign melanocytic naevus (compound naevus stage). Continuing junctional activity with epidermal melanocytic nests associated with dermal migration of cords of naevus cells.

Fig. 19.7a Intradermal naevus. Lightly pigmented, raised skin papilloma.

Fig. 19.7b Benign melanocytic naevus (intradermal naevus stage). Residual cords and nests of naevus cells in the dermis. No residual junctional activity.

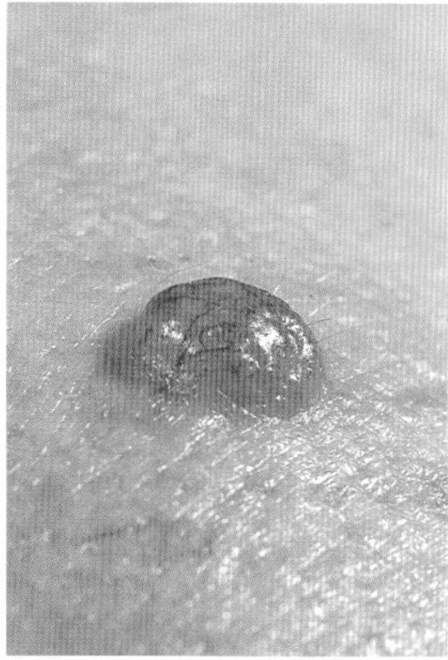

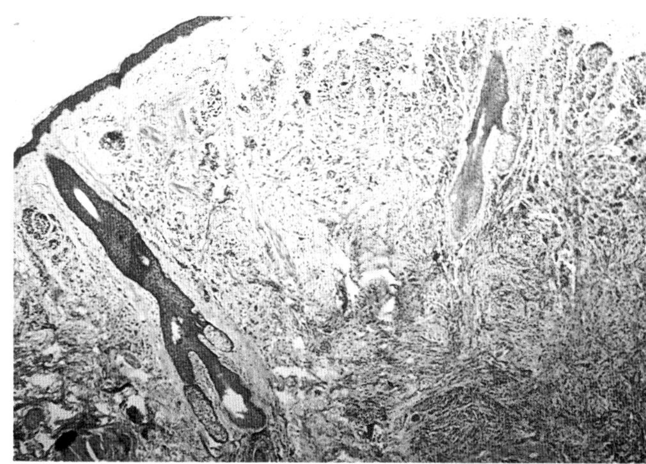

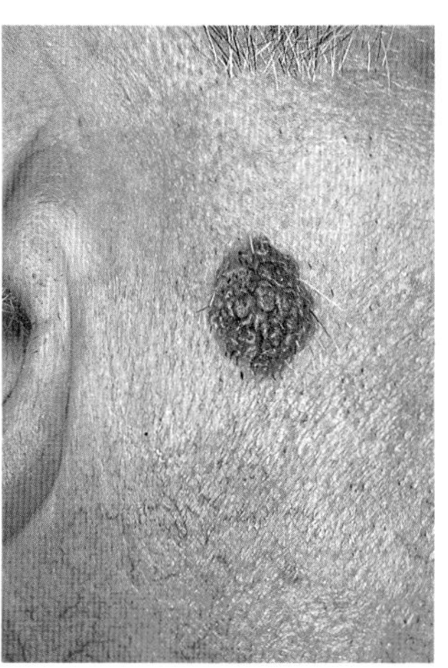

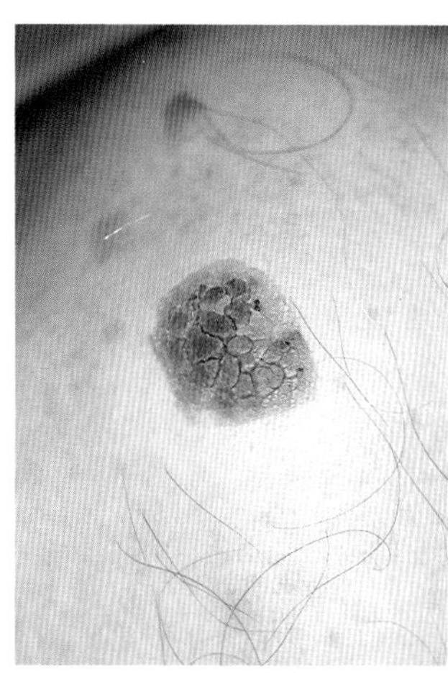

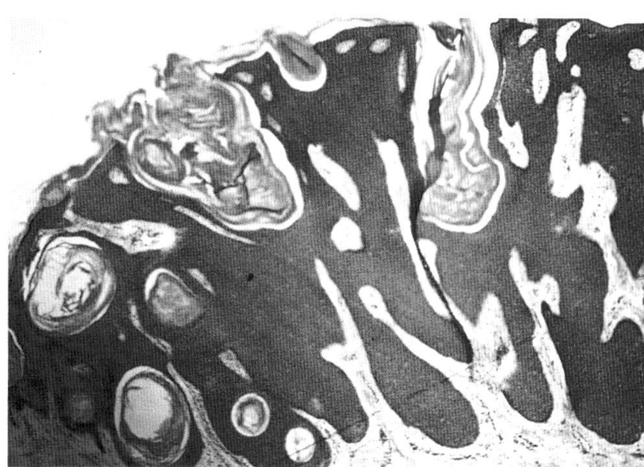

Fig. 19.8a, b Seborrhoeic wart (basal-cell papilloma). Note raised, multiple brown/black lesions with a stuck-on appearance.

Fig. 19.8c Seborrhoeic wart (basal-cell papilloma). Note epidermal thickening featuring basal-cell proliferation, horn cysts, and surface keratosis.

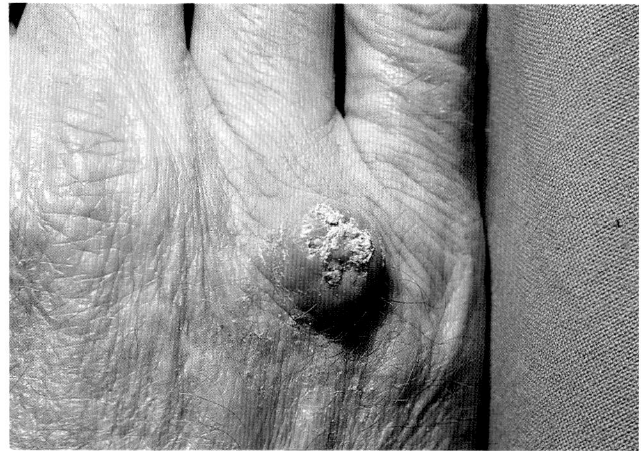

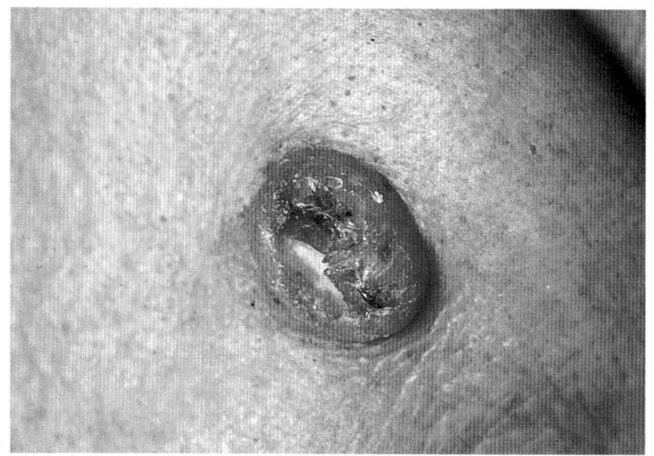

Fig. 19.9a, b Keratoacanthoma. Rapidly growing, spontaneously resolving lesion, with central ulceration and keratin plug.

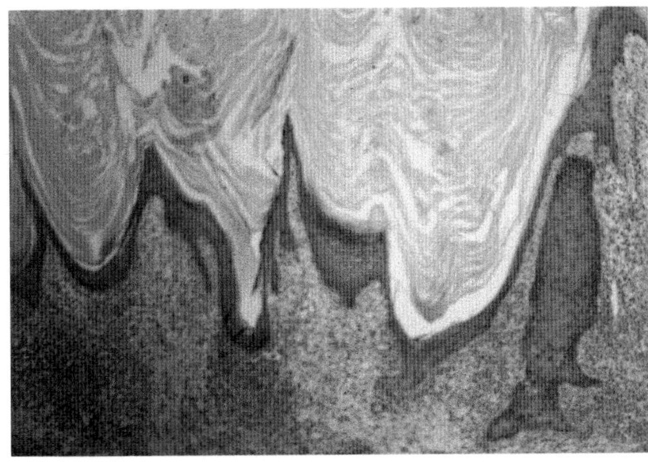

Fig. 19.9c Keratoacanthoma (low-power magnification). Part of keratin cup of keratoacanthoma with underlying squamous cell proliferation.

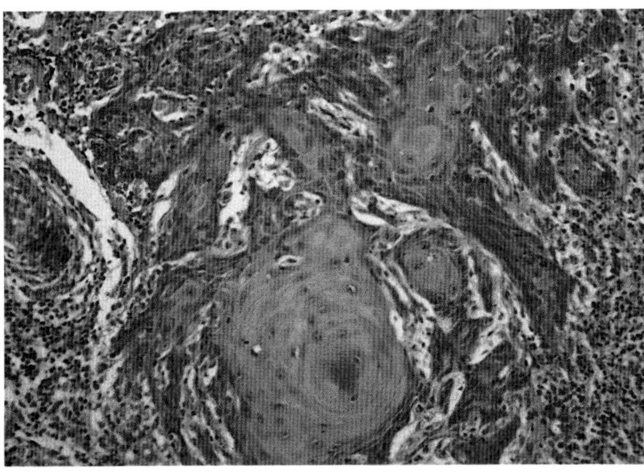

Fig. 19.9d Keratoacanthoma (high-power magnification). Note base of lesion showing irregular squamous cell proliferation. Note also close similarity to squamous cell carcinoma. (Therefore history is important.)

Fig. 19.10a, b Basal cell carcinoma (rodent ulcer). Common, slowly growing, non-metastasizing lesion, locally destructive, and on exposed sites. Note surface capillaries and pearly appearance. Eventual ulceration and rolled-over edges.

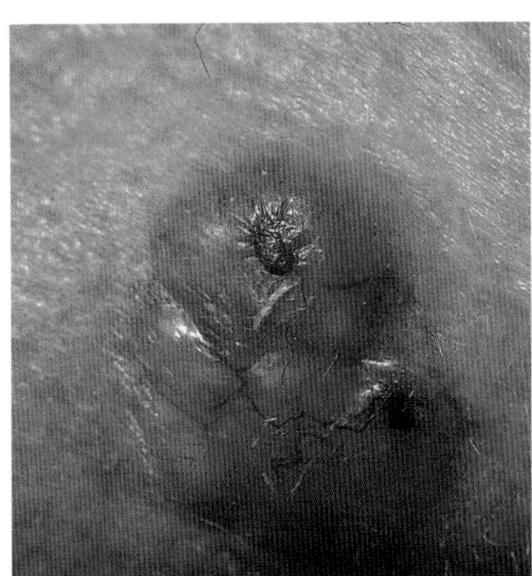

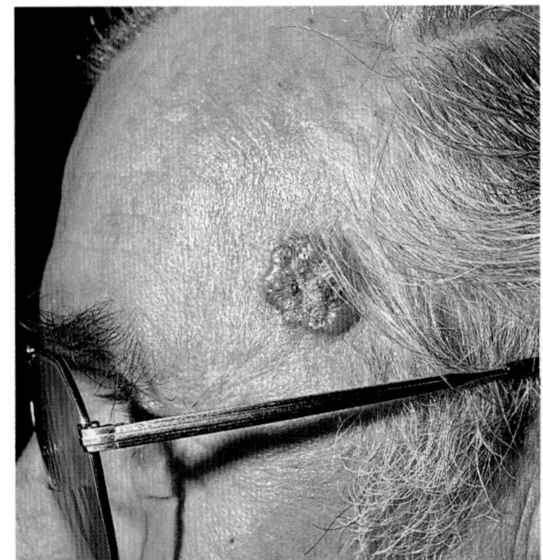

Fig. 19.10c Basal cell carcinoma (rodent ulcer). Histological appearance showing clumps of neoplastic epidermal basal cells infiltrating the dermis. Surface ulceration.

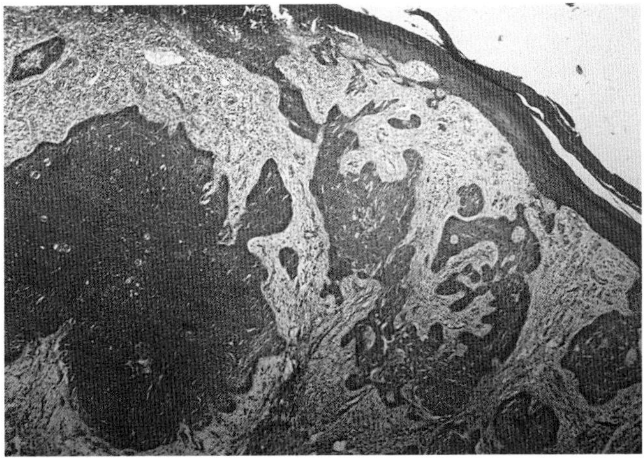

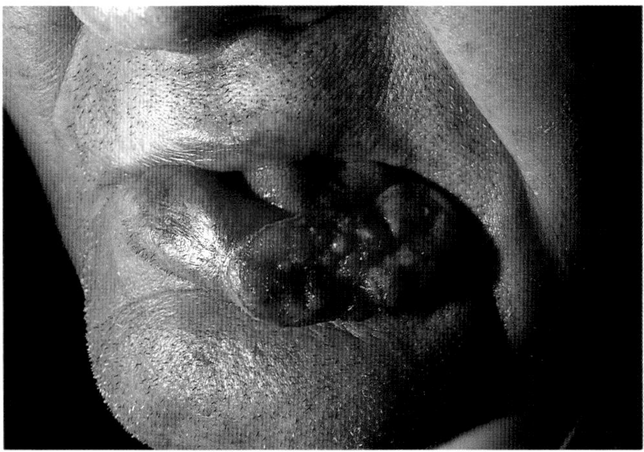

Fig. 19.11a Squamous cell carcinoma of lower lip. Note hyperkeratotic, ulcerated, rapidly growing lesion, which can metastasize.

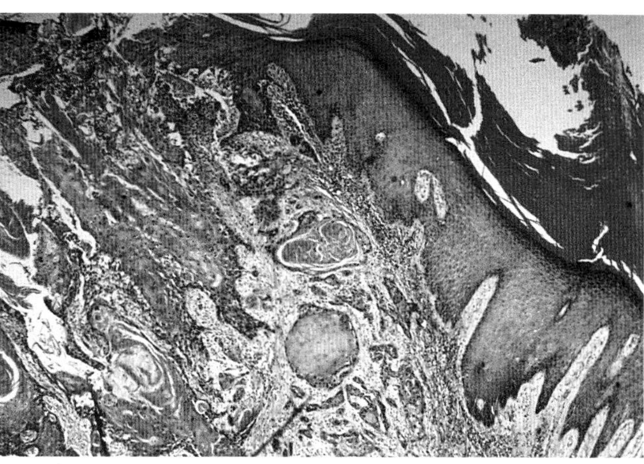

Fig. 19.11b Squamous cell carcinoma. Histological appearance. Note irregular proliferation of neoplastic squamous cells with ulceration and underlying infiltration of the dermis. Horn pearls present.

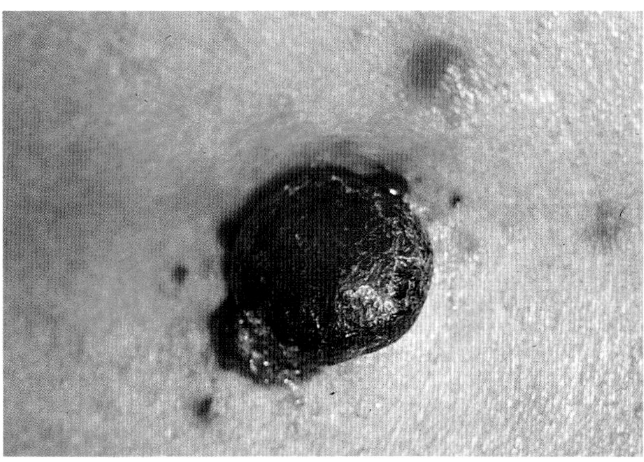

Fig. 19.12a Malignant melanoma. Note irregular margin, and variations in colour brown/black/red. Prognosis depends on thickness and depth of infiltration of lesion. Can metastasize and be very aggressive.

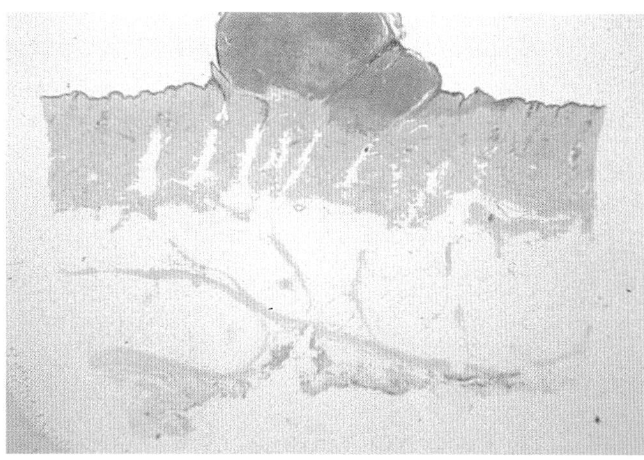

Fig.19.12b Polypoid malignant melanoma showing surface ulceration and infiltration of upper one-third of the dermis. (The Breslow thickness was 4.2 mm.)

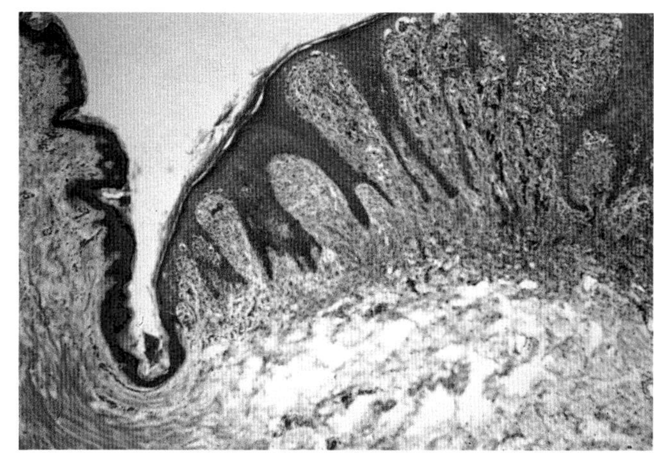

Fig. 19.12c Malignant melanoma. Histological appearance. Irregular groups of variably pigmented malignant cells infiltrating the epidermis and dermis.

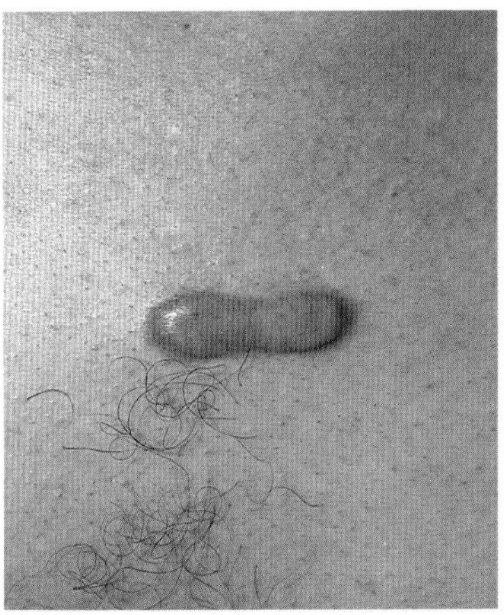

Fig. 19.13a Keloid scar. Note pale, hypertrophied area

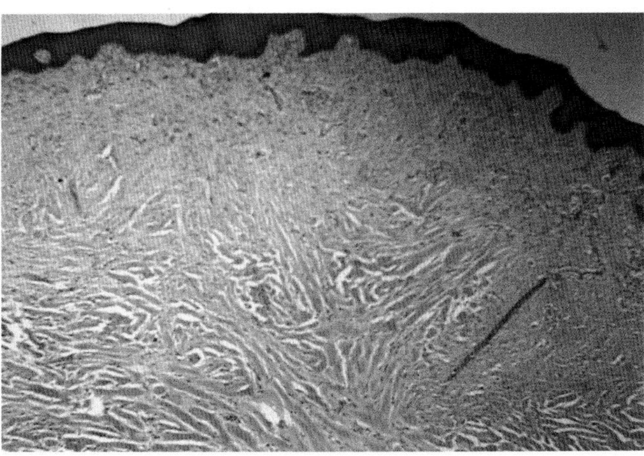

Fig. 19.13b Keloid scar. Note coarsely thickened hyalinized collagen bundles in the dermis.

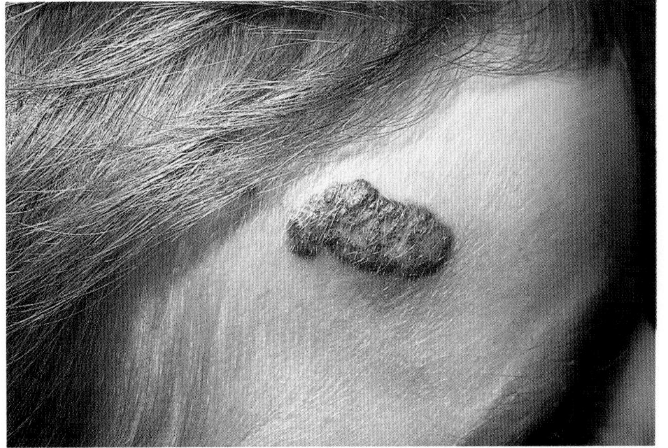

Fig. 19.14a Haemangioma.

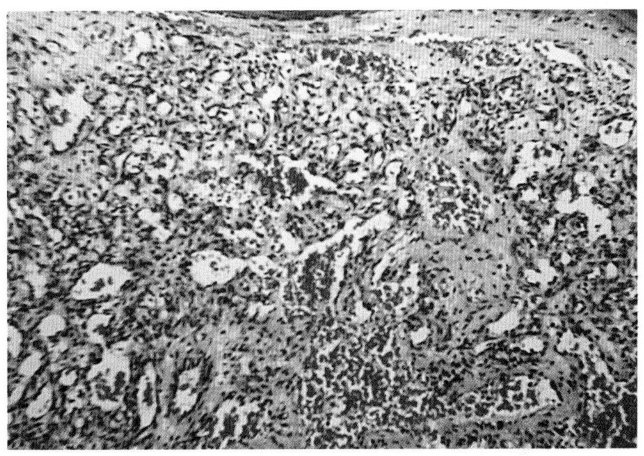

Fig. 19.14b Haemangioma – histological appearance. Note numerous small vascular channels, mainly of capillary structure, in the dermis.

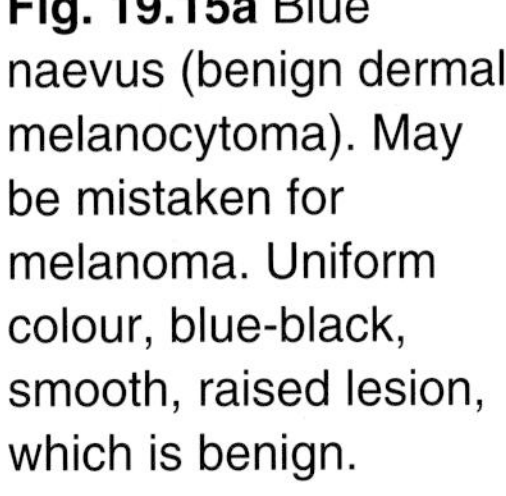

Fig. 19.15a Blue naevus (benign dermal melanocytoma). May be mistaken for melanoma. Uniform colour, blue-black, smooth, raised lesion, which is benign.

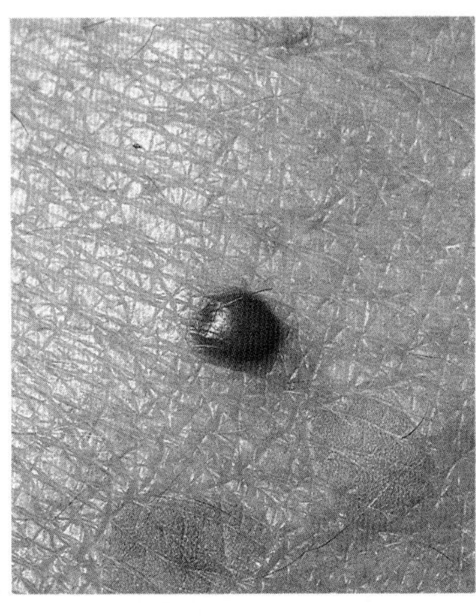

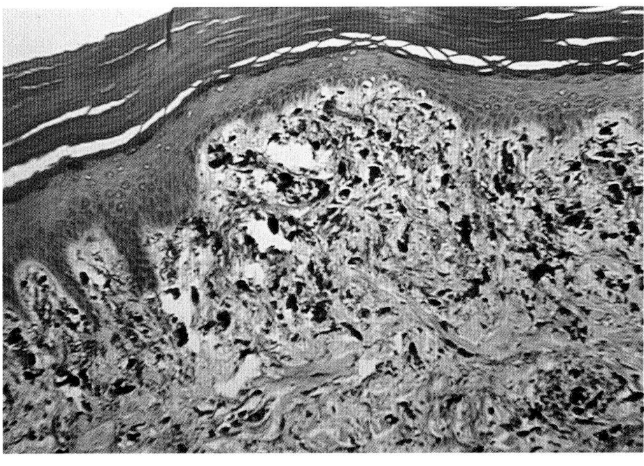

Fig. 19.15b Blue naevus – histological appearance. Note deeply pigmented melanocytes in the dermis. The overlying epidermis is normal.

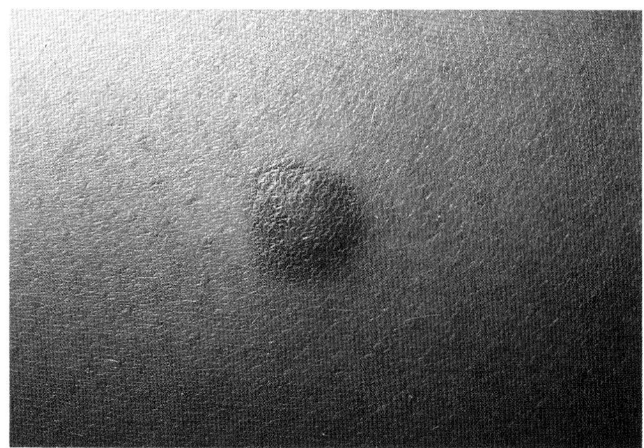

Fig. 19.16a Histiocytoma (dermatofibroma). Firm, pale, fibrous nodule commonly on lower limbs following trauma. Benign.

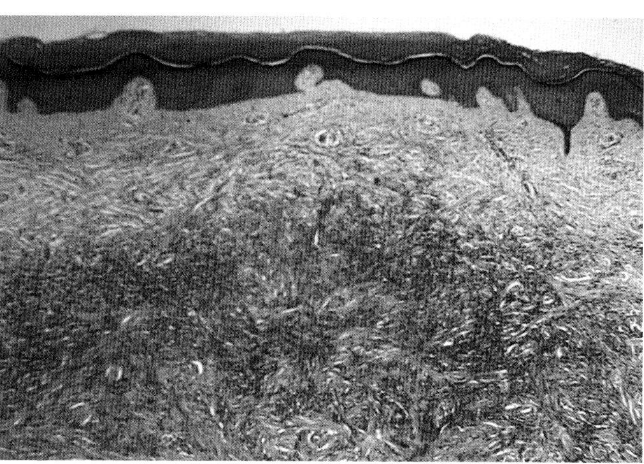

Fig. 19.16b Histiocytoma (dermatofibroma) – histological appearance. Note fibroplastic and histiocytic proliferation in the dermis in variable proportions in different lesions.

Fig. 19.17 A histological specimen being put into formol saline. It is good practice to send every specimen for routine histological examination.

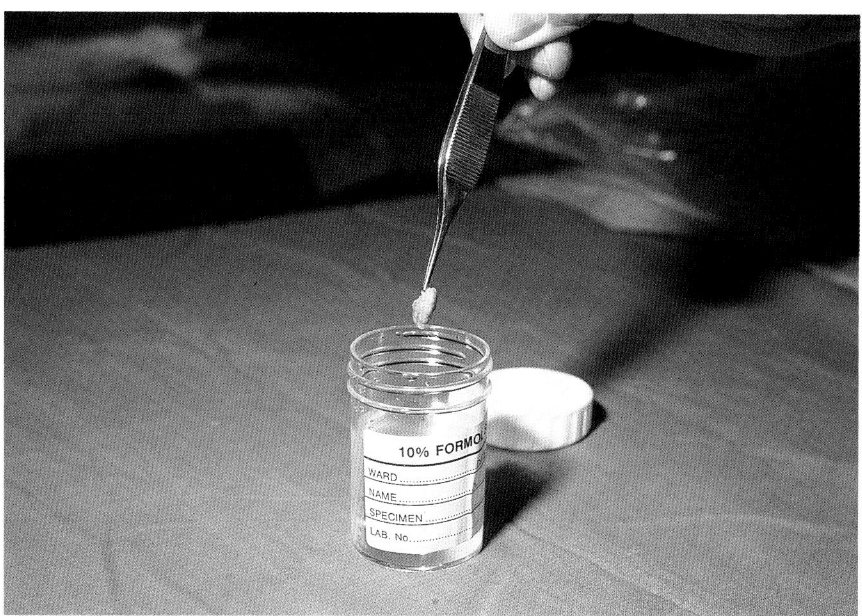

19.2 THE HISTOLOGY BOOK

For medicolegal reasons as well as audit it is important not only to send specimens off for histology (Fig. 19.17), but also to have personally seen every report when they return.

One way of ensuring that no reports are lost is to use a histology book (Fig. 19.18). In this are recorded the date, patient's name and address, and clinical diagnosis; and when received, the final histological diagnosis. Any missing reports are easily spotted, and action taken.

Fig. 19.18 Sample page from histology book. Note that the histology report for Lee Black has not been returned or noted by the doctor, and will need to be followed up.

Fig. 19.18 Sample page from histology book

Date	*Name*	*Address*	*Diagnosis*	*Histology*	*Received*
1.1.96	John Smith Senior	12 South St London	Sebaceous cyst	Sebaceous cyst	√ √
1.1.96	Alice Green (Mrs)	Southcot 23a High St	Intradermal naevus	Intradermal naevus	√ √
8.1.96	Christopher Braston	24 Acorn Rd E. Hosting	?Melanoma ?Naevus	Junctional naevus (benign)	√
8.1.96	Lee Black (12.10.04)	Rose Cott 12 West St	?B.C.C.		
15.1.96	Ann Gray (23.5.21)	245 High Rd Larkhill	Seborrhoeic wart	Seborrhoeic wart	√
15.1.96	Dr. Philip Hoaking	The Mount E. Bradshaw	?Fibroma R. thigh	Histiocytoma	√

20

Statistical analysis

You know, my children, that Surgical Operations are divided into two classes: those that benefit the patient, and those that more often kill ... abstain from undertaking dangerous and difficult treatments'

Albucasis, AD *1013–1106*

By keeping simple records of every operation performed, valuable statistical analysis is possible, which in turn may be of help in planning future requirements for the practice. A register of operations may be compiled using a hard-back book in which is entered the date, patient's name, address, age and sex, together with the type of operation. This list may be numbered chronologically or include a code for additional data retrieval or computer storage. At the end of each year, a breakdown of the year's operations is made, from which can be compiled a summary and analysis (Table 20.1).

20.1 RECORD KEEPING

The importance of keeping accurate comprehensive and legible records of every operation cannot be emphasized enough. Details should be written down immediately the operation is finished, and not committed to memory; such details as which digit, whether left or right, which joint, whether infected or not, size, situation and extent of the lesion, history, signs and symptoms, findings at operation, method of anaesthesia, dose of anaesthetic used, skin preparation, method of excision, whether histology was requested, haemostasis, closure, type and number of sutures used, type of dressings used, estimated date of suture removal and subsequent management – all these should be entered on the patient's notes and signed and dated. At this stage the doctor should personally check that any specimen which is being sent for histology is correctly labelled and corresponds to the histology request form.

20.1.1 Pre-printed information leaflets which may be given to the patients after their operations (see Chapter 50 for full list)

(a) Liquid nitrogen
(b) Ingrowing toe-nails
(c) Injection ganglion
(d) Injection varicose veins
(e) Electrocautery
(f) Meibomian cysts

Table 20.1 Analysis of minor operations performed over 5 years by the author

Category	*Operation*	*Year 1*	*Year 2*	*Year 3*	*Year 4*	*Year 5*
Injections	Tennis elbow	52	56	45	45	54
	Intra-articular	23	38	38	41	41
	Carpal tunnel	22	18	23	42	53
	Piles	26	27	48	22	36
	Hormone implant	37	30	47	51	68
	Others	6	2	9	21	29
Aspirations	Cysts and bursae	24	23	48	33	25
	Hydrocele	5	6	5	8	15
	Abdominal paracentesis	1	4	2	3	3
	Breast cysts	10	18	19	13	27
	Bartholin's cysts	3	3	3	3	2
	Aspirate and sclerose ganglion	14	22	22	16	16
	Others	5	5	2	3	8
Incisions	Abscesses	39	38	32	30	37
	Meibomian cysts	11	16	13	25	19
	Thrombosed external piles	33	29	17	9	20
	Others	2	2	7	9	5
Excisions	Suture lacerations	58	50	41	31	27
	Sebaceous cysts	44	51	68	76	69
	Intradermal naevi	93	67	97	131	165
	Lipoma	6	6	9	13	20
	Basal cell carcinoma	14	6	17	12	10
	Others	15	12	25	15	17
Curette	Warts and verrucae	115	136	90	81	93
	Others	66	48	35	29	17
Toes	Ingrowing toe-nails	45	34	48	57	42
	Removal of toe-nails	9	5	6	12	2
	Others	2	4	2	16	3
Tourniquet	Decompression carpal tunnel	2	3	12	22	21
	Release trigger finger	0	2	2	1	0
	Others	0	2	0	0	0
Diagnostic	Proctoscopy	98	137	192	187	259
	Sigmoidoscopy	85	77	154	137	172
	Needle biopsy	6	7	3	6	20
	Skin biopsy	14	4	8	17	14
	Rectal biopsy	3	3	5	3	2
	Others	1	1	2	8	12
Miscellaneous	Pinch graft to ulcer	3	3	2	2	3
	Varicose veins	11	8	24	42	44
	Cervical erosions	7	4	1	7	8
	Cryocautery	280	216	416	428	604
	Others	5	21	25	14	26
Totals for the year		**1295**	**1244**	**1664**	**1721**	**2108**

20.2 ORGANIZING A MINOR OPERATING LIST

It is much better to set aside a time each week for a minor operating list rather than doing each as it arises. Not only can the patient make preparations, but the surgery staff and nurses can prepare instruments, equipment and forms in advance, clean the room and generally anticipate what will be needed. It is also a more efficient use of everyone's time, the only disadvantage of arranging a list is the risk of cross-infection, particularly if an unsuspected abscess or heavily infected lesion is treated at the beginning of the list before the remaining 'clean' cases. With scrupulous attention to aseptic technique, and the use of CSSD packs, cross-infection should not occur; nevertheless it is good practice to put 'clean' operations such as vasectomy or excision of ganglion, where infection could be disastrous, first on the list, and arrange 'dirty' cases such as infected ingrowing toenails and abscesses at the end.

Having decided to reserve a set time regularly for minor operations, an appointment book should be made (Fig. 20.1), giving time and date, details of the patient's name and address, nature of operation and estimated time allowed. Initially, the doctor should keep this appointment book personally, and personally see every patient. With experience, an accurate estimate of the time each operation takes will be learned and at this stage the appointment book may be taken over by a receptionist or secretary, with clear instructions from the doctor about arrangements for transport and subsequent follow-up. Telephone numbers of patients should be recorded in case it is necessary to change the order of the list and contact the patient at short notice.

A typewritten list of the operations should be prepared with copies for the treatment room, nurses, receptionists, filing clerks, and doctor. By so doing, appropriate patient notes may be prepared, histology forms and containers labelled, and necessary instruments and dressings prepared.

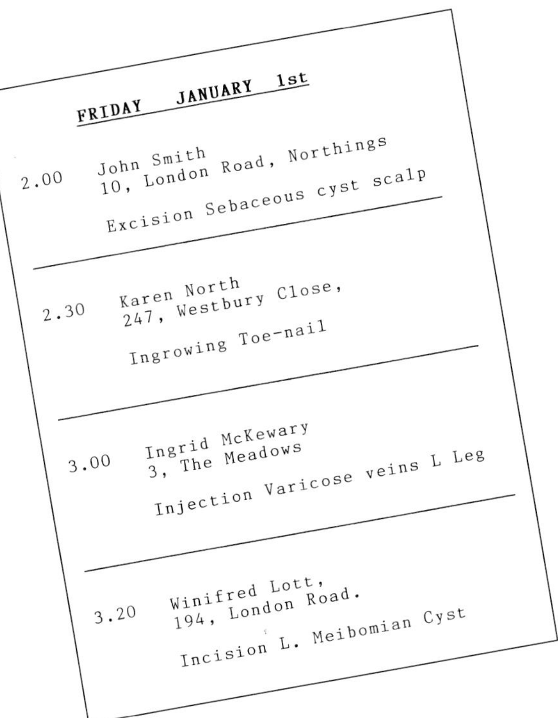
FRIDAY JANUARY 1st

2.00 John Smith
10, London Road, Northings
Excision Sebaceous cyst scalp

2.30 Karen North
247, Westbury Close,
Ingrowing Toe-nail

3.00 Ingrid McKewary
3, The Meadows
Injection Varicose veins L Leg

3.20 Winifred Lott,
194, London Road.
Incision L. Meibomian Cyst

Fig. 20.1 An appointment book can also be used for the 'operating list' each week.

20.3 INFORMING THE PATIENT

The doctor should personally discuss with the patient every detail of the operation: what is involved, the type of anaesthetic, the site and size of any scar, the removal of any sutures, how long the procedure will take, whether transport will be required to take the patient home or whether they will be able to drive or walk home, alone or accompanied. It is important to give an estimate of how long the patient may need to be away from school or work, and any risks of the operations should be carefully explained. It is also important to advise patients whether the operation will be 100% curative (e.g. excision of simple naevus or cyst) or whether recurrence may be expected and what proportion can be expected to recur (e.g. varicose vein sclerotherapy, excision of ganglia, ingrowing toe-nails). It is well known that much of the information given to patients is not remembered; consequently it is helpful to have pre-printed leaflets to give to the patients to take away with simplified details of their operation, appointment times and any necessary arrangements. These leaflets may also act as an *aide mémoire* for the doctor and staff (Fig. 20.2).

Fig. 20.2 Pre-printed information leaflets which may be given to the patients after their operation (see Chapter 50 for full list).

Postoperative instructions following liquid nitrogen treatment

1. Liquid nitrogen destroys tissues by freezing to −196°C. This results in ice forming inside the cells, and as this thaws, it causes cell death.
2. Immediately following treatment, apart from a slight discomfort, it will look as if nothing has happened to the skin.
3. Gradually, over the next few days, swelling, reddening, and sometimes blistering will occur.
4. Following this stage, healing occurs, which is usually remarkably pain-free, and leaves only a very slight scar, or none at all.
5. In dark skins, there is usually an area of depigmentation following cryotherapy; this normally recovers over the next year.
6. Reaction to liquid nitrogen is very variable; in some patients quite alarming looking blistering can occur, together with swelling of the surrounding tissues. Despite this, satisfactory healing still occurs.
7. Keep the treated area dry for 6 days if at all possible; it does not need any dressing unless blistering has occurred, in which case a simple non-stick dressing may be applied.
8. It is important to check with your doctor whether you need to be seen again, as more than one session is occasionally needed to cure some lesions.
9. If you have any queries, please do not hesitate to contact the surgery.

Ingrowing toe nails postoperative instructions

1. A small strip of nail, including the nail has been removed, and the base treated with pure phenol to prevent this narrow strip from regrowing.
2. When you arrive home, please rest on a settee with the feet elevated on a cushion for the remainder of the day; this reduces the discomfort and the tendency to bleeding.
3. A simple analgesic tablet such as paracetamol may be taken for any postoperative discomfort.
4. Please make an appointment to see nurse on

   ______________________ at ______________________

   and a second appointment to see nurse on

   ______________________ at ______________________
5. If you have any queries, please do not hesitate to contact the surgery.

Injection treatment for ganglion

A ganglion is a cyst filled with clear jelly; it is often situated near a joint, and may cause pain, and slowly increase in size. Some eventually rupture spontaneously and disappear, but this may not happen for up to 3 years.

1. Injection treatment consists of drawing off the jelly from the ganglion, and then injecting an irritant fluid into the empty cyst.
2. This causes an inflammation within the ganglion. A pressure bandage is then applied with the object of compressing the inflamed surfaces and thus obliterating the cyst.
3. Please keep the bandage in place for 2 weeks.
4. If it works loose, you may reapply it firmly, but do not disturb the pressure-pad overlying the ganglion.
5. At the end of 2 weeks, you may remove the pad and bandage, and normally no further follow-up visits are required.
6. If, however, you have any queries, please do not hesitate to contact the surgery.

Injection treatment for varicose veins

Injection treatment for varicose veins consists of injecting an irritant fluid into the vein and applying a firm dressing over the injection site. The object of the treatment is to create an inflammation inside the vein, and then by compressing the inflamed surfaces together, hope that they will adhere to each other, thus obliterating the lumen of the vein.

The following simple instructions should be followed:

1. The bandages should be left on (day and night) for 3 weeks. Some discomfort should be expected during the first few days; in a small number of patients it is very painful, in which case you should take any simple analgesic tablets such as paracetamol, aspirin, or codeine at regular intervals until the pain subsides.
2. If the outer layers of bandage work loose or begin to dig into the skin, it is helpful to carefully remove the outer bandage whilst lying down, and to then reapply it firmly from the toes up to the knees, making sure not to disturb the pressure pads overlying the injection sites in the veins.
3. Walk at least three miles every day.
4. If you wish to have a bath, the bandaged leg may be kept dry by putting it inside a large watertight polythene bag (e .g. a bin-liner) with two elastic bands around the top.
5. After 3 weeks, please make an appointment to see the doctor to have the bandages removed.
6. If you have any queries, please do not hesitate to contact the surgery.

Postoperative instructions – Electrocautery

1. Many warts, moles, naevi, and keratoses can be removed by planing off with a sharp blade or curette.
2. Following removal, the base of the lesion is treated with either the electro cautery or diathermy.
3. This seals any bleeding vessels and leaves a dried crust on the surface.
4. Healing will occur over the next 2–4 weeks on average.
5. It is helpful to keep the area completely dry for at least 2 days, and preferably longer.
6. If you have any queries, please do not hesitate to contact the surgery.

Meibomian cysts – Postoperative instructions

1. A Meibomian cyst occurs in the eyelid and is caused by a blockage of the little lubricating duct inside the eyelid.
2. Treatment consists of incising the cyst under a local anaesthetic.
3. This is done from inside the eyelid, so you will not have a visible scar.
4. After the operation, eye ointment is applied, and a pad and bandage put on; this is to protect the eye against dust, etc. on the way home, as the eye is still anaesthetized.
5. The pad and bandage may be removed after 4 hours.
6. Do not be alarmed when you remove the pad – there will be a mixture of ointment, secretions and blood, which can look alarming!
7. Gently clean the eyelids with warm water.
8. Thereafter, apply the eye-drops three times a day for 1 week.
9. It is not normally necessary to see you again, but if you have any queries, please do not hesitate to contact the surgery.

20.4 COMPLICATIONS

With careful selection, good operating technique and the provision of sterile instruments and dressings, complications from minor surgical procedures are rare. The commonest complication is sepsis – this may be unavoidable if the lesion is already infected (e.g. ingrowing toe-nails, infected sebaceous cysts and abscesses) or may occur as a result of cross-infection during the operation or postoperative period.

Tissues should be handled as little as possible, a no-touch technique developed by doctor and assistant, breathing and coughing over the wound avoided, sterile drapes utilized to keep the operating field as free from contamination as possible, and careful application of skin antiseptics should be made, making sure not to miss any areas. The widespread use of powerful antibiotics as a 'cover' is unnecessary and should be condemned as bad practice; however, the judicious use of antibiotics in a few carefully selected patients is justified and may result in healing by first intention. These may be given orally, by injection, or directly into the lesion (e.g. Fucidin inserted in abscess cavities prior to closure).

20.4.1 Haemorrhage

This is rarely a problem; most is venous and can be controlled by firm pressure and the use of diathermy or electrocautery. Small arteries can be clipped with curved mosquito artery forceps and tied if necessary, but most can be controlled by skin sutures alone.

20.4.2 Damage to nerves, tendons and arteries

Again, all these complications are extremely rare; knowledge of the underlying anatomy is essential, the awareness of variations from normal and the use of bloodless operating fields for such operations as carpal tunnel decompression are mandatory. Should damage occur to any nerve, tendon or artery, this fact should be carefully recorded, accurate measurements taken, and a decision taken whether to attempt repair or refer to a specialist colleague. Provided the blood supply to the affected part is adequate, closure and referral at a later date is recommended unless immediate help is available. It is wise that the patient be informed and any action to be taken discussed with him or her (Chapter 51).

20.5 'BRAVERY CERTIFICATES'

Some procedures inevitably will be uncomfortable or even painful despite all measures at pain relief.

Where children are involved, a 'Bravery Certificate' (Fig. 20.3) signed by the doctor and staff and given to young patients at the end of the procedure helps to take their mind off the discomfort, restores trust, and often makes a return visit less traumatic to parents, child, and doctor!

Thornhills Medical Group
To certify that
aged:
was very brave at the surgery
signed :
date :

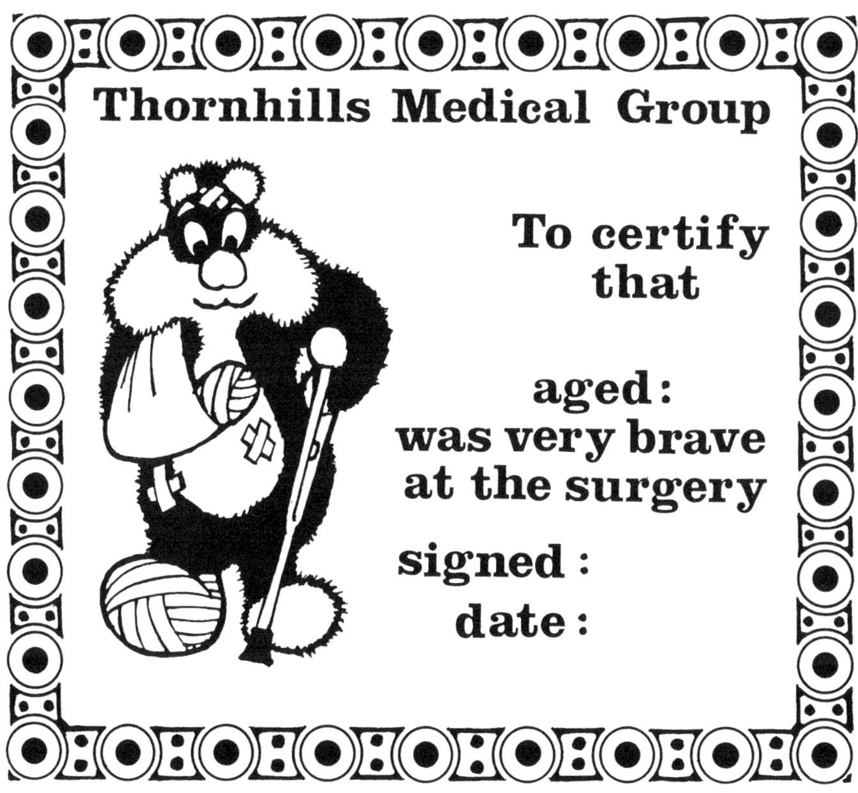

Fig. 20.3 'Bravery certificates', which are popular with young patients.

21

Audit

Minor surgery lends itself admirably to audit, i.e. the monitoring and appraisal of care against predetermined standards, with the aim of improving overall standards of care. It is a valuable exercise for the surgeon; without regular assessment even the best doctor has only an anecdotal impression of what his results are as far as his patients are concerned.

We should be saying to ourselves: 'Is what I think I am doing what really gets done, and if not, why not?'

It is very simple to count the numbers and types of minor operations done each year and to analyse these in groups: what also needs to be examined is:

Am I getting it right?
Are my diagnoses accurate?
What is my success rate?
What is my failure rate?
What is my infection rate?
How many patients do I then refer to specialist colleagues?
Is what I am doing, cost-effective?
What are my scars like?
Am I offering a good service; is it better than the local hospital service?
Are my patients satisfied with the service?
What are the waiting times?
Am I satisfied with methods of pain relief?
Are all histology reports seen, noted, and acted upon?
Am I becoming a specialist in complications?
Is there always a trail of blood to the waiting room from my treatment room?
Should I give up minor surgery?

It is helpful to consider a series of criteria to be satisfied before any audit process is undertaken [22, 23]:

1. There should be potential benefits in terms of better care.
2. It should be ethically acceptable to both patient and doctor.
3. There should be a willingness to make changes in the light of the results of an audit.
4. Standards should be set and aims agreed by the participants.
5. There should be an appropriate sample size and selection.
6. Data collection must be accurate and honest.
7. The results must be confidential to the participants unless agreed otherwise.

Audit of minor operations in general practice may conveniently be divided into the following groups:

1. Method: What was actually done?
2. Results: Was the histological report the same as the clinical diagnosis?
3. Follow-up: Infection, Histology, etc.
4. Cost: Compare results with other centres
5. Outcome: Patient satisfaction
6. Implement changes
7. Then reaudit to analyse improvements.

For those doctors considering introducing some form of audit for their minor operations, a start can be made by counting and analysing the types of operation done over one year.

Secondly, introduce a Histology book (Chapter 14) to compare clinical diagnosis with histological diagnosis.

Thirdly, introduce a patient questionnaire to evaluate patient satisfaction.

Fourthly, keep an 'infection and outcome' book, recording both satisfactory and unsatisfactory outcomes.

By such means it is possible not only to monitor what one is doing, but also to identify areas where there are problems, and ultimately improve the service to patients, as well as increasing job satisfaction and enjoyment.

Part Two :

Routine minor surgery

22

Injections and aspirations

In the cure of ascitic hydropsy proceed thus: after having placed the patient on his back, draw the skin upward. Then take a knife and pierce as far as siphac (peritoneum). Have to hand a cannula and place it in the puncture and draw away as much of the watery matter as the patient may endure. But bear ever in mind that it were better to take too little than empty wholly for the loss of strength that cometh thereby.

Mundinus, Abdominal Paracentesis, AD *1275–1326*

With the availability of steroid and local anaesthetic injections the doctor now has a very effective treatment for many musculoskeletal and articular problems. Even when the exact diagnosis is in doubt, e.g. 'fibrositis' or 'lumbago', a carefully placed injection of steroid with local anaesthetic may dramatically relieve all the patient's pain. Similarly, an acutely inflamed joint in rheumatoid arthritis will respond very well to aspiration and injection of steroid.

22.1 CHOICE OF STEROID

There are many different steroid preparations available and nearly as many differing views on which is the most suitable. There is probably little to choose between the different preparations, but as a general guide, if a weaker preparation will give as good results as a stronger steroid, the weaker one should be used.

Similarly, if an exact point of tenderness can be identified it may be preferable to inject a small quantity of potent steroid into the lesion, but if a more diffuse area is involved it may be helpful to inject a larger volume of a more dilute preparation. Thus most soft-tissue lesions will respond adequately to hydrocortisone mixed with a larger volume of lignocaine, whereas most intra-articular injections seem to respond better to the smaller-volume potent steroids. Three preparations are commonly used:

1. Hydrocortisone acetate (Hydrocortistab) 25 mg/ml
2. Methylprednisolone acetate (Depo-Medrone) 40 mg/ml
3. Triamcinolone hexacetonide (Lederspan) 20 mg/ml.

Hydrocortisone and triamcinolone may be mixed with lignocaine, but methylprednisolone tends to flocculate in the syringe. It is, however, manufactured premixed as Depo-Medrone plus Lidocaine. Triamcinolone is relatively insoluble (0.0003% at 25°C) and consequently stays in the tissues for several weeks or months.

22.2 LANDMARKS

A good knowledge of surface anatomy is essential for accurate position of soft-tissue steroid injections, particularly to avoid damage to underlying structures such as nerves and tendons.

Where possible, as accurate a diagnosis as possible is desirable, and will improve overall results.

22.3 INDICATIONS FOR USE

Steroid injections are useful in the treatment of the following conditions:

1. Rheumatoid arthritis
2. Osteoarthritis
3. Traumatic arthritis
4. Gouty arthritis
5. Synovitis and bursitis
6. 'Fibrositis'
7. Tendinitis
8. Epicondylitis
9. Intermittent hydrarthrosis

22.4 CONTRAINDICATIONS IN THE USE OF STEROIDS

Because of the relative insolubility and the limitation of systemic activity, there are not many absolute contraindications, but the following situations should be considered carefully:

1. Active or recently healed tuberculosis
2. Ocular herpes simplex
3. In the presence of infection
4. Acute psychoses
5. Where there is a history of known hypersensitivity
6. Where previous injections have produced atrophy
7. Immunization procedures are better avoided in patients on high-dose steroids, because of the possibility of neurological complications
8. It is advisable not to inject more than three joints at one session
9. Too many repeated injections in one joint are inadvisable.

Following steroid injections it is advisable to ask the patient to rest the affected limb for 24–48 hours where possible.

22.5 TENNIS ELBOW (LATERAL EPICONDYLITIS)

This is one of the easier lesions to inject, but the results are often disappointing inasmuch that many recur after an apparently successful injection.

It is also worth noting that the natural history of lateral epicondylitis or tennis elbow is almost complete resolution in 2 or 3 years even without any treatment; therefore the doctor is dealing with a self-limiting condition and the effect of any injection is, hopefully, to accelerate healing. In the first instance it is important to establish a correct diagnosis, as cervical nerve root entrapment can cause similar pain, particularly C6 lesions referred to the lateral epicondyle. The patient usually complains of pain in the elbow, worse on attempting to pick up wide objects, and can usually localize the point of maximum tenderness. Gripping causes pain, but flexion and extension of the elbow is usually painless. On examination, there is marked tenderness on palpating the extensor insertion into the external (lateral) epicondyle, and pain on resisted dorsiflexion of the wrist. As would be expected the right elbow is affected much more than the left.

22.5.1 Technique

With the patient sitting comfortably facing the doctor and the elbow flexed to a right angle, the point of maximum tenderness is identified (Fig. 22.1).

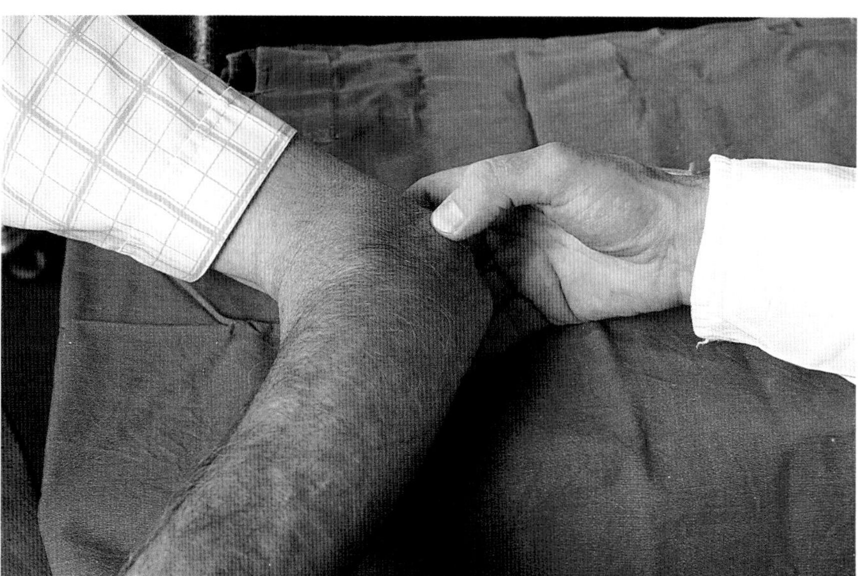

Fig. 22.1 Injection for tennis elbow (lateral epicondylitis), palpating the most tender spot.

The overlying skin is painted with povidone-iodine in alcohol (Betadine alcoholic solution) or similar antiseptic. A mixture of steroid and local anaesthetic is now drawn into a sterile 2 ml syringe using a no-touch technique. Three preparations are commonly used:

1. Methylprednisolone and lignocaine, marketed as Depo-Medrone 40 mg with Lidocaine 10 mg premixed in a 1 ml or 2 ml single-use vial. It should not be mixed with any other injection.
2. Triamcinolone hexacetonide, marketed as Lederspan 20 mg in 1 ml single-use vials. This may be mixed with saline or lignocaine as required.
3. Hydrocortisone acetate, marketed as Hydrocortistab 25 mg/ml in all-glass single-use ampoules; this too may be mixed with saline or lignocaine as required.

Having drawn the solution into the syringe, the needle is carefully removed and replaced with a new sterile 25 swg × 5/8 in. (0.5 mm × 10 mm) needle, fixing it very firmly; this reduces still further any risks of cross-infection. The patient and doctor should not talk or cough over the exposed needle, and for the same reason it is a good idea to routinely wear a mask.

Without touching the site of the injection or touching the needle, the point of maximum tenderness is located, and the injection made directly into it. Considerable pressure is needed, hence the reason for fixing the needle firmly to the syringe; the object is to distribute the injection around the bone interface where most of the pain nerve endings are found. The remainder of the injection is placed in the tissues adjacent to the epicondyle (Fig. 22.2).

Having given the injection, the patient is asked to 'work it in' during the next few hours by repeatedly extending the elbow joint pronating the wrist

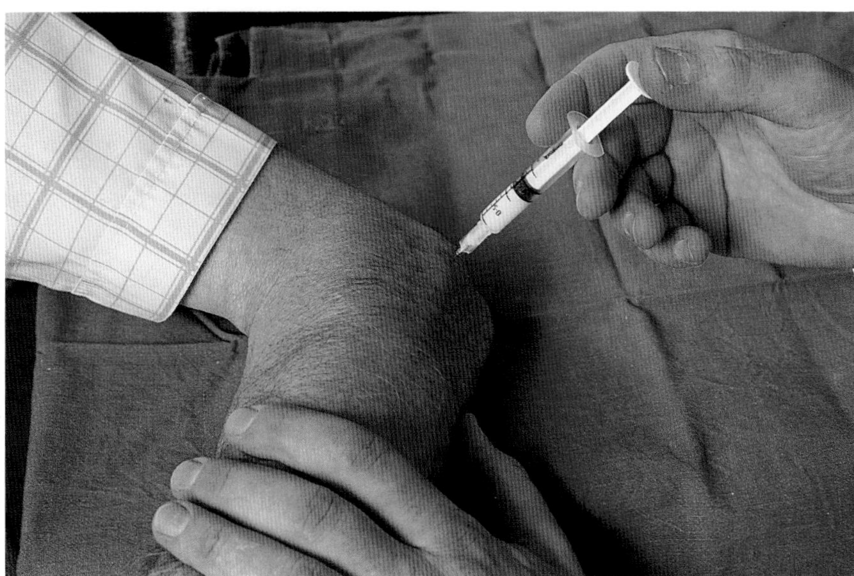

Fig. 22.2 Injection of steroid and local anaesthetic being given into the most tender spot for tennis elbow.

and at the same time palmar flexing the joint. It is also worth warning the patient that the injection site may be extremely painful during the first 24 hours, and thereafter relief may be expected. With meticulous technique there should be no danger of infection, but one of the commonest side effects to be seen is atrophy of tissues beneath the injection site, resulting in a small depression in the skin; this is seen in other situations where subcutaneous steroid injections are given, and is not confined to tennis elbow.

Aftercare is equally important, it is not a good idea to strenuously exercise the hand and fingers – 'to see if it has worked' – on the contrary, the lesion must be rested for several days to allow sound healing.

Despite this, recurrences are common, and the question of a second injection arises. This is unlikely to be as successful as the first, and most doctors therefore limit the number of injections to 2 or 3, preferring to let the condition cure itself spontaneously thereafter.

22.5.2 Alternative treatments

Relief may also be obtained from analgesics, physiotherapy in the form of friction and ultrasonics, and the application of a firm, non-stretch bandage or splint around the body of the forearm muscles just distal to the painful insertion.

22.6 GOLFER'S ELBOW (MEDIAL EPICONDYLITIS)

This has the same signs and symptoms as a tennis elbow except that the tenderness is over the medial epicondyle and is reproduced by resisted palmar flexion of the wrist. Treatment is exactly the same as that for tennis elbow, but the volume of injection may be slightly less. The most tender spot is located by extending the elbow and externally rotating the wrist; the overlying area painted with povidone-iodine in spirit (Betadine alcoholic solution) and the injection made from the anterior surface. It must be remembered that the ulnar nerve lies in a groove just behind the medial epicondyle and any injection should be accurately placed to avoid damage to this nerve. Likewise, it is important to look for any operation scars around the elbow joint in case the patient has had a transposition of the ulnar nerve from behind the epicondyle to in front, for previous nerve entrapment. Putting the patient's arm behind their back gives better access to the medial epicondyle.

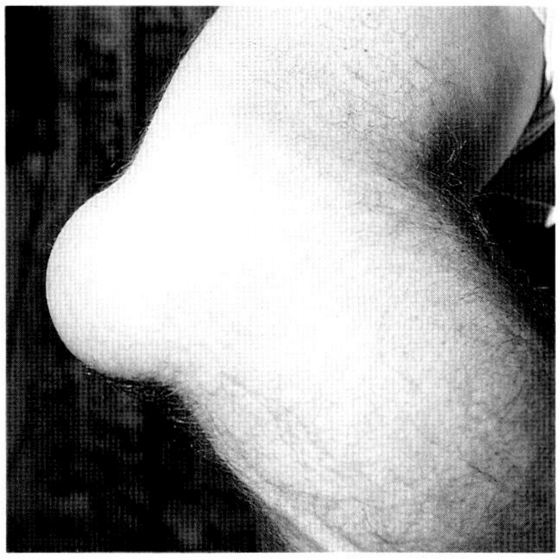

Fig. 22.3 Olecranon bursitis.

22.7 OLECRANON BURSITIS

This is commonly due to repeated trauma: most cases will resolve with firm support, but where the condition is giving discomfort or the bursa is unusually large, aspiration may be attempted, followed by the injection of one of the three steroid preparations, e.g. 1 ml Depo-Medrone, 1 ml Lederspan or 1 ml Hydrocortistab. Infection is not uncommon and extreme care needs to be taken to avoid introducing infection at the time of aspiration (Fig. 22.3).

22.8 INTRA-ARTICULAR INJECTIONS

Any joint in the body may become inflamed or develop an effusion or arthritis, and the majority may be entered with a sterile needle either to withdraw fluid or inject steroids, or both.

Certain points need to be borne in mind:

1. An absolute sterile technique is mandatory as a septic arthritis is a disaster.
2. A knowledge of the anatomy of the joint is essential, together with the best method of approach.
3. It should always be remembered that steroid injections rarely cure the underlying pathology – they merely suppress the active inflammation.
4. Repeated injections in any one joint are inadvisable unless all other measures have failed.

22.8.1 The elbow

Pain can arise at either the true elbow joint or the radio-humeral joint. Injection of the true elbow joint is performed with the elbow flexed and the needle inserted posteriorly, whereas the radio-humeral joint is approached laterally (Fig. 22.4).

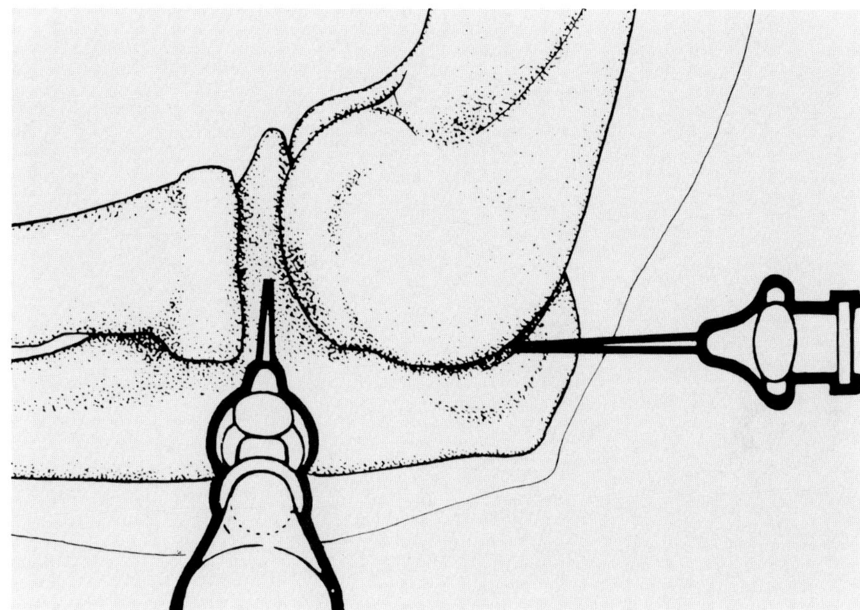

Fig. 22.4 Injection sites at elbow.

22.9 THE PAINFUL SHOULDER

This is a common complaint, and accurate diagnosis of the exact cause is often difficult. Many are due to referred pain from the cervical spine, others from inflamed bursae, tendons, or capsule, and it is in this latter group that steroid injections offer much relief.

The six common lesions are supraspinatus tendinitis, subacromial bursitis, infraspinatus tendinitis, subscapularis tendinitis, 'capsulitis', and arthritis. Fortunately each can be treated by a common approach, namely the posterior aspect of the shoulder.

22.9.1 Technique

With the patient sitting with his or her back to the doctor, the spine of the scapula is palpated and followed laterally until it becomes the acromial process; using the index finger, the coracoid process is located anteriorly; the line joining these two points gives the direction of injection. The overlying skin is painted with povidone-iodine in spirit (Betadine alcoholic solution) and 2 ml methylprednisolone 40 mg with lignocaine 10 mg (Depo-Medrone with Lidocaine) drawn into a 2 ml syringe. The needle is discarded and replaced with a new 21 swg × 1½ in. (0.8 mm × 40 mm) needle. The needle is inserted about 1 in. (2.5 cm) so that it runs below the acromial process towards the coracoid process. There should be no

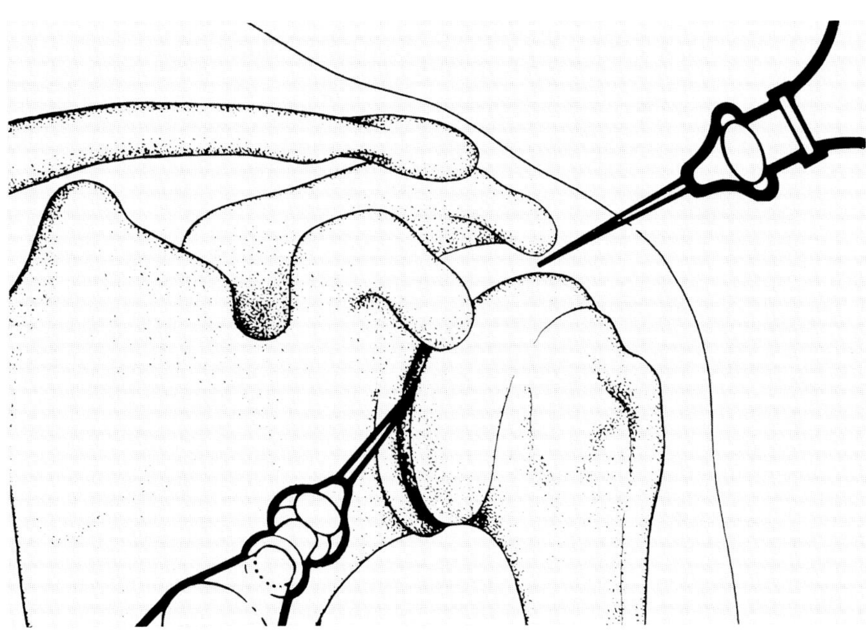

Fig. 22.5 Injection sites for the painful shoulder.

resistance to injection as the needle is in the upper recess of the shoulder joint (Fig. 22.5).

As with tennis and golfer's elbows, the patient should rest the joint for one or two days, then gently exercise; likewise he or she should be warned that the pain may be exacerbated during the first 24 hours before relief is obtained. Injection may often be combined with physiotherapy to achieve maximum benefit.

22.9.2 Acromioclavicular joint

Injury to this joint is common in sportsmen, and subluxation or dislocation can occur, as can degenerative arthritis and even a 'spur'.

The joint is of the plane variety, and it is possible to enter it with care from the front, centrally. Using a fine-gauge needle (25 swg or 23 swg) up to 0.5 ml may be injected.

22.9.3 Glenohumeral joint

This is the true shoulder joint: signs of disease are limitation of external rotation and pain. The joint is best approached by the posterior approach as described (22.9.1), and the ease of injection usually indicates that the needle is in the right place.

22.9.4 Bicipital tendinitis

This is due to an inflammation of the synovial sheath surrounding the tendon of the long head of the biceps in the bicipital groove. It can be successfully treated by injection.

Technique

The tender area is palpated with the patient reclining and the palm externally rotated and facing upwards. The overlying skin is cleaned using povidone-iodine in spirit.

The needle is introduced alongside the tendon in the bicipital groove and the injection made. If there is doubt, inject some local anaesthetic first which should relieve the pain. Care should be taken not to inject into the tendon as this could cause it to rupture.

22.10 INJECTION OF THE CARPAL TUNNEL

Symptoms from compression of the median nerve in the carpal tunnel are very common and consist of numbness or pain over the middle three fingers which is worse at night when the patient typically hangs the arm out of bed or shakes the hand in an attempt to alleviate the discomfort. Pain may also radiate from the wrist proximally to the elbow. Eventually, wasting of the thenar muscles occurs (Fig. 22.6). The injection of steroids into the carpal tunnel often relieves all the symptoms permanently, and even if the symptoms recur following injection, at least the doctor will know that the original diagnosis was correct and that surgical decompression will be successful.

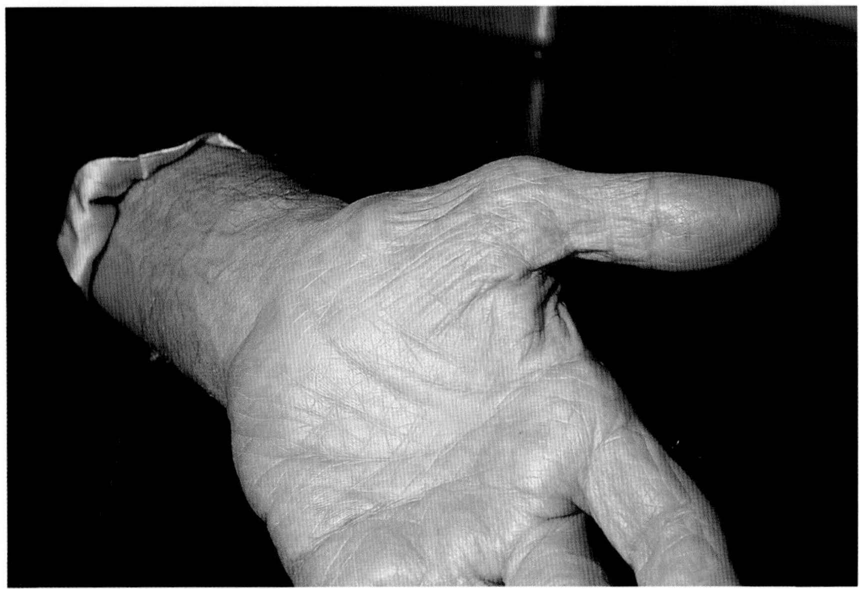

Fig. 22.6 Untreated, compression of the median nerve may result in severe wasting of the thenar muscles.

22.10.1 Establishing the diagnosis

The typical history is paraesthesia affecting the middle three fingers, but occasionally paraesthesia occurs in the whole hand which suggests that the superficial branch of the ulnar is also involved. It is commoner in pregnancy, myxoedema, rheumatoid arthritis, acromegaly, osteoarthritis and obesity.

The following tests may be used:

1. Tinel's test – percussion over the flexor retinaculum reproduces the symptoms.
2. Phelan's sign – forcibly flexing the wrist for up to a minute reproduces the symptoms.
3. Electrophysiological tests – if still in doubt, electromyography can be done which will give an accurate diagnosis.

22.10.2 Technique

The injection site is on the palmar surface of the hand, just lateral to the midline in the line of the skin crease dividing the forearm and hand. The median nerve lies just beneath the tendon of the palmaris longus muscle (Figs 22.7 and 22.8).

With the patient sitting by the side of the doctor, his or her hand is placed palm upwards on a sterile sheet from a sterile dressing pack. The overlying area is liberally painted with povidone-iodine in spirit (Betadine alcoholic solution). Neither patient nor doctor should speak or cough over the injection site.

A 2 ml sterile syringe is used to draw in 1 ml of methylprednisolone acetate (Depo-Medrone), the needle is then discarded and replaced with a

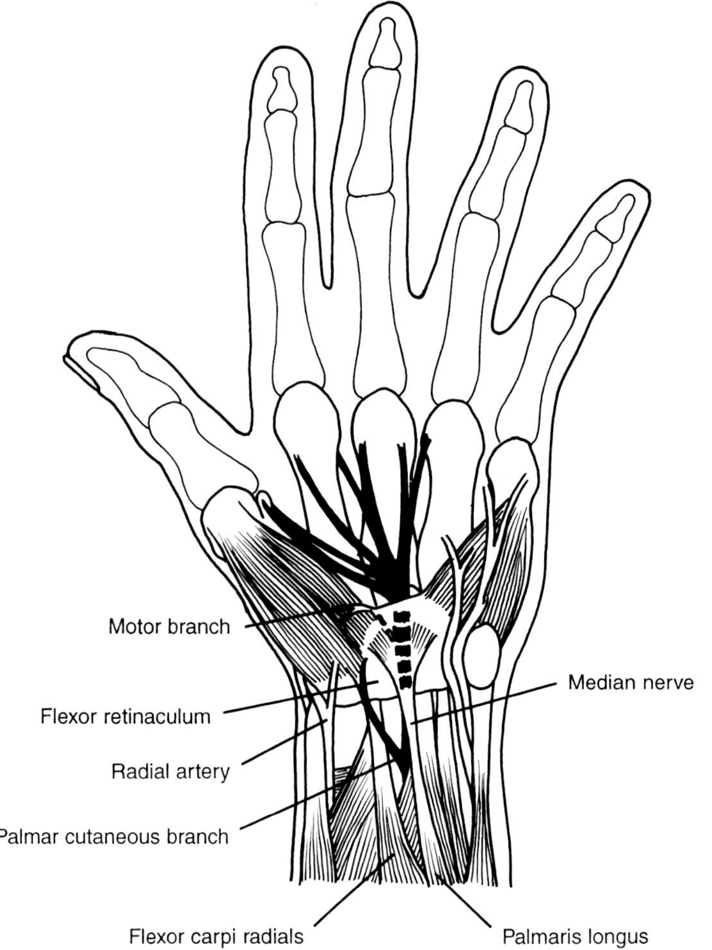

Fig. 22.7 Anatomy of wrist, and median nerve in relation to the carpal tunnel.
(Redrawn from *Gray's Anatomy, 30th edition,* by permission of Churchill Livingstone, Edinburgh.)

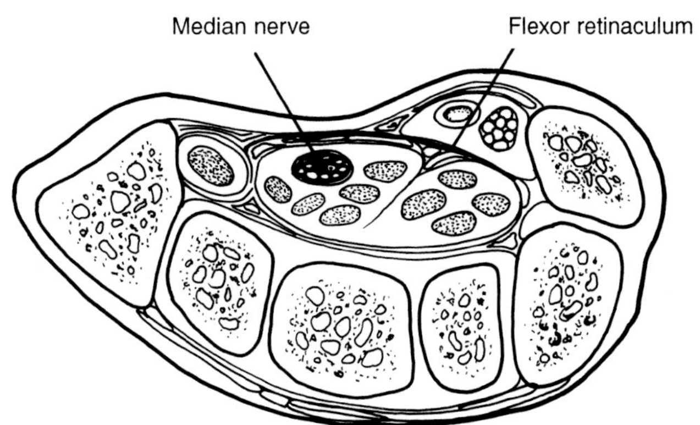

Fig. 22.8 Cross section of the wrist showing the median nerve in the carpel tunnel surrounded by tendons.

new, sterile 25 swg × 5/8 in. (0.5 mm × 16 mm) needle. Lignocaine is not added on this occasion as local anaesthetics injected around the median nerve would produce unacceptable anaesthesia of the fingers and in most cases the injection of steroid alone is not painful.

The patient is told to flex the wrist against the resistance of your hand. This will demonstrate the palmaris longus tendon (present in over 60% of the population). Make a mark with a pencil tip or your thumb-nail just lateral to the tendon at a level of the distal palmar crease. This is the site of the injection. The patient is asked to relax the wrist, and the needle is inserted at an angle of approximately 45° pointing towards the fingers. The needle tip should now be lying behind the flexor retinaculum.

Aspirate to check you are not inside a blood vessel, then slowly inject up to 0.5 ml steroid (Figs 22.9 and 22.10). Normally there is little resistance

Fig. 22.9 Injection of the carpal tunnel showing angle of needle and level in relation to the median nerve. (Kindly provided by Dr. Trevor Silver.)

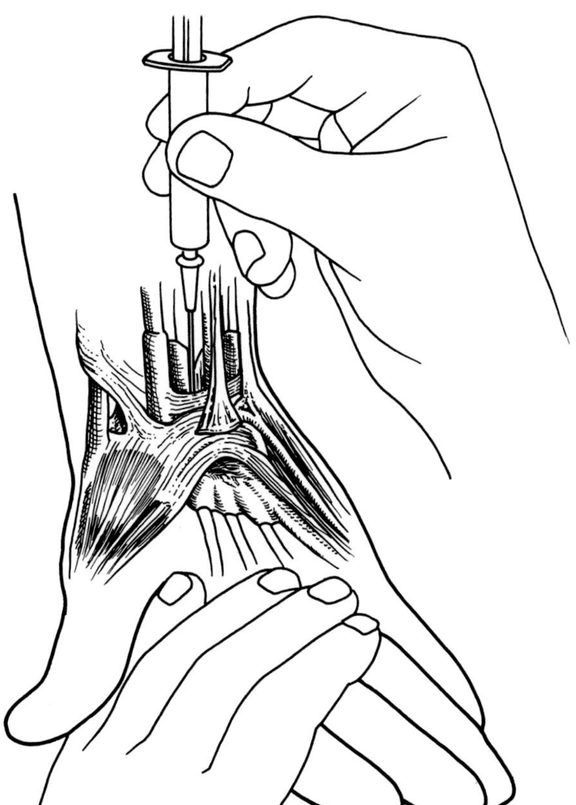

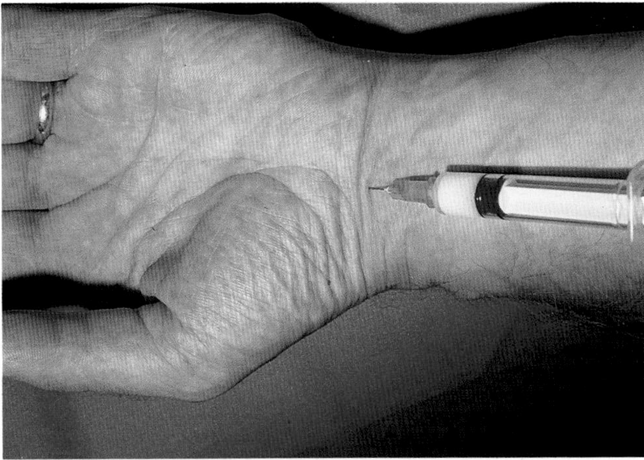

Fig. 22.10 Injection of the carpal tunnel, facing away from the patient; entry point of the needle is in the thinner skin of the wrist.

and only slight discomfort to the patient. Any severe pain or 'electric shocks' in the fingers which might indicate irritation of the median nerve should be reported. Should this occur, the needle is withdrawn slightly and repositioned more laterally, away from the nerve. Warn the patient that the symptoms may be aggravated for 24–48 hours, and to take a mild analgesic such as paracetamol.

22.11 INJECTION OF TRIGGER FINGER

Trigger finger is due to a tenosynovitis of the flexor tendons of the fingers with a nodular expansion of the tendon which catches in the tendon sheath. The patient complains of locking of one finger or thumb in flexion, which then gives a click when forcibly extended. Treatment by injection is often very successful; the injection is made into the tendon sheath and not the tendon itself.

22.11.1 Technique

The fourth finger is commonly affected and is injected as follows: the patient sits facing the doctor with the hand, palm upwards, resting on a sterile sheet on the desk. Povidone-iodine in spirit (Betadine alcoholic solution) is applied, and 1 ml of methylprednisolone acetate (Depo-Medrone) drawn into a 1 or 2 ml syringe. The needle is discarded and a new, sterile, 25 swg × 5/8 in. (0.5 mm × 16 mm) needle attached. The injection is made over the site of the triggering, which is commonly in line with the flexor tendon where it crosses the distal palmar crease (Fig. 22.12). As with carpal tunnel injection, the needle should be inserted at an angle with the bevel pointing downwards, parallel to the underlying tendon, applying

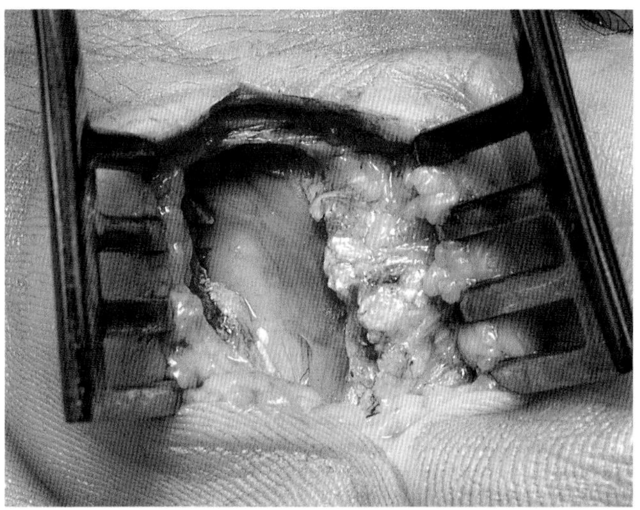

Fig. 22.11 The median nerve is considerably larger than is generally realized. This shows the flexor retinaculum divided at operation.

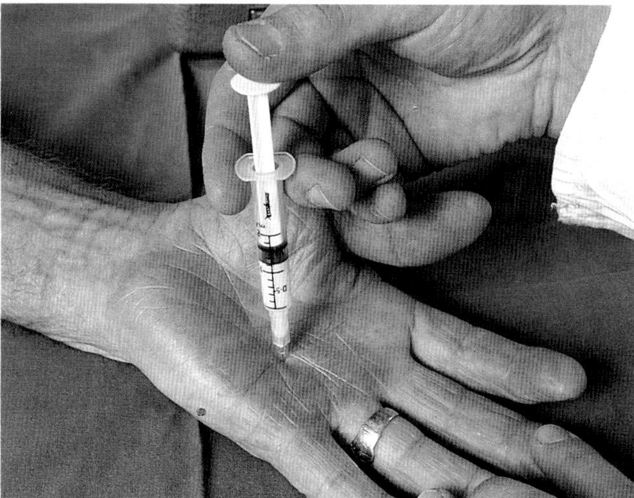

Fig. 22.12 Injection site for trigger finger.

gentle pressure to the syringe plunger as the needle is advanced. By palpating the tendon sheath with the fingers of the opposite hand, the doctor can usually feel when the injection fluid has entered the tendon sheath. An injection of 0.5 ml of solution is made, the needle is withdrawn, and the patient asked to exercise all the fingers for a minute to evenly distribute the steroid. Improvement usually occurs after 48 hours and may be permanent. Where triggering recurs, surgical division of the sheath is recommended.

22.12 INJECTION FOR DEQUERVAIN'S DISEASE (stenosing tenosynovitis of the short extensor and long abductor thumb tendons)

DeQuervain's stenosing tenosynovitis is a common cause of wrist pain. It is often due to over-use of the fingers and thumb, resulting in pain on using the wrist and on gripping, and in a few patients can be very resistant to treatment and cause much discomfort. Often there is visible swelling over the line of the tendons, and palpable crepitus can be elicited in many cases.

22.12.1 Technique of injection

The skin is cleaned using povidone-iodine in spirit. The needle is inserted tangentially alongside the tendon, into the tendon sheath. Injection should offer no resistance, and the fluid may be felt or seen to travel along the tendon sheath.

If doubt exists about the placing of the needle, disconnect the syringe, and ask the patient to move his thumb. If the needle tip is in the tendon itself, movement of the thumb will cause tilting of the needle.

Ten milligrams of hydrocortisone in 2 ml 1% lignocaine is injected; alternatively 4 mg triamcinoline in 2 ml 1% lignocaine, or 1 ml Depo-Medrone plus lidocaine may be used.

It is preferable to offer injection earlier rather than later, as the longer the condition has existed, the less effective is steroid injection. In fact, if it has existed for longer than 6 months, surgical decompression is usually required.

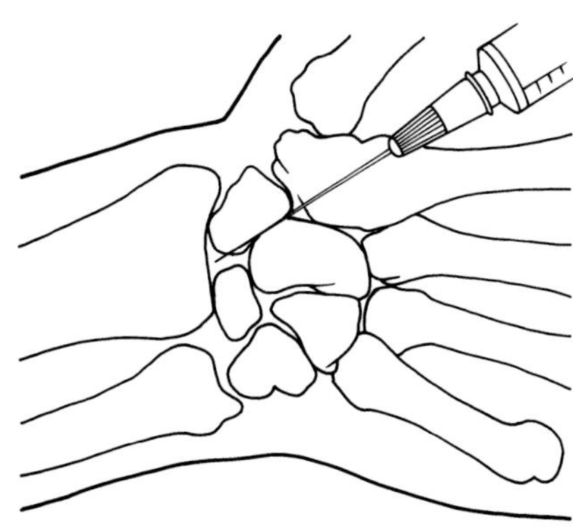

Fig. 22.13 Site of injection for radiocarpal joint.

22.13 RADIOCARPAL JOINT

This joint is commonly involved in early rheumatoid arthritis, and often responds well to a carefully placed steroid injection. The easiest site for injection is over the dorsum of the wrist, in the gap between the end of the radius and the lunate and scaphoid bones (Fig. 22.13). Gentle palmar flexion opens up the joint and assists injection. If the needle is in the correct space, it enters easily and injection may be done easily. With advanced rheumatoid arthritis, normal surface landmarks are lost, and entry into the joint space may be more difficult. After cleaning the skin with povidone-iodine in spirit, 10 mg hydrocortisone acetate in 5 ml of 1% lignocaine may usually be injected. As an alternative 4 mg triamcinolone in 5 ml 1% lignocaine or 1 ml DepoMedrone plus Lidocaine may be used.

22.14 FIRST CARPOMETACARPAL JOINT (thumb base)

This joint is commonly involved in both osteoarthritis and rheumatoid arthritis. It is also unusual that steroid injections in this joint are equally effective whether the diagnosis is osteoarthrosis or rheumatoid arthritis. The reason for this is not clear.

The diagnosis may usually be made by pressing over the joint in the 'anatomical snuff box' and by forced adduction of the thumb into the palm.

22.14.1 Technique of injection

Feel for the joint line with the tip of the index finger, and mark it with a felt-tip pen. By applying countertraction, the joint space is opened up, and the needle inserted into the joint space, having first cleaned the skin with povidone-iodine in spirit (Fig. 22.14).

Only a very small volume can be accommodated, i.e. 0.5 ml or less of Depo-Medrone with Lidocaine.

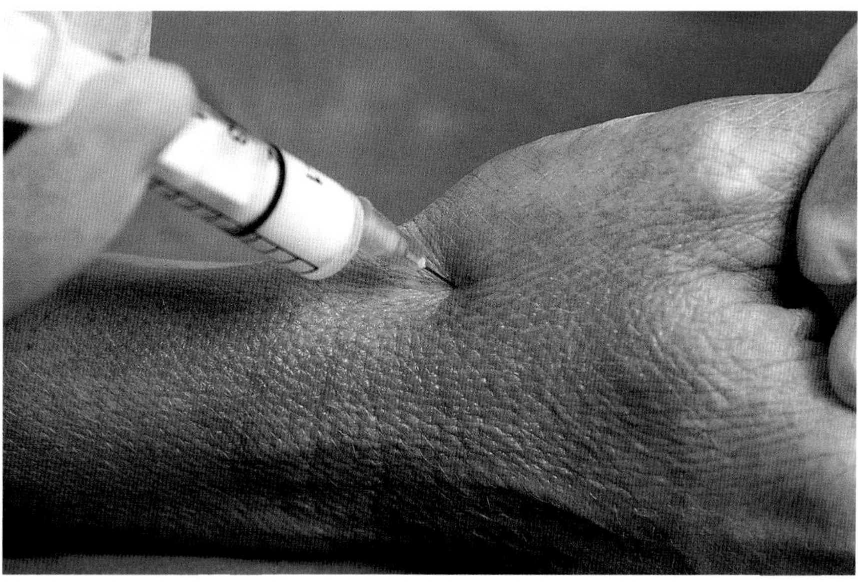

Fig. 22.14 Injecting the first carpometacarpal joint.

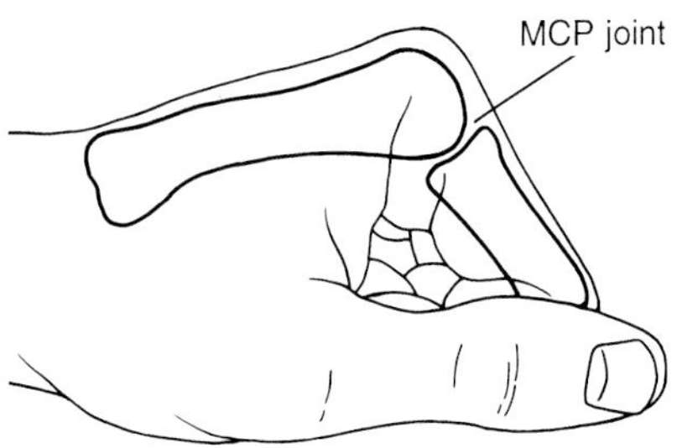

Fig. 22.15 Site for injection of the metacarpophalangeal joint.

22.15 METACARPOPHALANGEAL JOINTS

The metacarpophalangeal joints are less easy to inject, but respond well to intra-articular steroid injections, particularly in rheumatoid arthritis.

The line of the joint needs to be identified. This is normally about 1 cm distal to the crest of the knuckle, and may be made more obvious by gentle subluxation of the joint (Fig. 22.15).

22.15.1 Technique of injection

Apply traction to the patient's finger with one hand while injecting with the other. By putting his index finger on the opposite side of the joint, the doctor can feel the distention of the joint as the injection is being made. Clean the skin with povidone-iodine in spirit.

About 0.25–0.5 ml Depo-Medrone with Lidocaine is all that the average metacarpophalangeal joint will take.

22.16 INTERPHALANGEAL JOINTS

Again, commonly affected by rheumatoid arthritis, the interphalangeal joints may be helped by carefully placed steroid injections. The method is similar to that used for injecting metacarpophalangeal joints, but a lateral approach is preferable, and the needle just inserted at the joint line. It is not possible to insert it further due to the shape of the joint. Counter-traction helps to open the space. 0.1–0.3 ml Depo-Medrone and Lidocaine is used.

As with all steroid injections, the patient is advised to rest the joint for 24–48 hours after injection.

22.17 INJECTION OF TENDON SHEATHS IN THE HAND

(see 22.11, Trigger finger)

The indications for injections in the tendon sheaths are triggering of nodules, effusion, or recent adhesion formation.

The tendon sheaths are arranged as shown in Fig. 22.16.

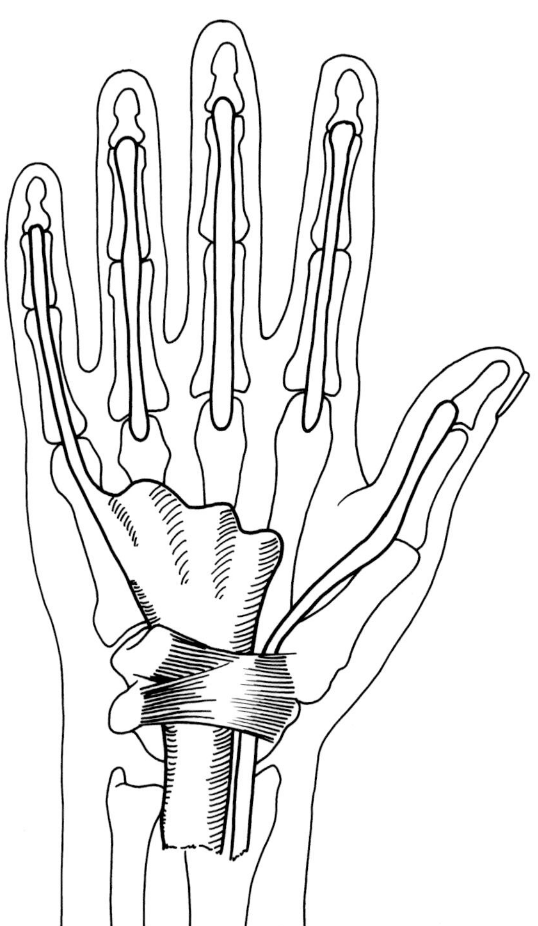

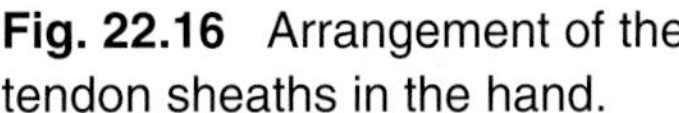

Fig. 22.16 Arrangement of the tendon sheaths in the hand.

22.17.1 Technique

First clean the overlying skin with povidone-iodine in spirit. Where there are palpable nodules, these may be infiltrated with a mixture of steroid and local anaesthetic, e.g. Depo-Medrone and Lidocaine. Where the whole of the tendon sheath is distended, it is preferable to inject directly into the sheath itself.

With the patient seated or lying down with the palm of the hand uppermost, the needle is inserted over the tendon sheath and slowly advanced until a space is found where little resistance to injection is encountered. If in doubt, disconnect the syringe and gently push the needle until it is in the tendon itself, as shown by tilting of the needle on movement of the finger. Slightly withdraw, reattach the syringe and make the injection.

22.18 INJECTION OF SMALL GANGLIA

Ganglia are jelly-filled cysts lying adjacent to joints or attached to tendon sheaths. They often appear to be connected to the joint by a valve mechanism, which allows fluid to enter but not leave the cyst. The fluid in the ganglion therefore gradually concentrates.

Small ganglia may often respond to a steroid injection placed directly in the cyst itself. Larger ganglia should either be excised surgically, or more easily aspirated and sclerosed (Chapter 43).

22.19 INJECTIONS AROUND THE HIP JOINT

Steroid injections into the hip joint itself are beyond the scope of this book, but periarticular soft-tissue injections in the structures adjacent to the hip joint give very rewarding results.

22.19.1 Subtrochanteric bursitis

This condition is commoner than realized. The patient, and sometimes the doctor, ascribe the pain in the 'hip' to be due to osteoarthritis. The patient complains of pain, worse when lying on the affected side in bed, and a point of tenderness can usually be found by asking the patient to lie on the couch, painful side uppermost, hip flexed, and identifying the most tender area alongside the greater trochanter.

Mark the spot, cleanse the skin with povidone-iodine in spirit, and inject a large volume (10–15 ml) of 1% lignocaine containing 50 mg hydrocortisone or the equivalent amount of triamcinolone 10–15 mg, using a 21 swg needle.

Advance the needle until it touches the greater trochanter, slightly withdraw, and inject into the area of the tough fibrous insertion of the gluteal fascia.

22.20 MERALGIA PARAESTHETICA

This is a superficial entrapment neuropathy due to compression of the lateral cutaneous nerve of the thigh as it passes through the deep fascia about 4 in. (10 cm) below and medial to the anterior superior iliac spine. Classically the patient complains of pain and paraesthesia over the antero-lateral area of the thigh.

If the patient's symptoms have lasted less than 2 weeks, it is worth waiting to exclude a diagnosis of herpes zoster. Having identified a local tender spot at the site of the penetration of the nerve, local anaesthetic and steroid is infiltrated around the area, e.g. 5 ml 1% lignocaine with 5–10 mg hydrocortisone.

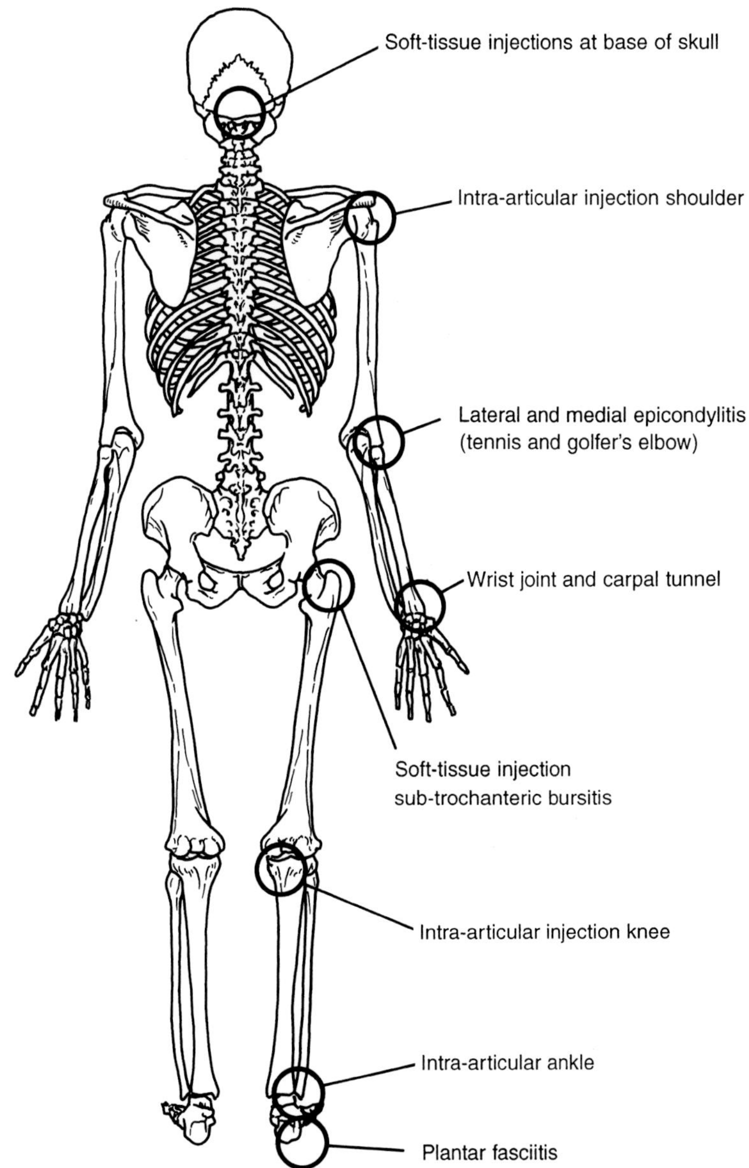

Fig. 22.17 Sites of the most common soft tissue and intra-articular steroid injections.

22.21 ASPIRATION AND INJECTION OF THE KNEE

Generally an effusion will be present; the best approach to the knee is laterally at the junction of the upper pole of the patella and the patellar tendon.

Povidone-iodine in spirit (Betadine alcoholic solution) is liberally applied, and three separate syringes prepared: the first is a 2 ml syringe loaded with 2% lignocaine and 25 swg × 5/8 in. (0.5 mm × 16 mm) needle with which to infiltrate local anaesthetic; the second is a 20 ml sterile syringe with 21 swg × 1 1/2 in. (0.8 mm × 40 mm) needle for aspirating the effusion, and the third is a 2 ml syringe loaded with 2 ml triamcinolone hexacetonide 20 mg/ml (Lederspan), the needle on this third syringe is disconnected.

After painting with skin antiseptic, the skin and subcutaneous tissues down to the joint are infiltrated with lignocaine (Fig. 22.18). Using the same track and the 20 ml syringe, any effusion is aspirated, put in a container for laboratory examination, and the colour noted; it may be clear, cloudy or blood-stained. If clear, this suggests osteoarthritis, and if bloodstained, a recent haemarthrosis; in both it is safe to inject steroids. This may be done simply by disconnecting the 20 ml syringe from the needle, and connecting the loaded 2 ml syringe. Gentle aspiration to confirm the needle is still inside the joint is followed by injection of steroid. The needle is then withdrawn, and a sterile dressing applied together with a firm compression bandage. If the aspirate is cloudy, it is not safe to inject steroids before excluding a septic arthritis; the fluid should be examined by Gram's stain and culture, and by polarized light for birefringent crystals found in gout.

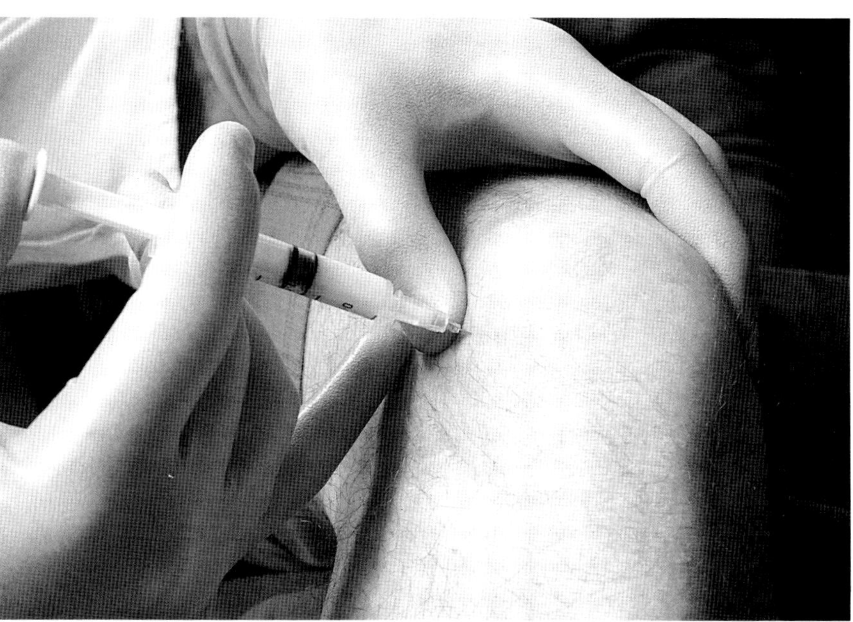

Fig. 22.18 Intra-articular steroid injection – the knee.

It is a good idea to routinely send any fluid aspirated for culture; not only can the unsuspected infection be diagnosed but, if subsequently any infection occurs, it is helpful to know that it was there at the time of the injection and not introduced by the operator.

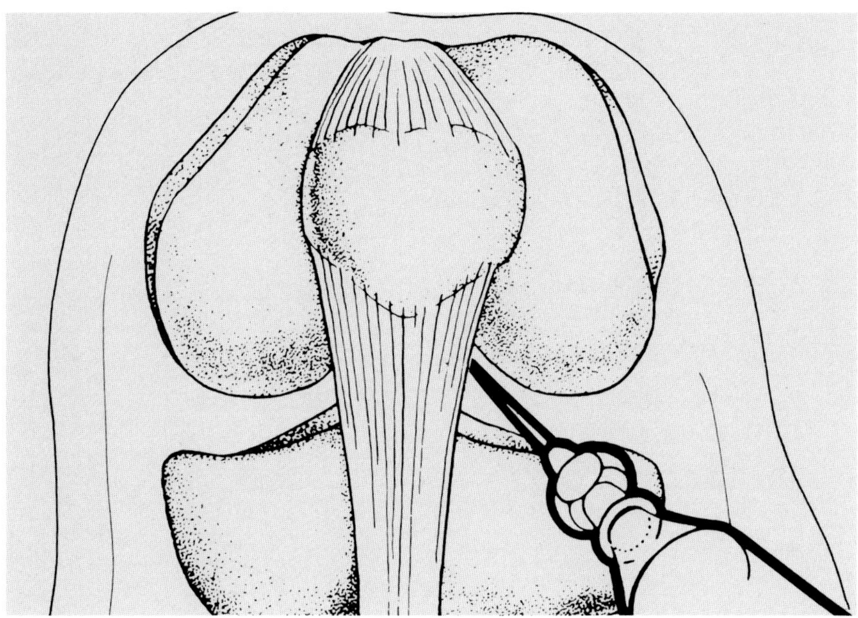

Fig. 22.19 Injection of the knee joint; relationship of needle to underlying structures.

22.22 SEMIMEMBRANOSUS BURSITIS (popliteal or baker's cyst)

This is a distention of the semimembranosus gastrocnemius bursa, and usually occurs whenever there is disease within the knee joint causing an effusion. Due to a one-way valve mechanism, fluid can track from the knee to the bursa, but not back again.

Treatment of a semimembranosus bursitis is therefore treatment of the underlying knee problem. There is no point in injecting the cyst with steroids, but a judiciously placed injection in the knee joint, by reducing the effusion, will often cure the cyst.

22.23 PREPATELLAR BURSITIS (housemaid's knee, clergyman's knee, coalminer's beat-knee, carpet-layer's knee, etc.)

This is a common condition caused by trauma to the prepatellar area as a result of excessive kneeling.

Most resolve spontaneously and give little trouble. If, however, it is judged necessary to treat the condition, an injection of Depo-Medrone 1 ml usually results in a rapid resolution.

22.24 THE FOOT

The main indications for steroid injections at the ankle are rheumatoid arthritis and seronegative arthritis.

It is always important to exclude any infection as a cause of swelling and pain, and particularly in the foot, gout.

22.24.1 The ankle

The ankle is relatively easy to inject. By asking the patient to dorsiflex the foot, the tendon of tibialis anterior can be identified, and the needle introduced just lateral to this, in the space between the tibia and the talus.

Inserting a needle directly into the ankle joint can be very painful: therefore an advance injection of local anaesthetic is given (Fig. 22.20).

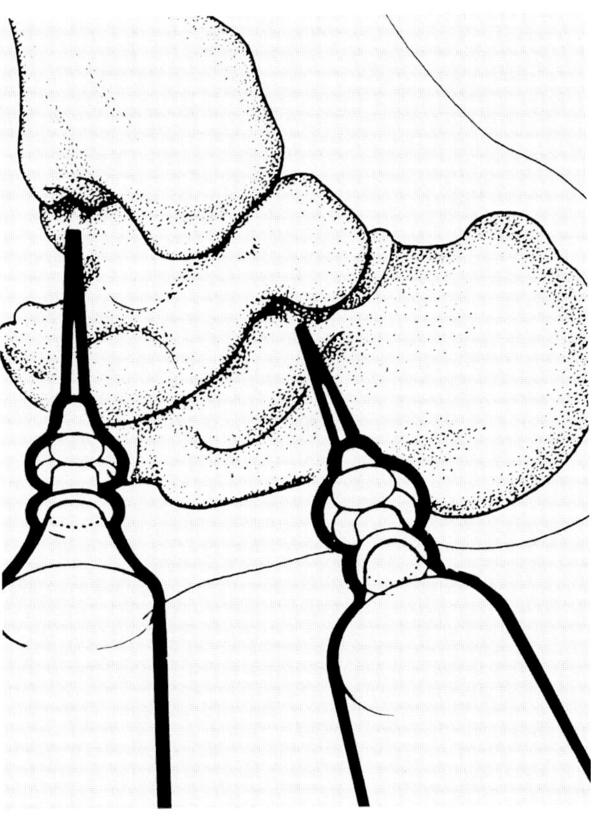

Fig. 22.20 Injecting the skin over the ankle joint with local anaesthetic, prior to aspiration and injection of the joint.

When the needle is in the joint, it is often possible to aspirate fluid, confirming that the needle is in the correct place, and also enabling a sample of fluid to be sent for bacteriology and biochemical examination.

Injections of 20 mg triamcinolone (1 ml), 100 mg hydrocortisone acetate, or 40 mg Methylprednisolone may now be given.

Scrupulous aseptic technique is mandatory to avoid any possibility of introducing infection, and the overlying skin should be thoroughly painted with povidone-iodine in spirit prior to any injection being given.

22.24.2 Plantar fasciitis

This is a common condition, causing extreme pain under the calcaneum. A localized tender spot can always be found, and X-rays frequently show the presence of a calcaneal spur, which is correctly more a transverse ridge rather than a spur. The presence or otherwise of a spur on radiological examination does not alter the decision to inject a plantar fasciitis, particularly as the results of any surgical treatment for calcaneal spurs are not good.

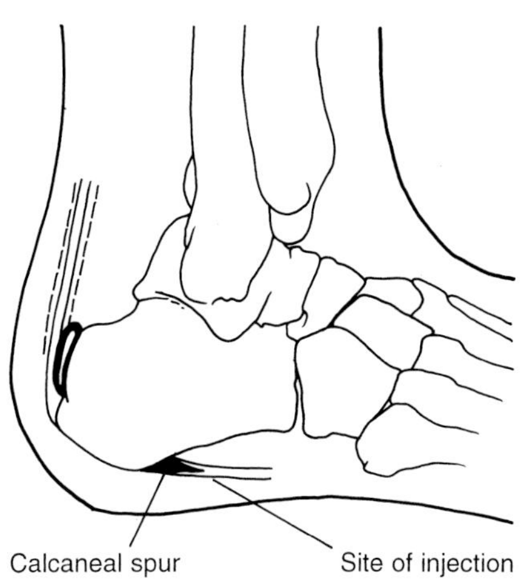

Fig. 22.21 Plantar fasciitis: site of injection.

Technique

With the patient lying on the couch, the point of maximum tenderness is identified and marked (Fig. 22.21). The overlying skin is painted with povidone-iodine in spirit, and the injection made either from the medial side of the foot, or directly through the sole of the foot. Because the exact site of pain is not always easy to identify accurately, it is preferable to use a larger volume of a dilute solution of hydrocortisone or triamcinolone in 1% lignocaine than a small volume of stronger steroid. Having said this, it is not always possible to inject more than 1 ml due to discomfort. If the injection has been made in the correct site, the local anaesthetic causes rapid relief of pain.

22.24.3 Tendo achilles tendinitis

This is mentioned largely to advise against injection. Although pain and swelling around the Achilles tendon is common, steroid injections have been known to cause rupture of the tendon with disastrous consequences. It is, therefore, not recommended to be done by the general practitioner.

22.24.4 First metatarsophalangeal (MTP) joint

The 1st MTP joint is commonly affected by crystal synovitis of gout, and by osteoarthrosis and rheumatoid arthritis.

The joint is best injected from the medial side, siting the point of entry in the joint line, below the extensor tendon.

Technique

The overlying skin is painted with povidone-iodine in spirit and the injection given using either 1 ml Depo-Medrone with Lidocaine or 2–5 mg triamcinolone in 1 ml 1% lignocaine or 5–10 mg hydrocortisone, also in 1% lignocaine 1–2 ml.

22.25 MISCELLANEOUS JOINT INJECTIONS

22.25.1 Temporomandibular joint

Pain in the temporomandibular joint may frequently be relieved by a carefully placed steroid injection using a 25 swg needle. Failing this, a temporary 'denture' may be made to alter the angle of bite.

22.25.2 Sternomanubrial joint

This joint may cause pain, and be palpably swollen. The patient will experience sternal pain and be worried they have heart disease. If a localized tender spot can be found, and pressure reproduces the pain, it may be helpful to inject a small quantity (2–5 mg triamcinolone) directly into the joint.

22.25.3 Tietze's syndrome (costochondritis)

This is a common finding, particularly in women between the ages of 30 and 65. Steroid injections are disappointing, but worth attempting if the patient is in much pain. Better results may be expected when there is visible and palpable swelling over the joint.

22.26 MISCELLANEOUS SOFT TISSUE INJECTIONS

Injection of steroids, with or without local anaesthetic, is often a valuable treatment even when the exact diagnosis is unsure. Up to 10 ml of 1% lignocaine with added hydrocortisone 25 mg is used, and infiltrated widely around the most tender spot [24].

22.27 ABDOMINAL ASCITES

By far the commonest cause of ascites seen by the general practitioner is intra-abdominal malignancy. By this stage of their illness, such patients are ill, weak, nauseated, and breathless. It is therefore very much kinder to 'bring the mountain to Mohammed' by taking the instruments and equipment to the patient's bedside, rather than transporting an already terminally ill patient to the surgery or hospital, particularly as the procedure will weaken the patient still further. Additionally, by draining the ascites in the patient's own bedroom, an intravenous 'premedication' injection of fentanyl 100 μg and midazolam 2–6 mg may be given so that the patient actually sleeps throughout the procedure and has no recollection of it afterwards; consequently the patient will have no apprehension should it need to be repeated at another date subsequently.

With modern diuretics, abdominal paracentesis is not performed as frequently as formerly; nevertheless there are significant numbers of patients who obtain good relief of their symptoms by judicious aspiration. It is not necessary, nor desirable, to draw off all the ascites – such a manoeuvre would be likely to precipitate a severe hypotensive reaction and would rapidly deplete the patient of large quantities of protein; the aim should be to remove enough fluid to make the abdomen feel soft, and to alleviate dyspnoea, vomiting, and discomfort. If doubt exists about the exact cause of the ascites, a diagnostic aspiration is easily performed, and the fluid sent for analysis, culture, and cytology. If this reveals malignant cells, the diagnosis may be easier, and the need for an exploratory laparotomy avoided.

In addition to aspiration, cytotoxic drugs may be injected into the peritoneal cavity through the same cannula.

Instruments required for abdominal paracentesis:

- 1 5 ml syringe with 23 swg × 1 in. (0.6 mm × 25 mm) needle with fentanyl 100 μg and midazolam 2–6 mg
- 1 5 ml syringe with 25 swg × 5/8 in. (0. 5 mm × 16 mm) needle loaded with lignocaine 1% and adrenalin 1:200 000
- 1 needle 21 swg × 1 1/2 in. (0.8 mm × 40 mm)

sterile dressing pack
abdominal paracentesis pack (comprising trocar and cannula or intravenous cannula, connecting tubing, connector, adjustable screw clamp)
self-adhesive tape 1 in. (0.6 mm) = 25 mm
Povidone-iodine in spirit (Betadine alcoholic solution)
1 standard sterile urine collecting bag with drainage tap
sterile universal containers if required for culture, examination of cytology
1 many-tailed bandage (optional)
4 large safety pins.

22.27.1 Technique for abdominal paracentesis

The patient will already be in bed and preferably with three or four pillows so that he or she is semirecumbent. A premedication intravenous injection of fentanyl 100 μg and midazolam 2–6 mg may be offered; some patients will appreciate being asleep for the aspiration, others will prefer to remain awake. Certainly with careful attention to detail while infiltrating with local anaesthetic, the procedure is totally without discomfort.

Depending on the underlying intra-abdominal pathology, a site is chosen away from any masses, usually in the lower abdomen towards the flank; the diagnosis of ascites is verified by gentle percussion, and the patient turned very gently towards the chosen side. Repeat percussion should confirm the presence of shifting dullness. A waterproof dressing sheet (Inco-sheets are ideal) is placed under the patient to protect the lower sheet, and the area chosen liberally painted with povidone-iodine in spirit (Betadine alcoholic solution). Using the 25 swg × 5/8 in. (0.5 mm × 16 mm) needle on the 5 ml syringe with lignocaine and adrenaline, a small bleb of local anaesthetic is raised in the skin. Very gradually the needle is advanced through the skin and underlying tissues, injecting all the time. If the 25 swg needle is not long enough to reach the peritoneal cavity, it is exchanged for a 23 swg × 1 in. (0.6 mm × 25 mm) or 21 swg × 1 1/2 in. (0.8 mm × 40 mm) needle, and the injection continued (Fig. 22.22) . The peritoneum is particularly sensitive, and great care should be used to infiltrate and advance the needle very slowly, allowing adequate time for anaesthesia to develop before advancing the needle. As this is the only part of the procedure which can be uncomfortable if poor technique is used, it is worth spending time to ensure that it is completely painless. This will also increase the patient's confidence and help to allay any anxiety. If the first paracentesis has been painless, the patient will not mind any subsequent aspirations.

Having completely anaesthetized the track from skin to peritoneum, the abdominal trocar and cannula is inserted exactly through the same track (Fig. 22.23). A little pressure is usually necessary, accompanied by a rotating action. Once the peritoneal cavity is entered, the trocar is withdrawn 1 cm and the blunt cannula pushed in to its hub. The trocar is now withdrawn, ascitic fluid spurts from the cannula, which should be rapidly connected via the thin rubber tubing and connector directly to a sterile urine drainage bag with drainage tap (Figs 22.24 and 22.25); this in turn

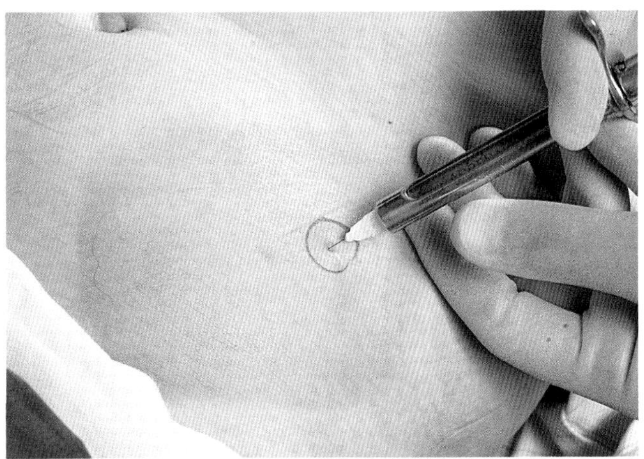

Fig. 22.22 Abdominal paracentesis, after preliminary skin antisepsis, local anaesthetic is infiltrated through the skin, down to peritoneum.

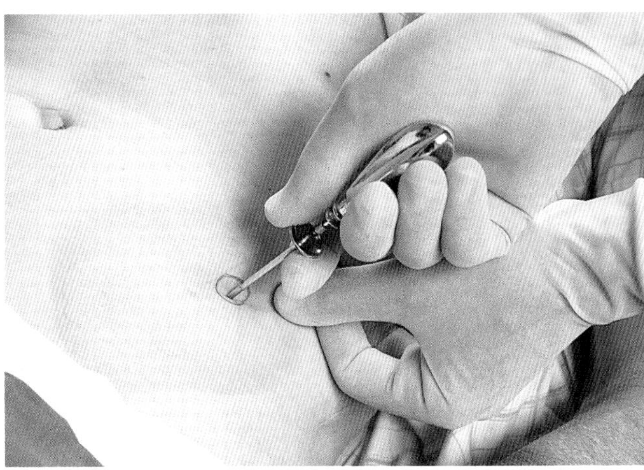

Fig. 22.23 Insertion of trocar and cannula.

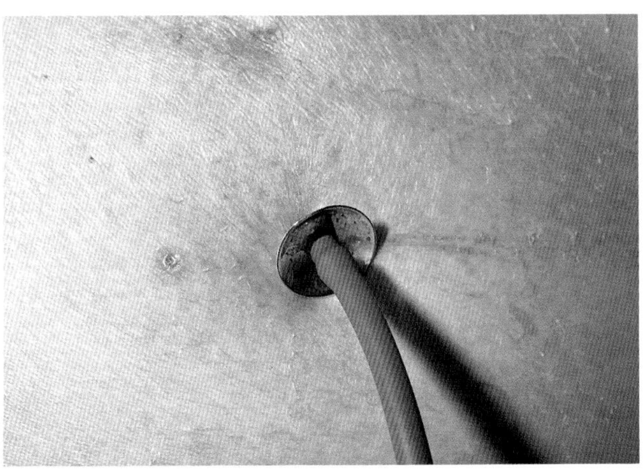

Fig. 22.24 The trocar is withdrawn, and the cannula connected by rubber tubing to a drainage bag.

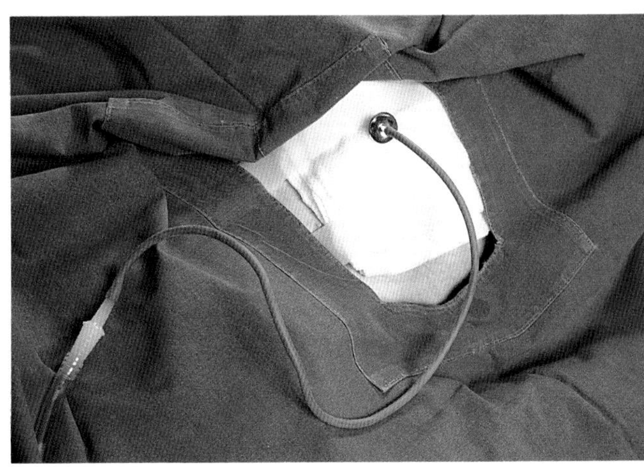

Fig. 22.25 Rubber tubing is connected to urine drainage bag.

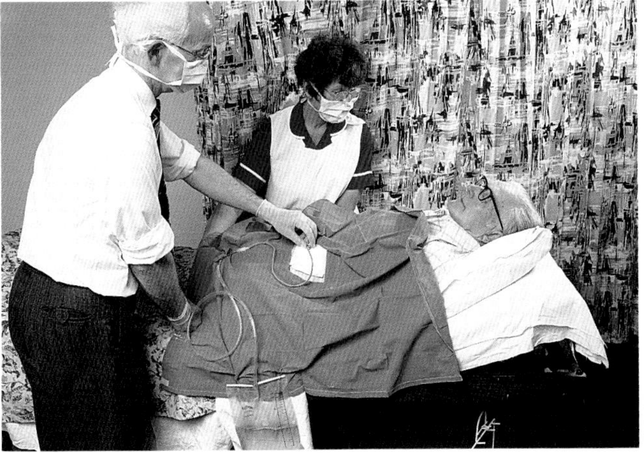

Fig. 22.26 Abdominal paracentesis. A procedure which may readily be performed in the patient's home.

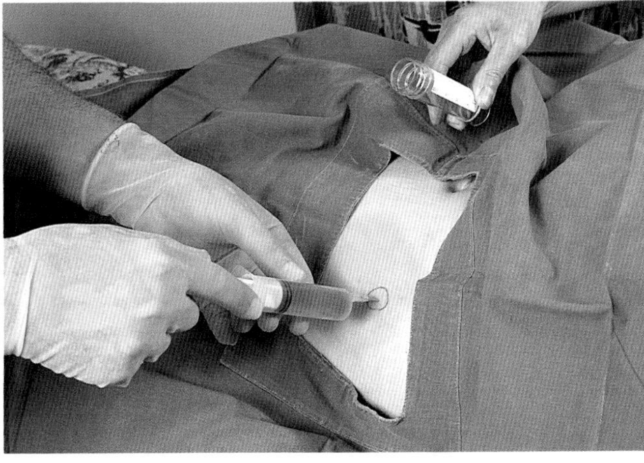

Fig. 22.27 Abdominal paracentesis; diagnostic aspiration. Fluid may then be sent for analysis and cytology.

can be attached to the patient's mattress with two large safety pins. The volume of ascites can be easily measured by reading the quantity on the marks on the urine drainage bag. When full, the bag can be emptied merely by opening the drainage tap into a basin beneath. If the rate of flow via the cannula is too rapid, it may be slowed by the application of an adjustable screw clamp to the rubber tubing (Fig. 22.26). Throughout the procedure, regular checks on the patient's pulse and blood pressure should be made.

Once sufficient fluid has been withdrawn to alleviate pressure effects, nausea, dyspnoea, discomfort and tightness, the cannula should be withdrawn, a self-adhesive dressing applied, and if thought necessary, a many-tailed abdominal bandage applied. Unless an excessive volume of fluid has been withdrawn this is probably unnecessary.

The patient should then remain in the bed for the next 12 hours to allow the circulation and blood pressure to reach equilibrium; should they need to get out of bed for any reason they should be accompanied.

The immediate relief of symptoms is generally followed by a gradual weakening of the patient, and on average it is rarely necessary to have to repeat an abdominal paracentesis more than three times.

The procedure for diagnostic 'tap' is exactly the same as for paracentesis, except that a 20 ml syringe attached to a 21 swg × 1½ in. (0.8 mm × 40 mm) needle is used instead of the trocar and cannula (Fig. 22.27).

If preferred, a size 14 swg (2 mm) intravenous cannula (Abbocath T) 14 may be used in place of the traditional trocar and cannula; this gives equally good results, and is probably slightly easier to insert, but a Luer type adaptor is necessary to connect to the tubing.

22.28 ASPIRATION OF PLEURAL EFFUSIONS

The majority of general practitioners will probably not need to aspirate pleural effusions, the main indication is diagnostic cytology; carcinoma of the lung is now replacing tuberculosis and empyema as the main indication for aspiration. A chest X-ray is desirable whenever possible, this will help to decide the best side for aspiration. With modern chemotherapeutic agents, radiotherapy, diuretics, and surgery, the need for large volume aspiration is far less than in previous years.

Instruments required:

10 ml syringe filled with 1% lignocaine and 1:200 000 adrenaline
25 swg × ⅝ in. (0.5 mm × 16 mm) needle
Two-way tap with Luer connectors
21 swg × 2½ in. (0.8 mm × 63 mm) needle
sterile universal containers.

Careful clinical examination and a recent chest X-ray will determine the best site for aspiration; this will usually be an intercostal space towards the back. As the intercostal blood vessels run along the underside of each rib, it is important to insert the needle just above the rib to avoid them.

A preliminary intravenous injection of fentanyl 100 µg and midazolam

2–6 mg may be offered if the patient is unduly apprehensive. The overlying skin is painted with povidone-iodine in spirit (Betadine alcoholic solution) and a small amount of lignocaine injected intradermally with the 25 swg (0.5 mm) needle to raise a weal. The needle is then changed for the longer 21 swg (0.8 mm) needle and two-way tap and the subcutaneous tissues, intercostal muscles, and pleura infiltrated with local anaesthetic. As with abdominal paracentesis, the local anaesthetic should be given very slowly, injecting a little before advancing the needle, and allowing time for the area to become anaesthetized. The doctor should be fully conversant with the working of the two-way tap and should test it before use; it should be possible to inject local anaesthetic through the needle, aspirate fluid back, and by turning the tap, isolate the needle in the pleural cavity while injecting the aspirated fluid into the universal container. It is essential that air is not accidentally allowed into the chest.

Normally the practitioner can feel the various layers through which the aspirating needle is passing; as soon as the pleural cavity is entered, fluid should be withdrawn into the syringe and transferred to the universal container (Fig. 22.28). If it is intended only to withdraw a small quantity of effusion for cytology, the two-way tap may be omitted and a 20 ml sterile syringe with 21 swg × 2½ in. (0.8 mm × 63 mm) needle used instead. In this case, just 20 ml of fluid are taken and the needle and syringe are withdrawn. A collodion dressing is immediately applied.

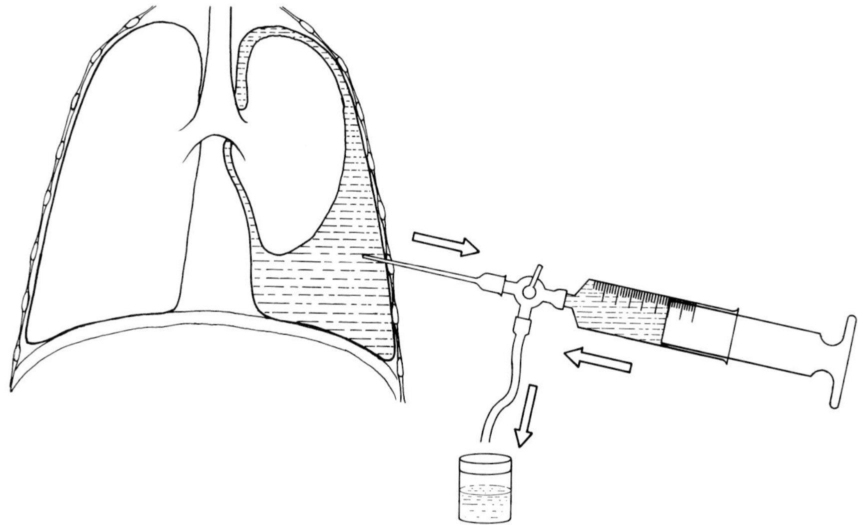

Fig. 22.28 Aspiration of pleural effusion. The needle should be inserted above a rib to avoid the intercostal blood vessels.

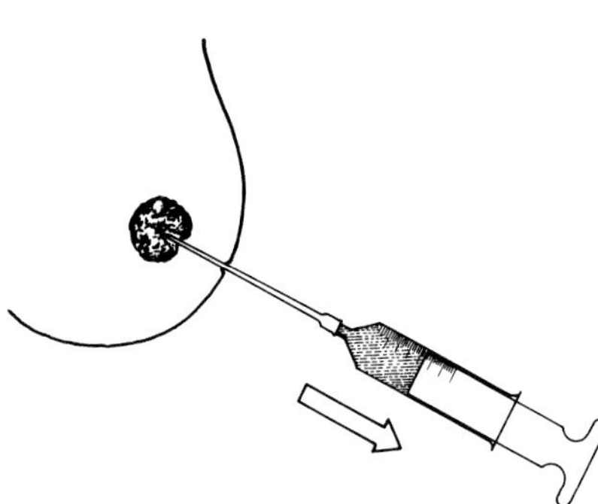

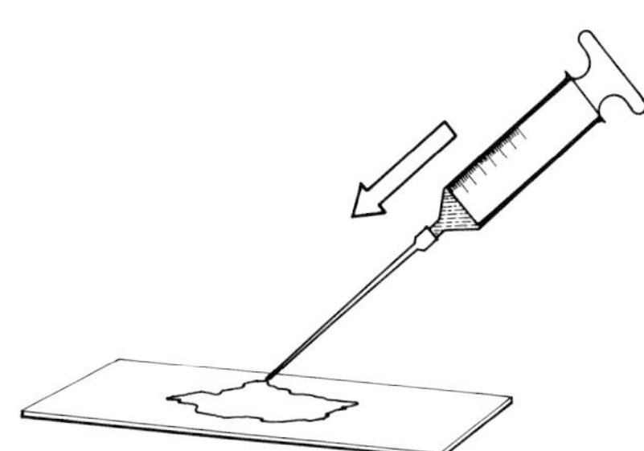

Fig. 22.29 Needle aspiration of breast lump.

22.29 NEEDLE BIOPSY

Histological diagnosis of certain tumours may be obtained by needle biopsy. Its use in general practice is limited, but it has a particular place for swellings in the breast which the practitioner feels are probably cystic and which, when aspiration is attempted, produce no fluid and feel hard, indicating the possibility of a tumour. By applying strong traction to the syringe plunger to create a vacuum and at the same time rotating the syringe and needle in a clockwise and anticlockwise direction as the needle is slowly withdrawn, a small piece of tissue will be left in the needle (Fig. 22.29).

By carefully 'blowing' the contents of the needle onto a microscope slide and fixing with preservative (the fixative used for cervical cytology is suitable) a sample may be sent for histological or cytological examination. Although not giving 100% positive accuracy, nevertheless a diagnosis may be made correctly in about 90% of needle biopsies. Obviously a swelling with a negative needle biopsy should still be referred to the surgeons for excision, but a swelling with a positive diagnosis on needle biopsy enables the patient and surgeon to plan the most appropriate treatment. Biopsy specimens may also be taken using a Tru-cut biopsy needle (Fig. 22.30); this is manufactured as a sterile disposable unit in various lengths and diameters.

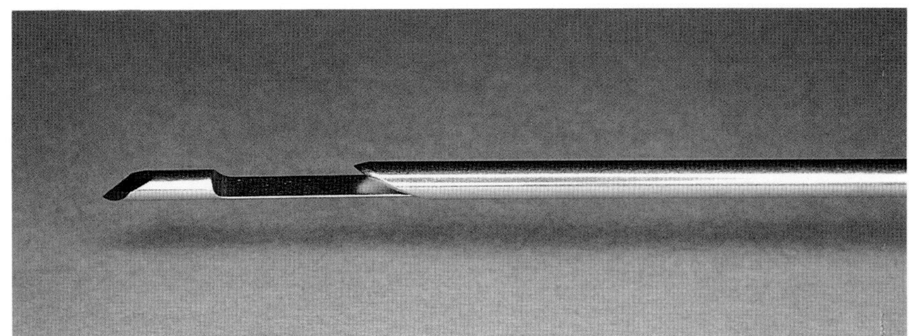

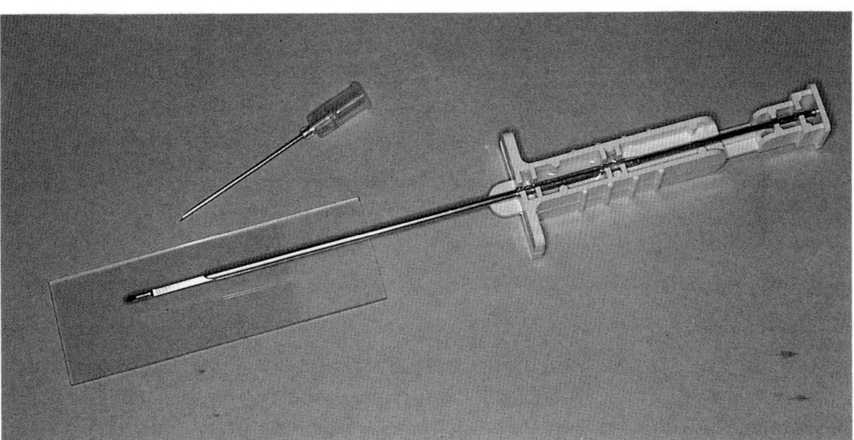

Fig. 22.30a, b The Tru-cut biopsy needle (Travenol Laboratories, Inc.).

22.30 ASPIRATION OF CYSTS AND BURSAE

Simple cysts may occur anywhere in the body, they may contain watery fluid which can be easily aspirated with a needle, or thick semisolid material which is quite impossible to aspirate through any needle. The two most commonly encountered cysts occur in the breast and thyroid; aspiration in these situations affords immense relief to patient and doctor alike and is often curative. As with all injection techniques, scrupulous asepsis must be observed, the minimum of trauma inflicted by the selection of the finest needle consistent with aspiration, and all fluid aspirated should be sent for cytological examination. Where any possibility of infection exists, the fluid should, in addition be sent for bacterial culture.

22.30.1 Aspiration of breast cysts

The typical breast cyst is smooth, round, very mobile, slightly tender, and not adherent to skin or deep structures. Diagnosis may be helped by the use of ultrasonography and mammography, but ultimately the only way to establish an accurate diagnosis is by aspiration. It follows that there will be occasions when a 'typical' breast cyst is found on aspiration to be solid, in this situation, the needle should not be immediately withdrawn, but used for needle biopsy.

To carry out the aspiration it is more comfortable for the patient to be lying down; the skin overlying the cyst is liberally painted with povidone-iodine in spirit (Betadine alcoholic solution) and the injection site anaesthetized using lignocaine and a fine 25 swg × 5/8 in. (0.5 mm × 16 mm) needle. A 20 ml sterile syringe with 19 swg × 1 1/2 in. (1.1 mm × 38 mm) needle is used for aspiration. The cyst should first be fixed with finger and thumb of the left hand, and the aspirating needle pointed towards the centre of the cyst. By applying gentle traction to the syringe plunger as the needle is advanced, the practitioner will know when the cyst has been entered. Typically the fluid aspirated is a dark green colour; as much as possible should be removed, hopefully emptying the cyst, and sent for cytology. Even if a negative cytology is obtained, the patient should be seen again in 4 weeks to check that the cyst has not reformed.

22.30.2 Thyroid cysts

Although not as common as breast cysts, thyroid cysts are just as easy to aspirate. It is advisable to confirm the diagnosis by ultrasonography or scan, and the technique, precautions, cytological examination, and follow-up are identical to those for breast cysts.

22.30.3 Aspiration and injection of hydrocele

A primary hydrocele is an excessive collection of serous fluid in the tunica vaginalis within the scrotum; it occurs at any age, but most commonly in adult life. The diagnosis is usually straightforward, particularly if the swelling transilluminates, but it must be remembered that a hernia in an infant also transilluminates.

Aspiration alone rarely cures a hydrocele, but aspiration and the injection of dilute aqueous phenol on two or three separate occasions can offer up to 90% cure [25]; failing this, surgical treatment of the tunica vaginalis is recommended.

A secondary hydrocele occurs as a result of infection or inflammation within the scrotum, thus it is always important to first examine the testis, epididymis, and cord to exclude any disease in these orders. The treatment of a secondary hydrocele is the treatment of its cause.

Instruments required:

2 ml syringe with 25 swg × 5/8 in. (0.5 mm × 16 mm) needle
2 ml 1% lignocaine
18 swg (0.9 mm) intravenous cannula, e.g. Abbocath T18

10 ml ampoules of 2.5% aqueous sterile phenol
20 ml syringes for aspiration and injection.

An injection of 2.5% aqueous phenol is not a standard preparation, therefore it needs to be ordered specially; however, it has a good shelf life and a small number may be kept in store ready for use.

The technique for aspiration and injection of hydrocele is as follows: the patient should lie on the couch or operating table; good illumination is important, a sterile sheet should be placed under the scrotum and between the legs. Povidone-iodine in spirit (Betadine alcoholic solution) is applied to the scrotum – this may cause a slight stinging sensation – and a point is chosen for aspiration. This point should be on the lower side, away from the testicle and avoiding any blood vessels on the surface of the scrotum. Local anaesthetic is carefully injected through the scrotal wall and underlying tissues, down to the hydrocele sac. This may be confirmed by gently withdrawing the syringe plunger and noting straw-coloured fluid entering the syringe. In a relatively small hydrocele it helps to hold the neck of the hydrocele, this makes it tense and prevents it extending into the inguinal canal, it also ensures that the operator has not missed an inguino-scrotal hernia.

The local anaesthetic needle is now withdrawn, and the 18 swg (0.9 mm) intravenous cannula inserted through the same needle track. By removing the central cannula needle, a soft, pliable catheter is now situated within the hydrocele sac: this is far less traumatic than the old steel trocar and cannula, and gives equally good results. The serous fluid may either be allowed to run out freely into a container, or aspirated by connecting a 20 ml syringe to the cannula, with or without a three-way tap. As the hydrocele empties, the sac is gently compressed with the left hand to remove most of the fluid, and the volume noted. If any doubt exists about the underlying pathology, the fluid should be sent for culture and cytology.

Keeping the cannula in place, a calculated volume of 2.5% sterile aqueous phenol is now injected according to the following formula:

Volume aspirated	Volume injected 2.5% phenol
Up to 50 ml	5 ml
Up to 200 ml	10 ml
Up to 400 ml	15 ml
Over 400 ml	20 ml

The cannula is now withdrawn and a simple collodion dressing applied.

After 6 weeks the procedure is repeated; most of the hydrocele will have recurred and it is important to have warned the patient that this is likely.

At the second aspiration, if it is noticed that the fluid appears darker or even blood-stained, success can be anticipated.

The patient is seen a third time 6 weeks later, and on this occasion the volume of fluid should be considerably less, or may not have recollected at all. For the elderly patient who would be a poor general anaesthetic and surgical risk, this is undoubtedly the treatment of choice, offering over 90% chance of complete cure.

22.30.4 Epididymal cysts

These are not as common as a primary hydrocele, nevertheless they can be aspirated and injected with 2.5% aqueous phenol exactly as described for hydrocele. Success is even higher, offering nearly 100% cure, provided the cyst is not multiloculated, in which case surgical excision is probably the treatment of choice. Aspiration and sclerosant injection should not be offered to men who intend having a family, as reductions in sperm counts have been reported following this treatment.

23

Incision of abscesses

Recent wounds if inflammation has set in, will result in fever with chills and throbbing. One should induce suppuration as soon as possible and not let the pus be blocked up. The flesh should be lacerated by the weapon. After that new tissue sprouts up

Hippocrates, 460–377 BC

Instruments required:

- scalpel handle size 3
- scalpel blade no. 11
- 1 malleable probe
- 1 pair sinus forceps
- assorted small drains
- Fucidin Gel
- sterile dressings
- wide-bore aspirating needle and syringe.

It is only within one generation that we have witnessed a dramatic reduction in the numbers of bacterial infections largely thanks to antibiotics. The image of the family doctor taking out his 'lancet' from his pocket to open a 'boil' is still in living memory! Large necrotic abscesses, so familiar in the last century, are now fortunately rarer, and in one year, the general practitioner will need to open only a few. Common sites for abscesses are the perineum, infected operation scars, and fingers. Small abscesses probably require little other than a dry dressing.

Spreading cellulitis and induration with lymphangitis is best treated with antibiotics, but once pus has collected it should be released, usually by incision. If the abscess is superficial and distending the overlying skin which has become thinned, incision using a pointed no. 11 scalpel blade on no. 3 handle is all that is necessary (Figs 23.1 and 23.2). Deeper abscesses, recognized by fluctuation, pain, fever, and rigors with leucocytosis will require incision, but because of the pain, will require some form of anaesthetic; this may best be managed with a general anaesthetic, but occasionally, where a general anaesthetic is considered inappropriate, careful local anaesthesia or Entonox inhalation may suffice. However, even this causes pain, is not always effective, and increases the risk of spreading the infection.

Having incised the abscess, the pus should be expelled by pressure, a bacterial swab taken for culture of the organisms, and a suitable drain inserted to prevent premature closure of the wound.

Recently good results have been obtained by incising the abscess,

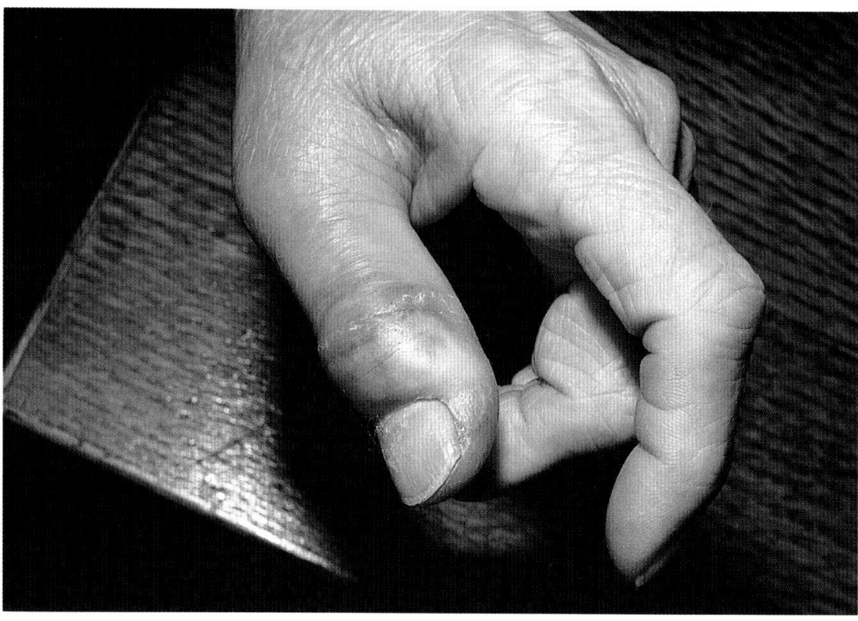

Fig. 23.1 Paronychia, thumb; simple incision and dressing is all that is required.

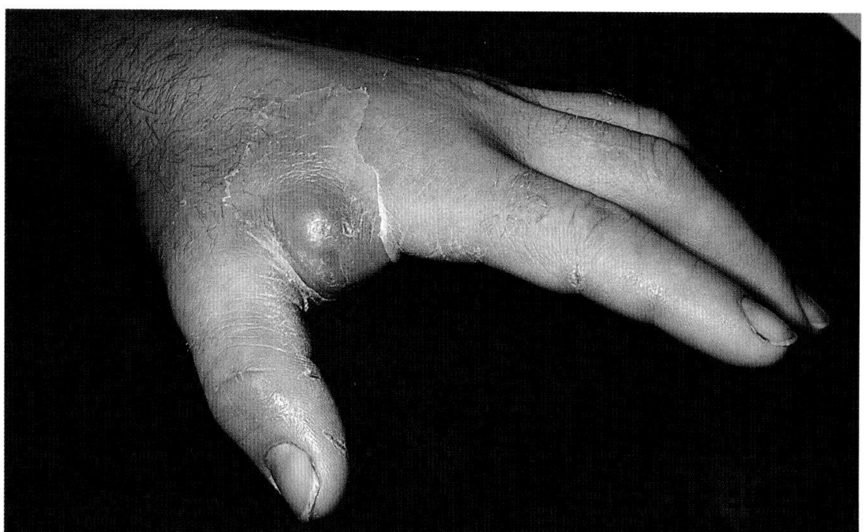

Fig. 23.2 Web-space abscess; incision and dressing required.

curetting the lining, and instilling Fucidin Gel. No drain is necessary, a dry dressing is applied, healing occurs rapidly and recurrence is rare. In some cases, even primary closure is possible.

Aspiration alone, using a wide-bore needle, often results in a cure, particularly with Bartholin's abscesses (Chapter 38) and may avoid the need for more radical surgery.

24

Dermatological minor surgery

24.1 NORMAL SKIN

As the majority of minor surgical operations are performed on skin, it is helpful to have a knowledge of simple skin biology and histology.

24.1.1 Anatomy (see Fig. 19.1)

The skin comprises epidermis, dermis, and skin appendages such as pilosebaceous follicles, eccrine, and apocrine sweat glands.

In the epidermis the basal or germinative layer is made up of small keratinocytes which gradually migrate to the surface over approximately 4 weeks. With the keratinocytes are smaller numbers of melanocytes whose function is to produce melanin pigment, which in turn finds its way to the keratinocytes and ultimately protects the cells against the effects of ultraviolet irradiation, which is known to damage nuclear DNA.

Naevus cells, found in pigmented naevi, are similar to melanocytes, and there is some evidence that melanocytes can differentiate into naevus cells.

Between the epidermis and the dermis is the basement membrane, which effectively cements the two layers together. Collagen is the main component of the dermis, with fibroblasts being the predominant cell, responsible for producing the three dermal proteins: elastin, reticulin, and ground substance.

Congenital capillary abnormalities may present as vascular naevi.

The pilosebaceous unit

This traverses both the dermis and epidermis and comprises the hair follicle, sebaceous glands, and erector pili muscle. The sebaceous glands produce sebum by disintegration of the glandular cells. Blockage of sebum in teenage adults results in acne.

Epidermal cysts occur following implantation of epidermis, or from the lining of pilosebaceous follicles and are filled with macerated keratin. The cysts seen commonly on the scalp are tricholemmal (pilar) cysts derived from the hair follicle; they occur in families, being inherited as an autosomal dominant gene, and are often multiple.

The nail

Nails are formed from epidermal invagination. The nail plate grows from

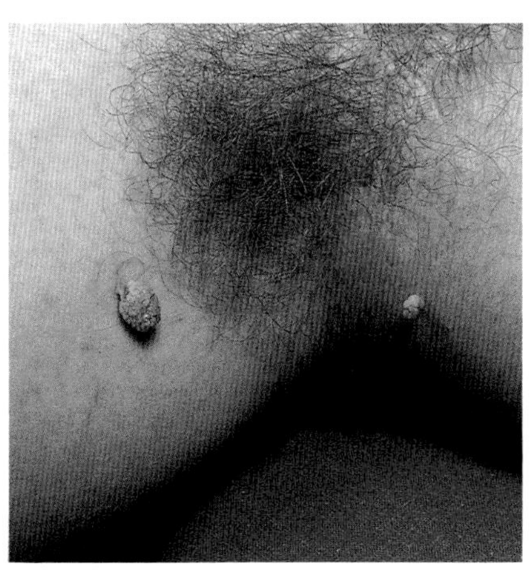

Fig. 24.1 Skin tags in axilla: easily removed by electrocautery.

the nail matrix and lies on the nail bed. The proximal part of the nail is the lunula, and the protective membrane covering the proximal part of the lunula is the cuticle. Damage to the cuticle may result in chronic infection around the nail bed. Ingrowing nails are a result of lateral pressure, chafing, and infection along the edge of the nail.

24.2 LESIONS SUITABLE FOR TREATMENT

Skin tags and papillomata

These are some of the easiest and most common conditions to treat. Small ones may merely be snipped off with scissors and the base cauterized either chemically or by heat (Fig. 24.1) or removed with a radio-surgery wire loop (Chapter 42).

Intradermal naevi

These are also extremely common and may be removed either by curette and cautery excision, radio-surgery or destruction by cryotherapy.

'Sebaceous cysts' (tricholemmal, pilar, epidermal)

These lend themselves admirably to minor surgery. Whichever method is used to treat them, the important point is to be sure the whole capsule has been removed, otherwise recurrence is likely.

Viral infections (warts and molluscum contagiosum)

Surgery has a limited role in the treatment of these troublesome conditions. Medical measures should always be tried first, but where these fail, and particularly where there are solitary lesions, treatment may be curette, radio-surgery, cautery, cryotherapy, or excision.

Vascular lesions

Certain vascular haemangiomata may be destroyed by electrocautery, diathermy, or cryotherapy. The granuloma pyogenicum is easily treated by curette and cautery; spider naevi are easily destroyed by the 'cold point' electrocautery, but strawberry naevi and port-wine naevi are generally not suitable for minor surgical treatment.

Hypertrophic and neoplastic lesions

Solar keratoses, seborrhoeic warts, keratoacanthoma and small basal cell carcinomata, histiocytomata and other small neoplastic lesions may be removed either by curette and cautery, radio-surgery, cryotherapy, or excision, depending on the experience and confidence of the operator.

24.3 LESIONS TO AVOID

Site

Avoid operating on the face, posterior triangle in the neck, axilla, and femoral triangle unless you are absolutely sure of the anatomy and can anticipate and deal with unexpected problems (Figs 24.2 and 24.3). Similarly avoid all but very superficial lesions in the breast as good local anaesthesia is often difficult to obtain and the incidence of malignancy is higher.

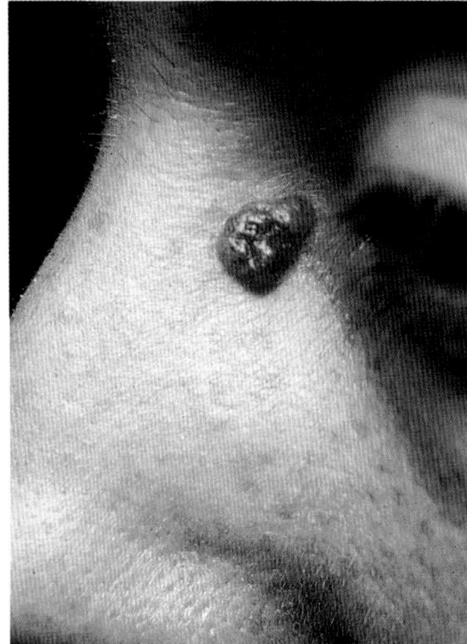

Fig. 24.2 Basal-cell carcinoma near inner canthus and nasolachrymal duct. Not suitable for minor surgery, and should be referred.

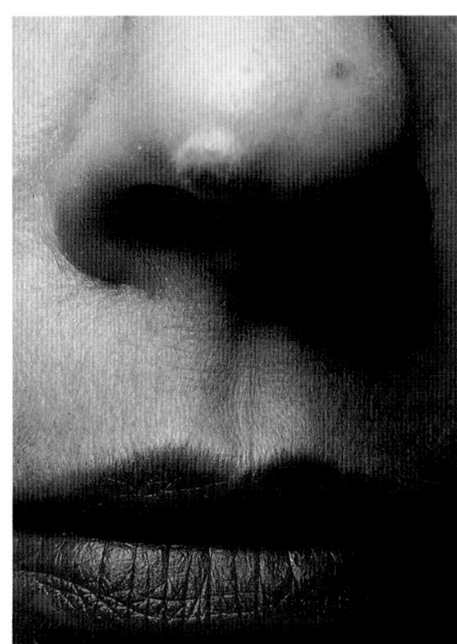

Fig. 24.3 Cellular naevus: tip of nose . This is a difficult site to obtain a good cosmetic result. Better referred or not treated.

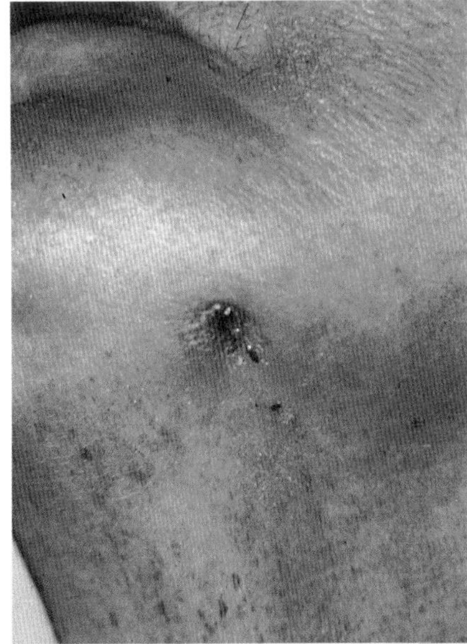

Fig. 24.4 Beware the small, innocent-looking weeping ulcerated lesion in this site. Excision will be followed by a recurrence. This is a dental sinus!

Size

Avoid removing large lesions where difficulty in skin closure might be anticipated. Also, larger lesions tend to have a larger blood supply!

Depth of lesion

Beware of the large, diffuse lipoma: this may extend to a deeper layer than expected, and be aware of the underlying anatomy, particularly nerves, tendons, and arteries.

Similarly, many ganglia need careful dissection down to a joint capsule, through tendons and vessels, in a bloodless operating field. Better not to start than find oneself in difficulties. (Consider alternative treatments for ganglia, Chapter 4.)

Beware of the discharging small ulcer on the face overlying the mandible: this could be a dental sinus, in which case simple excision will be followed by a recurrence. Examination inside the patient's mouth will reveal the source of the sinus (Fig. 24.4).

24.3.1 Malignant lesions

Excising a nodular malignant melanoma has no place in minor surgery. Where a thin, small, pigmented lesion is encountered, it may be judicious to excise it and allow a clear margin. Such a judgement depends on the experience and skill of the operator. Basal cell carcinoma and squamous cell carcinoma, particularly if on the face and especially if near the eye, should be referred to a specialist. Small tumours in other sites may be suitable for excision.

Age

Avoid operating on young children who either cannot co-operate, keep still, or endure a local anaesthetic.

If it pulsates, don't touch it!!!

24.4 LESIONS THAT DO NOT REQUIRE TREATMENT

Strawberry naevi resolve spontaneously, as do most warts, molluscum contagiosum, and even keratoacanthomata.

Small intradermal naevi are often better left alone in case the resulting scar is more unsightly than the original lesion, and histiocytomata are often better left untreated as they extend through full skin thickness and therefore require excision.

25

Skin lesions

> *Naevi Materni are those marks which frequently appear on the bodies of children at birth and which originate from impressions made on the mind of the mother during pregnancy*
>
> *Encyclopaedia Britannica, 1797*

Almost all dermal lesions can be removed in the surgery by a general practitioner, the two exceptions being any lesion which is too large to permit skin closure, and the malignant melanoma. Facilities for histological examination are essential, and it is good practice to send every specimen excised for histological examination; not only does this improve the doctor's diagnostic acumen, it avoids the pitfall of inadvertently removing an amelanotic malignant melanoma, and provides a permanent record of the tissues and pathology removed. Most of the lesions to be described can be removed leaving a neat inconspicuous scar; where the doctor anticipates otherwise the patient should be advised in advance.

One instrument set will be suitable for all the lesions described and the technique with slight variations is applicable to each.

Instruments required:

- scalpel handle size 3
- scalpel blade size 10
- Volkmann double-ended sharp-spoon curette
- Kilner needle holder 5¼in. (13.3 cm)
- pair standard stitch scissors, 5 in. (12.7 cm), pointed
- pair toothed dissecting forceps 5 in. (12.7 cm)
- pair Halstead mosquito artery forceps, curved, 5 in. (12.7 cm)
- povidone-iodine in spirit (Betadine alcoholic solution)
- 10 ml syringe
- 25 swg × ⅝in. (0.5 mm x 16 mm) needle
- 23 swg × 1 in. (0.6 mm x 25 mm)needle
- 21 swg × 1½in. (0.8 mm x 40 mm) needle
- ampoule 10 ml 1% lignocaine with or without added adrenaline 1:200 000
- skin closure strips (Steri-strips) 6 mm × 75 mm (Ref. 3M GP41)
- sterile monofilament nylon suture 4/0 Ethilon (Ref. W319) (Ethicon) 19 mm curved cutting needle
- electrocautery with platinum tip burner or equivalent unipolar diathermy for coagulation.

25.1 GENERAL TECHNIQUE FOR EXCISION

The first consideration with any dermal lesion is a provisional diagnosis; secondly, does it need to be removed? Lesions such as the infant's strawberry naevus should be left alone as it always resolves completely (Fig. 25.1 a–c). Similarly many warts and molluscum contagiosum may well regress spontaneously and be better left to nature (Fig. 25.2 a, b). The third consideration, once it has been decided to remove any dermal lesion, is to decide the line of the final scar, bearing in mind that scars in the line of skin creases and wrinkles are much neater, as are transverse scars across joints, and scars which lie at right-angles to the direction of pull of underlying muscles (Chapter 10). Picking up the skin and squeezing the lesion between finger and thumb will demonstrate skin creases and also help to assess whether excision will result in too much skin tension. The fourth consideration is the method of removal – is this lesion better excised, or

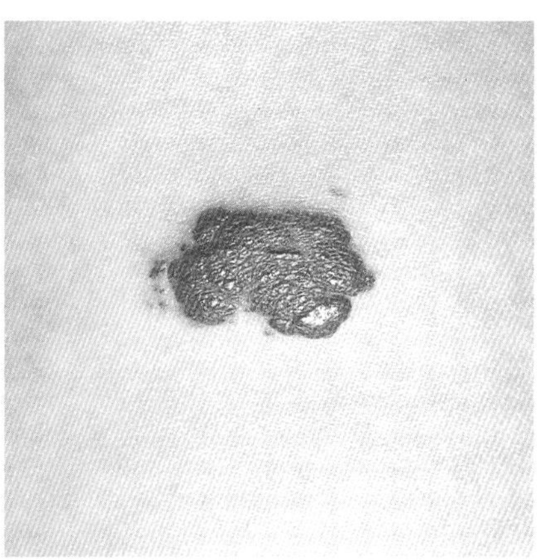

Fig. 25.1a The strawberry naevus, which will disappear completely without any treatment; it should never be excised or cauterized.

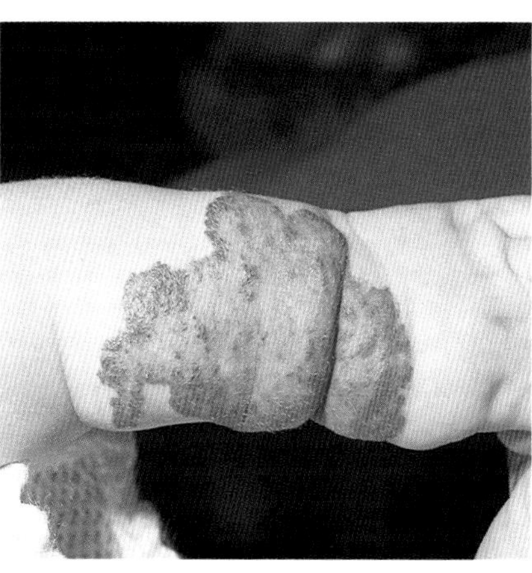

Fig. 25.1b Large strawberry naevus (superficial angioma) on forearm.

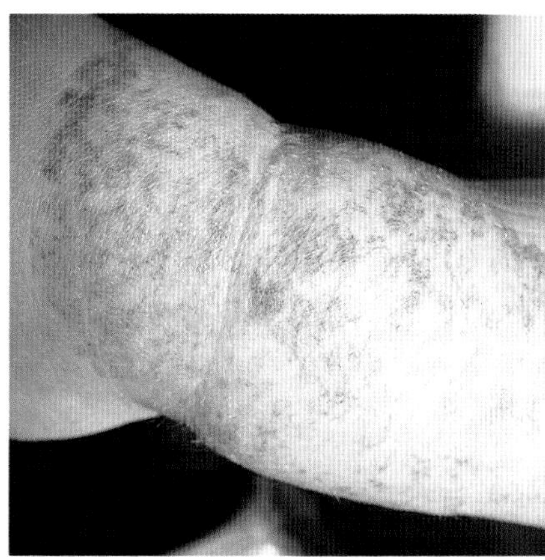

Fig. 25.1c Strawberry naevus (superficial angioma) showing spontaneous resolution.

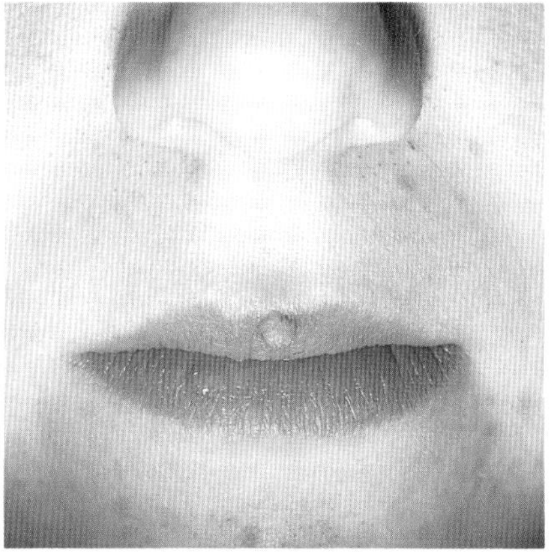

Fig. 25.2a Many viral warts disappear spontaneously without leaving a scar.

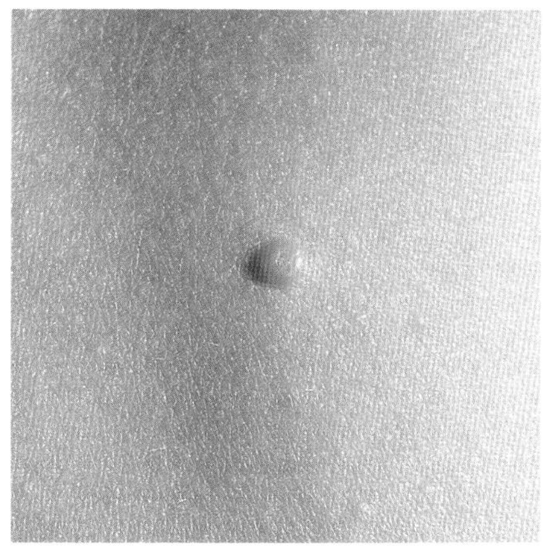

Fig. 25.2b Solitary molluscum contagiosum. Many will clear spontaneously.

curetted and cauterized, desiccated, fulgurized, treated with the diathermy or cryoprobe or radio-surgery, or is the diagnosis such that a preliminary skin biopsy should be taken?

Assuming excision is the method of choice, the lesion and surrounding skin is liberally painted with povidone-iodine in spirit (Betadine alcoholic solution) and the area anaesthetized using infiltration of local anaesthetic.

For small lesions, a skin bleb of lignocaine is raised at either end of the proposed scar using either a 30 swg needle and dental syringe or a 25 swg × 5/8 in. (0.5 mm × 16 mm) needle (Fig. 25.3a). The needle is then changed for a larger one, either 23 swg (0.6 mm) or 21 swg (0.8 mm) and inserted through the skin bleb, infiltrating the underlying skin in a fan shape distribution from either end. A sterile 'lithotomy type' drape is put over the skin, leaving just the lesion exposed. After washing and scrubbing the hands thoroughly with chlorhexidine in detergent (Hibiscrub) they are dried, and a pair of sterile surgical gloves applied.

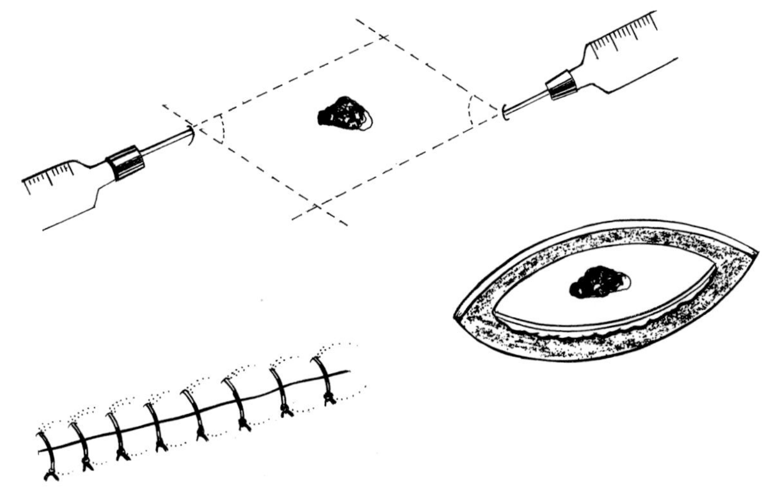

Fig. 25.3a Method for infiltrating skin with local anaesthetic for excision of intradermal lesion, and skin closure with interrupted sutures.

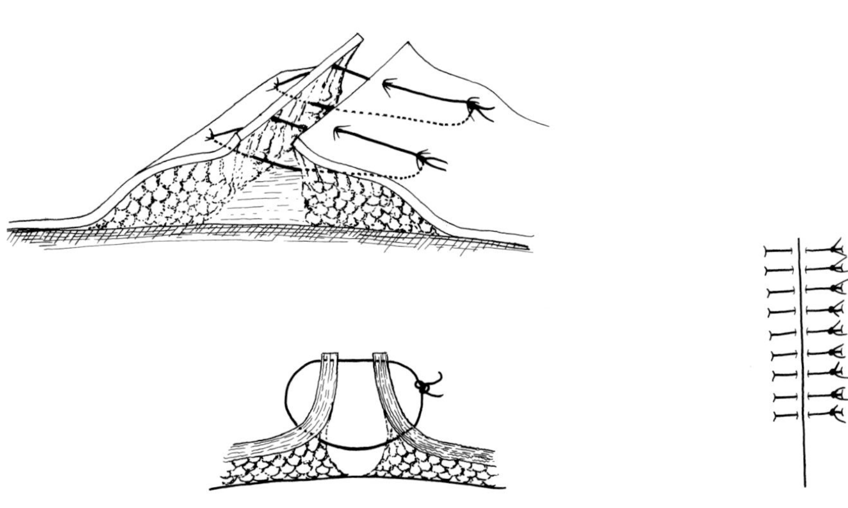

Fig. 25.3b Method of skin closure to avoid inversion of the skin edges (vertical mattress suture).

From now on a completely aseptic technique must be used, preferably no-touch, with the minimum of tissue trauma and handling. The wearing of a face-mask is optional – provided the operator does not cough, sneeze, or talk continuously over the wound, it is probably not essential. However, wearing a mask does protect the patient from droplet infection, and does enable the doctor to hold a conversation with the patient, explaining the procedure. Similarly if the patient has any upper respiratory infection, or is liable to cough, sneeze, or talk, he or she should likewise wear a mask, as should any assistant.

The lesion is now excised using an elliptical incision through skin and subcutaneous tissues, attempting to excise a triangular wedge of tissue rather than leaving a flat base. Any small bleeding points can be controlled with pressure alone using a sterile gauze swab. The excised wedge/ellipse of tissue is placed immediately in a histology container and covered with 10% formol-saline as fixative. This container should be promptly labelled with the patient's name, date, and nature of specimen, and if appropriate, which side or digit. The resulting wound is generally much bigger than expected due to retraction of the skin edges; bleeding vessels usually stop spontaneously, any brisk bleeding can be controlled by artery forceps.

It is a good idea at this stage to ascertain whether the skin edges will approximate without undue tension. If they can be brought together easily, the wound may be stitched forthwith; if tension is present, it is worth undercutting the edges with a scalpel so that the skin will slide over the subcutaneous tissues, and then suturing the wound.

The two reasons for poor healing are dead spaces and undue skin tension. Dead spaces fill with blood and serum and produce a subcutaneous haematoma which can become infected, while undue tension on skin edges produces ischaemia, non-union, and necrosis.

Both dead spaces and skin tension can be dealt with by the judicious use of absorbable subcutaneous sutures such as catgut or coated vicryl, but only the minimum number necessary should be used as too many act as foreign bodies and increase the risks of infection.

Generally the wound is best closed using interrupted monofilament nylon sutures, spaced closely together, supported if necessary by the application of self-adhesive skin closure strips (Steri-strips). When inserting sutures, the aim should be to slightly evert the skin edges; this can be achieved by taking slightly more of the subcutaneous tissue in the bite of the needle than skin. If the edges still tend to invert despite this manoeuvre, the suture should be passed through the skin 1 mm from each edge (vertical mattress) (Fig. 25.3b). This is an excellent stitch, but can be difficult to remove. Depending on the site of the scar, the sutures may be removed on the 5th to 10th day, leaving the Steri-strips to give additional external support.

All that remains is the application of a dry, sterile dressing and the instructions to the patient to leave the dressing completely undisturbed until the sutures are removed, unless there is a specific reason to inspect the wound earlier. It is also helpful to rest the limb or part of the body containing the scar for at least 48 hours to initiate healing. Thereafter, gentle activity is beneficial.

25.2 CURETTE AND CAUTERY

As an alternative to surgical excision, many lesions may successfully be removed with a sharp-spoon Volkmann curette, afterwards cauterizing the base with the electrocautery to control bleeding. The technique is exactly as described under the section on warts and verrucae (Chapter 27). As with warts, it is important to find the correct plane of cleavage when using the curette; it is also helpful to have a selection of curettes of various sizes corresponding to the size of the lesion (Fig. 25.4a–c).

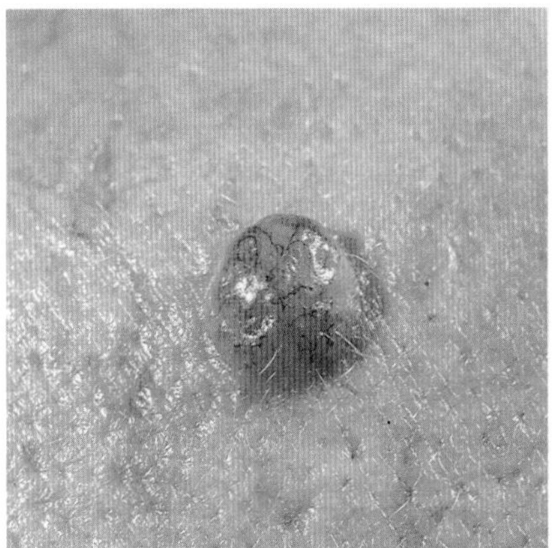

Fig. 25.4a Simple intradermal naevus, suitable for removal with curette.

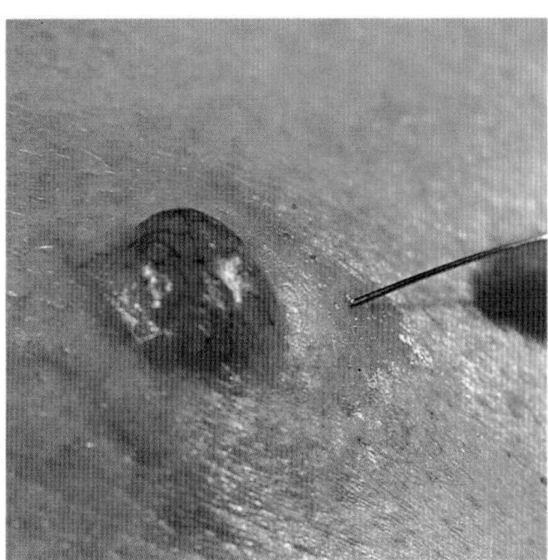

Fig. 25.4b Intradermal naevus. Infiltrating the base with local anaesthetics.

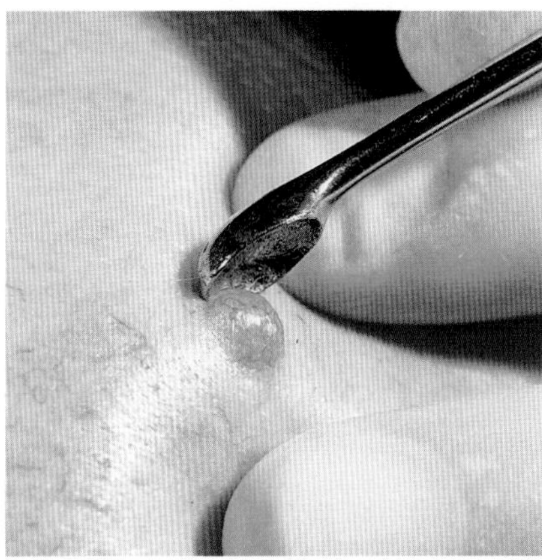

Fig. 25.4c Intradermal naevus. Removal with Volkmann sharp-spoon curette (see also Chapter 42).

25.3 INTRADERMAL NAEVI AND PIGMENTED NAEVI

Pigmented naevi are lesions characterized by a proliferation of epidermal melanocytes, later migrating downwards into the dermis. They can be divided into flat lesions, slightly raised lesions, verrucous lesions, dome-shaped lesions, and pigmented hairy lesions. The main indication for removal is any suspicion that it may be turning malignant, as suggested by sudden enlargement, alteration in the pigment, ulceration or bleeding. Most patients request removal for cosmetic reasons, or because the lesion is catching on clothing or razors when shaving. Surgical excision or radiosurgery is the treatment of choice for all pigmented naevi (Fig. 25.5).

25.4 HISTIOCYTOMA (DERMATOFIBROMA)

These are fairly common tumours found frequently on the legs, cause unknown, but may be related to trauma. They occur in the dermis and present as a smooth, firm nodule. They are benign, commonly multiple, and the treatment is surgical excision (Fig. 25.6).

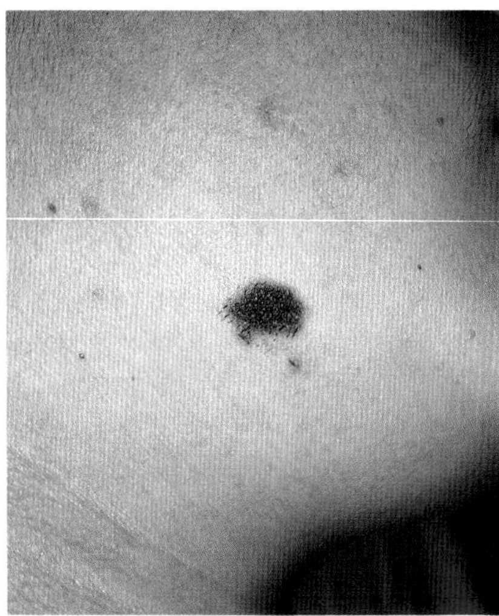

Fig. 25.5a Pigmented intradermal naevus which bled regularly after shaving.

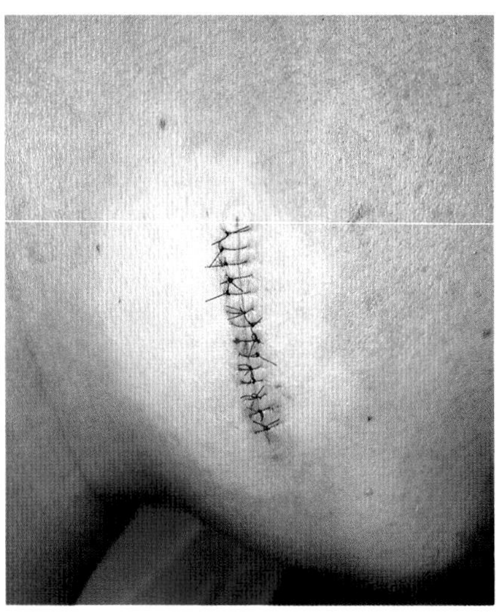

Fig. 25.5b Excised; closure with fine, interrupted sutures. (Blanching of surrounding skin is from adrenaline in the local anaesthetic.)

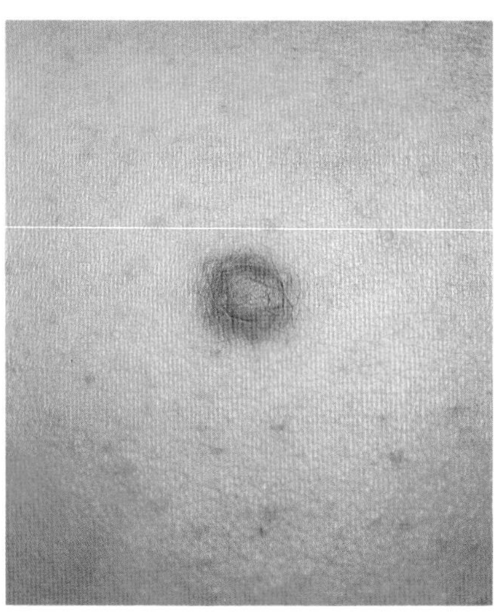

Fig. 25.6 Typical fibrous histiocytoma. Excision is the treatment of choice.

25.5 CYLINDROMA (TURBAN TUMOUR)

This is a rare tumour, also benign, occurring commonly on the scalp and initially may be mistaken for a sebaceous cyst until excision is attempted, when a firm, granular, adherent lesion is found. Treatment is surgical excision.

25.6 SOLAR KERATOSIS

As the name implies these lesions are found in areas of skin exposed to light; they are discrete and raised with a crumbling surface. As they are purely epidermal, they may be treated with radio-surgery, curettage and electrocautery or cryotherapy, using a nitrous oxide or liquid nitrogen cryoprobe, or simply shaved off with a scalpel blade and the base cauterized (Figs 25.7, 25.8–25.11).

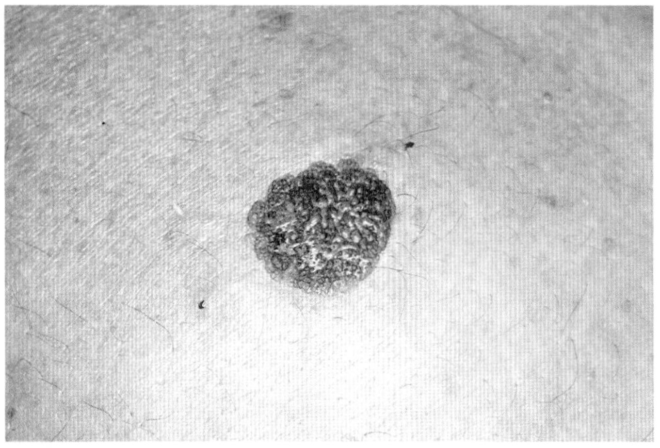

Fig. 25.7a Solar keratosis.

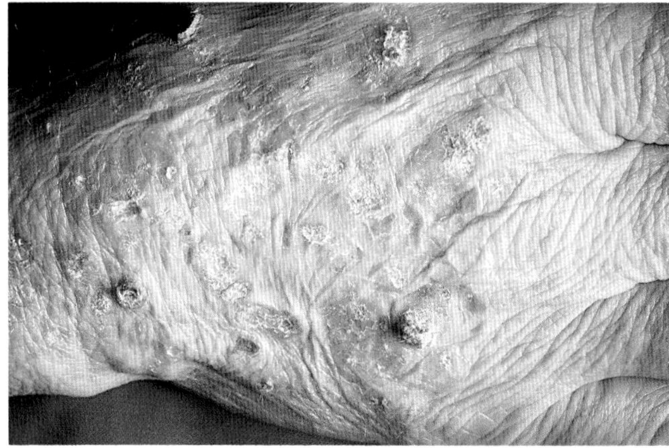

Fig. 25.7b Multiple solar keratoses, back of hand.

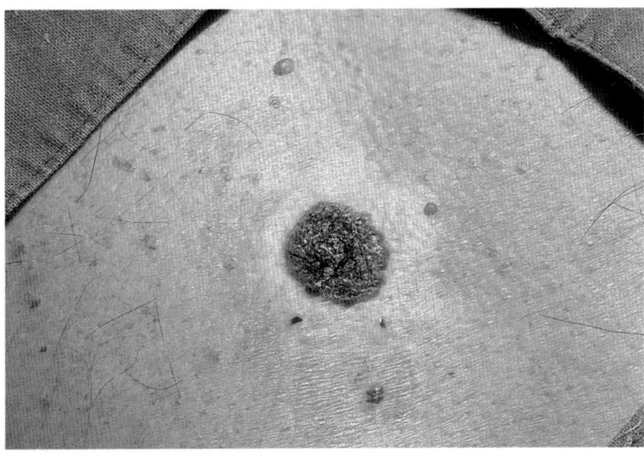

Fig. 25.8 Seborrhoeic wart on back. Infiltrate base with local anaesthetic.

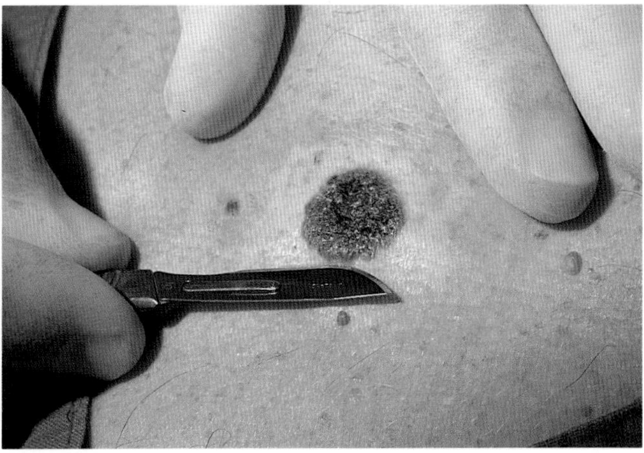

Fig. 25.9 Holding scalpel blade parallel to the skin, cut through the base of the wart.

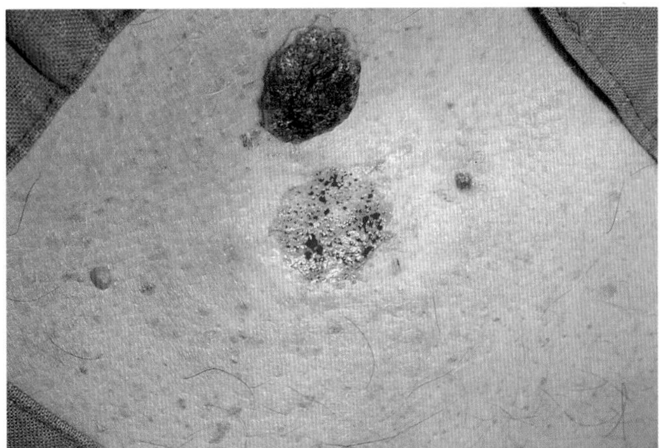

Fig. 25.10 Bleeding vessels in base.

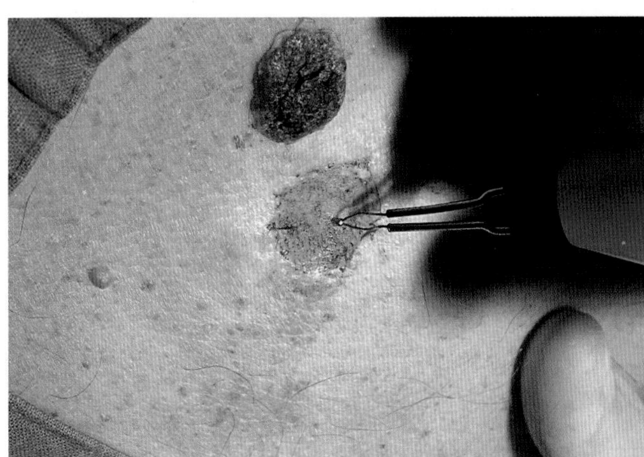

Fig. 25.11 Bleeding vessels cauterized with electro-cautery.

25.7 SEBORRHOEIC WARTS

These are due to a benign proliferation of epidermal cells: they become commoner with increasing age. They present as multiple, raised, brown or black lesions, often looking as if they had been stuck on the skin. Curettage and cautery, radio-surgery or shaving and cautery is the treatment of choice (Figs 25.8–25.13).

25.8 KERATOACANTHOMA

These are not uncommon lesions, which can be mistaken for basal and squamous cell carcinomata; they present as a small papule which grows rapidly in size over a period of 2 or 3 months. The edges are rolled over with a central depression and a thickened keratin plug. Interestingly, they gradually involute over a period of 6 months. The cause is still unknown.

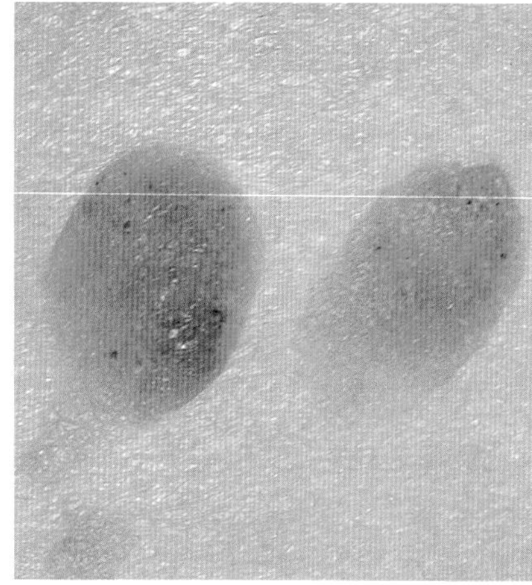

Fig. 25.12 Seborrhoeic wart, abdomen. Easily removed by curette, or shaving with scalpel, followed by cautery to the base.

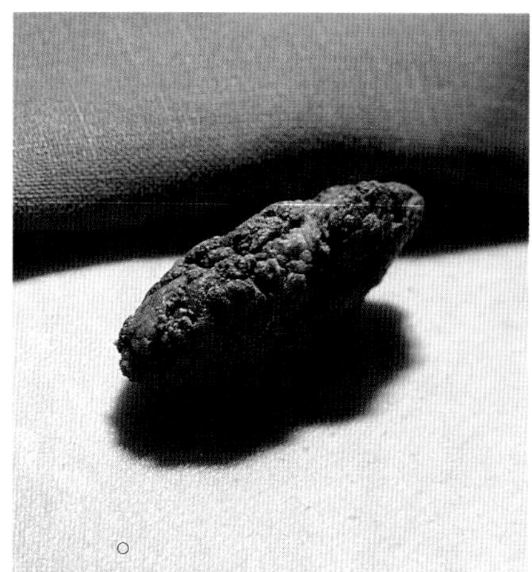

Fig. 25.13 Larger seborrhoeic wart (basal cell papilloma), equally suitable for removal.

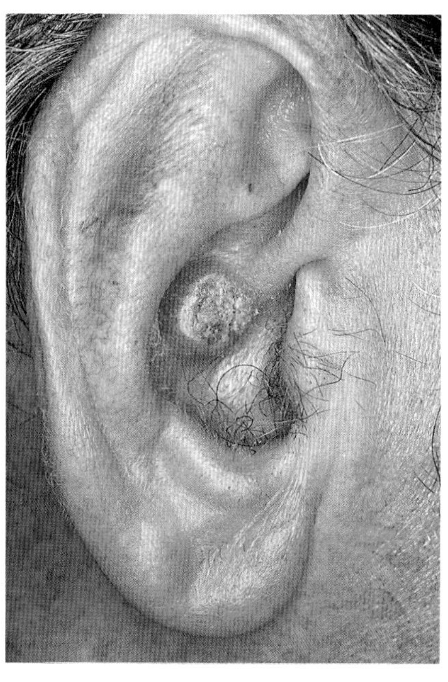

Fig. 25.14 Typical keratoacanthoma inside ear; present for 3 months, enlarging rapidly.

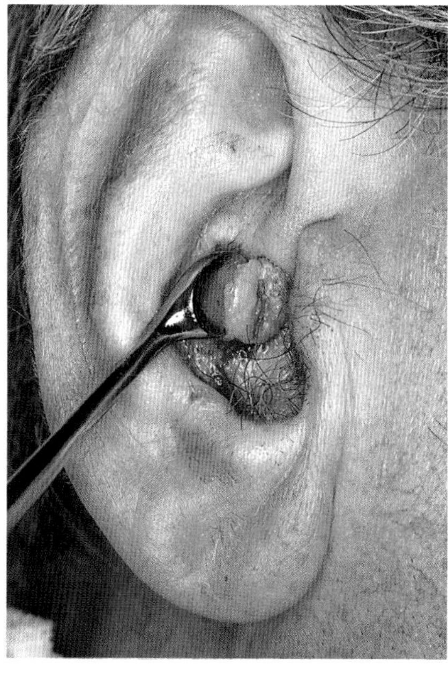

Fig. 25.15 Keratoacanthoma. Easily curretted with sharp-spoon curette.

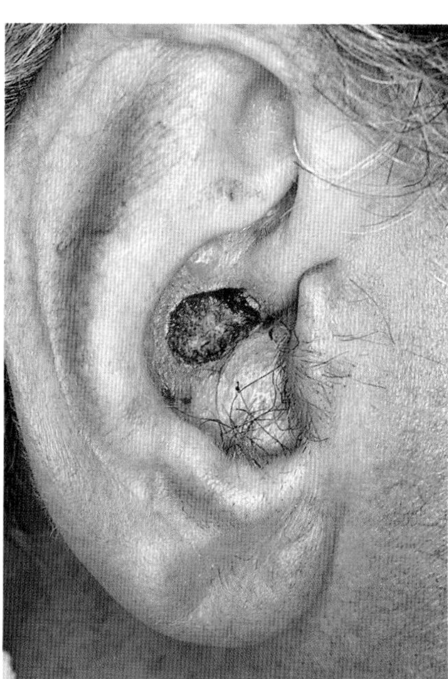

Fig. 25.16 The base of the lesion is cauterized with the electrocautery.

Treatment is by curettage and cautery or complete excision biopsy (Figs 25.14–25.18).

25.9 GRANULOMA PYOGENICUM (ERUPTIVE ANGIOMA)

This is a type of haemangioma, so called because it was originally thought to be due to infection by a staphylococcus. It presents as a solitary raised swelling, bright red in colour, and bleeds profusely. The most effective treatment is curettage and cautery under local anaesthesia (Figs 25.19–25.21).

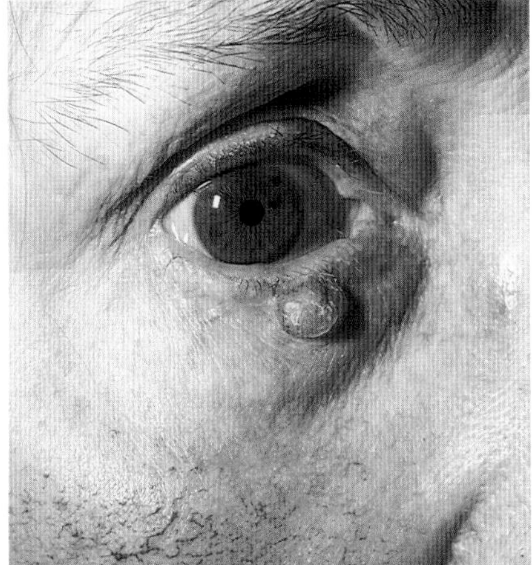

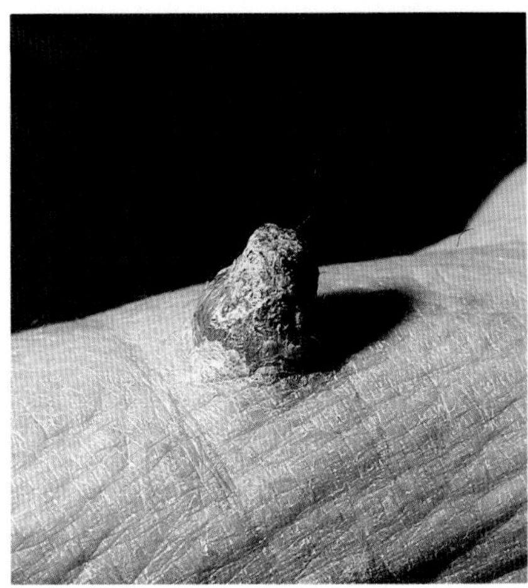

Fig. 25.17 An atypical, early keratoacanthoma; this could have been mistaken for a basal cell carcinoma.

Fig. 25.18 A typical keratoacanthoma, easily curetted and base cauterized.

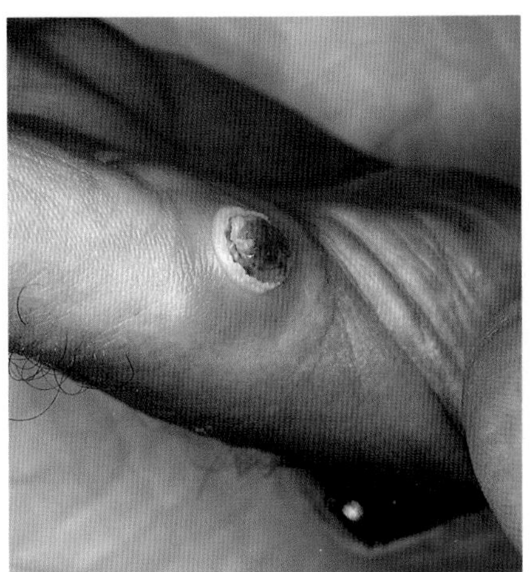

Fig. 25.19 Granuloma pyogenicum on palmar surface of hand. Treatment by curette and cautery.

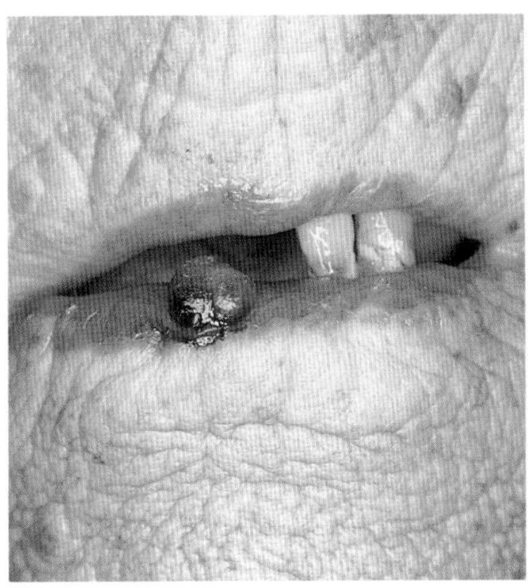

Fig. 25.20a Granuloma pyogenicum on lower lip.

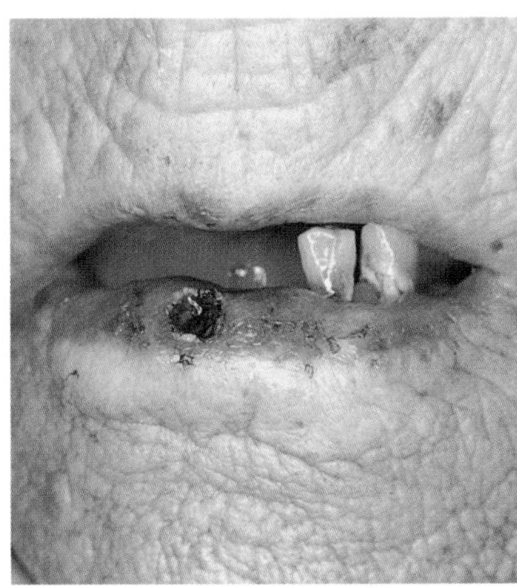

Fig. 25.20b After removal with curette, and with base cauterized under infiltration local anaesthesia.

Fig. 25.21 Granuloma pyogenicum on tongue. Treatment by either curettage or cautery or radio-surgical excision using wire loop. Bleeding, which can be brisk, is controlled by pressure and coagulation electrode.

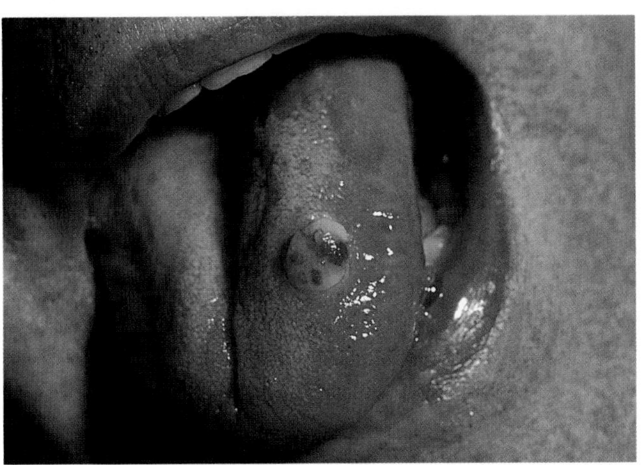

25.10 SPIDER NAEVI

These are common vascular lesions typified by a very small central red arteriole from which radiate fine, superficial blood vessels. The most effective treatment is radio-surgery or electrocautery to the central arteriole without anaesthetic, or inserting the needle electrode of the Hyfrecator into the arteriole, also without anaesthetic (Figs 25.22–25.25).

25.11 HAEMANGIOMA

Various vascular tumours and lesions are seen on the skin. Cavernous haemangiomata frequently occur on the lower lip and face. The problem with excision is that of haemorrhage, but good cosmetic results may be obtained by desiccation or coagulation using the unipolar diathermy. Treatment consists of inserting either the single needle electrode or a pair

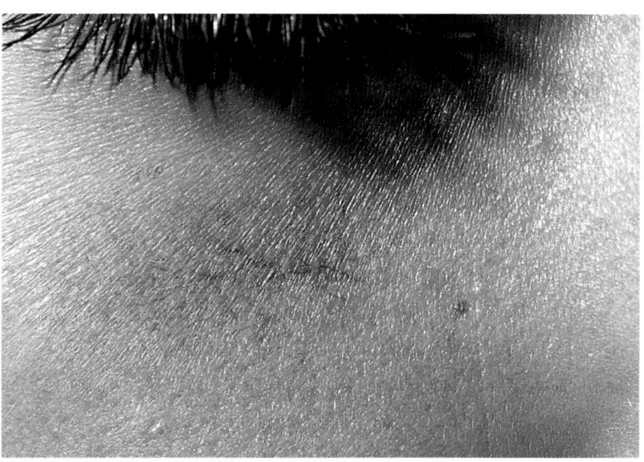

Fig. 25.22 Typical spider naevus on face.

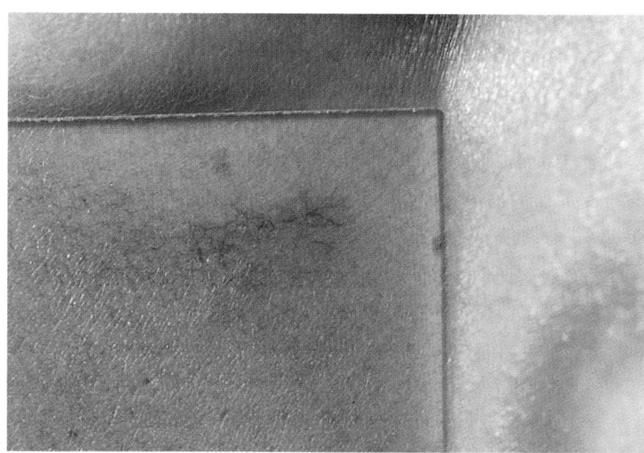

Fig. 25.23 Using pressure with a microscope slide demonstrates the feeding arteriole.

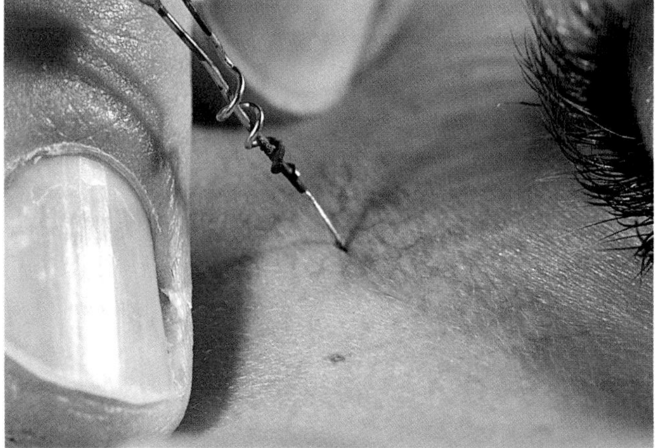

Fig. 25.24 Using the cold point electrocautery burner, or needle diathermy electrode, the arteriole is coagulated.

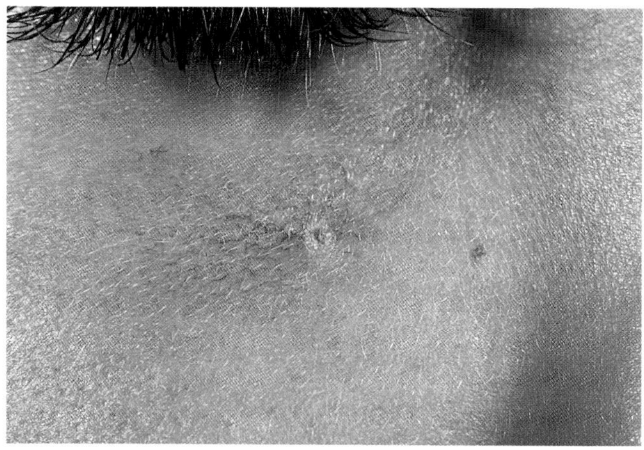

Fig. 25.25 The appearance immediately following cautery.

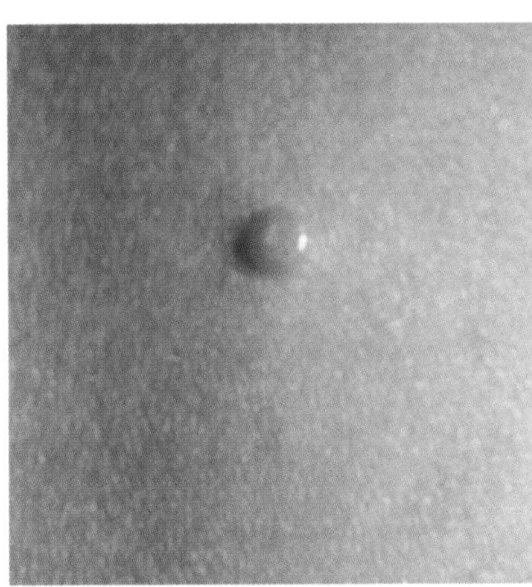

Fig. 25.26 Single lesion of molluscum contagiosum. Easily treated, but difficult to anaesthetize in young children.

of bipolar electrodes into the centre of the lesion and passing a high-frequency current through the haemangioma. Coagulation rapidly occurs, the procedure is virtually bloodless, and healing occurs rapidly over the ensuing 3–4 weeks. Larger vascular lesions may require more than one treatment.

25.12 MOLLUSCUM CONTAGIOSUM

This is a viral tumour of the skin, commonly seen in children. It has a typically pearly appearance with an umbilicated centre. Treatment is either pricking each lesion with a pointed stick soaked in phenol, or destruction using the electrocautery or diathermy, following anaesthesia with Emla cream or local infiltration (Fig. 25.26). Good results have also been reported using a fine liquid nitrogen cryoprobe.

25.13 REMOVAL OF TATTOOS

Many patients request the removal of tattoos which have been self-inflicted or professionally performed; small tattoos are excised exactly as any intradermal lesion, larger tattoos are better referred to a plastic surgeon or treated with the laser.

25.14 JUVENILE MELANOMA

This is a lightly, or non-pigmented naevus which appears in childhood and grows rapidly. Histologically, juvenile melanomata may resemble malignant melanomata, but they are always benign. (Pigmented naevi rarely undergo malignant change before puberty.) Treatment, therefore, is surgical excision (Figs 25.27 and 25.28).

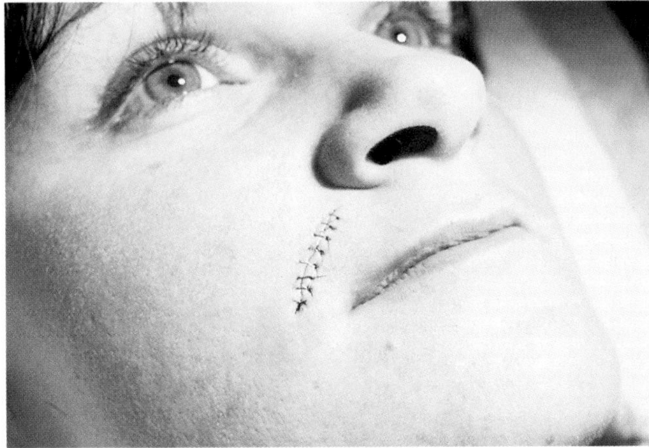

Fig. 25.27 Suture line following excision of dark pigmented naevus. Note line of scar to coincide with skin crease and numerous fine interrupted Prolene sutures.

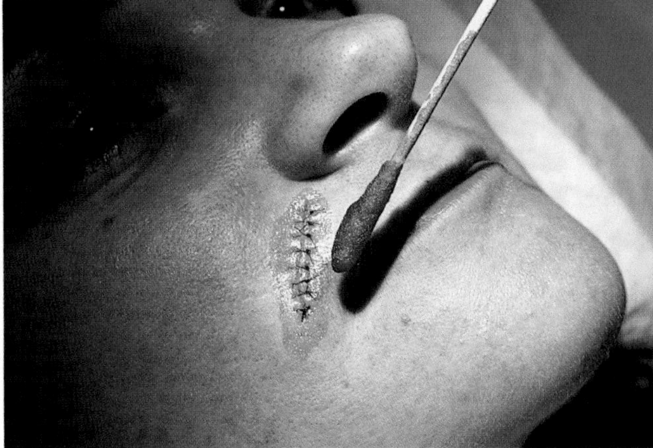

Fig. 25.28 Tincture Benzoin Co. being applied to the fine sutures to prevent knots 'slipping'. These sutures will be removed after 4 days and the wound supported with Steri-strips.

25.15 MALIGNANT MELANOMA

This is a tumour of epidermal melanocytes, and the incidence throughout the world is rapidly rising. The exact cause is not fully understood, but appears to be related to increasing exposure to sunlight, particularly short sharp bursts resulting in burning of the skin.

In the UK the female: male ratio for melanoma is 2:1, and in women 50% occur on the legs, while in males, the trunk is the commonest site.

Three common varieties are seen in general practice:

1. Superficial spreading melanoma. This is the commonest lesion, presenting as irregular, brown/black/bluish lesions with intermingled reddened areas (Fig. 25.29a, b, c).
2. Lentigo maligna melanoma usually occurs on the sun-exposed skin, commonly on the face in the elderly (Fig. 25.29b).
3. Nodular melanoma is the most rapidly growing and most malignant. It can occur anywhere on the body, often does not have much melanin, is often very vascular, and ultimately ulcerates (Fig. 25.29c).

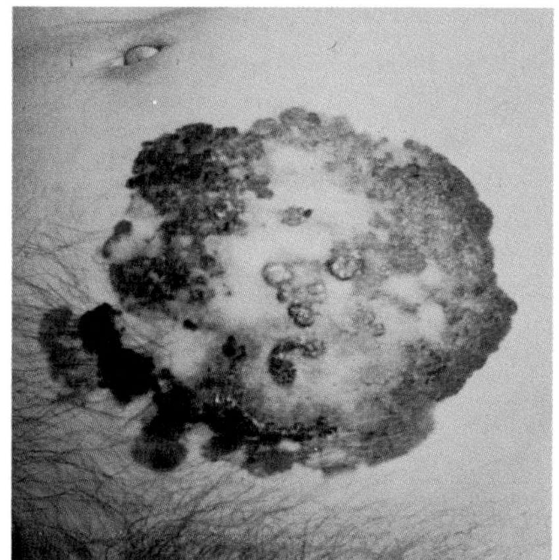

Fig. 25.29a Superficial spreading malignant melanoma.

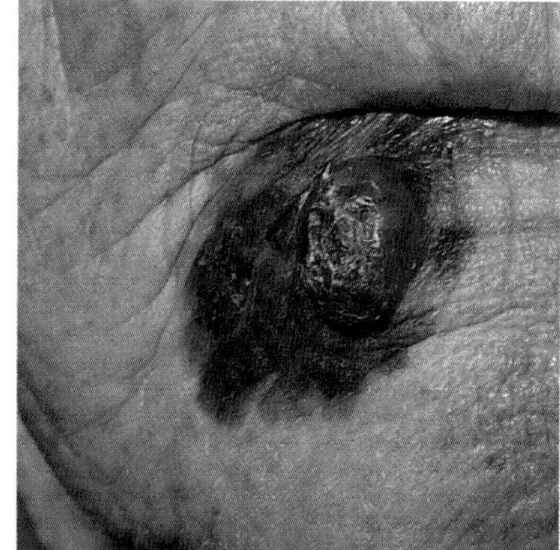

Fig. 25.29b Lentigo maligna melanoma.

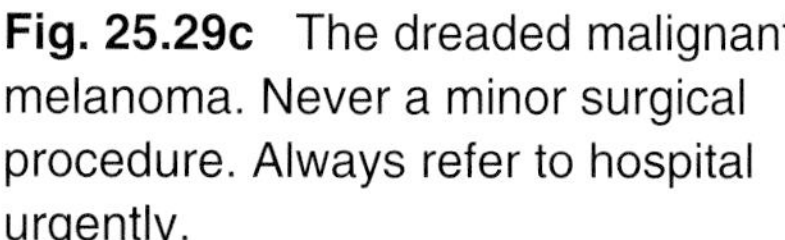

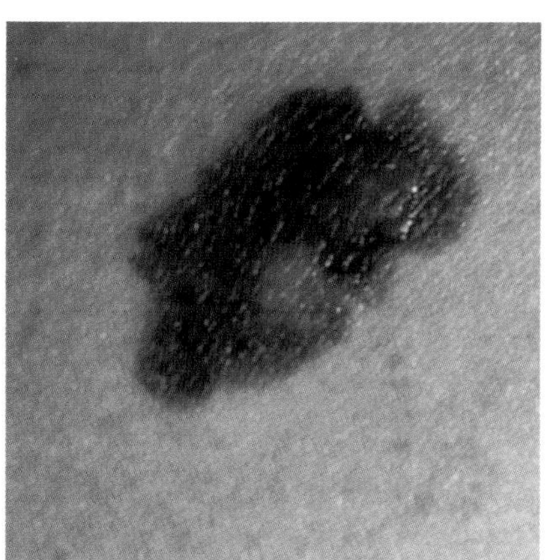

Fig. 25.29c The dreaded malignant melanoma. Never a minor surgical procedure. Always refer to hospital urgently.

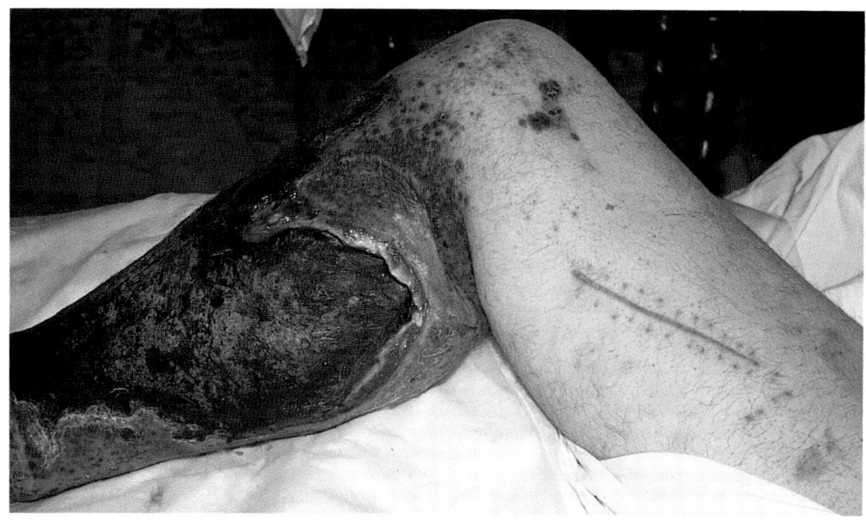

Fig. 25.30 Malignant melanoma. Six months after Fig. 25.29c. Despite wide excision in hospital and chemotherapy, metastatic spread ensued. (Patient died 3 months later.)

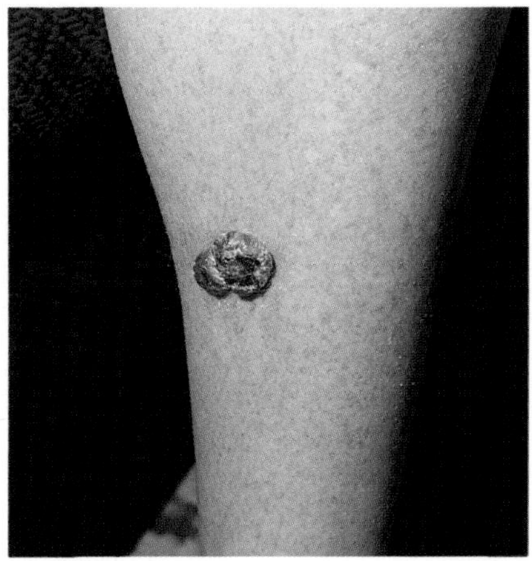

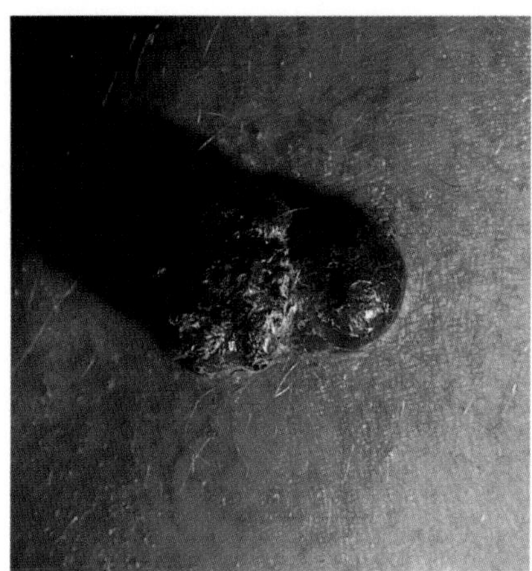

Fig. 25.31a Another malignant melanoma on the leg. Widely excised; patient still alive 20 years later.

Fig. 25.31b Close-up of same malignant melanoma. Prognosis totally unpredictable.

Occasionally there may be no pigment – the 'amelanotic malignant melanoma' which can be extremely difficult to diagnose (Fig. 25.32).

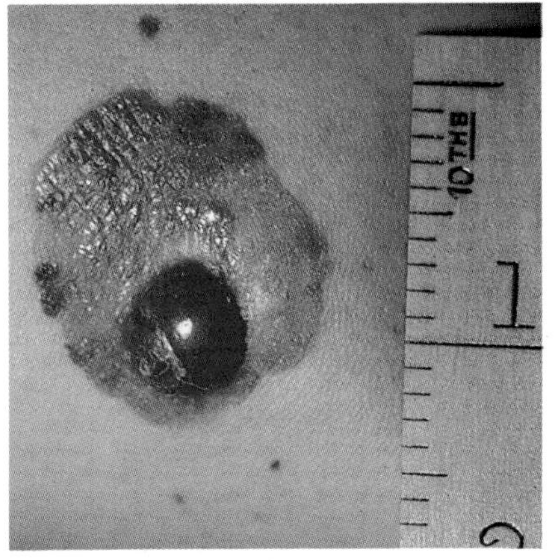

Fig. 25.32 Superficial nodular amelanotic malignant melanoma.

25.15.1 Prognosis of malignant melanoma

Our understanding of the natural history of malignant melanoma has changed in the last 10 years, and it is now recognized that it is the histological depth of the lesion that determines survival or otherwise. This measurement, in millimetres, from the overlying granular layer of the epidermis to the deepest identifiable tumour cells is known as the tumour thickness or Breslow thickness. An alternative classification is the Clarke grading I–IV which is also related to tumour thickness.

If the Breslow thickness is less than 1 mm, there is a 90% 5-year survival rate, whereas lesions measuring 3–3.5 mm or more carry a 40% 5-year survival rate. This knowledge now means that it is not necessary to always widely excise and skin-graft all malignant melanomas, but a more selective approach may be adopted.

If the patient presents with a thick, nodular malignant melanoma, the prognosis is already bad and the chance of metastases is very high. In these patients, wide excision, skin grafting, and chemotherapy should be tried, with or without lymph node dissection, and treatment offered in a centre specializing in malignant melanomata.

If, however, the patient presents with a shallow, small melanoma, excision with a 5 mm border is all that is probably required for cure.

Furthermore, if a melanoma is inadvertently excised, and the histological report received in less than 10 days, it is safe to reoperate and perform a wider excision without prejudicing the outcome.

Thus, two requests should be made to the histopathologist if a suspected melanoma has been excised.

1. May the histology report be given to you within 10 days.
2. If positive, could you be told the Breslow thickness in millimetres.

As a general guide, malignant melanomas should never be removed by the general practitioner, but referred to a specialist unit.

25.16 BASAL CELL CARCINOMA (BCC OR RODENT ULCER)

This is the commonest malignant tumour of the skin, usually occurring on the face and appears to be induced by exposure to ultraviolet light. It starts as a small papule which spreads, leaving a central ulcer. The edges are pearl-coloured with fine telangiectasia; left alone they slowly increase in size but never metastasize. Treatment is by radiotherapy (95% cure), surgical excision (95% cure) or curettage and cautery (80% cure). Small basal cell carcinomata are easily treated by the general practitioner and although curettage and cautery gives a lower cure rate than radiotherapy, it gives a better cosmetic result.

When treating small basal cell carcinomata by curette and cautery, improved results are obtained if the curette/cautery sequence is repeated three times to ensure eradication of the basal layer. Surgical excision is the treatment of choice to give the neatest scar (Figs 25.33–25.35).

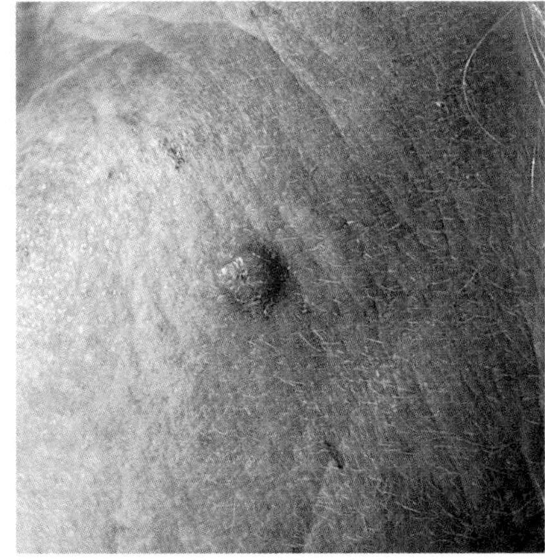

Fig. 25.33 Basal cell carcinoma (rodent ulcer) on typical site. Line of eventual scar marked with two green dots in skin crease.

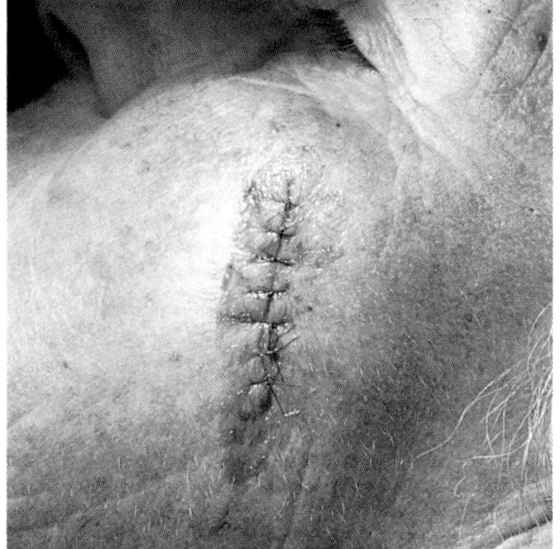

Fig. 25.34 Line of excision to coincide with skin crease.

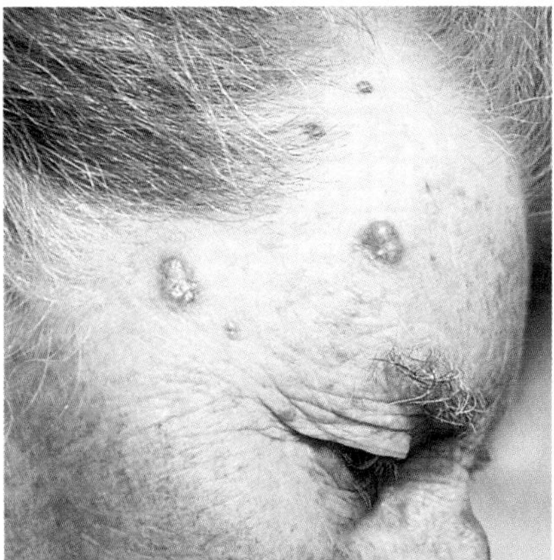

Fig. 25.35a Patient with multiple basal-cell carcinomata on face.

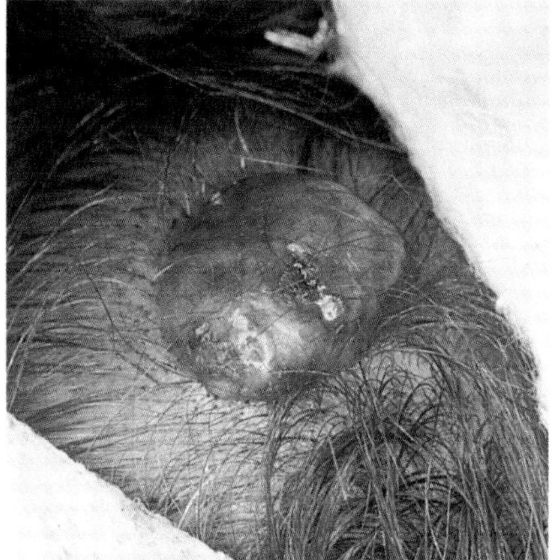

Fig. 25.35b Unusually large basal-cell carcinoma occurring on scalp of patient aged 93. Removal was by electrocautery dissection in view of age. Completely cured.

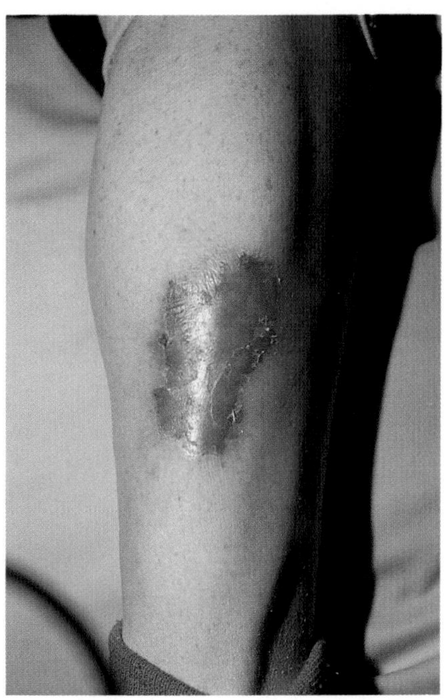

Fig. 25.36 A large deceptive area of Bowen's disease (carcinoma-in-situ) on the lower leg, present for 18 months, confirmed by biopsy and treated successfully with liquid nitrogen cryosurgery.

25.17 SQUAMOUS CELL EPITHELIOMA

This, too, is thought to be due to over-exposure to ultraviolet light. It can occur anywhere on the body and can affect the mucous membranes, particularly lips and tongue. Unlike the basal cell epithelioma, squamous celled carcinomata have the ability to metastasize, but nevertheless if treated early the prognosis is excellent. Treatment is by surgical excision, radiotherapy, or both.

25.18 CARCINOMA-IN-SITU (BOWEN'S DISEASE)

This is a form of intraepithelial carcinoma-in-situ which can occasionally metastasize and or progress to an invasive squamous cell carcinoma. Originally many Bowen's lesions were thought to be due to arsenic.

It presents as an isolated, scaling, erythematous plaque, not dissimilar to psoriasis. Surgical excision is the treatment of choice, but in carefully selected cases nitrogen cryosurgery is successful (Fig. 25.36).

25.19 KELOIDS

Despite meticulous care in skin closure, certain patients develop hypertrophic or keloid scars. These occur more frequently in dark-skinned individuals and in certain sites of the body, particularly in front of the sternum.

If a patient gives a history of developing hypertrophic or keloid scars in previous surgery, serious consideration should be given as to the advisability of performing surgery, as the likelihood of another keloid scar is high. Similarly, a request from a patient to excise a keloid scar should be resisted, as an even larger keloid scar is likely to be the end result.

Faced with a keloid scar, intralesional steroids, e.g. triamcinolone, should be tried monthly, and often give good results. When operating on a patient with a tendency to keloid scar formation, it may be helpful to apply a strong steroid cream during the postoperative healing phase, in an attempt to prevent the hypertrophic reaction. For medicolegal reasons it would be prudent to advise the patient about the risks of hypertrophic scarring, and to record this advice in the patient's notes.

25.20 SKIN BIOPSY

One of the advantages of general practitioner minor surgery is the ability to establish a rapid diagnosis of any suspect skin lesion by a simple biopsy. The technique is not difficult and, where histology facilities exist, a firm diagnosis is possible in a matter of days. The object is to choose a representative lesion, including the margin, together with a piece of adjacent healthy skin, and to remove a narrow ellipse, closing the wound with one or two fine interrupted Prolene sutures. Neater results may be obtained by the use of a skin punch-biopsy instrument (Downs Surgical). These are manufactured in different sizes and consist of a sharpened steel tube mounted on a handle. They may be disposable (Stiefel Laboratories) or reusable (Downs Surgical and Chas Thackray Ltd) (Figs 25.37a, b, c and

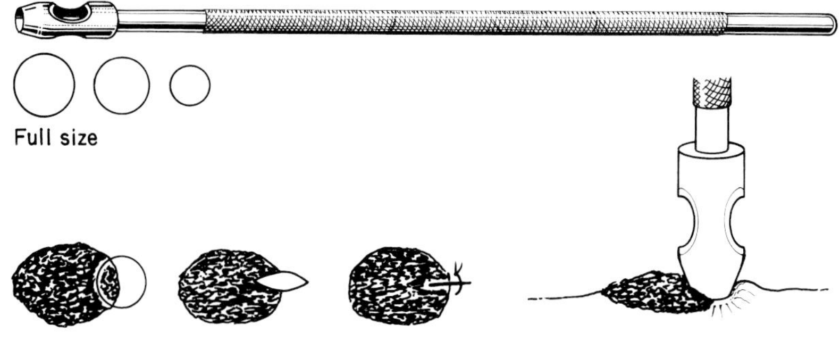

Fig. 25.37a Skin biopsy: the Hayes Martin skin punch biopsy instrument (Chas F. Thackray Ltd) with three interchangeable heads. Closure is usually with just one stitch.

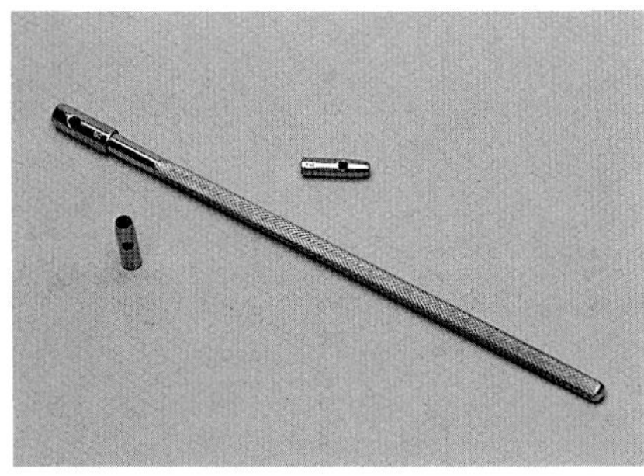

Fig. 25.37b Hayes Martin skin punch biopsy instrument.

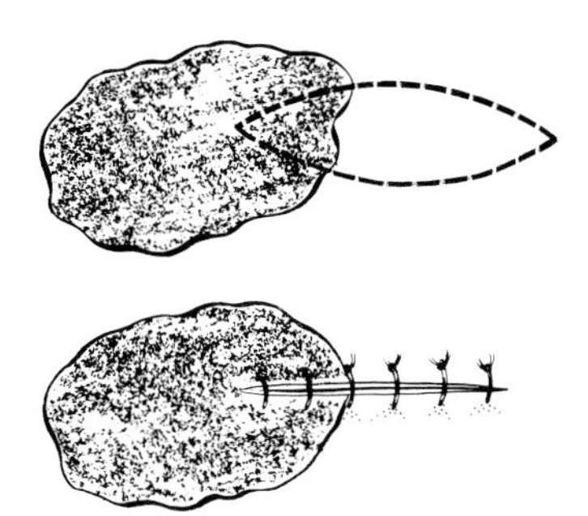

Fig. 25.37c Incision and closure for skin biopsy using scalpel.

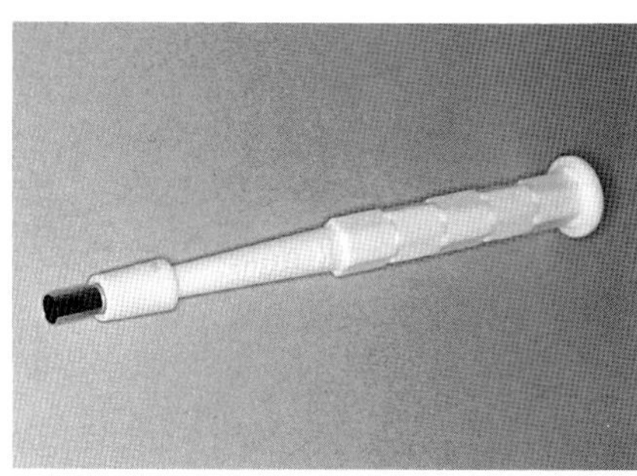

Fig. 25.38 Disposable, sterile skin biopsy punch (Stiefel Laboratory).

25.38). It is good practice to send every specimen for routine histological examination.

After choosing a representative area, which is then anaesthetized, the skin is stretched taut, and the punch pressed firmly against the skin. By rotating the handle a core of skin and subcutaneous tissue is obtained. Closure is usually with just one stitch.

26

Skin tags and papillomata

Polypi are pendulous fleshy indolent tumours, so-called from their supposed resemblances to the animal of that name. A ligature is passed round it and daily tightened till the tumour drops off

Encyclopaedia Britannica, 1797

It is surprising how many patients have lived with their assorted skin tags and squamous papillomata, feeling they were too trivial a condition to seek medical advice; yet they have caused much anxiety and embarrassment. The majority are easily removed in a matter of minutes, the diagnosis confirmed histologically, and the patient's anxiety allayed.

Instruments required:

- 5 ml syringe
- 25 swg × 5/8 in. (0.5 mm × 16 mm) needle
- ampoule 1% lignocaine with 1:200 000 adrenaline
- pair toothed dissecting forceps 5 in. (12.7 cm)
- electrocautery with pointed platinum tip burner
- Nobecutane spray or equivalent
- small adhesive plaster dressings
- histology container with 10% formol-saline.

Very small tags may be picked up with the toothed dissecting forceps and separated at the base using the electrocautery. No bleeding occurs, the procedure takes one second, a small adhesive dressing is applied, the specimen can be sent for histology, and healing takes a matter of days.

Larger skin tags or papillomata can still be removed with the electrocautery but it is better to infiltrate the base with local anaesthetic first (Figs 26.1, 26.2, 26.3 and 26.4). Where the base of the lesion is very broad, and particularly where a neat cosmetic result is desired, it is preferable to excise the papilloma under local anaesthesia, using an elliptical incision, and suturing the skin edges.

As an alternative method, if the practitioner does not possess an electrocautery, most small skin tags and papillomata may be tied off using a fine thread and allowed to drop off. This is perfectly acceptable but separation can take 1 or 2 weeks.

Fig. 26.1 Typical squamous papilloma; easily removed with the electrocautery.

Fig. 26.2 Numerous small skin tags in axilla. Easily removed with the electrocautery.

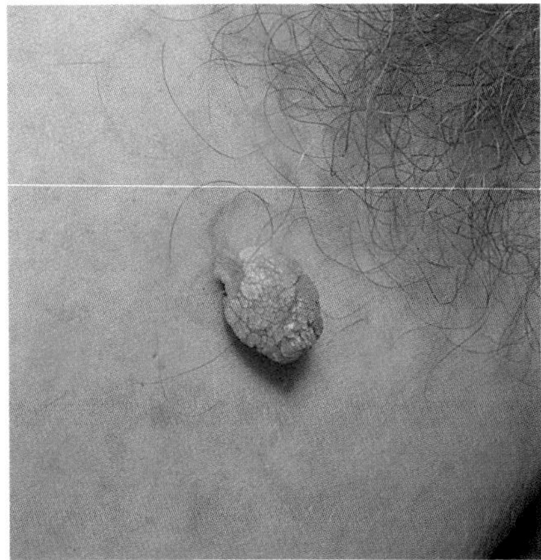

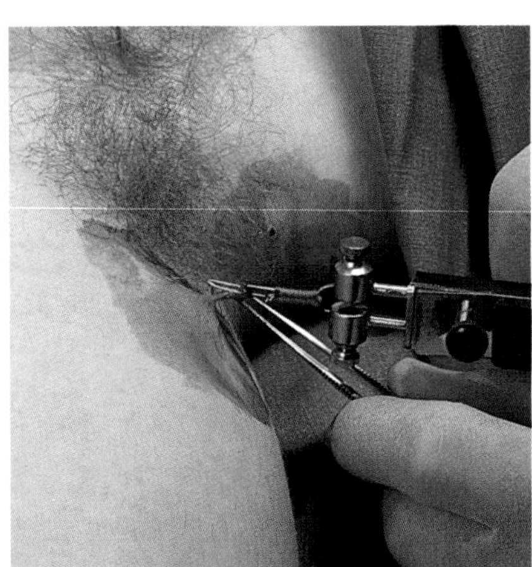

Fig. 26.3 Large fleshy fibrolipoma, base of back. Narrow base; easily removed just with electrocautery.

Fig. 26.4 Fibrolipoma. Base infiltrated with local anaesthetic and removed with the electrocautery.

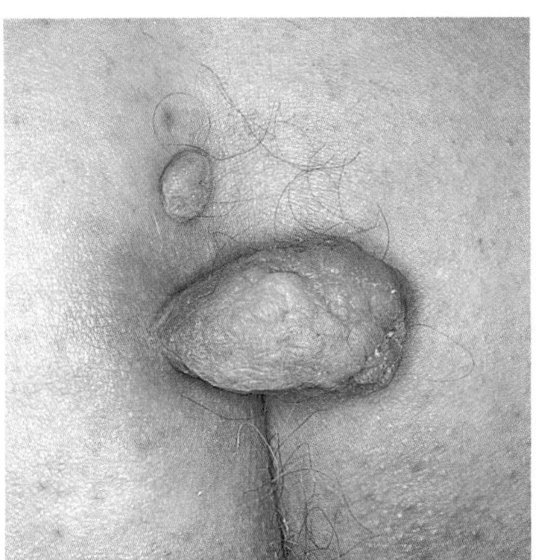

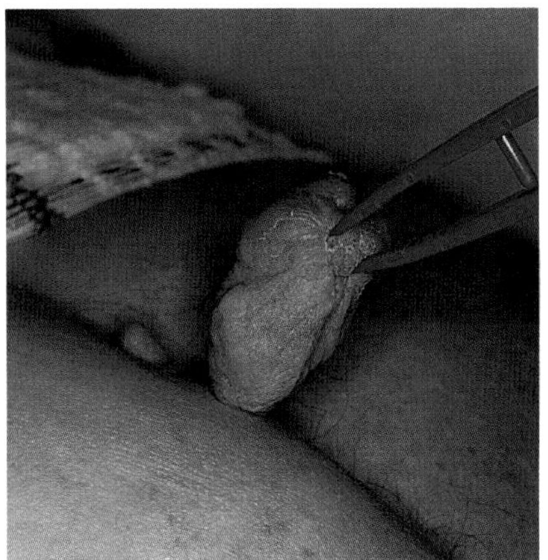

Fig. 26.5 Squamous papilloma on the posterior pillar of the fauces.

Fig. 26.6 Squamous papilloma on the tongue. Curetted and base cauterized after local infiltration of anaesthetic.

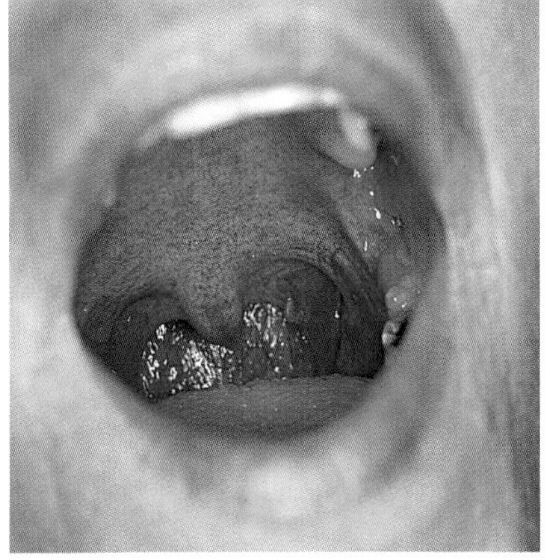

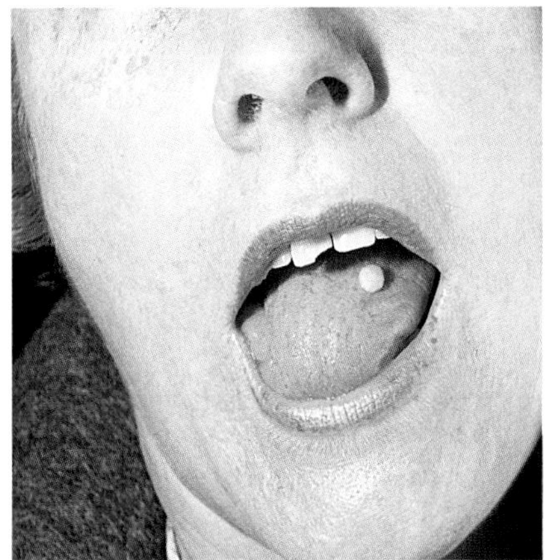

Fig. 26.7 Small cutaneous 'horn'. Easily curetted and base cauterized.

Fig. 26.8 After removal: base cauterized with the electrocautery; rapid healing.

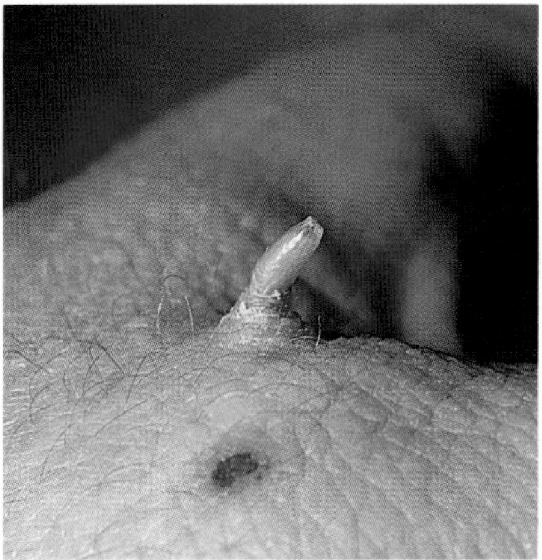

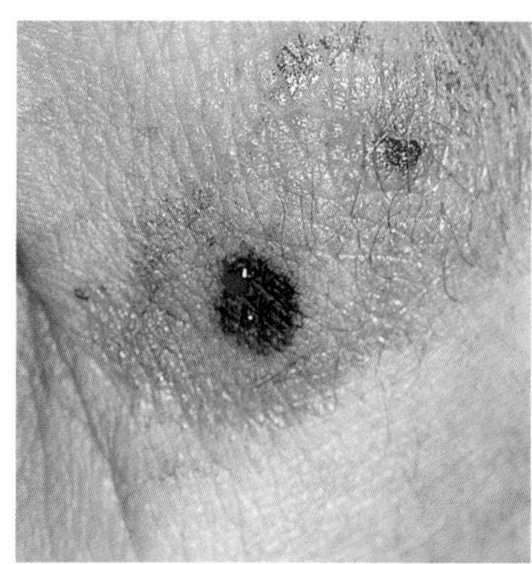

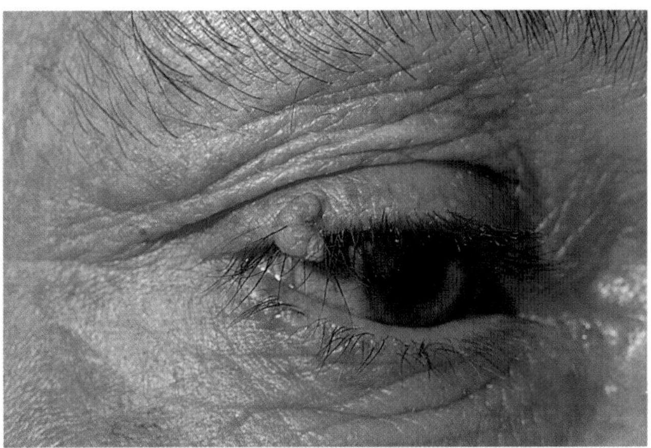

Fig. 26.9 Small, warty papilloma on upper eye-lid removed with small curette and base cauterized.

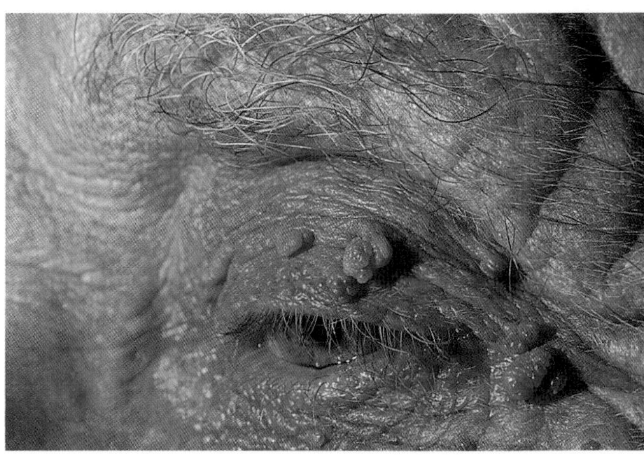

Fig. 26.10 Multiple skin tags on eye-lids. Easily removed with electrocautery 'cutting' burner. Anaesthesia by infiltration using 30 swg needle and 1% lignocaine.

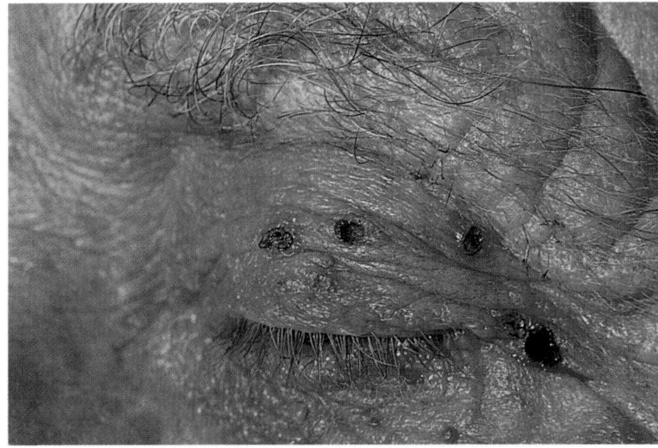

Fig. 26.11 Following removal with electrocautery. Healing occurs rapidly. No dressing is required.

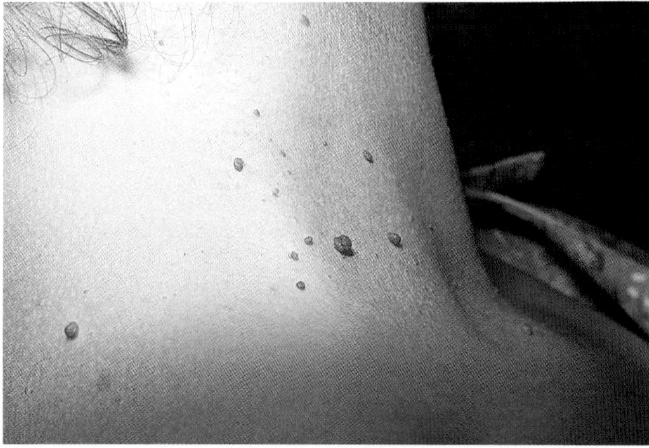

Fig. 26.12 Numerous filiform 'warts' on neck. Very common. Can be easily picked up with forceps and removed using just the electrocautery, or snipped off with scissors and any bleeding vessels touched with the cautery.

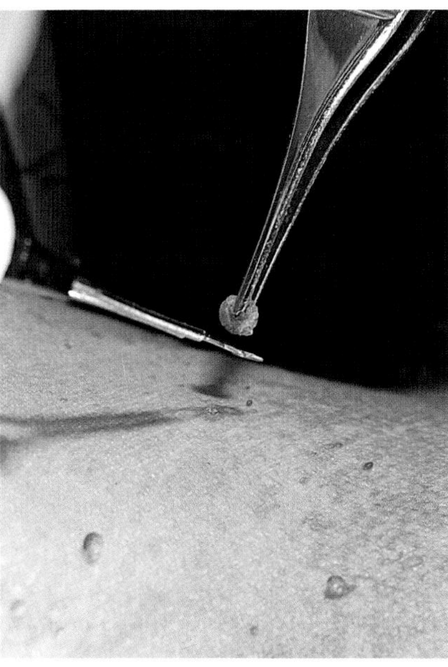

Fig. 26.13 Picking up skin tags with fine-toothed forceps and dividing with electrocautery.

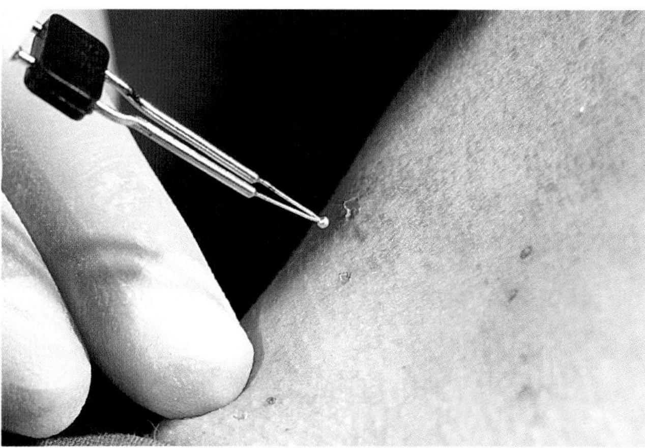

Fig. 26.14 Any bleeding points or shallow skin tags may be touched with the ball-end electrocautery burner.

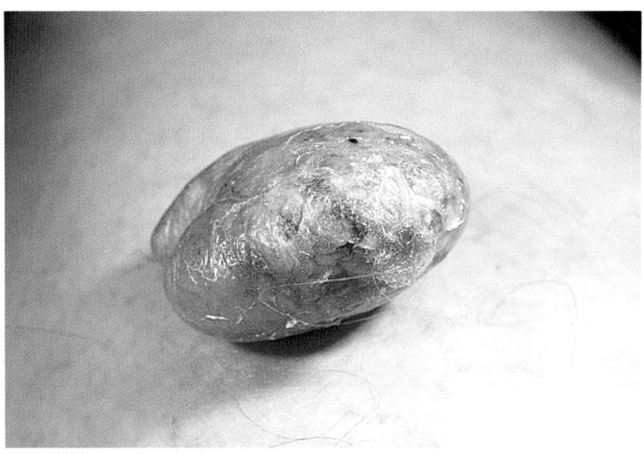

Fig. 26.15 Large fibrolipoma at back of leg. Narrow base, so suitable for division with just electrocautery.

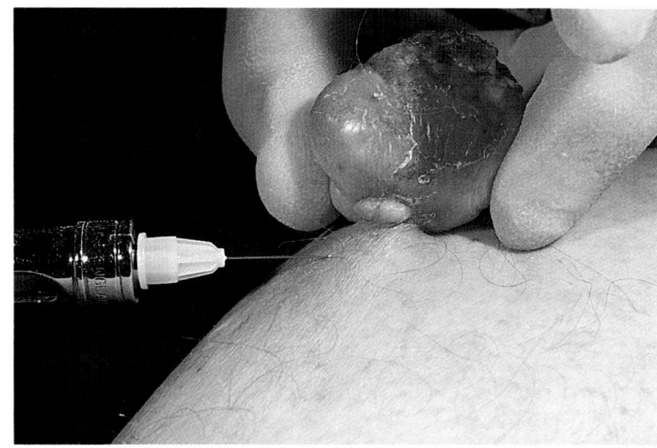

Fig. 26.16 Infiltrating the base with lignocaine 1%.

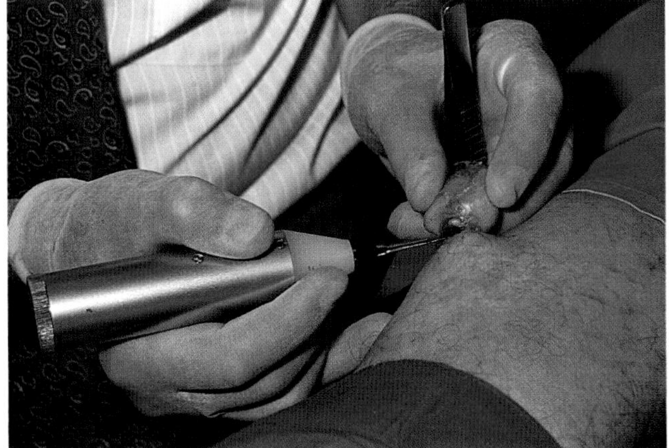

Fig. 26.17 Separating the fibrolipoma from leg using just electrocautery.

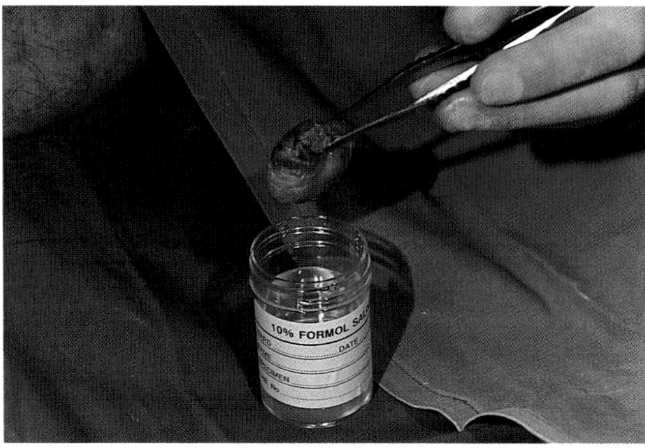

Fig. 26.18 Specimen sent for histological examination.

27

Warts and verrucae

Regardless of this, small morbid swellings arise in the skin such as myrmicia (flat warts) achrocordones, psydraces, and epinytides (herpes zoster) ... All of these are well-known diseases

Galen of Pergamum, AD *129–99*

Warts and verrucae are extremely common; they affect children and young adults primarily, are caused by the wart virus and are therefore infectious. They may be single or multiple, painless or painful, slowly growing or rapidly growing, disappear spontaneously after a few weeks, or remain stubbornly resistant to all treatments for years, the multiplicity of treatments and so called 'cures' give an indication of how ineffective most are! They can cause despair in doctor and patient alike! Fortunately, practically all warts and verrucae eventually disappear spontaneously, never to return, but as this may take several years, most patients seek treatment in an attempt to cure them in a shorter time. Some treatments are undoubtedly harmless and worth trying – others definitely carry certain well-recognized risks and may leave permanent scarring. In a self-limiting condition, therefore, the practitioner must not let his or her surgical enthusiasm inflict a treatment which is worse than the original condition. Neither should the treatment be painful as the majority of sufferers will be young children unlikely to forget or forgive.

Treatments for warts and verrucae fall into two categories: medical and surgical. No apology is made for including a selection of medical treatments before considering surgical approaches.

27.1 MEDICAL TREATMENTS

27.1.1 Psychological therapy

Although warts are known to be caused by a virus infective agent, they can be made to disappear by psychological treatments. This fact was known for centuries by the 'wart charmers' and in recent years by hypnotherapists. If a patient believes that their warts are going to disappear as a result of any treatment, a significant proportion do in fact regress and disappear!

27.1.2 Monochloroacetic acid

Solitary warts or verrucae respond well to a saturated solution of monochloroacetic acid pricked into the wart using a sharp-pointed wooden applicator (Figs 27.1 and 27.2).

One drop of acid is placed on the surface of the wart, and with a

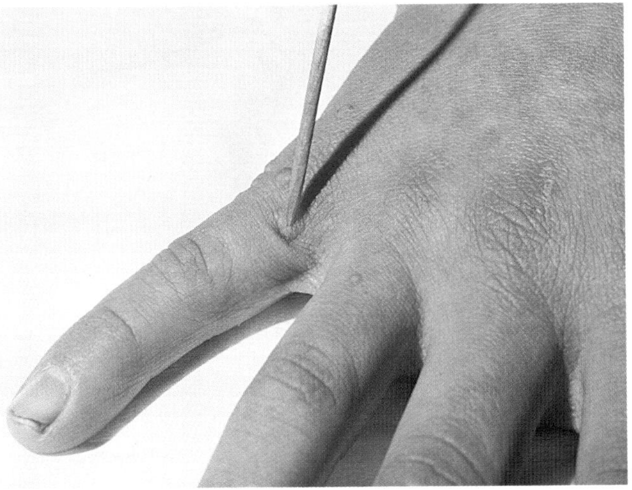

Fig. 27.1 Solitary warts may be effectively treated with a saturated solution of monochloroacetic acid, pricked in with a wooden applicator until no more is absorbed.

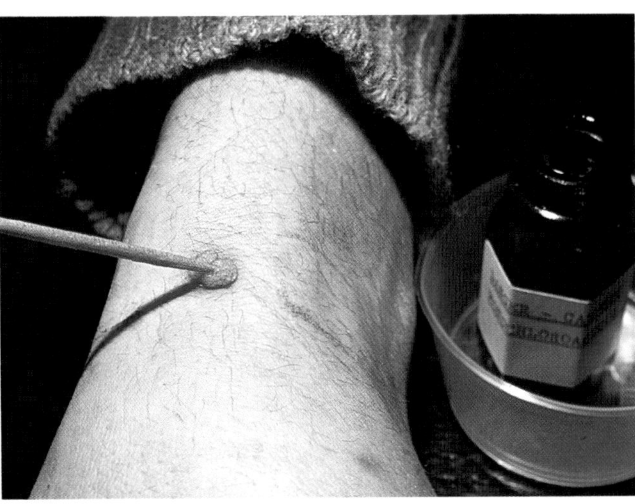

Fig. 27.2 Monochloroacetic acid being applied to solitary wart on wrist.

wooden applicator is pricked through the horny outer layer. Often the acid appears to soak into the wart very much like absorbent paper. Further drops of acid are applied and pricked into the wart until no more will soak in. It is most important not to allow any acid on the surrounding skin or a painful burn will result. Should any spread from the wart, it should be immediately removed with a soft paper tissue. Following the application of monochloroacetic acid, there is normally a reddening of the skin over the next 4 or 5 days, and signs of healing after 8 days. One application is often successful, and the treatment may be repeated if necessary. Ointments containing podophyllin and/or salicylic acid are equally effective.

27.1.3 Podophyllin and/or salicylic acid

The risk of podophyllin is over-enthusiastic treatment in a desperate attempt to cure the verruca; this results in painful burns to the surrounding skin, often the verruca is cured, but at the expense of considerable discomfort (Fig. 27.3). If using podophyllin and salicylic acid ointment (Posalfilin) only enough to cover a pin-head should be used; this should be placed in the centre of the verruca, covered with a plaster dressing and repeated daily until cured. A simple way by which the patient can tell if the verruca is cured is by compressing the skin on either side of the verruca: if painful it is still present, if painless, it is cured (Fig. 27.4). Plasters with 40% salicylic acid are an effective means of dealing with multiple plantar warts; they macerate the top layers of skin, including the wart.

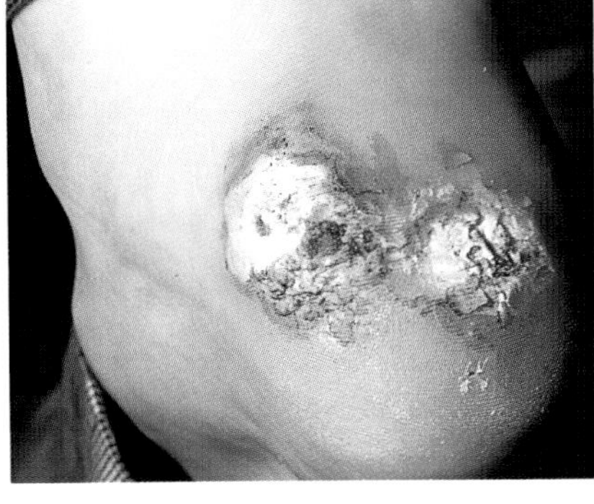

Fig. 27.3 Over enthusiastic treatment of verrucae with podophyllin and salicyclic acid.

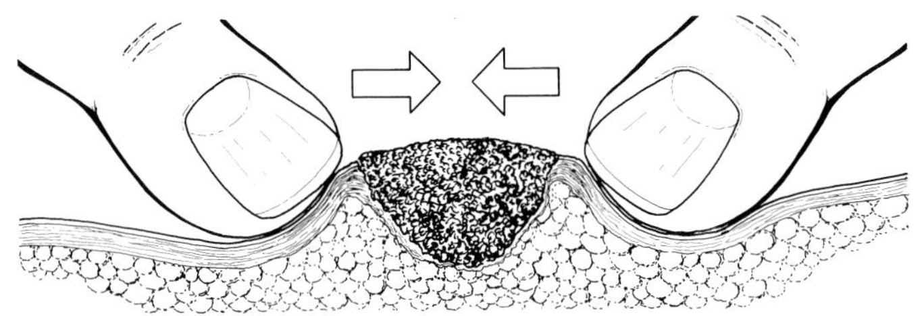

Fig. 27.4 A simple method to determine whether a wart or verruca is cured: compress laterally between finger and thumb, if no pain – cured!

27.1.4 Aqueous formalin or glutaraldehyde solution

Multiple verrucae may also be treated by soaking the whole foot in 20% aqueous formalin solution for 10 min each day (Fig. 27.5). The skin becomes hard and like leather, and liable to crack, particularly between the toes if the solution is not washed off. Using a similar principle, glutaraldehyde solution may be applied just to the wart or verruca daily until it is cured.

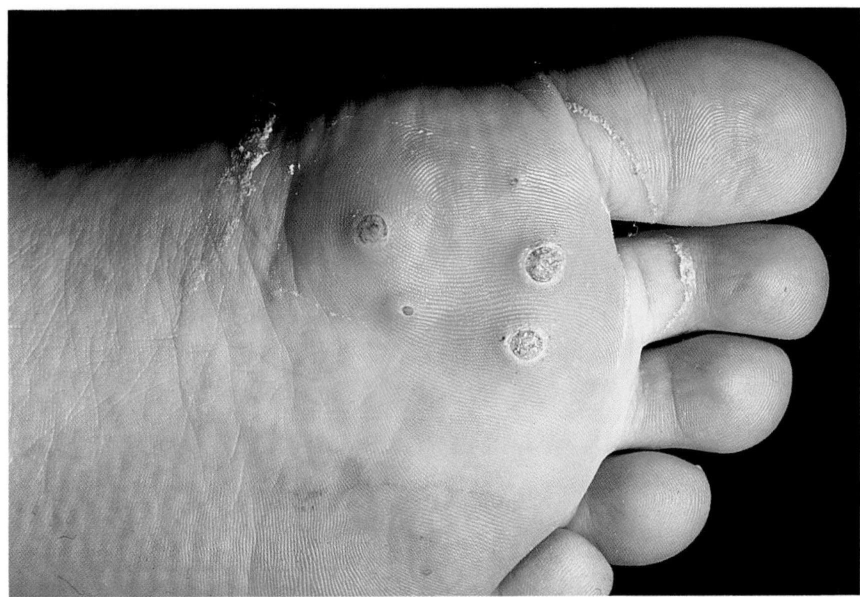

Fig. 27.5 Multiple verrucae; best treated medically with salicyclic acid or formalin.

27.1.5 Genital warts

Genital warts (condylomata acuminata) are more susceptible to treatment than the ordinary hard wart; in this case the treatment of choice is podophyllin in spirit or tinct. benz. co. applied very carefully to each wart. Traditionally 25% podophyllin was recommended, unfortunately this often burned the surrounding skin, and a trial using 0.5% podophyllin resin in 70% ethanol [26] applied twice daily for 3 days gave equally good results. Liquid nitrogen cryosurgery also gives excellent results with less scarring.

27.2 SURGICAL TREATMENTS

There are as many surgical as there are medical treatments for warts and verrucae, indicating again that no one treatment offers more than a reasonable chance of cure. Treatments involve burning, freezing, curetting and excision. There are various instruments which will destroy warts or verrucae by heat, the simplest is the standard electrocautery, by which a platinum electrode is heated to red heat by the passage of an electric current. It is first necessary to infiltrate the base of the wart with local anaesthetic (lignocaine 1% with or without adrenaline, depending on the site), the wart may then be destroyed using the electrocautery.

Another method of producing heat within tissues is by passing a high-frequency electric current through it; this is used regularly for coagulating bleeding vessels in the operating theatre; a large pad is strapped to the patient's thigh and connected to one side of the output of the machine while the other output lead is connected to a small pointed instrument such as a pair of artery forceps. This is a bipolar diathermy apparatus. Similar portable diathermy machines are now available which use just one electrode and these are the unipolar diathermy machines, or Hyfrecators. In use, the needle electrode is inserted in the centre of the wart and the electric current switched on. The heat generated within the wart destroys it; normally a local anaesthetic is used to infiltrate the base of the wart before applying the electrode. No further treatment is required apart from a sterile, dry dressing.

27.2.1 Curetting and cautery

Most solitary warts and verrucae can be removed with a curette and either this or radio-surgery is probably the treatment of choice (Chapter 42).

Instruments required (Figs 27.6–27.12):

dental syringe and 30 swg needle (0.3 mm)
cartridge of 2% lignocaine with 1:80 000 adrenaline
or
2 ml syringe
25 swg × 5/8 in. (0.5 mm × 16 mm) needle
ampoule 1% lignocaine with 1:200 000 adrenaline
Volkmann double-ended sharp-spoon curette
electrocautery and pointed burner or unipolar diathermy
histology container
dry dressing
povidone-iodine (Betadine aqueous solution).

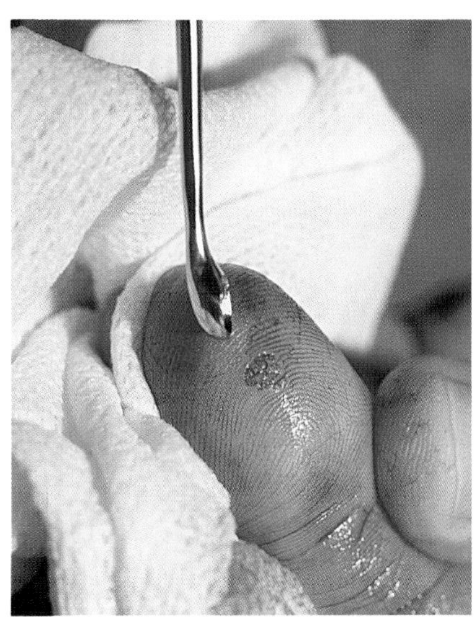

Fig. 27.6 Solitary wart on thumb; present for 1 year and painful. Curette and cautery offers high chance of permanent cure.

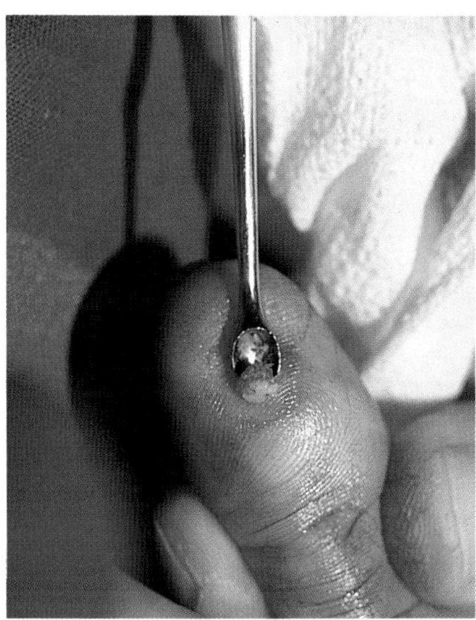

Fig. 27.7 Wart being curetted out. A tourniquet and ring block prevents bleeding at this stage.

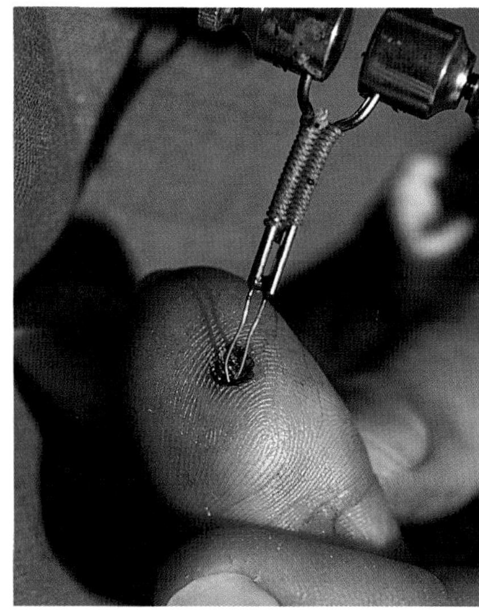

Fig. 27.8 The base of the wart is now cauterized with the electro-cautery.

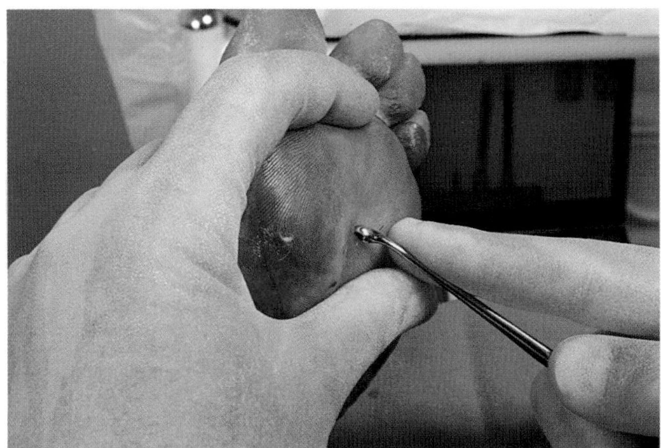

Fig. 27.9 Verruca on sole of foot. Anaesthesia by posterior tibial nerve block.

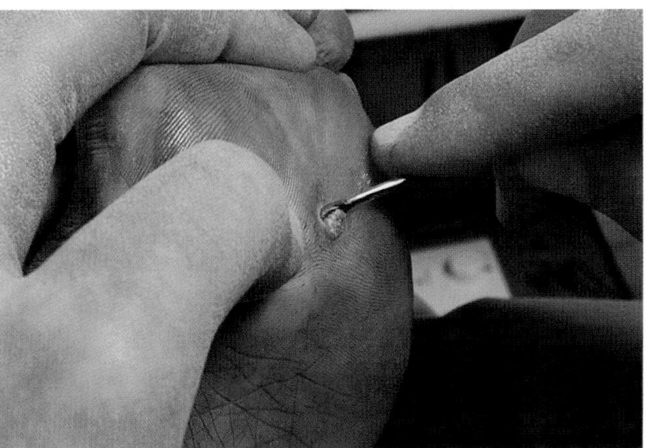

Fig. 27.10 Technique of using curette to remove verruca; firm pressure and a rotating action.

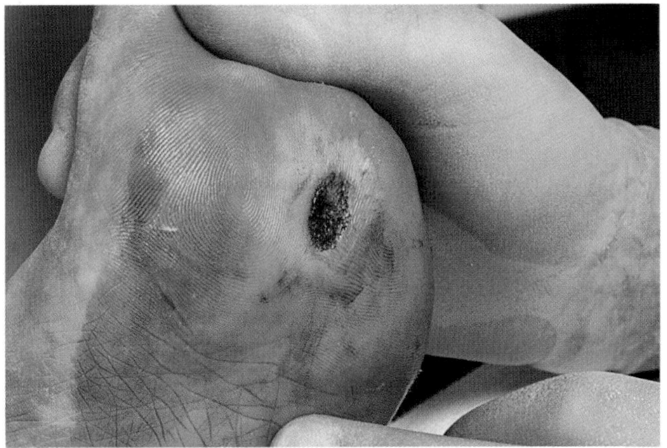

Fig. 27.11 After removing the verruca, the base is cauterized with the electrocautery.

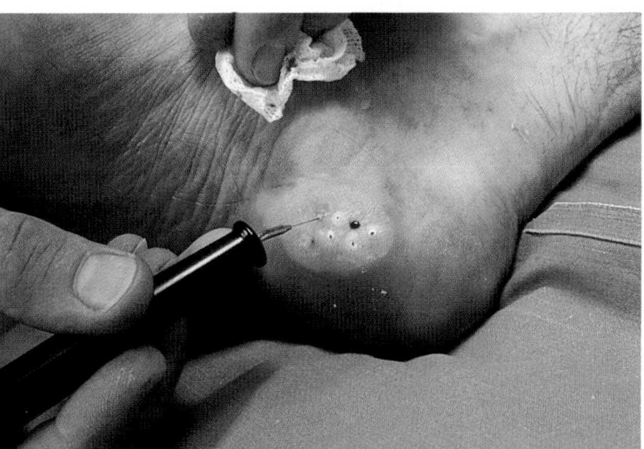

Fig. 27.12 A cluster of stubborn verrucae being individually treated with the Hyfrecator needle after preliminary paring of any hard skin.

The wart and adjacent skin is painted with povidone-iodine (Betadine aqueous solution). Using the dental syringe and 30 swg needle or the 2 ml syringe with 25 swg (0.5 mm) needle the base of the wart is infiltrated with local anaesthetic. It is now possible to curette the wart easily from the skin; this is best achieved by holding the handle of the curette firmly, perpendicular to the skin, pressing the curette firmly, against the edge of the wart, and then by a rotating action, shelling out the wart. When the correct tissue plane is reached the wart or verruca will readily separate, leaving a neat circular hole which bleeds easily despite the adrenaline in the local anaesthetic mixture. To control this bleeding the vessels are coagulated using the electrocautery, which additionally destroys any remaining fragments of wart. A dry dressing is applied; healing is usually complete in 3 weeks with freedom from pain after 2 days.

27.2.2 Excision of warts

Excision of warts is appropriate in certain sites such as the face where a neat scar is desirable, but as the majority of warts will disappear spontaneously without leaving a scar, excision should only be considered as a last resort.

Instruments required for excision of warts:

- 10 ml syringe
- 25 swg x 5/8 in. (0.5 mm x 16 mm) needle
- 21 swg x 1 1/2 in. (0.8 mm x 40 mm) needle
- scalpel handle size 3
- scalpel blade size 10
- pair toothed dissecting forceps
- pair stitch scissors
- Kilner needle holder
- suture: Mersilk Ethicon Ref. W533
- ampoule 10 ml, 1% lignocaine with adrenaline 1:200 000
- dressings
- povidone-iodine in spirit (Betadine alcoholic solution).

The wart and surrounding skin is painted with povidone-iodine in spirit and the base anaesthetized using first the 25 swg (0.5 mm) needle, followed by the 21 swg (0.8 mm) needle. An ellipse of skin is removed with the wart in the centre; this is sent for confirmatory histology and the wound closed using fine, interrupted Mersilk sutures. These are removed in between 5 and 10 days, depending on the site of the original lesion.

27.2.3 Cryosurgery for warts and verrucae

As well as destruction by heat, tissues can be destroyed by freezing, and in many situations this method offers a better treatment, free from pain, with an excellent cosmetic result. The different equipment and modes of use are described in Chapter 18 but there are three different machines, using carbon dioxide, nitrous oxide, and liquid nitrogen, in ascending order of efficiency. Liquid nitrogen gives the lowest temperature and has the highest success, carbon dioxide has only limited uses, while the nitrous oxide cryoprobe is valuable for superficial lesions. The technique is as follows:

The wart or verruca is pared down, moistened with water-soluble jelly or glycerine and the cryoprobe applied. As freezing progresses, the probe becomes frozen to the wart, which may now be lifted a few millimetres from subcutaneous tissues by gentle traction on the probe. When the wart is frozen solid, the probe is warmed, detached, and the wart allowed to thaw. The procedure is repeated as this second freeze appears to give improved results.

Immediately following freezing little can be seen, and the wart appears exactly as before treatment; slight throbbing is experienced during the next few hours, to be followed over the ensuing days by painless necrosis, and healing. It is the absence of pain and the very acceptable end result which makes cryosurgery so attractive.

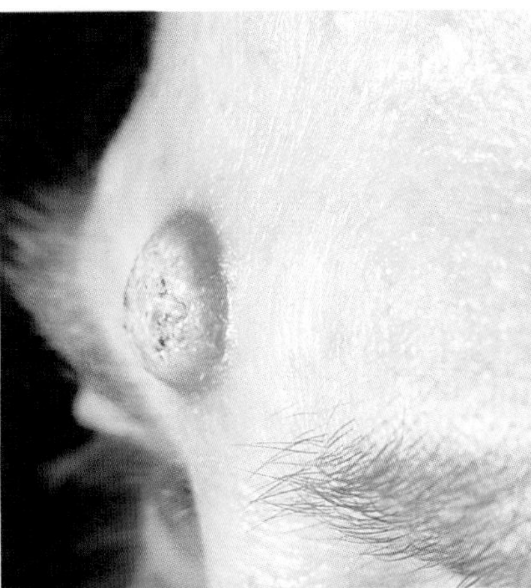

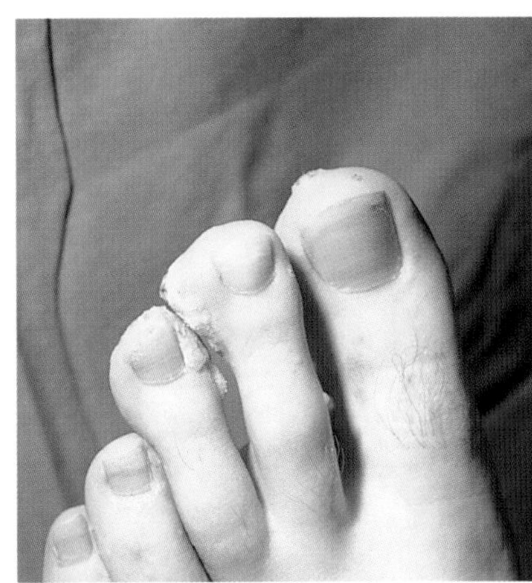

Fig. 27.13 Solitary wart on forehead, suitable for cryosurgery.

Fig. 27.14 Multiple warts on toes. Treatment either with formalin soaks or cryosurgery.

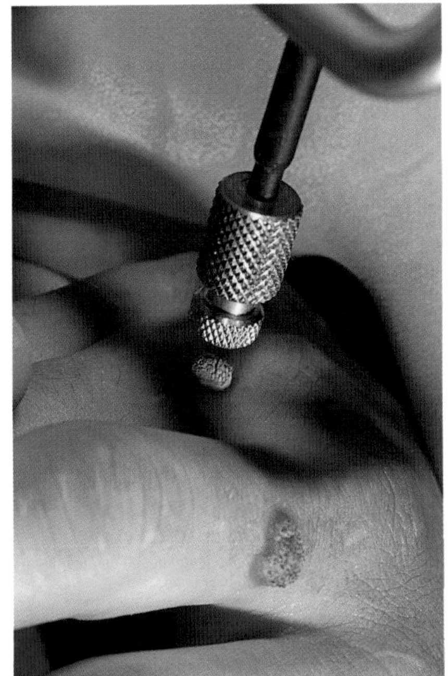

Fig. 27.15 Treatment of warts on hand by liquid nitrogen cryospray.

Condylomata acuminata are easily treated with a nitrous oxide cryoprobe. Larger warts are better treated with liquid nitrogen using a spray applicator (Chapter 18; Figs 27.13, 27.14 and 27.15) taking care to avoid damage to the underlying tendons, nerves and joints (Figs 27.16 and 27.17).

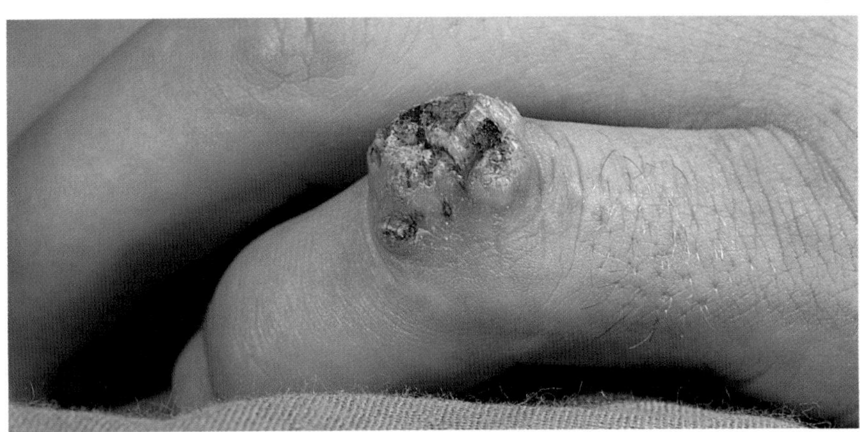

Fig. 27.16 Warts in certain situations require extra care. This wart overlies the joint capsule and extensor tendons. Over zealous treatment could result in damage to these structures.

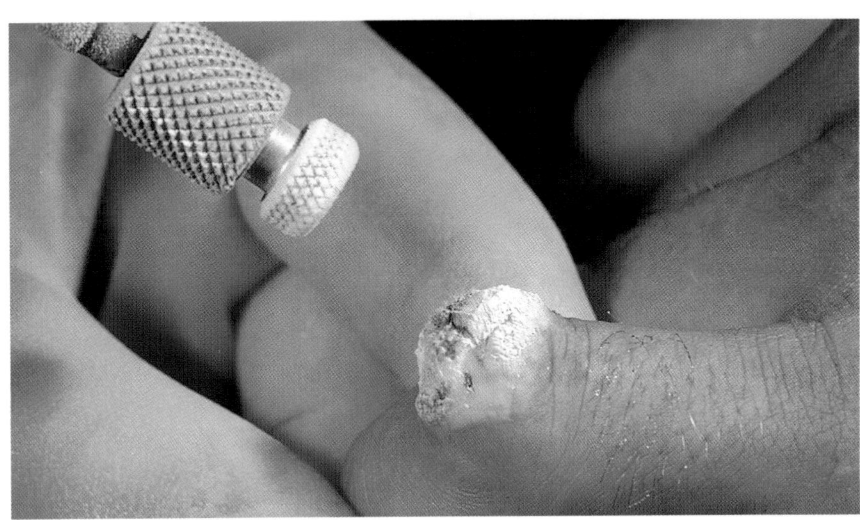

Fig. 27.17 Treatment with liquid nitrogen cryospray: several short treatments would be safer than one long freeze (Chapter 18).

27.2.4 Radio-surgical treatment of warts (see also Chapter 42)

Solitary warts and verrucae can also be removed using a radio-surgical instrument and wire loop. Treatment is very quick, simple and causes less tissue damage than electrocautery or diathermy. Local infiltration is still needed. Any bleeding may also be controlled with the radio-surgical unit.

28

Sebaceous cysts

I made an incision in the scalp, and upon the side on which I stood, which was about three-fourths of its size, I with difficulty detached it from the skin. ... The edges of the wound were brought together and lint and plaster applied. The King bore the operation well

Account by Sir Astley Cooper of the removal of a sebaceous cyst from the scalp of King George IV, 1820

True sebaceous cysts are very rare; epidermal and tricholemmal cysts are very common and usually referred to as sebaceous cysts.

Epidermal cysts occur following implantation of epidermis, or from the epidermal lining of pilosebaceous follicles, and are filled with macerated keratin; they can occur anywhere on the body, commonly fingers, from implantation.

The cysts commonly seen on the scalp are tricholemmal (pilar) cysts which are derived from the hair follicle; they occur in families, being inherited as an autosomal dominant gene, and are often multiple. Both types of cyst are ideal for removal in the doctor's treatment room under local anaesthetic. For the remainder of the chapter the term 'sebaceous cyst' will be used as it is better known for both epidermal and tricholemmal cysts.

Instruments required:

25 swg × 5/8 in. (0.5 mm × 16 mm) needle
scalpel handle size 3
scalpel blade size 15
pair stitch scissors 5 in. (12.7 cm)
pair McIndoe curved scissors 7 in. (17.8 cm)
pair toothed dissecting forceps
pair Halstead mosquito forceps 5 in. (12.7 cm) curved
Kilner needle holder 5 1/4 in. (13.3 cm)
surgical sutures, braided silk, metric
gauge 2 (3/0) on curved cutting needle (Ref. Ethicon W 533) or
equivalent monofilament nylon or Prolene
1% lignocaine with adrenaline 1:200 000
syringes and needles
povidone-iodine in spirit (Betadine alcoholic solution).

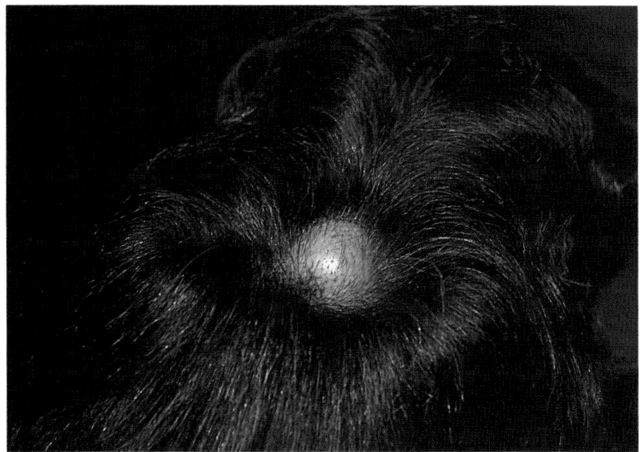

Fig. 28.1 Typical sebaceous cyst on scalp.

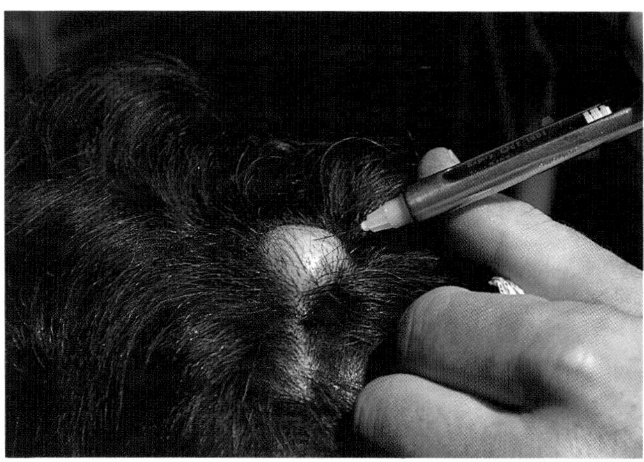

Fig. 28.2 The overlying skin is infiltrated with local anaesthetic and a small quantity injected into the base of the cyst.

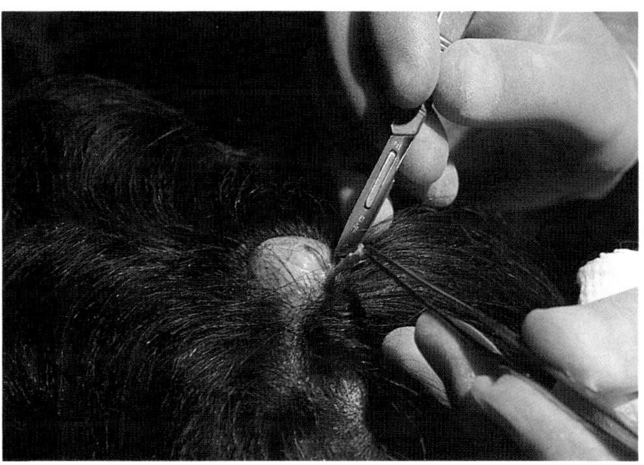

Fig. 28.3 An elliptical incision is made over the cyst, exposing the underlying cyst.

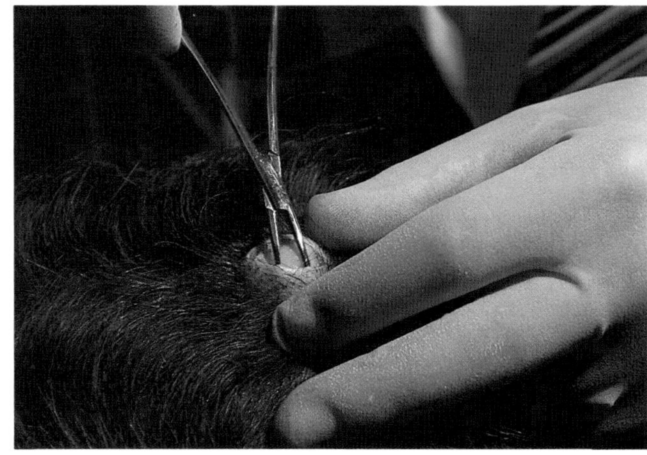

Fig. 28.4 Using curved mosquito forceps or curved McIndoe scissors, the cyst is dissected free.

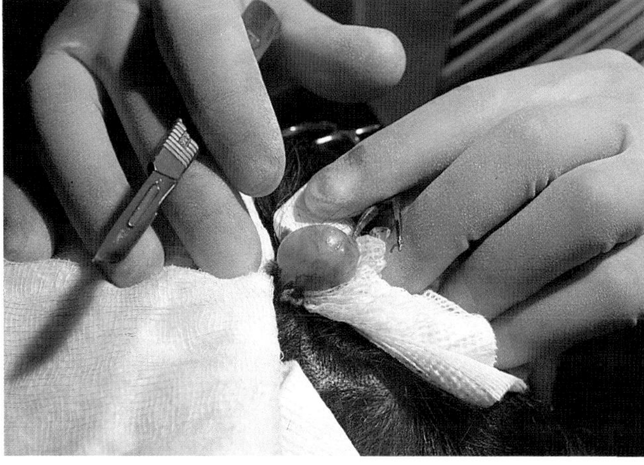

Fig. 28.5 With a little patience and careful dissection, the cyst may be removed complete.

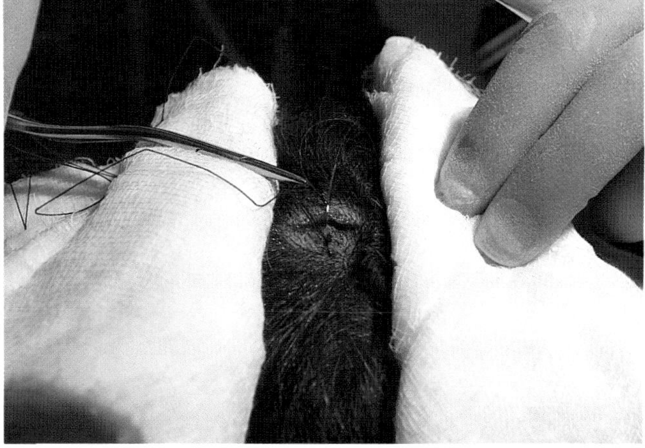

Fig. 28.6 Closure is with interrupted braided silk sutures.

28.1 TECHNIQUE FOR REMOVAL OF SEBACEOUS CYST ON THE SCALP (Figs 28.1–28.6)

The patient should preferably be lying down rather than sitting in a chair; even the most unlikely character is liable to faint, and it is embarrassing to have to complete the excision of a cyst on the floor!

Any overlying hairs are clipped with scissors (it is not necessary to shave large areas of scalp) and the overlying skin painted with povidone-iodine in spirit.

With the finger and thumb of the left hand fixing the cyst, local anaesthetic is injected through the skin using a 25 swg × 5/8 in. (0.5 mm × 16 mm) needle, with the bevel flat against the skin. Keeping pressure on the syringe plunger, the needle is slowly advanced, until it reaches the tissue plane between skin and cyst. At this stage, there is a loss of resistance in the syringe plunger, and distension of the cyst may be felt with the palpating finger and thumb of the left hand. Further pressure on the syringe plunger spreads the lignocaine and adrenaline around the cyst, causing the overlying skin to blanch (Fig. 28.2).

Done carefully, this technique separates the tissue planes and makes subsequent excision easier. One additional injection of local anaesthetic is made underneath the cyst before finally removing the needle. Occasionally the pressure of the local anaesthetic infiltration causes the cyst to eject some of its contents through the blocked punctum.

28.1.1 Incision

Very small cysts can be removed merely by a single incision and digital pressure, when the cyst will pop out (Figs 28.7 and 28.8). Closure with one stitch is all that is required. Larger cysts require dissection, and the excision of an ellipse of redundant skin. The ellipse of skin should be chosen to include the central punctum; it may be excised, exposing the underlying cyst. Using the blades of a curved McIndoe's scissors, the cyst is freed by gently inserting the closed blades and opening them. Any adhesions can be separated either by this method or cutting, using the same scissors (Fig. 28.4). At this stage the cyst may be grasped with the toothed

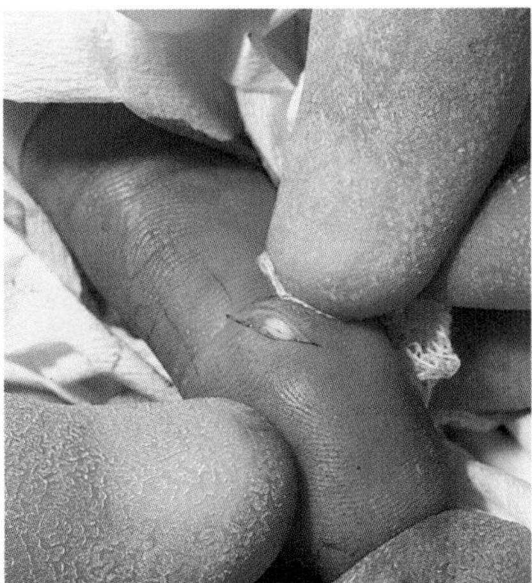

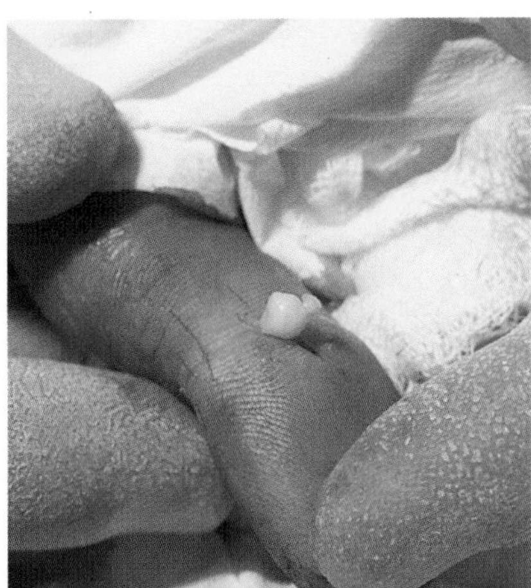

Fig. 28.7 Small inclusion or epidermal cyst in finger. Easily removed under ring block and tourniquet.

Fig. 28.8 The same cyst being expressed by the application of finger pressure on either side.

dissecting forceps, traction applied, and the remaining adhesions divided. Bleeding is not usually a problem, except perhaps with cysts at the back of the neck; it can normally be controlled with firm pressure and usually stops when the edges of the wound are sutured. The aim should be to remove the cyst complete, although this is not always possible, particularly with thin-walled cysts where the centre has become infected. Where there is evidence of infection, the cyst should still be removed, but before closure, a small quantity of fucidic acid gel (Fucidin Gel) should be instilled into the cavity and the skin then sutured in the usual way.

28.1.2 Closure

Interrupted braided silk sutures should be used, which may be removed on the 8th–10th postoperative day. Where there is redundant skin which tends to invert on skin closure, the edges should be picked up in the stitch as shown in Fig. 28.9.

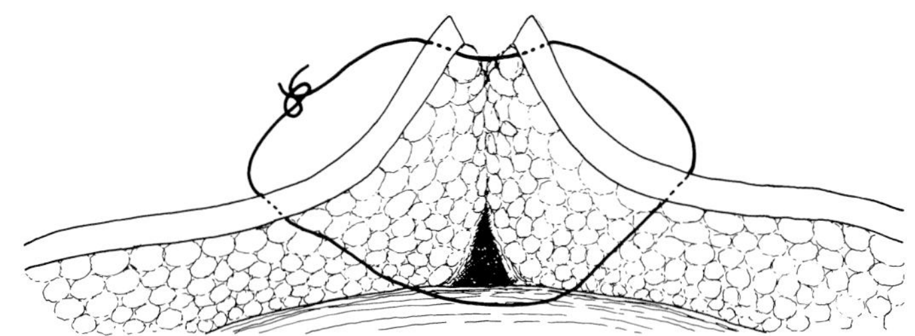

Fig. 28.9 Method of preventing skin edges inverting when suturing (vertical mattress suture).

28.2 ALTERNATIVE METHOD FOR REMOVAL OF SEBACEOUS CYST

Some practitioners prefer to bisect the cyst, squeeze out the contents with a gauze swab, and then pull out the lining of the cyst with a pair of artery forceps. This is a much quicker procedure than dissection, but has the disadvantage of being messy, carries a slightly higher infection rate, and the contents of a sebaceous cyst have a slightly unpleasant, persistent, odour. Nevertheless, it is a perfectly acceptable method of removal.

28.3 HISTOLOGY

As with all excised specimens, even the humble 'sebaceous cyst' should be sent for histological examination if at all possible; just occasionally an unsuspected squamous cell tumour, cylindroma or other rarity may be discovered.

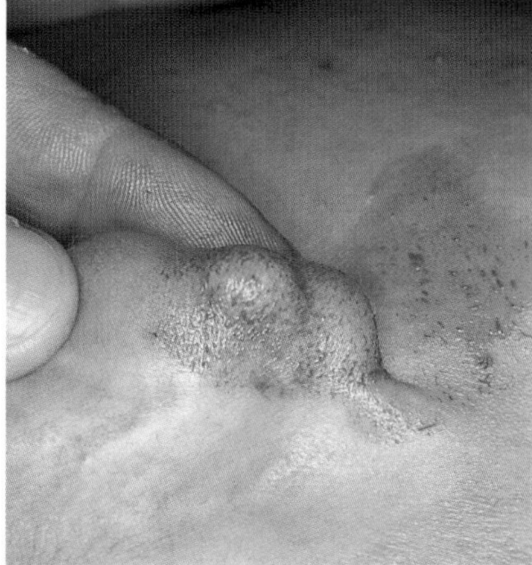

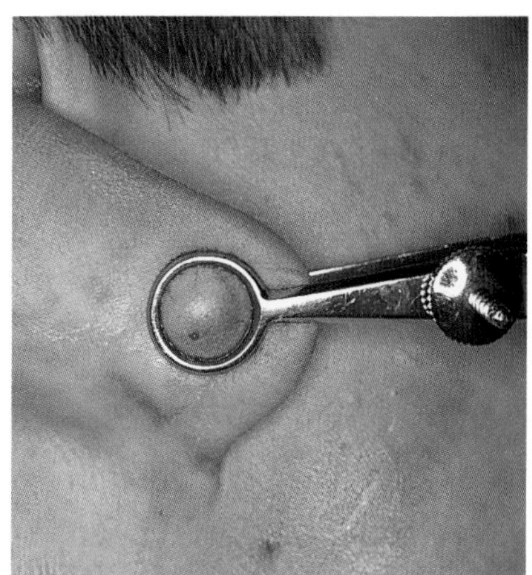

Fig. 28.10 Small ear-lobe cysts are very common.

Fig. 28.11 The application of ring forceps enables the cyst to be held and also controls bleeding.

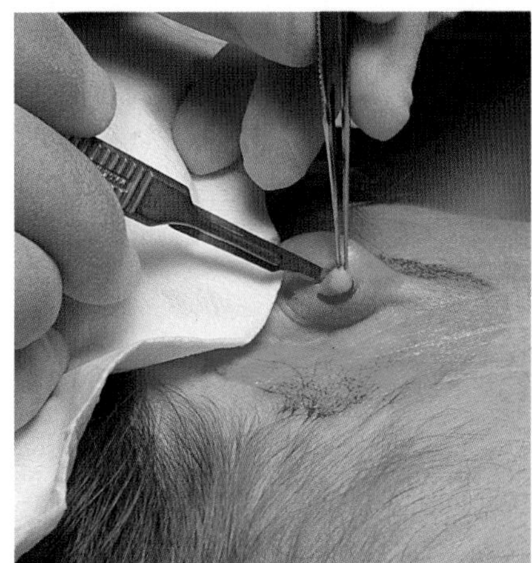

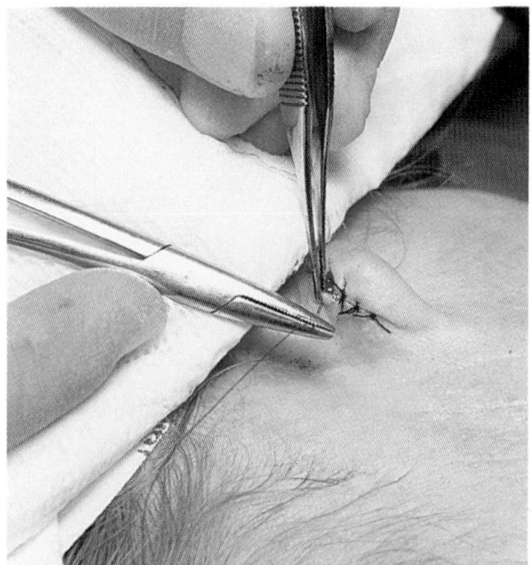

Fig. 28.12 Small epidermal cyst behind the ear; dissected free after infiltration with local anaesthetic.

Fig. 28.13 After removal of cyst, wound closed with fine, interrupted braided silk sutures.

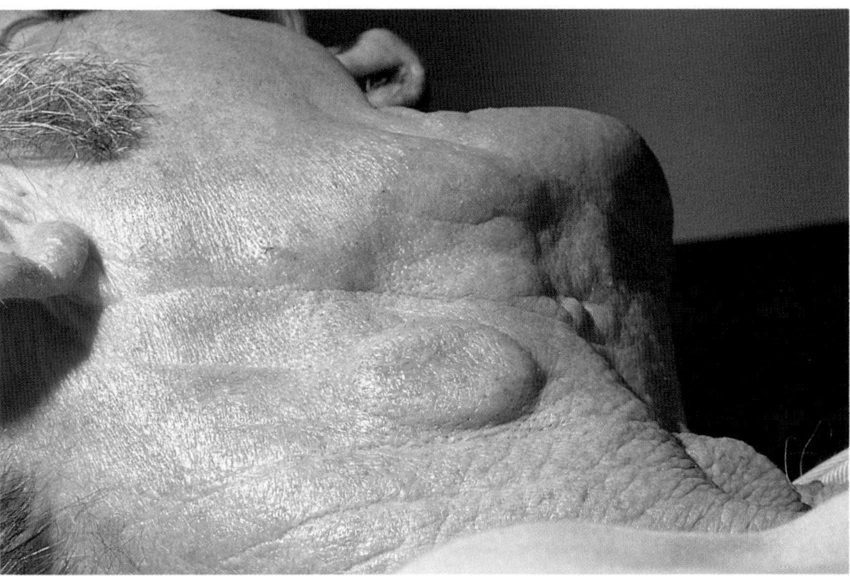

Fig. 28.14 Unusual shaped sebaceous cyst on neck.

29

Excision of lipoma

When thou meetest a fatty growth, in the neck ... then say thou 'He has a fatty growth in his neck – I will treat the disease with the knife, taking care of the blood vessels the while'

Ebers Papyrus, 1500 BC

A lipoma is a benign, fatty tumour which can occur anywhere on the body, varying in size from a small marble to larger than a football. On palpation a lipoma feels lobulated and semi-cystic – smooth in outline, and generally painless. Lipomata may be solitary or multiple and the most commonly given reason for requesting removal is cosmetic, although in some sites, pressure effects may cause symptoms. Although appearing to be quite superficial, many lipomata extend deeper than expected, and the doctor should be aware of this fact before embarking on excision.

Many lipomata can be enucleated using a gloved finger; others are tethered by fibrous bands which give the lipoma its typical lobulated appearance; these bands need to be dissected free with the curved McIndoe's scissors.

Instruments required:

- scalpel handle no. 3
- scalpel blade no. 10
- pair McIndoe's scissors 7 in. (17.8 cm) curved
- pair toothed dissecting forceps
- Kilner needle holder $5^1/4$ in. (13.3 cm)
- Halstead's artery forceps 5 in. (12.7 cm) curved
- Povidone-iodine in spirit (Betadine alcoholic solution)
- 10 ml 1% lignocaine with 1:200 000 adrenaline
- syringes and needles.

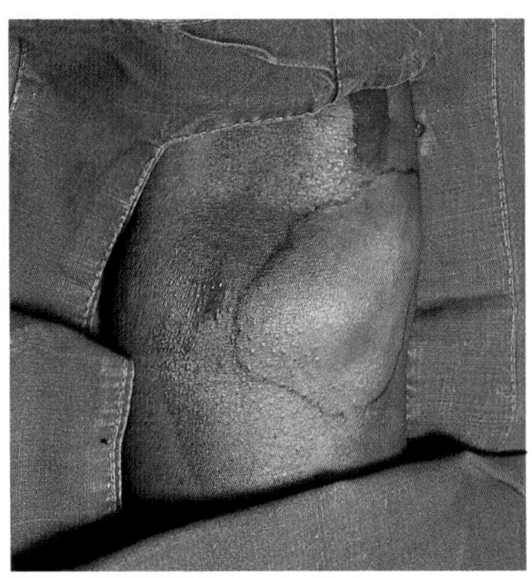

Fig. 29.1 Lipoma situated in antecubital fossa; the brachial artery is marked in red.

The size, shape and extent of the lipoma is first ascertained, and its relationship to any adjacent structures noted. The overlying skin is painted with povidone-iodine in spirit and the area infiltrated with 1% lignocaine with adrenaline 1:200 000, remembering to include the deeper part of the lipoma (Fig. 29.1). An incision is made boldly through the skin directly to the lipoma, which will bulge typically into the wound (Fig. 29.2). At this stage a gloved finger can be inserted between skin and lipoma to see whether it will shell out (Fig. 29.3); if not, further blunt dissection is carried out using the McIndoe's curved scissors and an opening action, dividing any fibrous bands tethering the lipoma to deeper tissues. With patience, the complete lipoma can be freed and removed (Fig. 29.4); it is

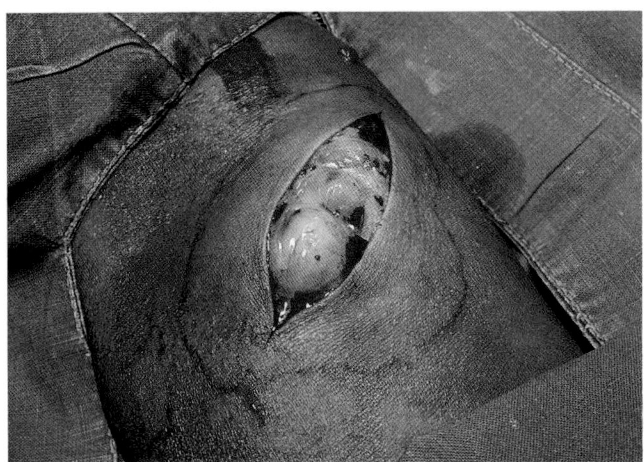

Fig. 29.2 Incising through the skin allows the lipoma to bulge through the wound.

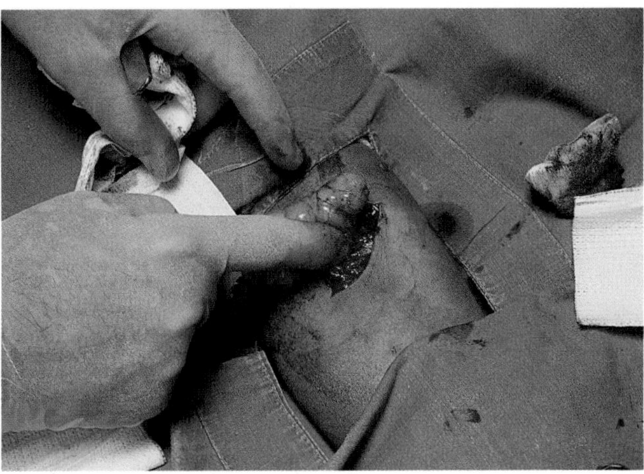

Fig. 29.3 Using finger dissection, the lipoma may be removed.

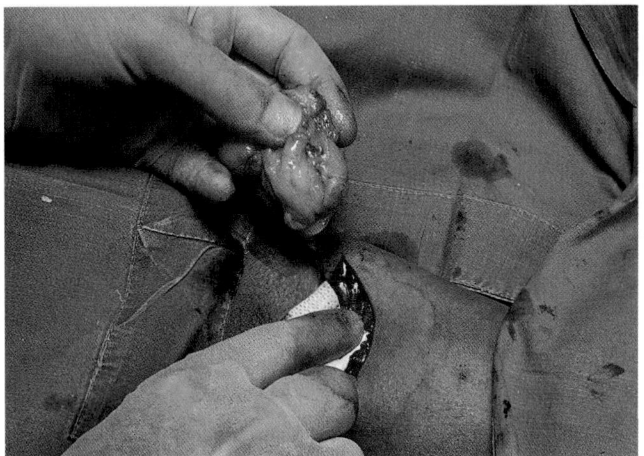

Fig. 29.4 Lipoma removed complete; any mild bleeding controlled with gauze swab.

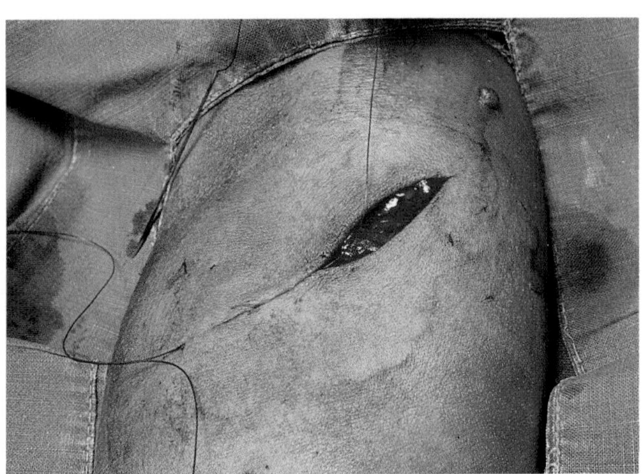

Fig. 29.5 Wound being closed with subcuticular nylon.

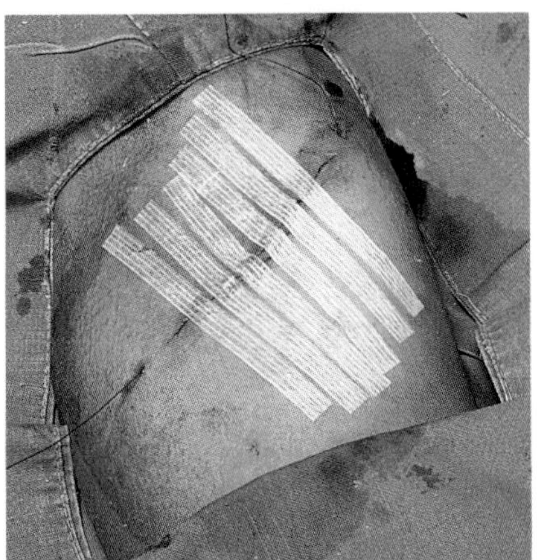

Fig. 29.6 Additional support may be given by the use of skin-closure strips.

then sent for routine histological examination. Following removal of a large lipoma, a substantial 'dead' space is left which might collect blood and delay healing; in this case it is advisable to close the space with interrupted catgut or Vicryl sutures. In excising larger lipomata, an ellipse of skin should also be removed to enable accurate closure with no redundant skin. Finally, skin closure should be with either interrupted sutures, or a subcuticular nylon suture, the latter being probably more acceptable to the patient who requested removal on cosmetic grounds (Figs 29.5 and 29.6).

30

Minor operations on the toes

To Heal the diseased Toes
Fennel Wax, Incense, Cyperus, Wormwood, Dried Myrrh, Poppy Plant, Poppy grain, Elderberries, Berries of the Uan tree, Resin of Acanthus, Dough of Acanthus, Resin of the Mafet tree, Grain of Aloes, Fat of the Cedar tree, Fat of the Uan tree, fresh Olive Oil, Water from the rain of Heavens. Make into one poultice and apply for 4 days

Ebers Papyrus, 1500 BC

30.1 THE TREATMENT OF INGROWING TOE-NAILS

Ingrowing toe-nails are extremely common, cause much discomfort and yet can be one of the most rewarding conditions to treat in general practice.

Surgical textbooks abound with scores of treatments, varying from quite minor procedures, often ineffective, to complete removal of the nail, ablation of the nail bed, and even amputation of the terminal phalanx resulting in weeks of painful, messy dressings and much time away from school or work. The cause is still not known; ill fitting shoes, and incorrect cutting of the nails have both been incriminated, but many patients are seen in whom these certainly do not apply and as the condition largely affects the big toe-nail on either foot, and appears to be cured by permanently narrowing the width of the nail, it may be that the width of the nail is an important contributing factor.

Three types of ingrowing toe-nail are seen. The first group is commonly seen in young patients between the ages of 10 and 20. Here, the nail is

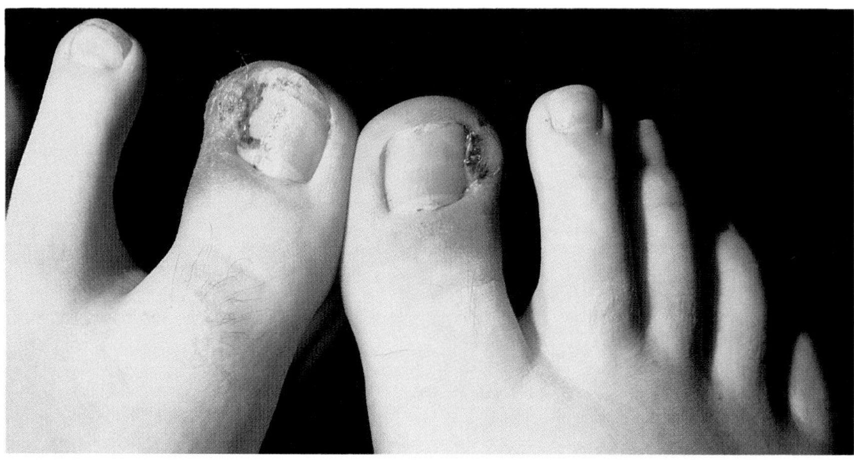

Fig. 30.1 Typical ingrowing toe-nails affecting the big toes on both feet.

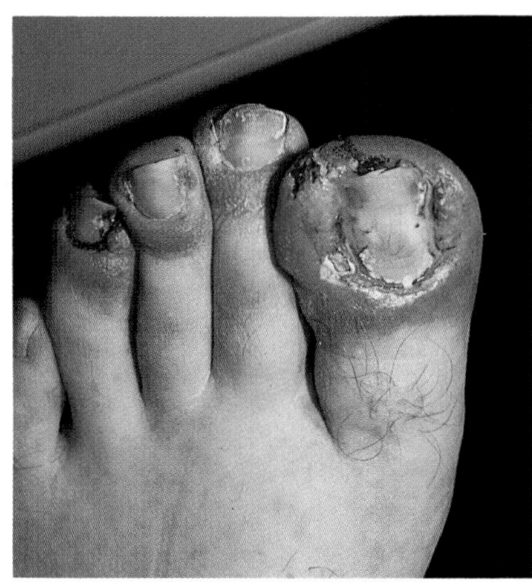

Fig. 30.2 A severely infected ingrowing toe-nail. Even one as bad as this can easily be cured with matrix phenolization.

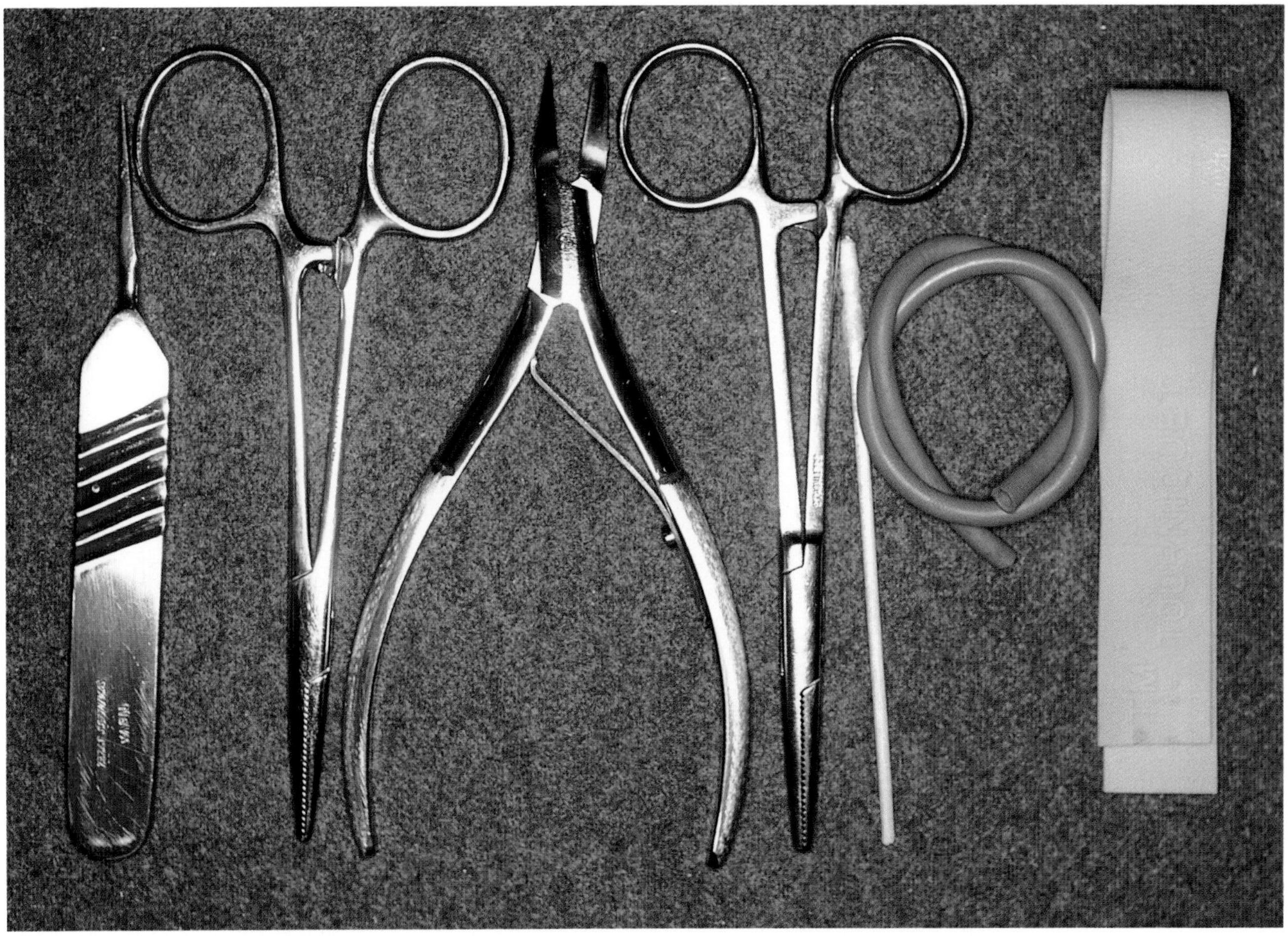

Fig. 30.3 Instruments required for ingrowing toe-nails; from left to right: nail chisel (Nova); artery forceps, straight; Thwaites nail nipper; artery forceps, straight; wooden applicator; rubber tube tourniquet.

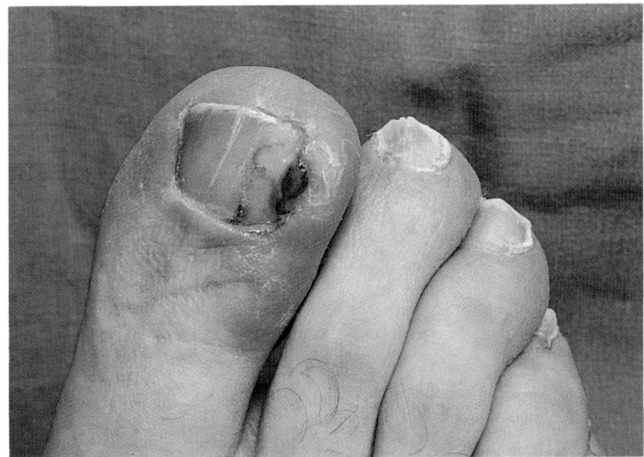

Fig. 30.4 Ingrowing big toe-nail.

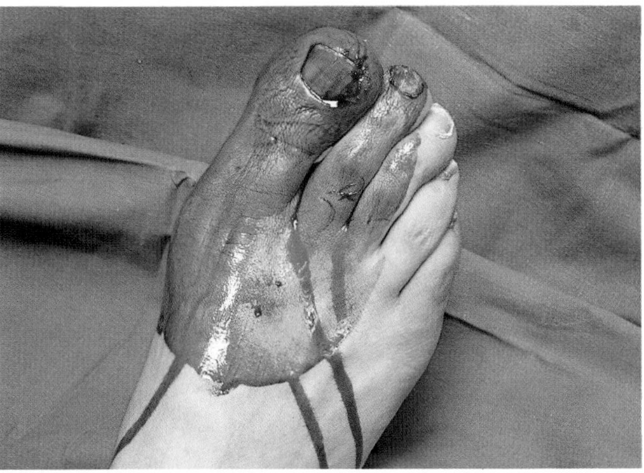

Fig. 30.5 The toe-nail and forefoot are liberally painted with povidone-iodine in spirit.

entirely normal in contour but the skin is hypertropied, often with granulations in the nail fold (Figs 30.1, 30.2 and 30.4). The second group is more likely to be seen in adults; here the nail has increased its convexity so that its edges press firmly on the shallow nail groove. In the third group, seen in all ages, the nail is incurving and ingrowing so that the nail plate has increased its convexity, particularly at the lateral edges so that the edge of the nail has curved through almost 180° and is digging into the lateral edge of the nail groove.

30.1.1 Medical treatments

Before embarking on surgery, medical treatments may be tried; one of the simplest for mild, early, ingrowing toe-nails is the application of Sofradex drops (dexamethasone 0.05% framycetin sulphate 0.5% and gramicidin 0.005%) four times daily for 1 week. If by the end of the time there has not been an obvious improvement, surgical treatment is indicated, offering nearly 100% cure.

The operation of choice is one which has been used by chiropodists for many years [27, 28, 29, 30], correctly described as nail matrix phenolization, and consists of removing a narrow strip of nail together with nail matrix on the affected side, and the application of liquefied phenol to cauterize the germinal epithelium. It is highly effective and gives rapid, painless healing, with virtually no recurrence [31].

Phenol appears to have a threefold action. First, it destroys the nail matrix and prevents that portion of nail regrowing. Secondly, it destroys the nerve endings, which explains the absence of pain during the healing phase. Thirdly, it destroys all pathogenic organisms, resulting in a sterile, cauterized area.

In the UK pure liquefied phenol containing 80% w/w in water is used; in the USA, liquefied phenol USP containing not less than 89% w/w in water is used. The higher strength used in America is unlikely to make any significant difference to the results, but it should be stored in brown glass bottles, ideally with a glass stopper as the solution changes from colourless to pink or brown when exposed to light, and the phenol can affect plastic caps and washers. Although it appears that phenol which has changed colour is nonetheless effective, it is probably wise to use a relatively fresh and colourless solution.

Wooden applicators with a wisp of cotton wool tightly wound around the tip are the best way of applying the phenol. They must be narrow enough to be easily inserted into the matrix cavity, and only enough phenol to saturate the space should be used, avoiding spilling the solution on adjacent skin.

30.1.2 Nail matrix phenolization

Instruments required (Fig. 30.3):

- syringes and needles
- local anaesthetic without adrenaline
- povidone-iodine in spirit (Betadine alcoholic solution)
- paraffin tulle with 0.5% chlorhexidine (Bactigras)

2 in. Kling bandage (5 cm)
Thwaites nail nipper or sharp-pointed, stitch scissors 5 in. (12.7 cm)
25 swg (0.5mm) needle
two pairs straight artery forceps 5 in. (12.7 cm)
nail chisel (Nova Instruments)
wooden applicator sticks
Volkmann sharp-spoon curette
rubber strip tourniquet
rubber tube tourniquet
pure liquefied phenol (BP) (USP).
30 swg (0.3mm) needle

It is helpful to advise the patient to arrange transport home and to bring a large shoe or slipper to accommodate the bandaged toe. Povidone-iodine in spirit is liberally applied to the toe (Fig. 30.5) extending proximally at least 1 in. beyond the interdigital clefts. A ring block or digital nerve block is performed using plain lignocaine or prilocaine: under no circumstances should adrenaline or any other vasoconstrictor be added to the local anaesthetic, otherwise ischaemia and possible necrosis could occur (Fig. 30.6).

For greatest comfort, and particularly in children, a 30 swg (0.3 mm) needle should be used with a dental syringe and cartridge. Unfortunately most dental anaesthetic cartridges contain adrenaline, but prilocaine 4% (Citanest) containing 40 mg/ml is manufactured in 2 ml cartridges (maximum adult dose prilocaine 400 mg). Failing this, a standard 5 ml syringe with 25 swg × 5/8 in. (0.5 mm × 16 mm) needle may be used with 1% lignocaine.

The digital nerves to the toe lie on the plantar side of the coronal plane; each should be infiltrated with 0.5 ml local anaesthetic, followed by a 'bridge' of solution across the dorsum of the toe, plus a similar bridge on the plantar surface, producing a complete ring block (Fig. 30.7).

Toes which are very reddened and inflamed are more difficult to anaesthetize, but it is well worth taking additional time and effort to achieve complete anaesthesia before operating.

A sterile gauze swab is now wrapped around the toe (Fig. 30.8) and over this is applied a rubber strip tourniquet or 1 in. cotton non-stretch bandage to exsanguinate the toe. (The rubber strip included in the butterfly intravenous cannulae kits makes an ideal tourniquet for fingers and toes.) Next, a fine rubber tube tourniquet is tied tightly around the base of the toe, and fixed with one of the pairs of artery forceps (Figs 30.9 and 30.10). The rubber strip and gauze swab are now removed, leaving a bloodless, anaesthetized toe (Fig. 30.11).

More povidone-iodine in spirit is applied, and a sterile paper drape is placed over the foot, with the toe protruding through a small hole cut in the paper.

Using the Thwaites nail nipper or pointed stitch scissors, the operator cuts a thin strip of nail adjacent to the granulations, approximately 2–3 mm away from the nail fold, and extending to the base of the nail (Fig. 30.12). This cut is then extended to the nail matrix or germinal epithelium, using a special nail chisel which splits the nail, using firm pressure, until resistance is encountered (Fig. 30.13).

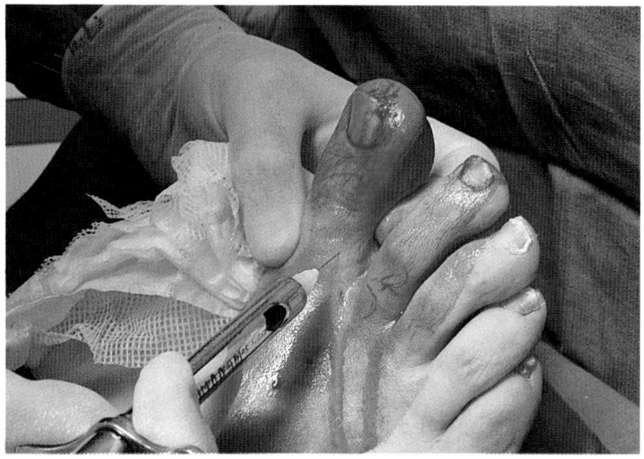

Fig. 30.6 The digital nerves are blocked with local anaesthetic (never use added adrenaline).

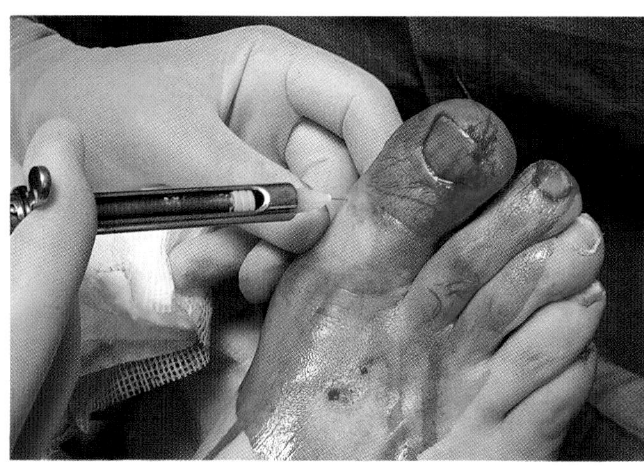

Fig. 30. 7 A complete ring block anaesthetic is performed.

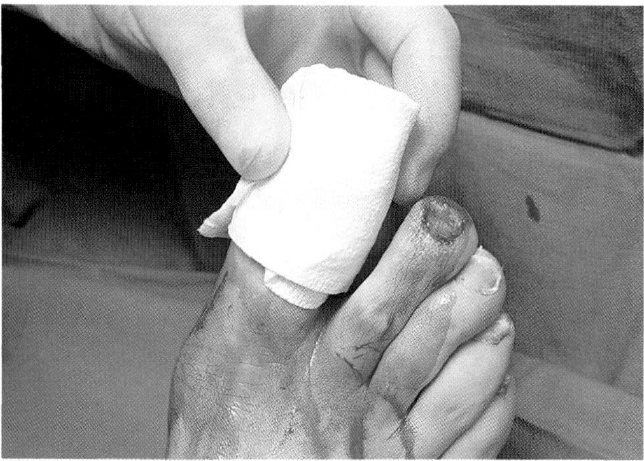

Fig. 30.8 A sterile gauze swab is wrapped around the toe.

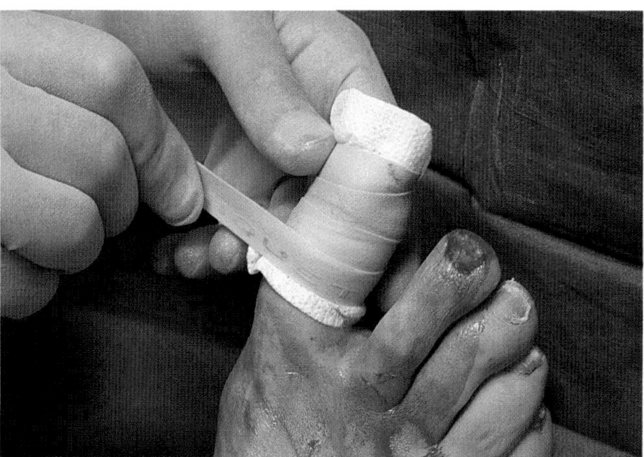

Fig. 30.9 A rubber strip tourniquet is wrapped over the gauze swab to exsanguinate the toe.

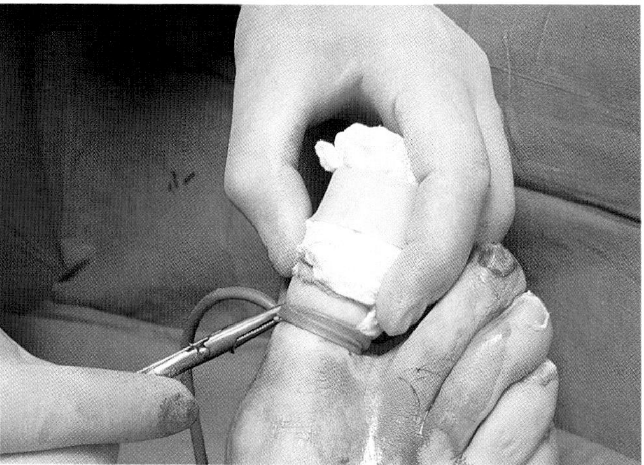

Fig. 30.10 A rubber-tube tourniquet is tied round the base of the toe and secured.

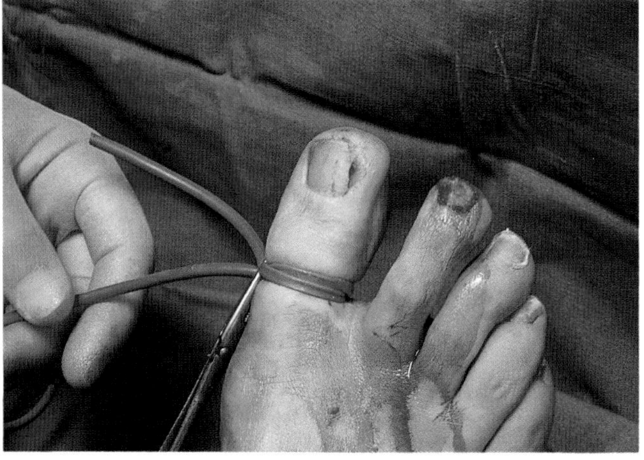

Fig. 30.11 The rubber strip and gauze swab are removed, and more povidone-iodine applied.

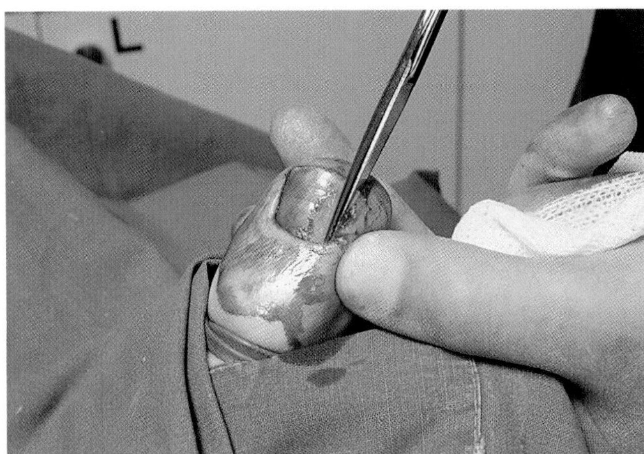

Fig. 30.12 Using either stitch scissors or Thwaites nail nippers a strip of nail is cut out as shown.

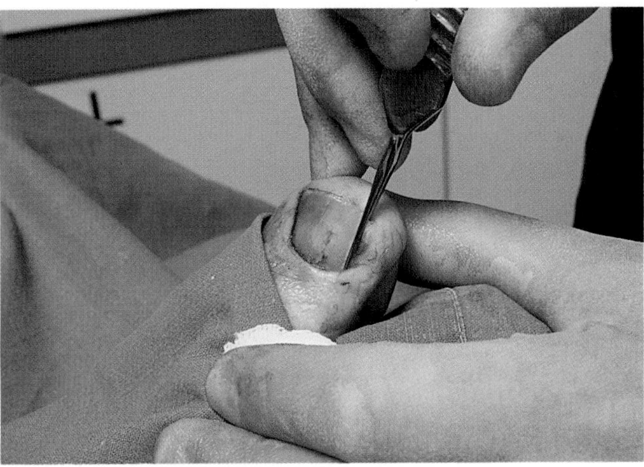

Fig. 30.13 The cut is deepened using the nail chisel, pushing it firmly down to the nail root.

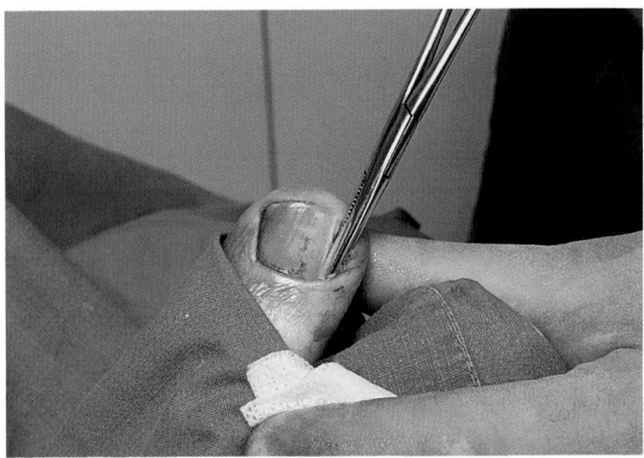

Fig. 30.14 The strip of nail is grasped with artery forceps and removed.

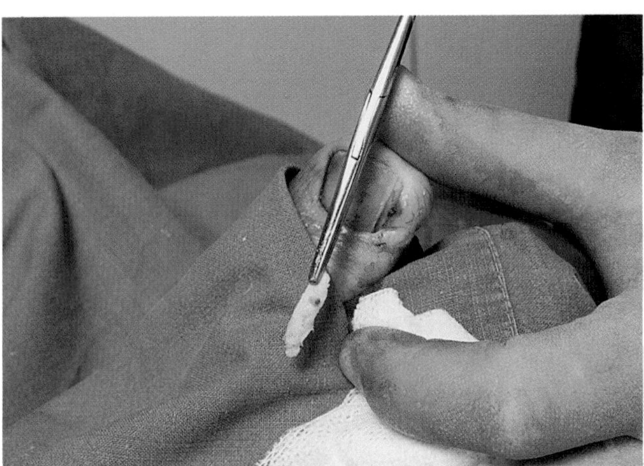

Fig. 30.15 The strip of nail which has been removed.

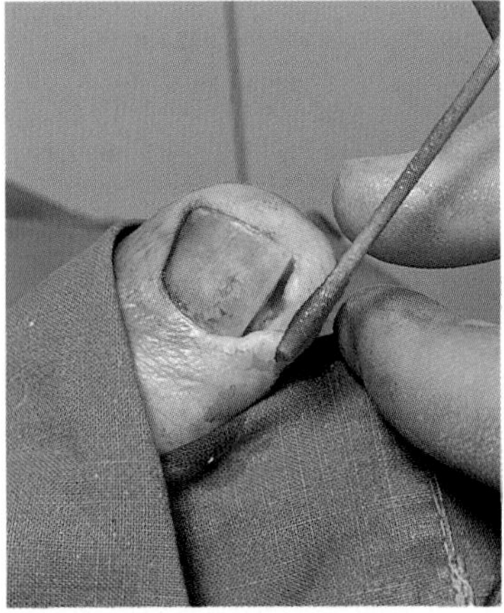

Fig. 30.16 Pure phenol is now applied, using a wooden applicator and cotton wool.

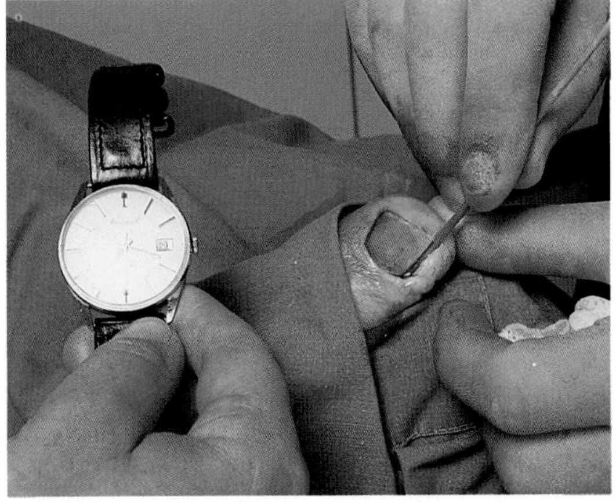

Fig. 30.17 The phenol must be applied for a minimum of 3 min by the clock.

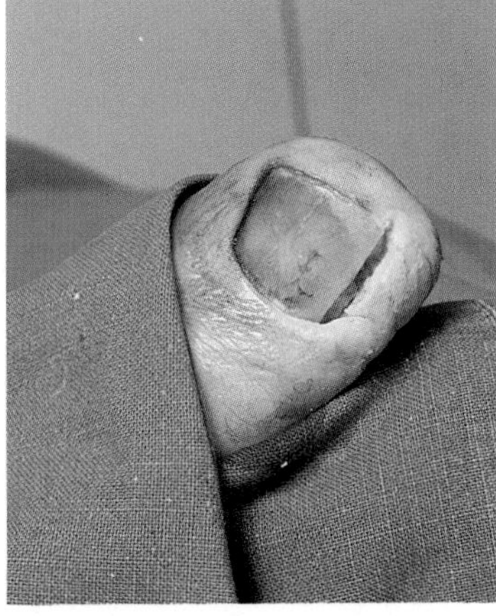

Fig. 30.18 The appearance of the nail bed after applying the phenol.

The chisel is removed, and the strip of nail is grasped with a pair of straight artery forceps and gently removed using a combination of traction and rotation, making sure not to tear the base of the strip, nor leave any fragments in the groove (Figs 30.14 and 30.15). Any excess granulations are now removed with the curette, although most can be left, and the phenol applied with the wooden applicator using a massaging action to ensure complete absorption, particularly in the matrix cavity (Fig. 30.16). The phenol is applied for exactly 3 min; if less than this, recurrence is likely. Sufficient is used to cauterize the groove formerly occupied by the strip of nail, but care is taken not to use too much which might spread over the adjacent skin and delay healing (Figs 30.17 and 30.18). After 3 min, a dry swab is used to mop away any surplus phenol; earlier accounts of the technique described the use of 5% chlorhexidine in spirit to 'neutralize' the phenol, this is now thought not to be necessary.

A dressing of paraffin tulle impregnated with 5% chlorhexidine is now applied, covered with one square of sterile absorbent gauze, and the toe bandaged (Figs 30.19 and 30.20).

The tourniquet is released, and the patient allowed home with instructions to rest the foot for 6 hours. Two follow-up dressings are necessary, the first on the third postoperative day, the second 1 week later on the tenth day, and this is usually all that is necessary. Frequently on the tenth day dressing the toe is found to be moist and 'messy' – this is thought to be due to a delayed 'phenol reaction', is quite common, and needs no special treatment. If discharge or granulations persist, an application of povidone-iodine spray powder (Disadine DP) is helpful, covered with a dry dressing.

Incurving, ingrowing nails are treated in an identical manner, removing a narrow strip from either edge of the nail, and phenolizing both sides simultaneously.

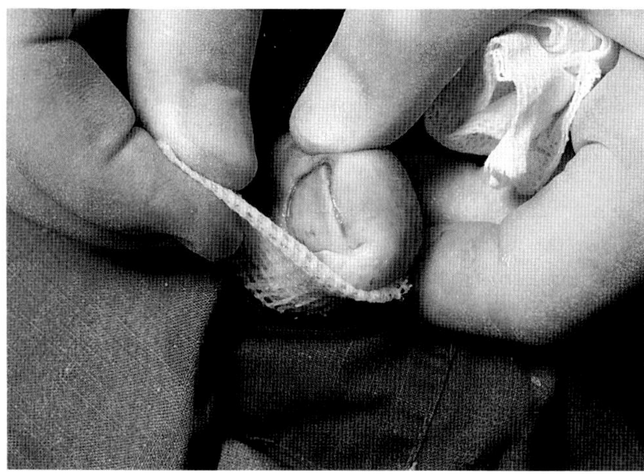

Fig. 30.19 A dressing of Bactigras or fucidin-tulle is now applied.

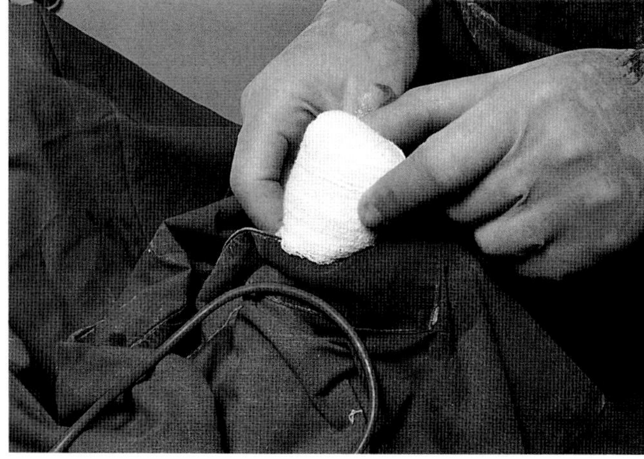

Fig. 30.20 This is now covered with a gauze swab and cotton bandages and left for 3 days.

30.1.3 Cryotherapy for ingrowing toe-nail

Destruction of the granulations of moderately severe ingrowing toe-nails is possible if the doctor possesses a liquid nitrogen cryospray unit.

Technique of cryotherapy

Because treatment may be painful, analgesic tablets taken 1 hour prior to freezing is advised, and in some patients, infiltration anaesthesia using lignocaine as a ring block will enable the freezing to occur painlessly. The spray is held about 1 cm away from the granulations and liquid nitrogen sprayed on the edge of the nail and toe until ice is seen to extend about 2 mm beyond the edge of the granulations. This normally occurs after thirty seconds of spraying.

Dermovate-NN cream or similar potent steroid cream is now applied under a dry dressing to minimize the reaction to the liquid nitrogen. Healing is usually complete in 6 weeks.

30.1.4 Wedge excision for ingrowing toe-nail

Many surgeons prefer a simple wedge excision of the granulation tissue to cauterization with phenol. Done carefully, it has the same high cure rate, but demands slightly more surgical skill and experience to judge the amount of tissue to be removed may require the insertion of one suture, and is occasionally accompanied by brisk bleeding when the tourniquet is released. For the doctor starting to treat ingrowing toe-nails, nail matrix phenolization is probably an easier technique to master initially.

Technique for wedge excision

As with nail matrix phenolization, the toe is first liberally painted with povidone-iodine in spirit and a ring block performed using plain lignocaine or prilocaine. A rubber tourniquet is next applied to exsanguinate the toe, and a rubber tube tourniquet then applied to the base of the toe.

A strip of nail is cut using a no. 15 scalpel blade on a no. 3 handle with the back of the blade adjacent to the nail-bed as shown (Fig. 30.21). This cut is extended to the base of the nail to include the germinal epithelium (Fig. 30.22a, b).

A second incision is now made on the lateral side of the toe, down to the first incision, thus removing a wedge of granulation tissue including a thin strip of nail (Fig. 30.23).

The nail bed and germinal epithelium are now curetted using a Volkmann sharp-spoon curette. This needs to be done thoroughly to minimize the risks of leaving a small amount of nail matrix behind (Fig. 30.24).

The proximal parts of the wound are now brought together with Steri-strips or a single 4/0 Prolene suture (Fig. 30.25), and a non-adherent Inadine dressing applied, covered by a dry gauze swab, and finally bandaged with a cotton conforming bandage (Crinx, Kling or similar) (Figs 30.26 and 30.27). This dressing is left undisturbed for 7–10 days, when the suture is removed and a smaller dry dressing applied.

Healing usually occurs rapidly, but the immediate postoperative phase

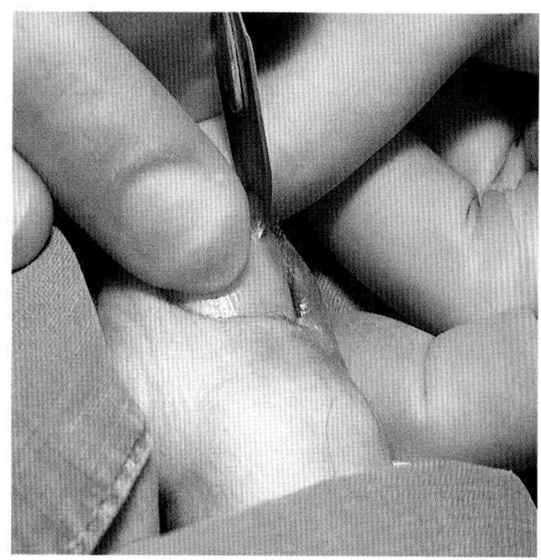

Fig. 30.21 Wedge excision of ingrowing toe-nail; initial incision, splitting the nail.

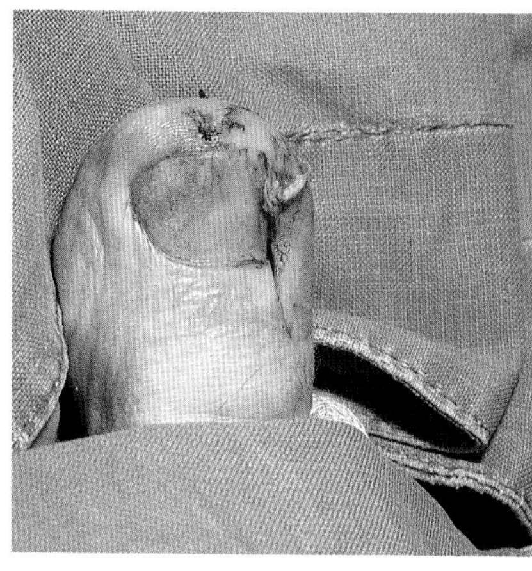

Fig. 30.22a Initial incision. A lateral incision would be made if many granulations were present.

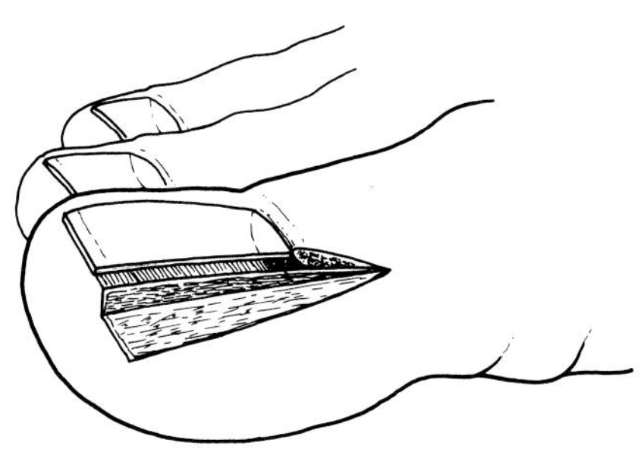

Fig. 30.22b Wedge resection of nail. (Redrawn from H.A.F. Dudley, J.R.T. Eckersley and S. Paterson-Brown, *A Guide to Practical Procedures in Medical Surgery,* by permission of Butterworth-Heinemann Ltd.)

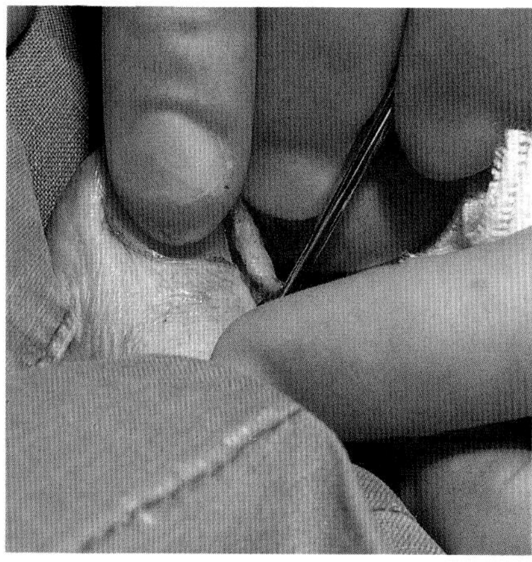

Fig. 30.23 Granulations being curetted together with any germinal epithelium.

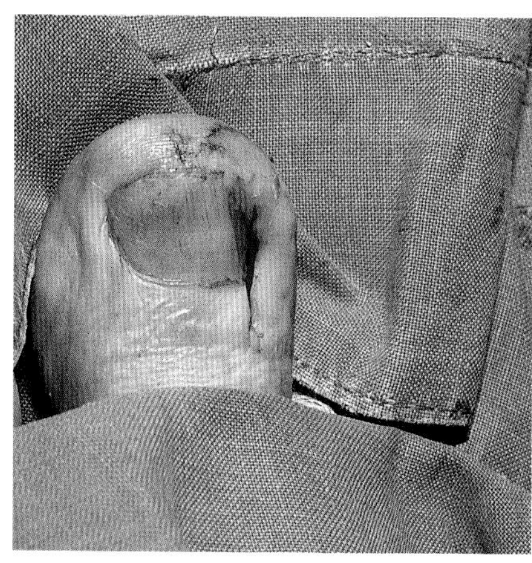

Fig. 30.24 Appearance after curetting granulations and nail matrix.

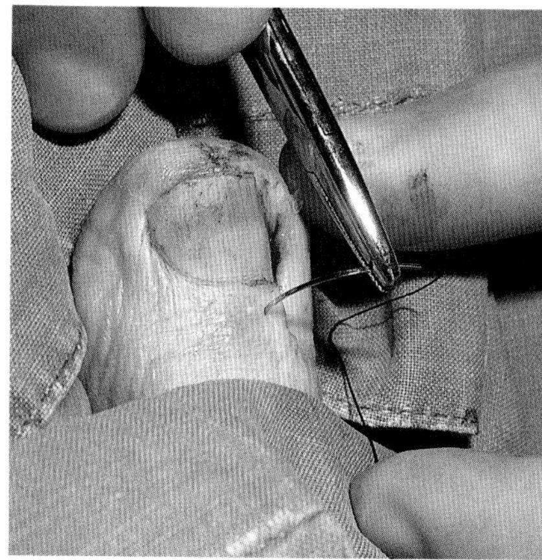

Fig. 30.25a Inserting fine suture. This is not always necessary and the edges may be held together with Steri-strips.

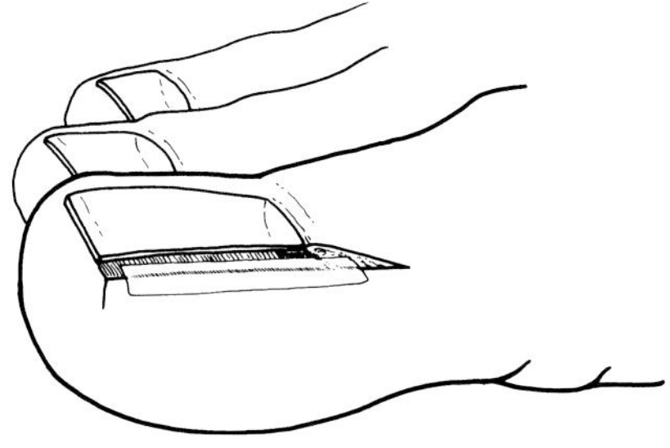

Fig. 30.25b Closure after wedge resection. (Redrawn from H.A.F. Dudley, J.R.T. Eckersley and S. Paterson-Brown, *A Guide to Practical Procedures in Medical Surgery*, by permission of Butterworth-Heinemann Ltd.)

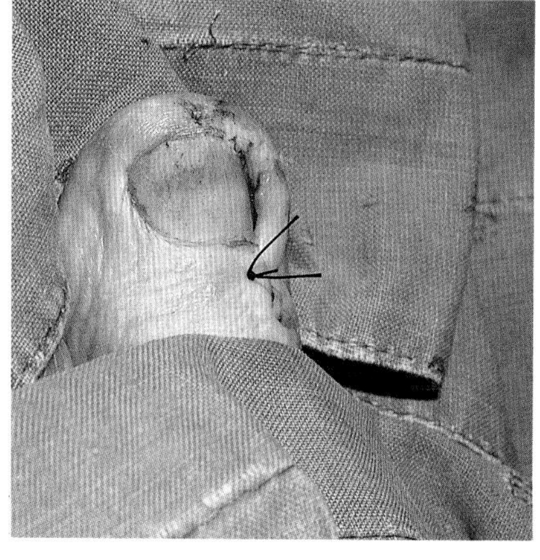

Fig. 30.26 One suture, if needed. This is removed on the 7th postoperative day.

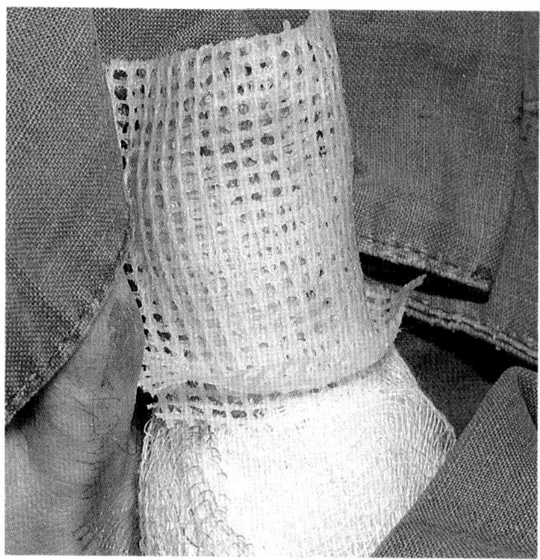

Fig. 30.27 Non-adherent dressing applied.

may be more uncomfortable than when using phenol, because of the anaesthetic effect of the latter.

30.1.5 Radio-surgical treatment of ingrowing toe-nails (see also Chapter 42)

The germinal epithelium may be destroyed very effectively using the radio-surgical unit and a specially designed nail matrixectomy electrode.

Technique

The preparation of the toe, anaesthesia and removal of the thin strip of nail on the affected side are identical to nail matrix phenolization, but instead of applying a swab soaked in pure liquefied phenol, the special electrode is inserted and a current passed for about 5 seconds (setting 2 on the Ellman Surgitron FFPF, Coagulation waveform). The toe is then dressed exactly as with the phenol treatment and reviewed three days later.

Healing is quicker than with phenol, and there is less reaction. Cure rates in excess of 98% have been reported by Hettinger (see Further Reading).

30.1.6 Nail-bed ablation

There are two situations when total ablation of the nail-bed may be the treatment of choice for the patient. The first is when recurrent ingrowing toe-nails fail to respond to either nail matrix phenolization or wedge excision, and the second is the patient with grossly distorted onychogryphotic toe-nails where simply removing the nail will result in the same situation recurring several months later.

Two techniques may be used:

1. Phenol
2. Surgical excision.

Technique of phenol ablation of nail-bed (see also Onychogryphosis, Fig. 30.28)

The preparation, ring block and application of tourniquet are exactly as described for the treatment of the ingrowing toe-nail. To remove the nail, it is first lifted away from the nail-bed with a McDonald's dissector or special nail elevator and then split in half using the Thwaites nail nipper. Each half may then be grasped with a strong pair of straight artery forceps and pulled off, using a combination of traction and rotation. If nail nippers are unavailable, the nail may be too thickened to be cut with any other instrument; accordingly it may be removed in toto using a strong pair of artery forceps.

Having removed the nail, the nail-bed and germinal epithelium are painted with pure phenol, paying particular attention to the groove containing the nail matrix. As with ingrowing toe-nails, the phenol is left in contact for at least 3 min (Fig. 30.29) then mopped dry and a paraffin-tulle dressing with 0.5% chlorhexidine (Bactigras) applied, covered with a sterile gauze swab and bandage.

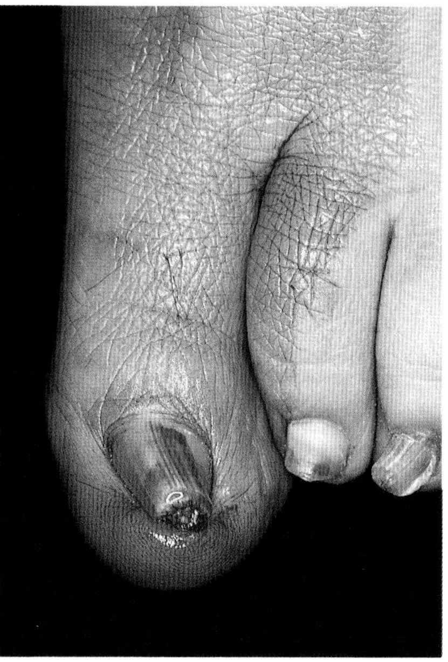

Fig. 30.28 Incurved, ingrowing, onychogryphotic nail causing much discomfort.

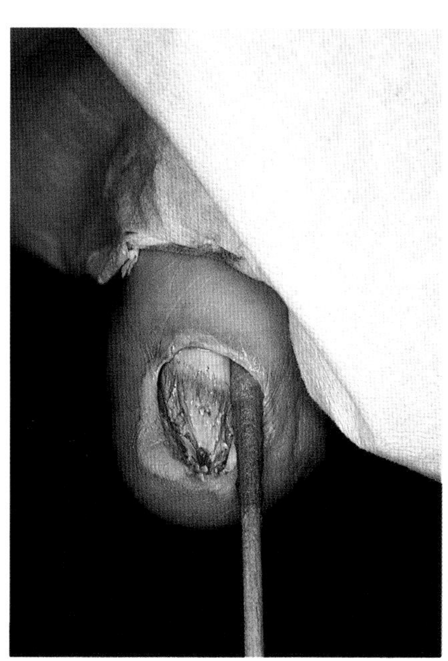

Fig. 30.29 After removal of the nail, the nail bed and germinal epithelium are treated with pure liquefied phenol for 3 min.

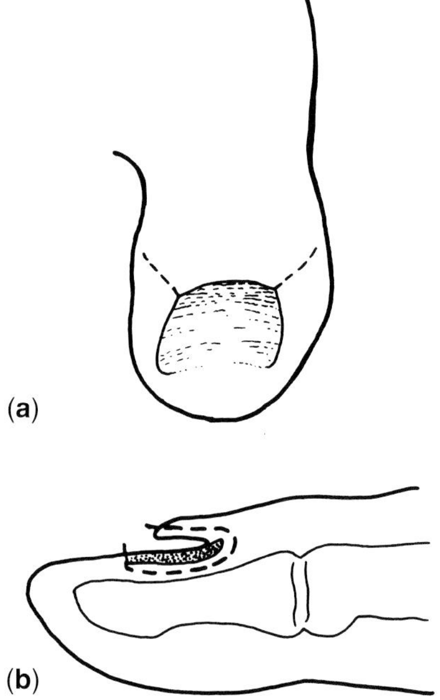

Fig. 30.30 Zadik operation. (**a**) Incisions; (**b**) block of tissue to be excised. (Redrawn from H.A.F. Dudley, J.R.T. Eckersley and S. Paterson-Brown, *A Guide to Practical Procedures in Medical Surgery,* by permission of Butterworth-Heinemann Ltd.)

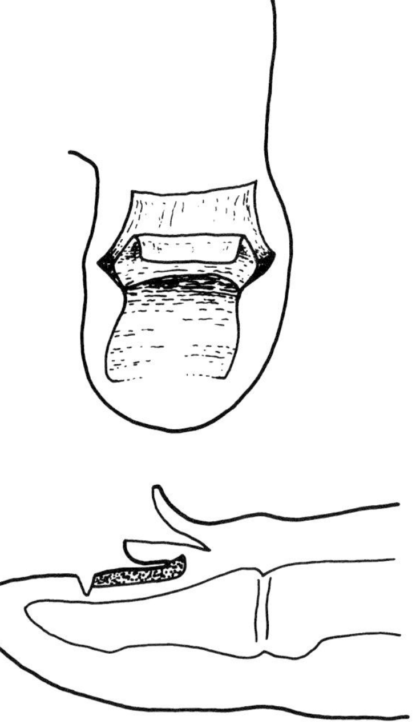

Fig. 30.31 Zadik operation: elevation of flap and incision into nail bed.

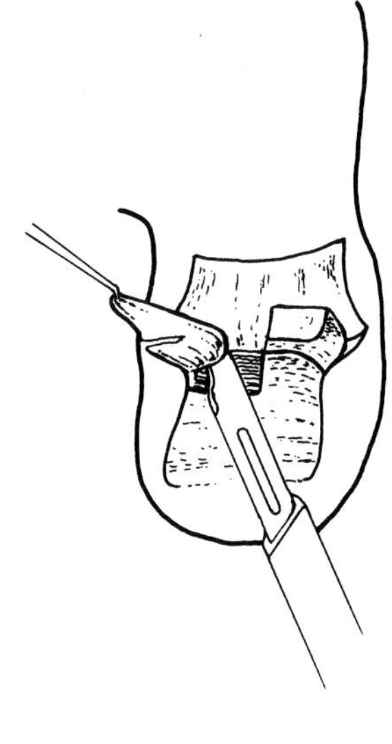

Fig. 30.32 Zadik operation. Dissection of the nail bed in two halves. (Redrawn from H.A.F. Dudley, J.R.T. Eckersley and S. Paterson-Brown, *A Guide to Practical Procedures in Medical Surgery,* by permission of Butterworth-Heinemann Ltd.)

Follow-up dressings are done on the third and tenth day and thereafter as necessary, any infection is treated with povidone-iodine powder spray. Healing takes 5–7 weeks, leaving a comfortable and cosmetically acceptable toe.

Nail-bed ablation by surgical excision (Zadik)

The toe is prepared exactly as with nail matrix phenolization, a ring-block performed, and tourniquet applied.

First the nail is completely removed. Two incisions 1 cm long are made, diverging proximally and laterally from each nail fold angle, ensuring that they do not extend as far as the interphalangeal joint (Fig. 30.30). Using skin hooks and a no. 15 scalpel blade, a skin flap overlying the nail germinal epithelium is raised and gently pulled back (Fig. 30.31). The block containing germinal epithelium is now removed in two halves as shown (Fig. 30.32). This leaves a defect, which may now be closed by advancing the flap of skin over it, and closing with 5/0 monofilament (Ethilon) sutures Ref. W 526.

A non-stick Inadine dressing is applied, covered by gauze and bandaged in place.

Any nail regrowth is always due to inadequate excision of the germinal epithelium: thus it is imperative to make a wide enough incision to see clearly the complete extent of the germinal epithelium.

30.2 ONYCHOGRYPHOSIS

... and his nails were like birds' claws

(Daniel, Chapter 4 verse 33 (RSV)

Onychogryphosis, or irregular thickening of the nail is commonly seen in the elderly; it may follow trauma, or arise secondary to a subungual exostosis, or following chronic hyperextension of the hallux. Once it has developed, it tends to be permanent, removal of the nail alone is followed by a

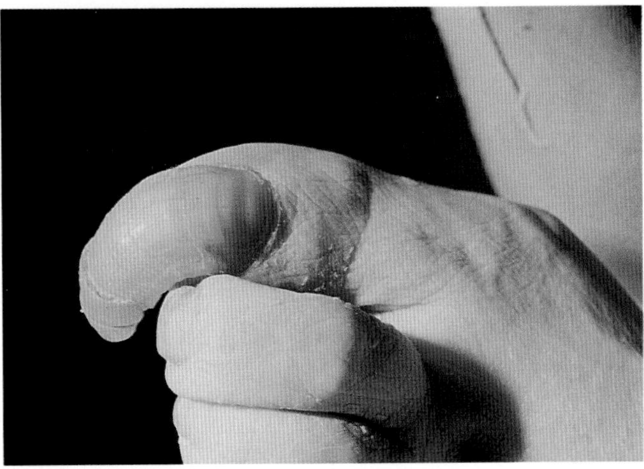

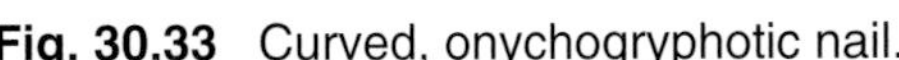

Fig. 30.33 Curved, onychogryphotic nail.

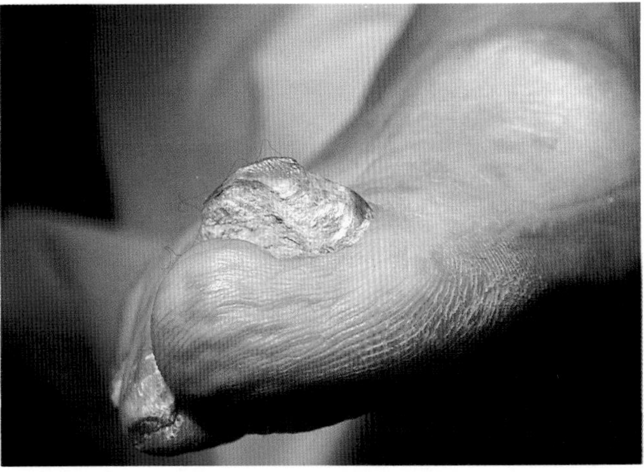

Fig. 30.34 Another onychogryphotic nail.

recurrence many months later; softening and burring of the nail likewise only give temporary relief (Figs 30.33 and 30.34). The only permanent cure, therefore, is removal of the nail and total nail-bed ablation.

If the condition is secondary to a subungual exostosis, removal of the nail may predispose to corn formation and further pain; it is therefore important to establish at the outset the possible aetiology of each case. Where total nail-bed ablation is chosen, the method is very similar to that used for ingrowing toe-nails.

A simple, immediate treatment for onychogryphosis is to break off the nail forcibly using thumb and finger (Fig. 30.35). Although such a technique sounds alarming, it is remarkably effective, and can be done under Entonox analgesia, 20 breaths, or digital anaesthesia using lignocaine. A loosening onychogryphotic nail may even be snapped off without any anaesthetic at all. As a percentage of such patients may have an impaired peripheral circulation, it causes less risk of trauma to avulse the nail under

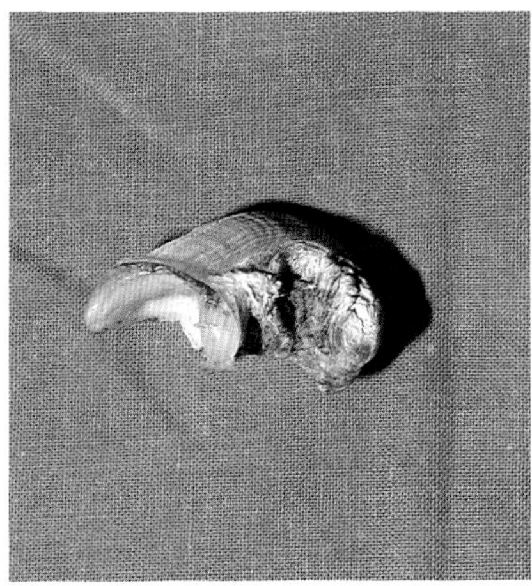

Fig. 30.35 Onychogryphotic nail removed simply by snapping it off.

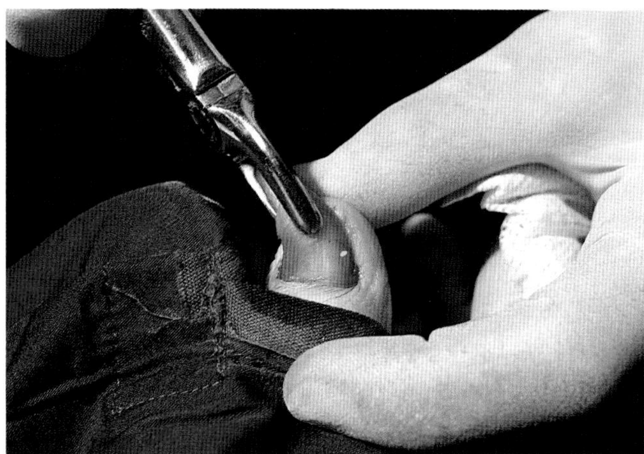

Fig. 30.36 The nail may either be split and removed in two pieces, or whole with a strong pair of forceps.

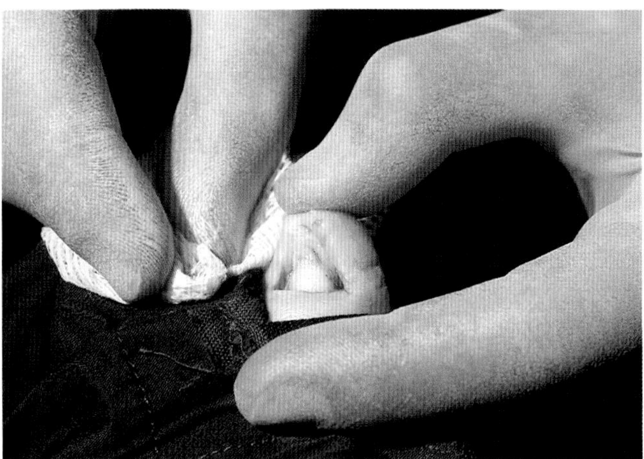

Fig. 30.37 The nail-bed after removal of the onychogryphotic nail.

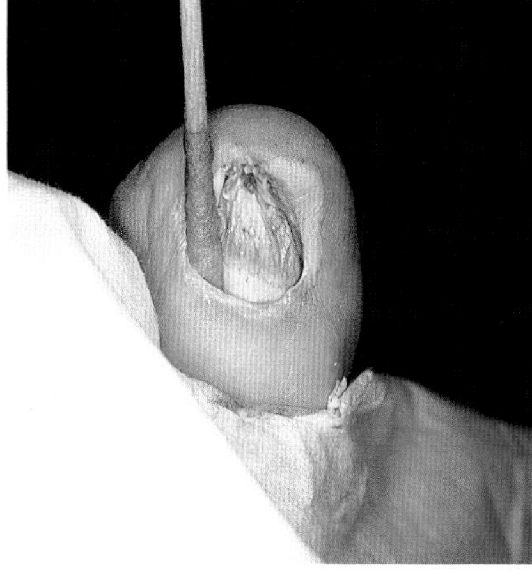

Fig. 30.38 Pure phenol is now applied to the nail bed and nail matrix for 3 min as for ingrowing nails.

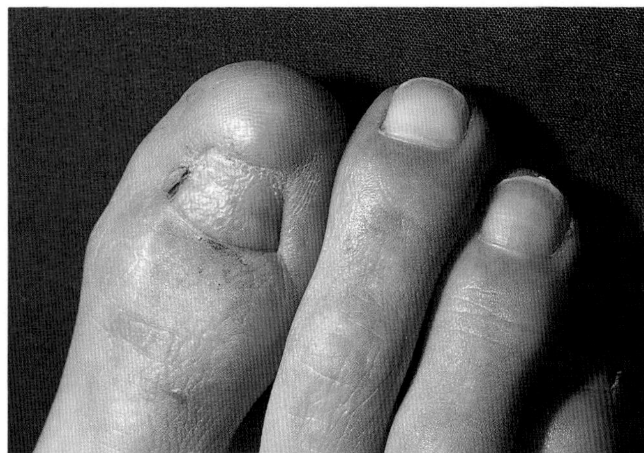

Fig. 30.39 Appearance of toe following phenol ablation of nail bed 3 months previously.

Entonox or even no anaesthesia rather than infiltrate the digit with local anaesthetic.

Having avulsed the nail, a simple, non-stick dressing, e.g. povidone-iodine (Inadine) is applied under a bandage, and the wound allowed to heal.

The chance of another onychogryphotic nail recurring is extremely high, and it may be judged preferable to destroy the nail-bed germinal epithelium to prevent any further nail growth (Fig. 30.36).

30.3 SUBUNGUAL EXOSTOSIS

Occasionally a patient presents with what at first sight appears to be a typical ingrowing toe-nail, or it may look like a subungual wart, but on closer examination (often after starting the operation!) the swelling is found to be bony hard, and further dissection reveals a subungual exostosis (Figs 30.40 and 30.41).

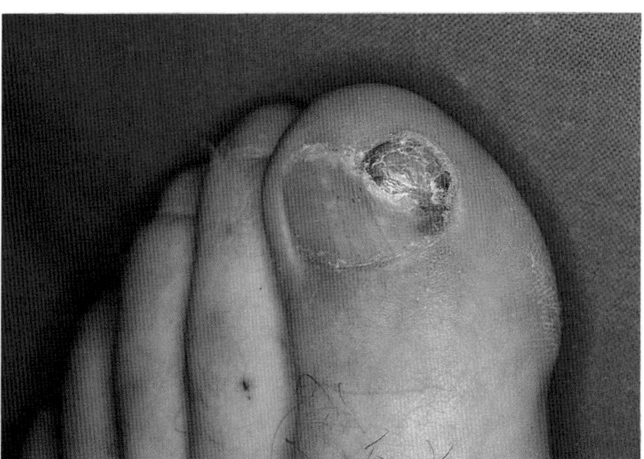

Fig. 30.40 Subungual exostosis presenting as atypical ingrowing toe-nail.

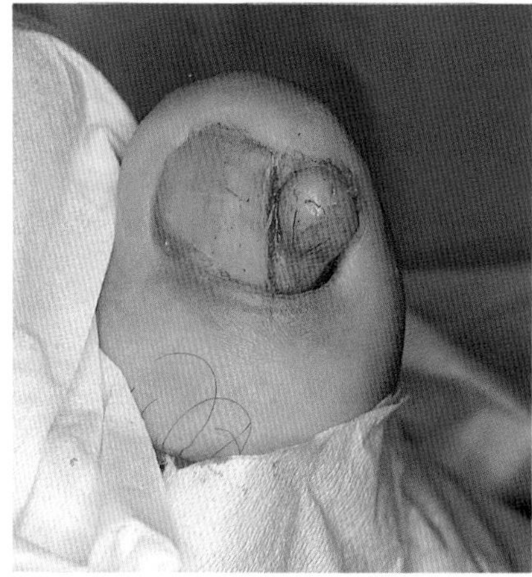

Fig. 30.41 At operation, the bony-hard swelling is seen to arise from the terminal phalanx.

It may be necessary to remove half or the whole nail to expose the exostosis. This may then be removed either with a nail chisel or by carefully cutting through with a scalpel blade. A firm, non-stick Inadine dressing is then applied, covered by gauze and a firm bandage. This may then be left undisturbed for 10 days.

30.4 SOFT CORN

This is a painful condition occurring in the web space between the toes: initially it looks like a wart, is very painful and fails to respond to wart cures.

Treatment consists of infiltrating the space with 1% lignocaine and then curetting the 'corn' using a Volkmann sharp-spoon curette, followed by cauterizing the base with the electrocautery or using phenol.

30.5 FUNGAL INFECTION OF THE TOE-NAILS

Established fungal infection of the toe-nails is almost impossible to eradicate: the best hope of cure consists in removing the toe-nail, sending it for mycological examination, and administering oral terbinafine (Lamisil) 250 mg daily while the new nail is growing.

As this may take from 12 to 24 months and entail daily terbinafine for 3–6 months it is even more important to establish the diagnosis mycologically beyond doubt.

31

Minor operations in ophthalmology

Now one eyelid must be held open by the assistant, the other by the surgeon. Thereupon the surgeon passes a sharp hook, the point of which has been a little incurved under the edge of the pterygium and fixes the hook in it ...

Celsus, AD *30*

31.1 REMOVAL OF FOREIGN BODIES IN EYES

Good illumination and magnification are essential. The standard ophthalmoscope with the +20 D lens gives good vision. The application of one drop of local anaesthetic eye-drops makes the whole procedure comfortable for the patient and easier for the operator.

If the object can be seen on the front of the eye-ball, it can usually be removed with a wisp of cotton wool wrapped around the end of a thin wooden applicator.

Failing this, an eye-spud may be used, or even a 19 swg (1.1 mm) needle, provided great care is taken. The possibility of a penetrating injury to the eye-ball should always be borne in mind, particularly if there is a history of high-speed grinding or the use of cold chisels.

It may be necessary to evert the upper eye-lid: this can be done by grasping the eye-lashes with finger and thumb of one hand and gently pressing down on the lid with a blunt, round rod.

31.2 MEIBOMIAN CYSTS

Meibomian cysts (tarsal cysts, chalazion) are extremely common and lend themselves admirably to general practitioner minor surgery, taking only a few minutes to cure. When large, and situated in the upper lid, the patient may complain of blurred vision owing to distortion of the cornea produced by pressure of the cyst on it, resulting in a temporary astigmatism of up to 3 dioptres. Spontaneous resolution is likewise common, but may take many months, and as surgical treatment is so quick and simple, it is to be preferred to waiting an indefinite time.

The diagnosis is usually straightforward; a small swelling can usually be seen on the outer surface of the affected eye-lid, eversion of this lid reveals a typical reddened spot with a paler centre, often pointing, and sometimes even discharging. The object of treatment is to incise the cyst, curette the cyst wall, and provide topical antibiotic cover until healing is complete, usually 7 days (Figs 31.1 and 31.2).

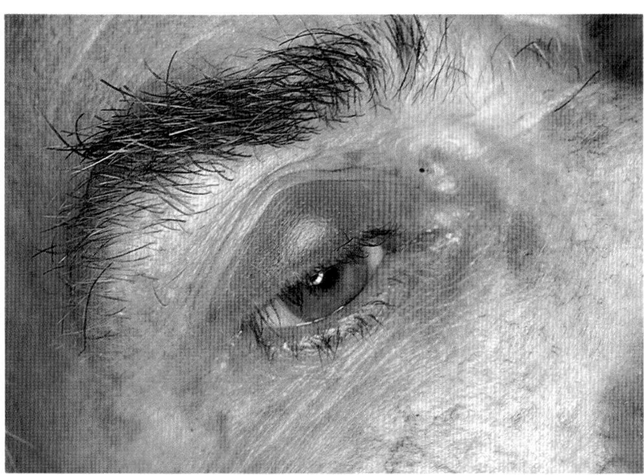

Fig. 31.1 External appearance of a Meibomian cyst on the upper eye-lid.

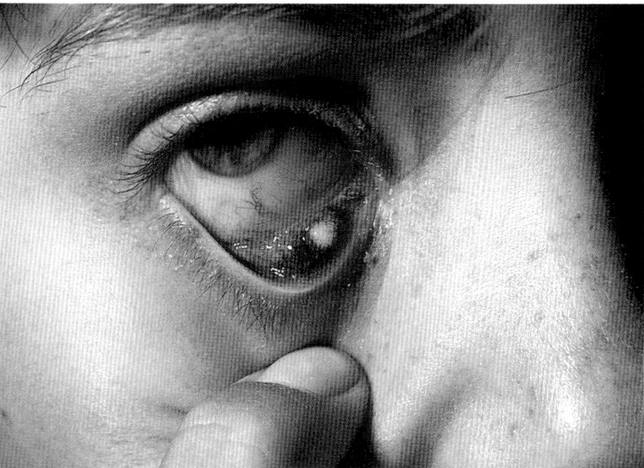

Fig. 31.2 A typical Meibomian cyst on the lower eye-lid.

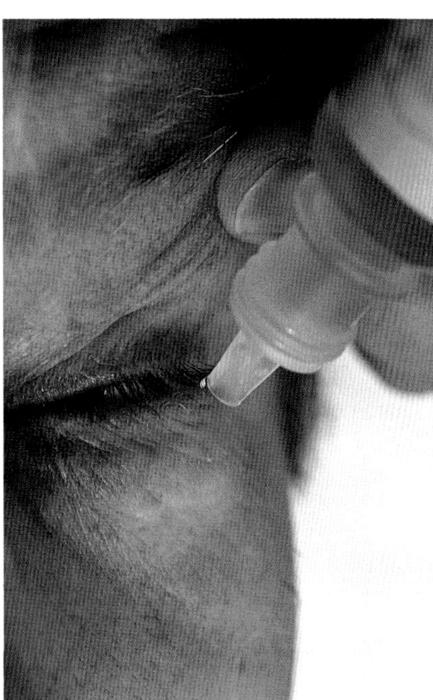

Fig. 31.3 Local anaesthetic eye-drops are applied.

Instruments required:

- dental syringe
- 30 swg (0.3 mm) needle
- cartridge of lignocaine 2% with 1:80 000 adrenaline
- anaesthetic eye-drops: amethocaine, lignocaine or Minims oxybuprocaine
- chalazion ring forceps (blepharostat)
- chalazion curette
- pair iris scissors $4^{1}/_{2}$ in. (11.4 cm) curved
- scalpel handle size 3
- scalpel blade size 11
- pair fine-toothed Adson dissecting forceps $4^{3}/_{4}$ in. (12 cm)
- chloramphenicol eye-drops and ointment
- eye pad and bandage.

The conjunctiva is anaesthetized using local anaesthetic eye-drops (Fig. 31.3) then with the fine 30 swg (0.3 mm) needle, lignocaine and adrenaline is injected into the skin over the cyst and a small quantity injected actually into the cyst itself (Fig. 31.4). Next, the chalazion ring forceps are applied to the eye-lid with the ring on the conjunctival surface exactly over the cyst, and the circular flat blade over the skin of the eye-lid. By tightening the screw on the ring forceps, the cyst is not only fixed and any bleeding controlled, but also the eye-lid may comfortably be everted, exposing the bulging cyst in the centre of the ring clamp (Fig. 31.5). Using the pointed no. 11 blade, a vertical incision is made in the cyst and the gelatinous contents released (Fig. 31.6). The cyst wall is then curetted using the small sharp-spoon chalazion curette, a small quantity of chloramphenical eye ointment applied, the ring forceps removed, and an eye-pad and bandage applied (Fig. 31.7).

This eye-pad is removed after 3 hours when the topical anaesthetic has worn off, and the patient is advised to clean away any blood, secretions and eye ointment with warm water. The patient is advised to use chloram-

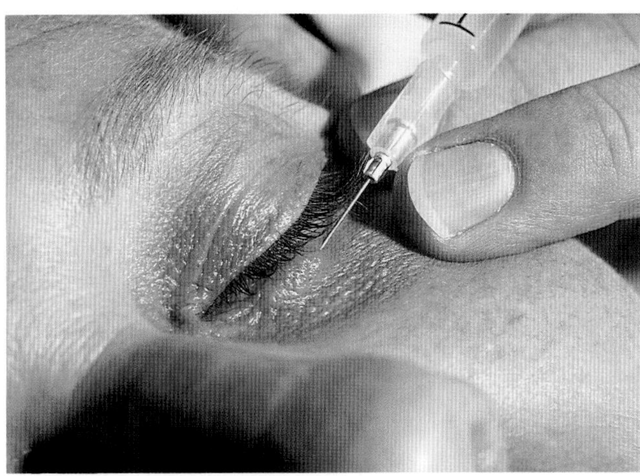

Fig. 31.4 After applying topical anaesthetic drops to the conjunctiva, the skin over the cyst is infiltrated with local anaesthetic, injecting a little into the cyst itself.

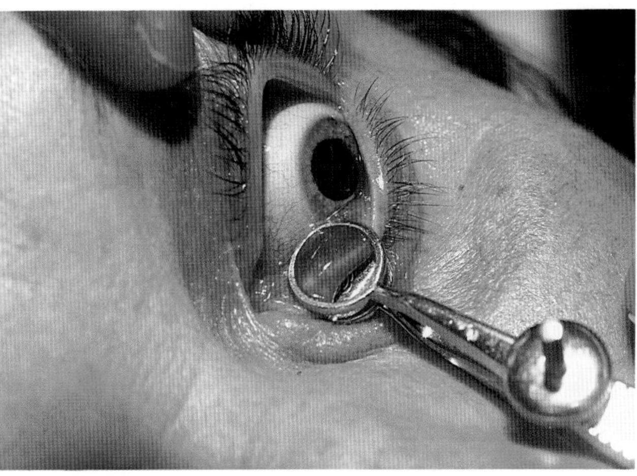

Fig. 31.5 The ring forceps are now applied so that the cyst lies in the centre of the ring.

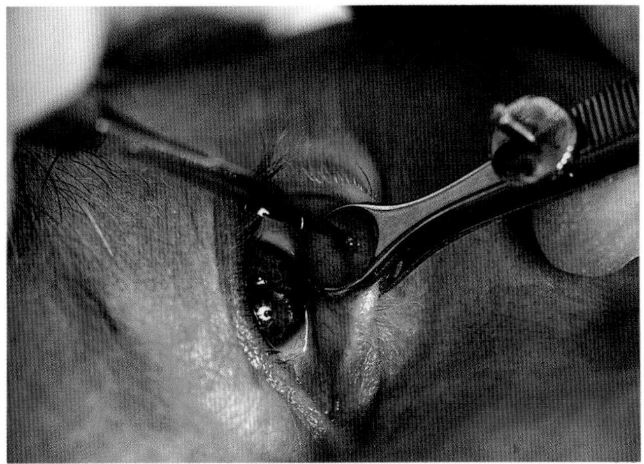

Fig. 31.6 The cyst is incised using a sharp-pointed scalpel blade.

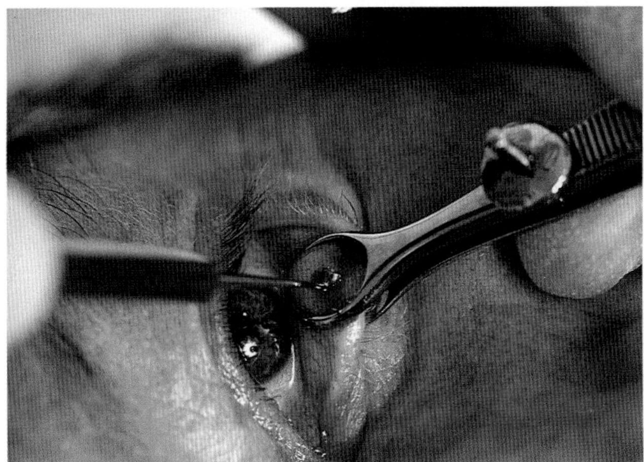

Fig. 31.7 Using a chalazion curette, the contents are removed, and the cyst wall curetted.

phenicol eye-drops three times a day for 7 days, when healing should be complete. Occasionally, in old cysts, most of the contents are fibrous and cannot be removed with the curette. In such cases the fibrous cyst should be grasped with a pair of fine toothed forceps introduced into the wound, and the mass removed using the curved iris scissors and scalpel.

31.3 ENTROPION

In the elderly, spasm of the orbicularis muscle results in inversion of the lower eye-lid which turns the eye-lashes so that they irritate the conjunctiva. This can be corrected by a simple 'skin and muscle' operation as follows: the conjunctiva is anaesthetized with topical 4% lignocaine or similar local anaesthetic. The skin over the lower eye-lid is next infiltrated using 1% lignocaine with 1:200 000 adrenaline and a pair of T-shaped forceps applied. A thin strip of skin, approximately 6 mm wide is excised, exposing the underlying muscle, a portion of which is also excised (Figs 31.8, 31.9 and 31.10). Any bleeding is controlled with the electrocautery. Equidistant spot burns are now placed along the margin to create scarring, fibrosis, and ultimate contracture, and the skin edges sutured with interrupted braided silk sutures 4/0 (metric gauge 1.5).

Careful judgement is needed – over-enthusiastic treatment could result in the production of an ectropion, a much more difficult condition to treat.

31.4 SYRINGING THE LACRIMAL DUCT

Blockage of the nasolacrimal duct is now relatively uncommon, but the patency can readily be checked by syringing. Two instruments are needed: a Nettleship's dilator for enlarging the lacrimal puncta, and a lacrimal cannula and syringe. First, pressure should be applied over the lacrimal sac on the side of the nose to see if any pus or mucus discharges through the punctum; then 4% lignocaine eye-drops are applied to the conjunctiva.

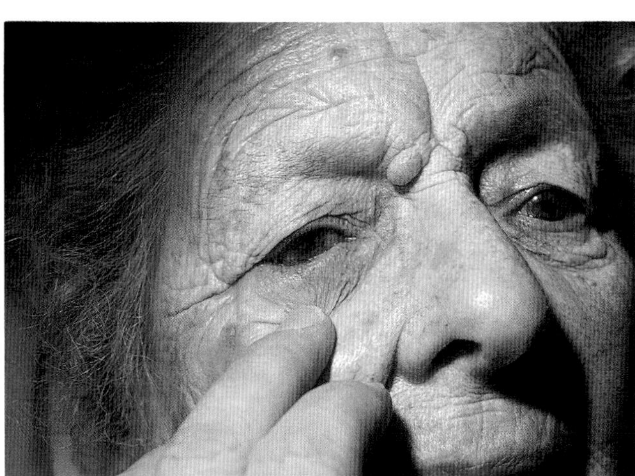

Fig. 31.8 Entropion.

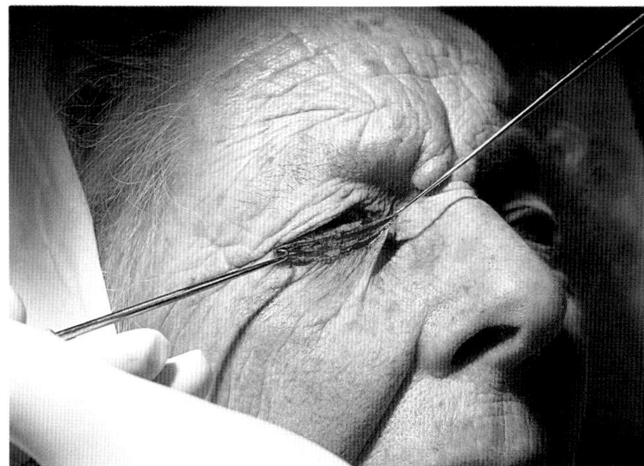

Fig. 31.9 A strip of skin is removed from the lower eyelid.

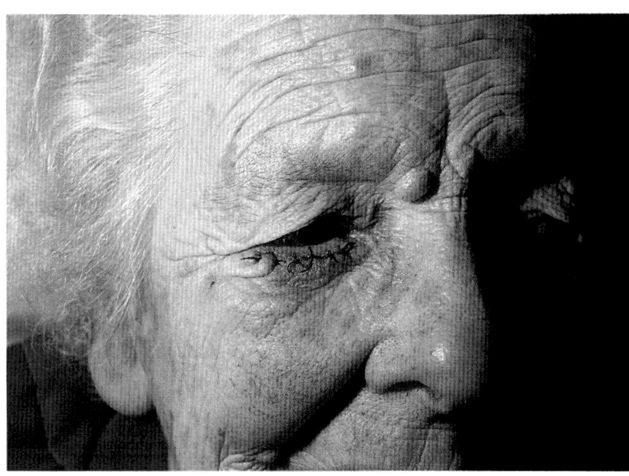

Fig. 31.10 After giving spot-burns to the underlying muscle, the skin is sutured.

Next the lower lid is everted to expose the inferior punctum, which is dilated with the point of the Nettleship's dilator. It should now be possible to insert the lacrimal cannula and syringe the duct using sterile normal saline.

31.5 THE USE OF THE TONOMETER TO DETECT GLAUCOMA

The eye be growne more solid and hard than it should be

Banister, describing 'absolute glaucoma' 1622

Glaucoma is the most preventable cause of blindness in this country; if detected early, medical treatment is 90% effective in reducing the intraocular pressure. It is estimated that in the UK, 300 000 people suffer from the disease, and it now accounts for 13% of all new blind registrations each year.

The intraocular pressure is measured in mmHg; the normal pressure in patients over the age of 40 is considered to be 15 mm; above 21 mm requires referral to a consultant ophthalmologist for further investigation, including charting of the visual fields.

Various instruments are available to measure the intraocular pressure; they vary in price from 50 pounds to several thousand pounds but the two most popular instruments in use are the Schiotz tonometer and the more recent Perkins applanation tonometer (Figs 31.11 and 31.12).

As it is not always feasible to screen the whole population for glaucoma, certain groups can be identified as being at special risk as follows:

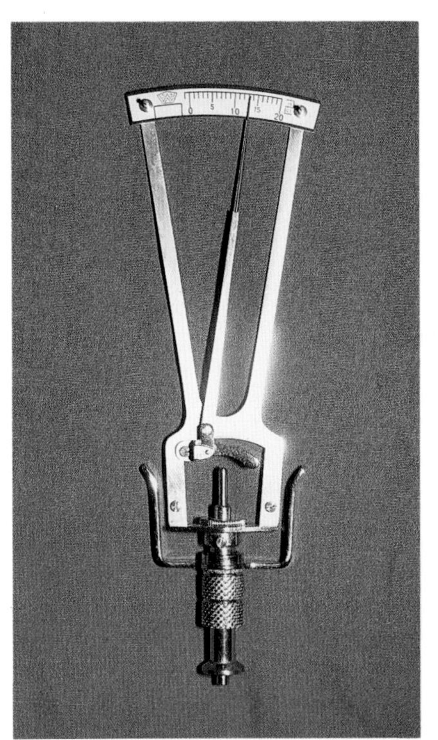

Fig. 31.11 The Schiötz tonometer; simple to use, and inexpensive.

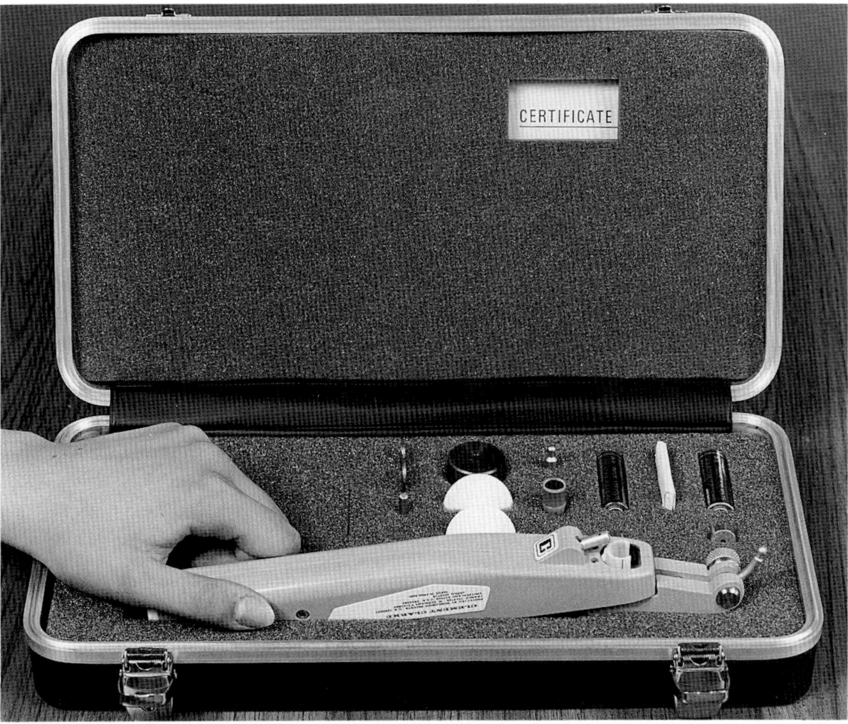

Fig. 31.12 The Perkins applanation tonometer (Clement Clarke International).

1. those patients over the age of 40;
2. patients with a family history of glaucoma;
3. patients with diabetes;
4. patients with a high degree of myopia;
5. patients with cardiovascular disease;
6. patients with a history of a bleeding episode requiring blood transfusion.

31.5.1 Technique of using the Schiotz tonometer

With the patient lying flat on the couch, local anaesthetic drops are instilled in each eye (Minims benoxinate 0.4% are suitable). Holding the tonometer as illustrated (Fig. 31.13), the scale is calibrated against a stainless steel spherical surface to check that the instrument reads '0'. It is now gently lowered on the centre of the eye as shown in the illustration, and the reading on the scale noted. (The scale has an inverse ratio to the intraocular pressure, i.e. the higher the reading the lower the pressure). The same procedure is carried out on the other eye, and the reading noted (Fig. 31.13). Using the conversion scale supplied with the instrument, the readings are translated into mmHg; the whole procedure taking less than one minute to perform.

Merely by using the criteria for screening as age – over 40 years – and a family history of glaucoma, the number of patients identified can be increased fivefold.

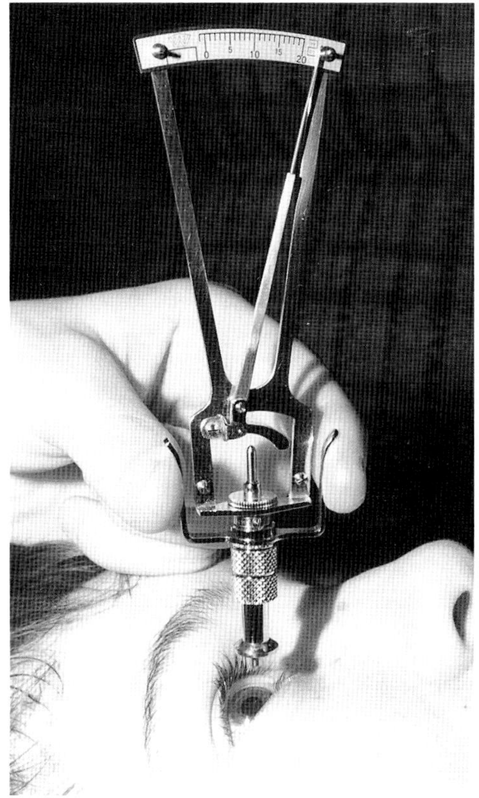

Fig. 31.13 Measuring the intraocular pressure with the Schiötz tonometer. After anaesthetizing the conjunctiva the instrument is gently lowered on the eye-ball and the reading on the scale noted.

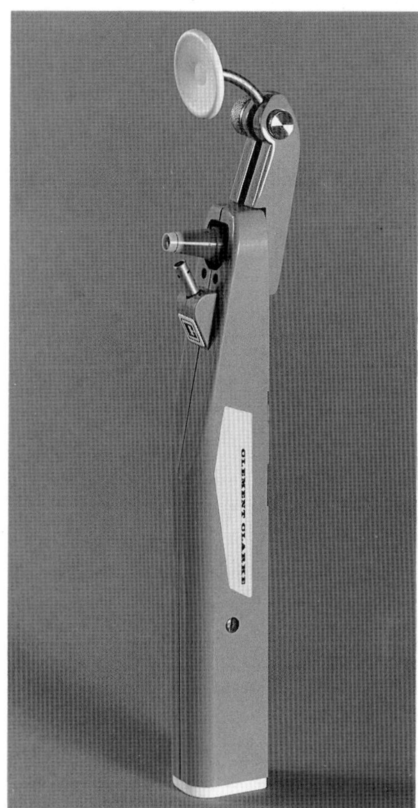

Fig. 31.14 To measure the intraocular pressure using the Perkins applanation tonometer, drops of fluoroscein and lignocaine are put into each eye, the instrument rested against the eye-ball and the reading noted when the semicircles coincide. The pressure, in mm of mercury, is obtained by multiplying this figure by ten.

31.5.2 Use of the Perkins applanation tonometer

This instrument is a hand-held tonometer designed by Professor E. S. Perkins, and has the advantage that it can be used to measure the intraocular pressure with the patient in any position (Figs 31.12 and 31.14). The principle is the same as that of the Goldmann applanation tonometer, in that an applanating surface is placed in contact with the cornea, and the force applied varied until a fixed diameter of applanation is achieved. A special doubling prism is used, through which the operator looks, and which rests directly against the cornea.

Method of use

The eyes are anaesthetized using eye-drops containing local anaesthetic and fluorescein. The Perkins tonometer should be held so that the thumb rests on the milled wheel which controls the internal spring as well as the switch for the illumination. The light is switched on by turning the wheel and the doubling prism gently pressed against the cornea, with the operator viewing through the prism. Two semicircles of fluorescein are visible through the viewing lens, and the force adjusted by turning the thumb-wheel until the inner margins of the semicircles coincide (Fig. 31.15).

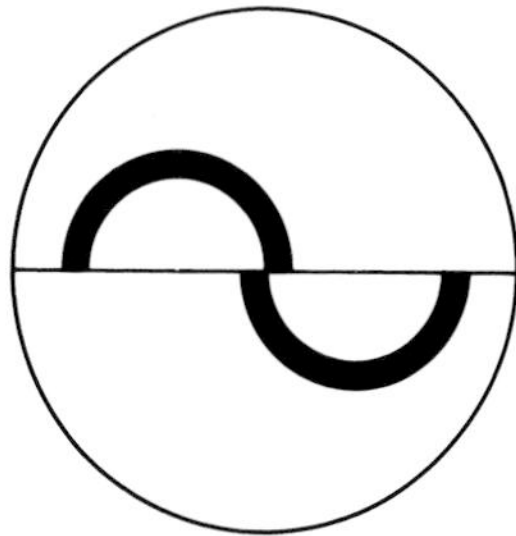

Fig. 31.15 The positions of the fluorescein semicircles when the pressure is correct.

The tonometer is removed from the eye, and the reading noted on the sliding scale. Multiplying the reading by 10 gives the tension in millimetres of mercury (mmHg).

The instrument is completely portable, can be held in the hand, has its own internal batteries and light, may be used in any position, and gives readings which are extremely reliable in less than one minute.

32

Epistaxis

Clean out for him the interior of both nostrils with two swabs of linen until every worm of blood which coagulates in the inside of his nostrils comes forth. Now afterwards thou shouldst place two plugs of linen saturated with grease and put into his nostrils

Edwin Smith, Surgical Papyrus, 3000–2500 BC

Most nose bleeds, particularly in children, are self-limiting; recurrent epistaxes often arise from a small collection of blood vessels in Little's area, just inside the nose on either side of the nasal septum. These can be successfully sealed by a variety of treatments, including the following.

32.1 SILVER NITRATE CAUTERIZATION

This is probably the simplest method. With the patient facing the doctor, and good illumination, Little's area is inspected on either side. Silver nitrate is now applied, using a disposable silver nitrate wooden applicator or using a pointed silver nitrate pencil stick held in an applicator (Figs 32.1, 32.2, and 32.3).

The treated area immediately turns white; some reflex watering of the patient's eyes always occurs. The patient is requested not to blow his or her nose for several hours, and normally only one treatment is necessary. No anaesthetic is required.

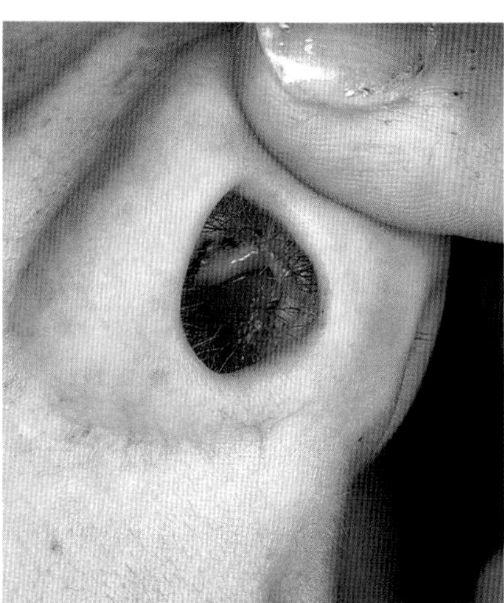

Fig. 32.1 The majority of nosebleeds occur from Little's area just inside the nostril, as shown.

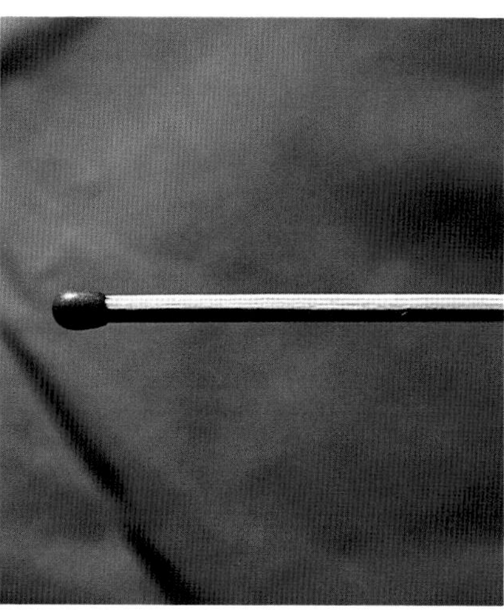

Fig. 32.2 Single-use silver nitrate applicators are ideal for cauterizing Little's area.

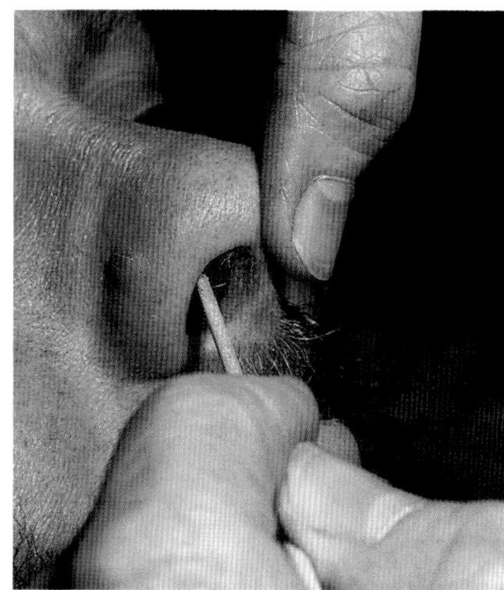

Fig. 32.3 Cauterizing Little's area with silver nitrate.

32.2 ELECTROCAUTERIZATION OF LITTLE'S AREA

More stubborn recurrent epistaxes may be treated with the electrocautery; but the nose must be anaesthetized. This is achieved by spraying the inside of the nose with xylocaine pressurized spray (lignocaine metered dose aerosol 100 μg per dose) or by the application of pledgets of cotton wool soaked in 4% lignocaine or similar topical anaesthetic.

With good illumination, the offending blood vessels are cauterized with the electrocautery. Only dull-red heat is used, and sparingly. Over-enthusiastic electrocauterization can lead to perforation of the nasal septum, and only one side should be cauterized at a time.

32.3 DIATHERMY OF LITTLE'S AREA

This may be achieved using the unipolar diathermy of Hyfrecator. As with electrocautery, the preliminary application of local anaesthesia is necessary. The area to be treated may be fulgurized by holding the needle electrode a very short distance away from the tissues and allowing a stream of sparks to play over the area. The current is turned down to minimum to avoid damage to the nasal septum.

32.4 CRYOSURGERY TO LITTLE'S AREA

Effective control may be achieved by freezing; the use of local anaesthesia is desirable but not always necessary. It is important to check that the probe will just cover the area to be frozen without accidentally touching any other part of the nose, otherwise this may become adherent to the probe and result in an additional 'frost-burn'.

32.5 PHOTOCOAGULATION OF LITTLE'S AREA

An infrared photocoagulator with narrow applicator may be used to control recurrent epistaxes. The topical application of local anaesthetic is necessary but the technique is simple and gives good results.

32.6 THE ACUTE BLEED

None of the aforementioned treatments is applicable during an acute nose-bleed, which must be controlled either by digital pressure or packing the nose with ribbon gauze soaked in 1:1000 adrenaline (plus 4% lignocaine if necessary). Should either of these fail, and particularly if the patient is elderly, where the source of bleeding is unlikely to be from Little's area, they should be referred to hospital.

33

The use of the proctoscope

The discharge of blood from the rectum is a disease chiefly confined to those advanced in life. It is occasioned by full living, abuse of purgatives, violent passions or habitual melancholy. To this effect, leeches and warm fomentations applied to the anus are the most efficacious remedies

Encyclopaedia Britannica, 1817

Examination of the anal canal in all patients with rectal symptoms is mandatory, but patients are still seen with inoperable cancers who missed having an early rectal examination.

Rectal bleeding is an extremely common symptom, fortunately in the majority it arises from haemorrhoids which can be visualized easily with a proctoscope. Instruments may be disposable or non-disposable, each having its own advantages and disadvantages.

33.1 DISPOSABLE PROCTOSCOPES

These consist of a plastic tube with central obturator; they may be presterilized in individual packs, and if sterilizing facilities are available (Chapter 6) they can be used on more than one occasion. External illumination is necessary for the majority of instruments, although some have provision for internal illumination.

33.2 NON-DISPOSABLE PROCTOSCOPES

These are generally made of stainless steel and consist of an outer tube and handle, together with a central obturator. Illumination can be from an external source, from in-built illumination in the form of a tungsten-filament or quartz bulbs, or from an external fibreoptic light source. They can be sterilized by autoclaving, dry heat oven or immersion (Chapter 6).

33.2.1 Technique

If the patient is lying in the left lateral position, with knees drawn up, the direction of the anal canal is upwards and forwards. A digital rectal examination is performed, and any abnormality in the rectum noted. The muscle tone of the anal sphincter is noted, as is the degree of discomfort caused by the examination. This may give a clue to the diagnosis of anal fissure, typified by pain and spasm. The examining finger is withdrawn, and the glove examined for any signs of blood. Next, the proctoscope is lubricated and very gently inserted into the anal canal; as soon as the instrument is felt to have passed through the sphincter, its direction is changed slightly posteri-

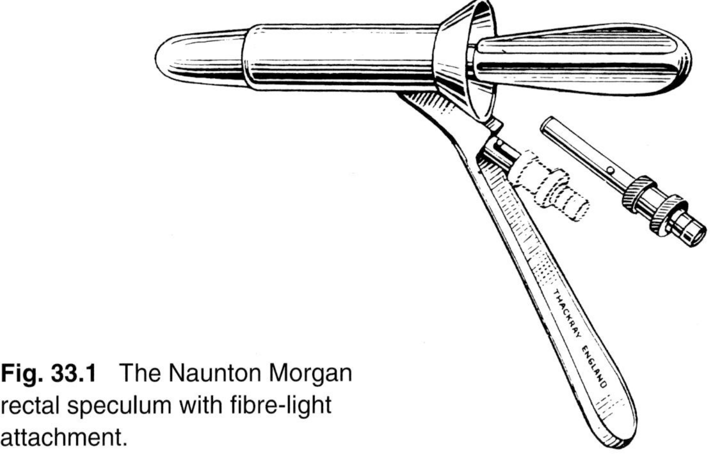

Fig. 33.1 The Naunton Morgan rectal speculum with fibre-light attachment.

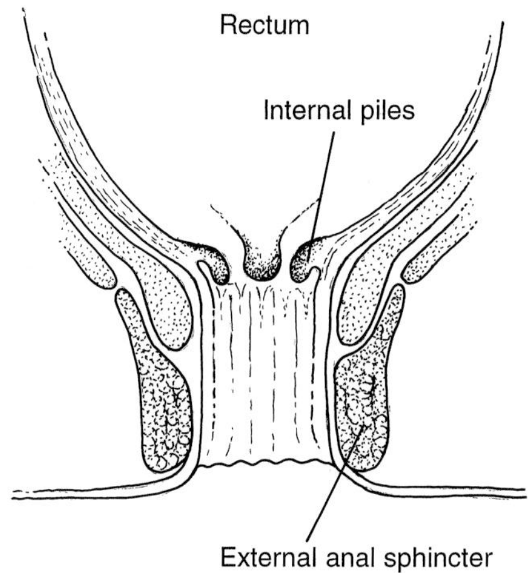

Fig. 33.2 Anatomy of the anus and rectum. (Redrawn from G.J. Hill, *Outpatient Surgery,* by permission of WB Saunders & Co.)

orly to take account of the direction of the rectum. The instrument is inserted fully to the flange, the obturator withdrawn, and the illumination switched on. The normal mucous membrane is pale, but capillaries and tributaries of the superior haemorrhoidal vein are visible. Any pathology is noted, and the proctoscope slowly withdrawn, during which the mucous membrane begins to close in. Prolapsing internal haemorrhoids become easily visible at this stage, and their positions may be noted for future reference. As the proctoscope is further withdrawn, lesions of the anal canal may be seen, such as proctitis or fissure.

Where the patient gives a history of bleeding on defaecation, it is worth reintroducing the proctoscope and asking the patient to strain down as the instrument is slowly withdrawn. In this way, a bleeding haemorrhoid or fissure can be identified. If suspected haemorrhoids are revealed on proctoscopy, it is often convenient to treat them at the time of the initial examination (Chapter 36).

34

Sigmoidoscopy

Signs, forsooth, of ulceration are these: the patient cannot abstain from going to the privy because of aching, and he passes a stinking discharge mixed with watery blood. Ignorant leeches will assure the patient that he has dysentery, when truly it is not. I never saw, nor heard of any man that was cured of cancer of the rectum, but I have known many that died of the aforesaid sickness

John of Arderne, 1306–90

Sigmoidoscopy is considerably easier to perform than is generally realized [32, 33]. It is not a difficult technique to learn, and with regular use the practitioner will quickly learn to recognize both the normal and abnormal appearances. The sigmoidoscope can be one of the most valuable instruments in general practice; combined with a pair of biopsy forceps, rapid diagnosis of carcinoma of the rectum, ulcerative colitis, rectal polypi, proctitis, and haemorrhoids can be made.

The first sigmoidoscope was invented by Bodenhamer in 1863 and consisted of a flexible tube of reflecting mirrors; unfortunately it was found to be impractical and it was not until 1895 that Kelly described a sigmoidoscope very similar to those found today. His instrument had the light bulb placed distally, which had the disadvantage of soiling by faeces and bulb failure. In 1912 Yeomans designed an instrument with proximal illumination and air insufflation, and apart from slight modifications today's instruments are very similar.

Improvements in illumination using fibreoptic light sources and cables have enabled better visualization to be obtained, and most recently, flexible fibreoptic sigmoidoscopes have been introduced which will examine more of the rectum and sigmoid colon than the conventional rigid instrument.

34.1 INDICATIONS FOR USE

Sigmoidoscopy forms an integral part of the routine investigation of all patients presenting with rectal bleeding, change in bowel habit, prolonged diarrhoea, and of the follow-up of patients who have had rectal surgery.

The standard adult stainless-steel Lloyd-Davies sigmoidoscope with proximal illumination gives good visualization, is easy to use, is well constructed and virtually indestructible (Fig. 34.1). A smaller diameter instrument is also available, but for the majority of examinations the adult size will be found to be more than adequate. Tungsten filament or quartz halogen bulbs give good illumination, but if a fibreoptic light source can be obtained this is even better and more reliable.

Reasonably priced disposable sigmoidoscopes are also available; these

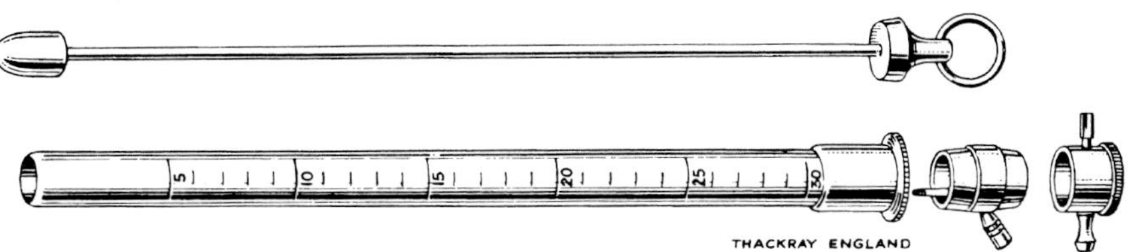

Fig. 34.1 The Lloyd-Davies stainless steel adult sigmoidoscope fitted with proximal fibre-light chamber.

have the advantage of not requiring repeated sterilization and cleaning, but will work out more expensive in the long run compared with the stainless steel models.

A telescope attachment with magnification is a valuable accessory, giving much improved views of the mucosa. Having assembled all the necessary instruments for sigmoidoscopy it is better to keep them all on a separate 'rectal trolley' ready for immediate use; this may then be taken from one consulting room to another at a moment's notice (Figs 34.2 and 34.3). Biopsy forceps, although expensive, are invaluable, and enable the doctor to take an immediate biopsy of any suspicious lesions. In order to take a biopsy, the window or telescope attachment at the operator's end of the sigmoidoscope needs to be removed in order to introduce the forceps, and this occasionally causes slight problems with loss of insufflated air, prolapse of mucosa, or poor visibility. Paterson's biopsy forceps (Figs 34.5 and 34.6), Chevalier Jackson's biopsy forceps (Fig. 34.6), or Yeoman's rectal biopsy forceps are all suitable for the taking of biopsies. Other instruments

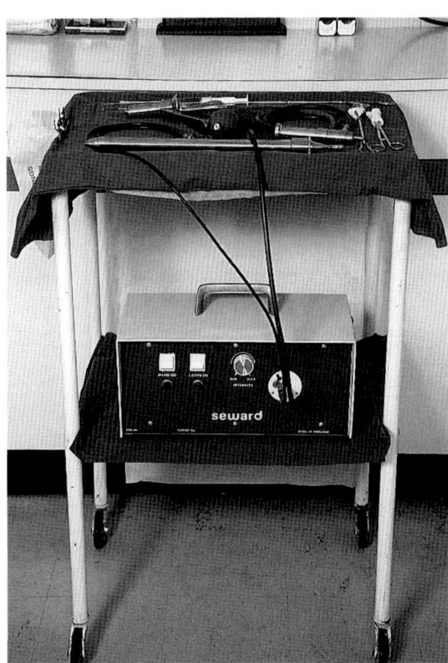

Fig. 34.2 It is a good idea to keep all instruments and accessories for sigmoidoscopy on one trolley for immediate use.

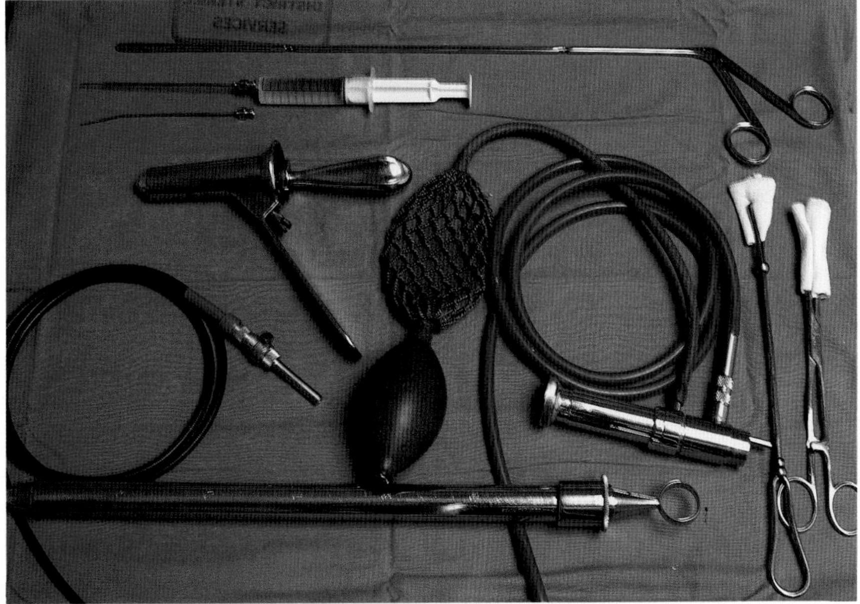

Fig. 34.3 Instruments ready for sigmoidoscopy.

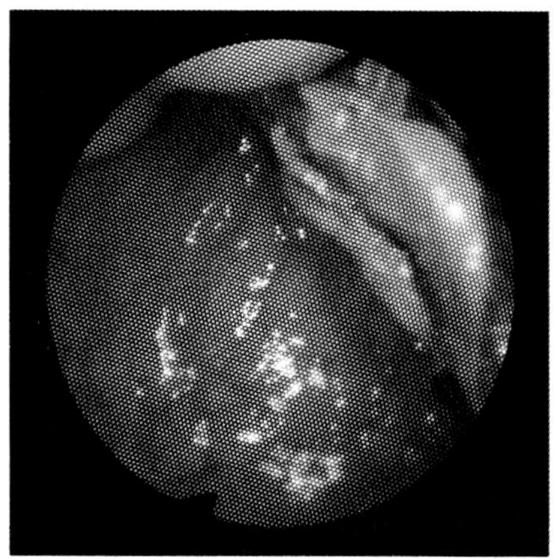

Fig. 34.4 View through sigmoidoscope on entering rectum. Small quantity faeces, which are negotiable.

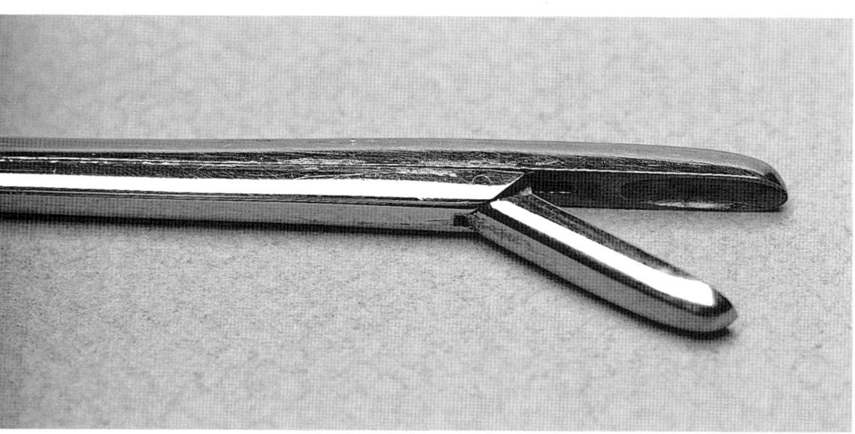

Fig. 34.5 Paterson biopsy forceps.

which may be kept on a 'rectal trolley' include a proctoscope, haemorrhoid injection syringe and needles, ampoules of 5% oily phenol, specimen containers with 10% formol-saline for histology, K-Y jelly, swabs, haemorrhoid ligator, grasping forceps, and neoprene bands, plus swab holder and swabs.

34.2 PREPARATION OF THE PATIENT

Normally no preliminary bowel preparation is necessary, nor desirable, as the instrument can usually be manoeuvred past any faeces (Fig. 34.4). Enemas or bowel wash-outs, as well as inflaming the mucosa, will wash away tell-tale blood-streaks or secretions. If the bowel is completely occluded with faeces, it is better to abandon the examination and attempt it on another occasion after defaecation.

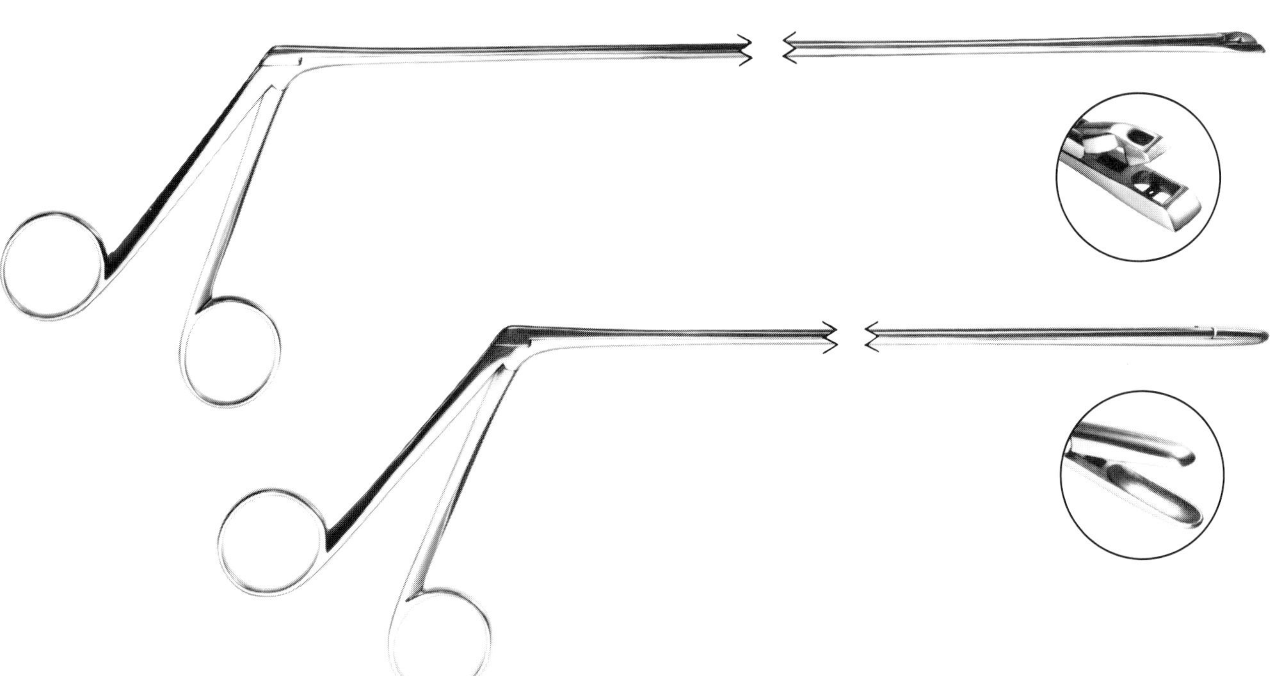

Fig. 34.6 Chevalier Jackson biopsy forceps (above) and Paterson biopsy forceps (below).

34.3 TECHNIQUE OF SIGMOIDOSCOPY

The actual sigmoidoscopic examination only takes a few minutes, thus, if the instruments are always ready assembled for immediate use, it may be included in the initial consultation. The left lateral position is both comfortable and adequate for most sigmoidoscopies. The patient should be positioned with the buttocks at the edge of the couch, and knees and feet at the opposite edge, curled up.

A careful explanation of what will be done should always be given to the patient, in particular they may feel embarrassed in case they lose faeces or blood and soil the examination couch; reassurance that the patient, and doctor, are protected by a glass window will allay much anxiety. The sigmoidoscope is assembled, the light checked, and the distal end lubricated with water-soluble K-Y jelly. Specimen containers and biopsy forceps are placed in an accessible position for the operator, and a digital rectal examination performed. This will reveal any low-lying masses, as well as lubricating the anal canal. Holding the sigmoidoscope, and with the palm of the hand covering the obturator to prevent it being extruded, the instrument is gently inserted into the anal canal, in the direction of the umbilicus. It helps at this stage to ask the patient to quietly breathe in and out of his or her mouth. As soon as the sigmoidoscope has entered the rectum, the obturator is removed, and the inspection window or telescope attached, together with the bellows; a little air is introduced, from now on the instrument is advanced under direct vision. The lower valve of Houston is seen on the left, then the middle valve on the right. The apex of the rectum often appears to be a blind end, but by gently withdrawing the sigmoidoscope and pointing it towards the left and slightly forwards, the entrance to the sigmoid can be seen. This is usually the most difficult part of the examination, but with gentleness and patience, it can usually be negotiated. The instrument may now be passed to 20–25 cm, provided the patient does not complain of pain. Any lesions or blood-stained discharges are noted, and the sigmoidoscope gradually withdrawn.

A better examination of the rectum is obtained as the instrument is being withdrawn than when it is being introduced. Any suspicious lesions can be biopsied and their exact distance from the anus measured on the scale printed on the side of the sigmoidoscope.

If blood or a blood-stained discharge is seen coming from further inside the bowel, a colonoscopy and/or barium enema should be arranged. Similarly if any infective lesion is suspected, rectal swabs can be taken for culture.

During the examination, air should be gently blown in with the bellows to keep the bowel lumen opened out, forcible air distension should be avoided as it may cause pain and spasm.

An analysis of sigmoidoscopies performed in general practice showed that the presenting symptom of bleeding occurred in 49%, and of those, 14% were found to have rectal cancer; 70% of these could not be felt on digital examination but could all be seen with the sigmoidoscope. Thus although the commonest cause of rectal bleeding is still haemorrhoids, nevertheless one in seven (14%) was found to have a carcinoma [34].

35

Thrombosed external haemorrhoids

But wit thou, ... that an abscess breeding near the anus should not be left to burst by itself ... be it boldly opened with a very sharp lancette so that ... the corrupt blood may go out

John of Arderne, 1306–90

More correctly described as perianal haematoma, the 'thrombosed external haemorrhoid' is a common condition, occurring spontaneously in young adults, sometimes associated with straining at defaecation, but often not. They are painful and can vary in size from a small pea to a large walnut; left untreated, they gradually absorb, leaving a small skin tag (Fig. 35.1). Surgical treatment offers a quick, effective cure, takes only a few minutes, and gives immediate relief of symptoms.

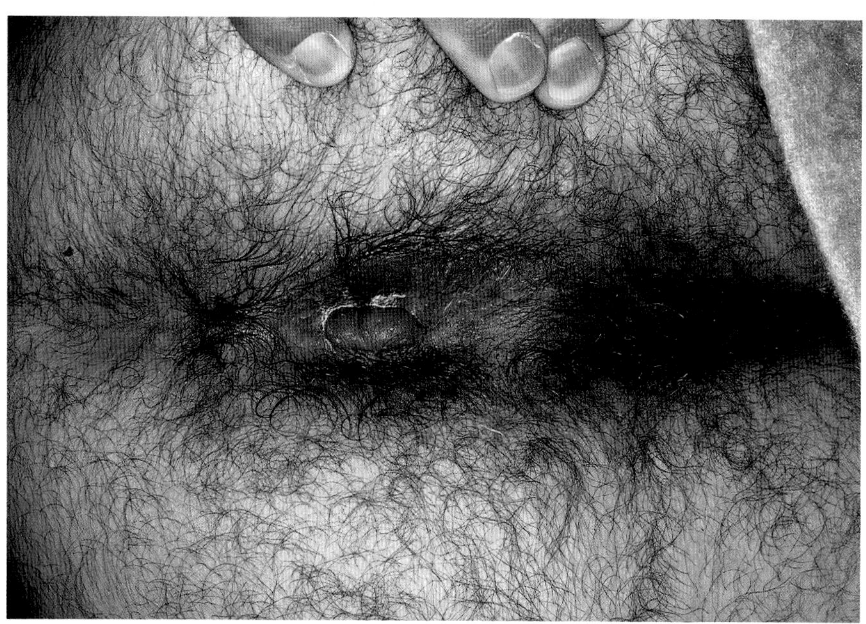

Fig. 35.1 Typical thrombosed external haemorrhoid.

Instruments required:

2 ml syringe
25 swg × 5/8 in. (0.5 mm x 16 mm) needle
1% lignocaine with adrenaline 1:200 000
pair toothed dissecting forceps 5 in. (12.7 cm)
pair iris scissors, straight 4 1/2 in. (11.4 cm).

With the patient lying on his or her left side, and knees drawn up, the base of the haematoma is infiltrated with local anaesthetic. If an assistant is available, he or she should be asked to pull the upper buttock upwards to expose the thrombosed haemorrhoid – if an assistant is not available, the patient may do this. An ellipse of skin is cut out using the iris scissors and dissecting forceps; this immediately reveals the typical black blood-clot inside the haemorrhoid, which may either be expressed by pressure or lifted out with the forceps. The wound is checked to make sure there is only one haematoma – occasionally two or three loculated clots are found and each should be removed. Generally there is only a little bleeding (Fig. 35.2), which can be controlled by the application of a sterile gamgee dressing. The patient is advised to have twice-daily salt baths until healing is complete.

Small perianal haematoma may conveniently be left to absorb spontaneously, but if surgery is contemplated, just a radial incision and expression of the clot may suffice.

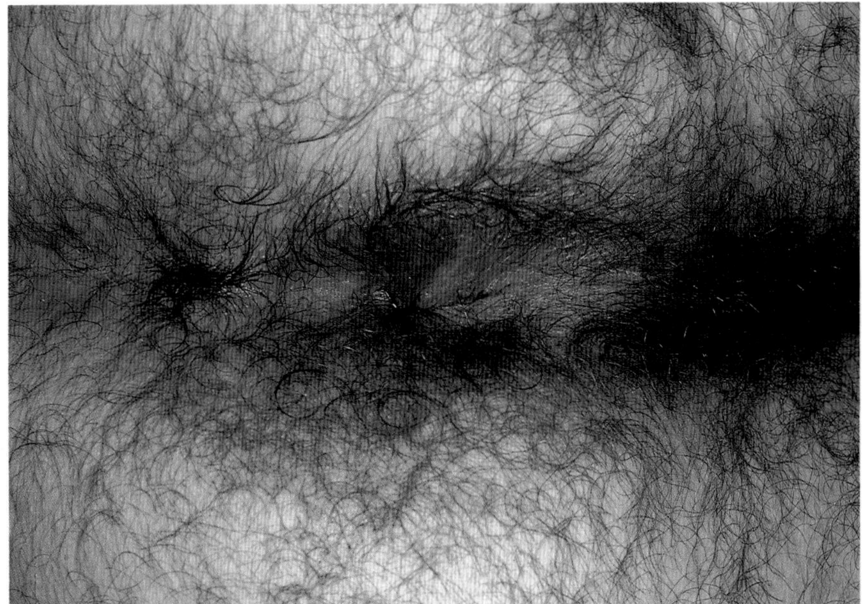

Fig. 35.2 Immediately after excising thrombosed external haemorrhoid; no stitch needed – the skin edges contract together. Bleeding is generally only slight.

36

Treatment of internal haemorrhoids

When there are chronic haemorrhoids in the anus, sear the patient with three cauterisations over the lower dorsal vertebra

Albucasis, 11th Century

It is a wise rule to suspect all haemorrhoids as being due to carcinoma of the rectum until proved otherwise. For this reason it is essential to examine every patient complaining of rectal bleeding with the proctoscope, and if possible the sigmoidoscope as well.

Three types of internal haemorrhoids can be recognized.

36.1 TYPES OF HAEMORRHOIDS

36.1.1 First degree

The haemorrhoids are small, bleed freely, especially after defaecation and, though not palpable with the examining finger, are visible when examined through the proctoscope. This type is eminently suitable for treatment in general practice by injection, photocoagulation, or cryotherapy.

36.1.2 Second degree

These haemorrhoids are larger, and tend to protrude after defaecation, but will generally reduce themselves. Bleeding may be less marked because fibrosis is developing in the pile. Treatment by injection, photocoagulation, and cryotherapy is still possible, as is neoprene-hand ligation, but the results are not consistently as good as first-degree haemorrhoids.

36.1.3 Third degree or prolapsing haemorrhoids

In this type, prolapse is severe, requiring digital replacement by the patient or doctor; strangulation is a common complication. Such haemorrhoids are not generally suitable for general practitioner treatment and should be referred to a general surgeon. Most uncomplicated haemorrhoids are painless; the presence of pain indicates inflammation, strangulation, thrombosis, or anal fissure.

36.2 TREATMENT OF INTERNAL HAEMORRHOIDS BY INJECTION OF SCLEROSING FLUID

This is still the method favoured by the majority of surgeons in the UK; the solutions used, and the technique employed, have changed little over the last 100 years and still give excellent results [35, 36].

Instruments required:

proctoscope with illumination
sigmoidoscope with illumination
haemorrhoid injection syringe and needle
5 ml ampoules of 5% oily phenol BPC.

With the patient lying in the left lateral position a digital rectal examination is performed to exclude any low-lying tumours, followed by a sigmoidoscopy. If there is any suspicion of blood coming from higher in the large bowel, either from the history or examination, colonoscopy and/or barium enema examination should be arranged.

A well-lubricated proctoscope is now inserted to its full length and the obturator removed. By gently withdrawing the instrument, any haemorrhoids will become easily visible; these are commonly situated at three o'clock, seven o'clock, and eleven o'clock positions corresponding with the termination of the branches of the superior haemorrhoidal artery.

It may be necessary at this stage to gently reinsert the proctoscope so that the base of each haemorrhoid can be seen. A submucosal injection of 5% phenol in almond oil is now given. This must be done at the upper end of the haemorrhoid and above the anorectal ring. Injections given below the anorectal ring are extremely painful. The bevel of the needle should be directed towards the mucosa rather than the lumen of the rectum, and the phenol injected slowly, until blanching is seen; the amount injected varies from 1 ml to 5 ml, or occasionally even more if the mucosa is very lax (Fig. 36.1).

All three primary haemorrhoids may be treated simultaneously, or if one is larger (commonly the right anterior) this may be given two injections, followed by subsequent treatments at a later visit.

The patient is given advice about avoiding constipation, put on a high-roughage diet, and allowed home. Follow-up examinations and injections can be at the discretion and preference of the doctor – weekly if other injections are anticipated, or after 6 weeks if routine follow-up is desired.

36.3 CRYOSURGERY TREATMENT OF INTERNAL HAEMORRHOIDS

Where a cryoprobe is available, satisfactory treatment of first- and second-degree haemorrhoids can be obtained, and if the patient is judged to be unfit for haemorrhoidectomy, even third-degree haemorrhoids can be treated [37]. The cryoprobe is applied to the haemorrhoid itself and a 2 min freeze given.

The nitrous oxide cryoprobe has the added advantage that it adheres to the tissue, so that gentle traction may be applied to prevent freezing of

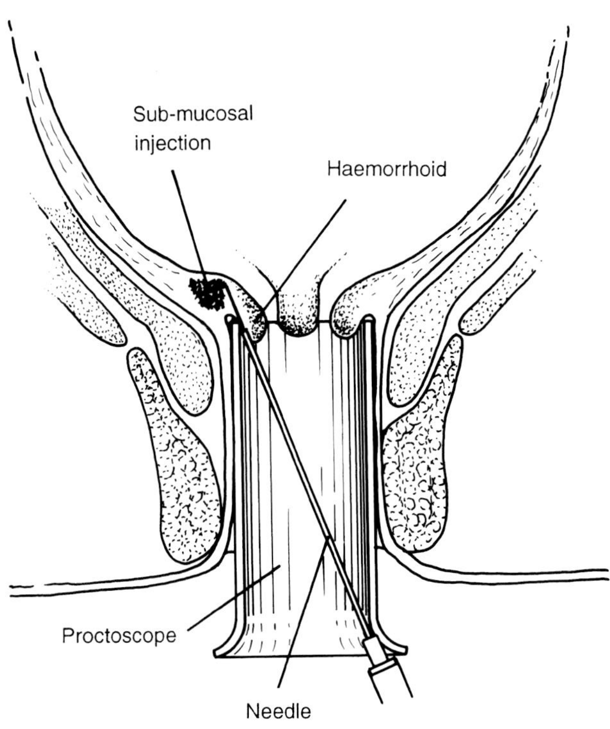

Fig. 36.1 Submucosal injection of haemorrhoid using 5% oily phenol.

deeper tissues. The probe must then be rewarmed before it can be separated from the pile. Treatment is well tolerated, some patients experience a dull ache during and immediately after freezing. The patient should be warned to expect a profuse watery, blood-stained discharge for many weeks following treatment.

36.4 INFRARED PHOTOCOAGULATION OF INTERNAL HAEMORRHOIDS

A relatively new and simple instrument for the treatment of internal haemorrhoids is the infrared photocoagulator. This consists of a low voltage quartz-halogen bulb with gold-plated reflector and a solid quartz rod which transmits infrared radiation to a Teflon-coated tip (Figs 36.2, 36.3, 36.4). A 1.5-s pulse of infrared radiation produces an accurately defined necrosis 3 mm deep and 3 mm in diameter. The probe may be used through the proctoscope in the same way as injection therapy, and is applied at exactly the same sites, i.e. above the base of each haemorrhoid. Three separate areas of coagulation are required at the base of each haemorrhoid for optimum results. Of all treatments currently available for internal haemorrhoids, photocoagulation is one of the simplest, safest, and quickest, and can be rapidly learned by any doctor [38].

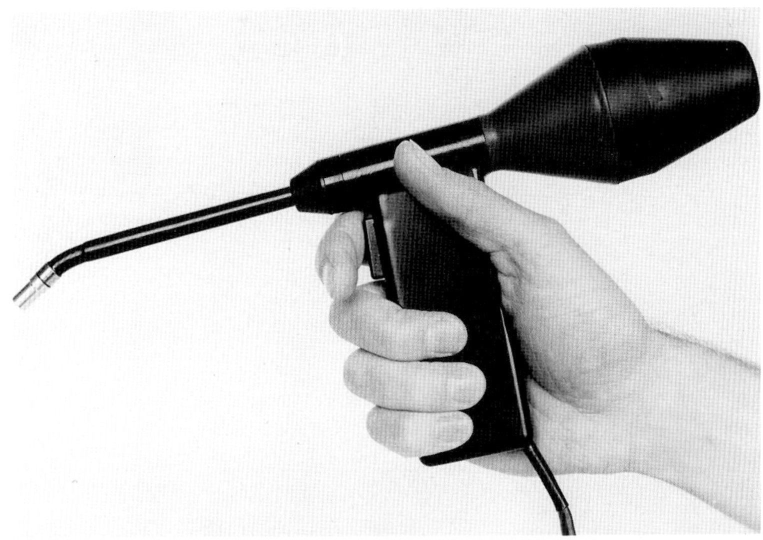

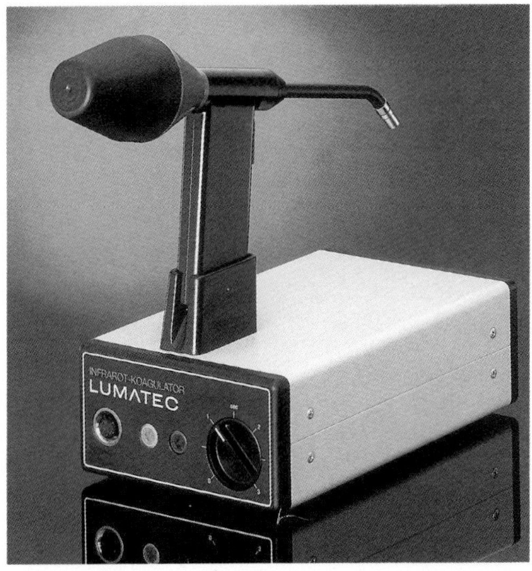

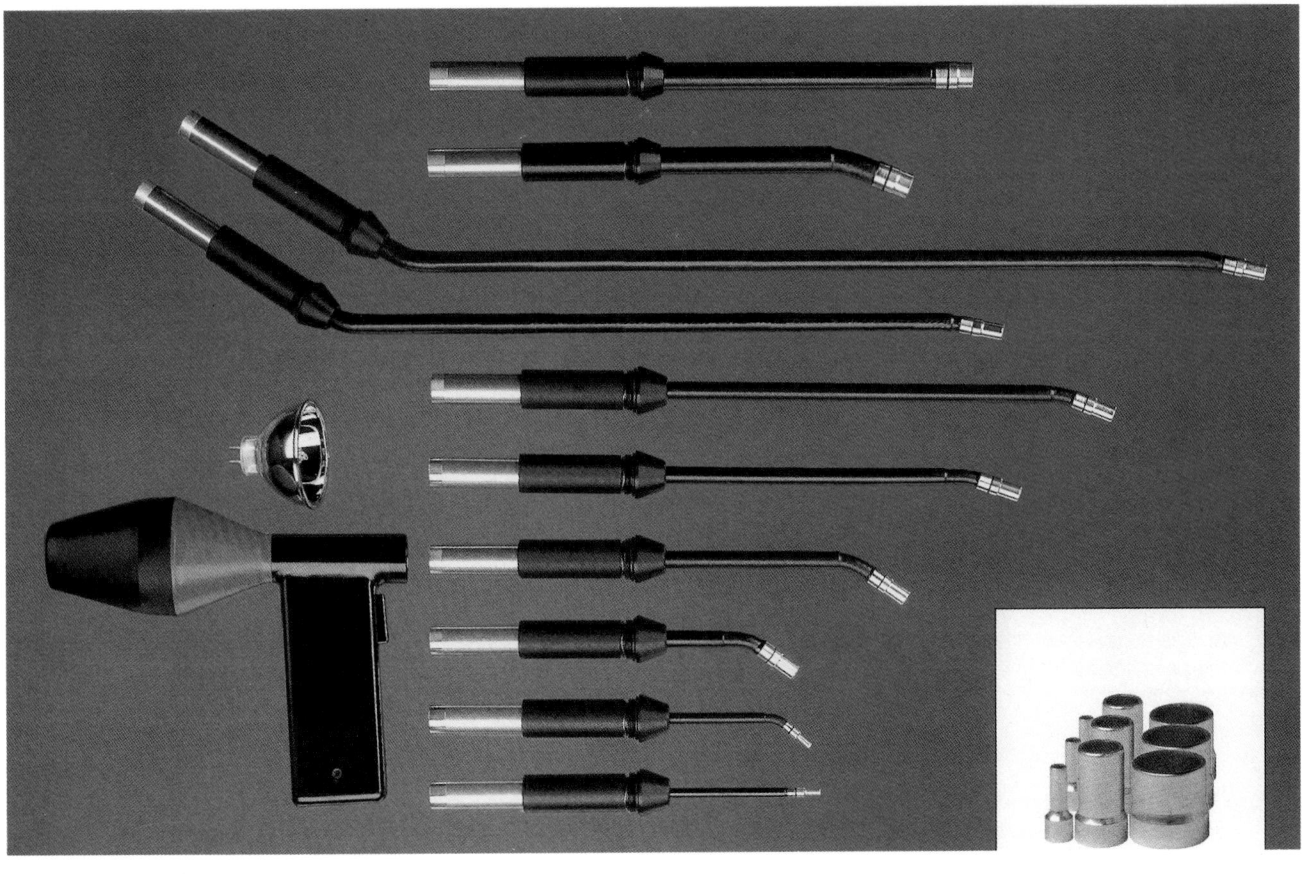

Fig. 36.2a The infrared coagulator: simple to use, three burns required at the base of each haemorrhoid (Chilworth Medicals Ltd). (**b**) The infrared coagulator on base with timer and transformer. (**c**) Selection of quartz glass light guides 2 mm, 6 mm and 10 mm.

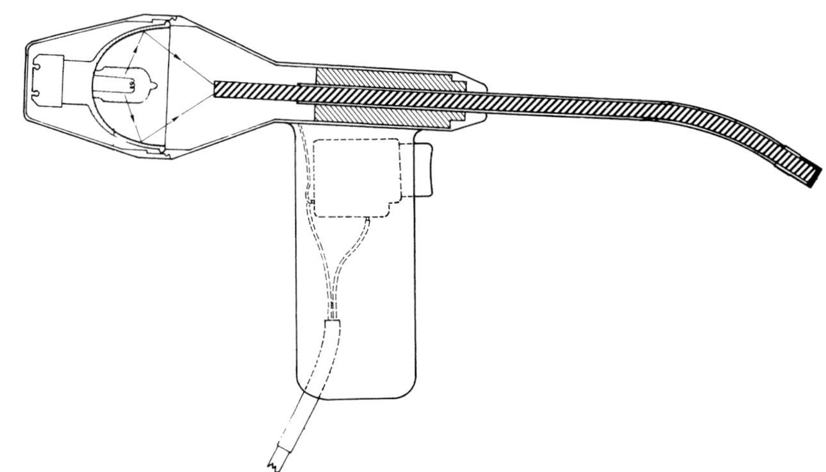

Fig. 36.3 How the photocoagulator works (Chilworth Medicals Ltd).

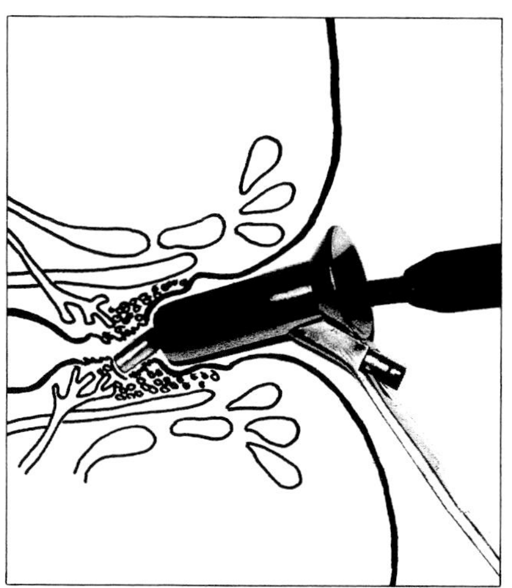

Fig. 36.4 Placement of photocoagulator within proctoscope (Chilworth Medicals Ltd.)

36.5 NEOPRENE BAND LIGATION OF INTERNAL HAEMORRHOIDS

Rubber-band ligation has been used successfully for the treatment of haemorrhoids, but the technique requires more skill and practice than injection or photocoagulation [39, 40, 41]. It is suitable only for haemorrhoids whose bases are more than 2 cm above the anorectal ring; if bands are applied below this level, severe pain is caused, and the removal of any constricting band is extremely difficult! An assistant is required to hold the proctoscope; the haemorrhoids are visualized, and the rubber band ligator, loaded with one band is passed through the proctoscope.

Using a pair of haemorrhoid-grasping forceps, the mucosa above the base of the haemorrhoid is pulled through the ring of the applicator, and the band slipped over the base by pressing the handle on the instrument (Figs 36.5, 36.6, 36.7). Secondary haemorrhage occurs in 1% of patients and can be severe.

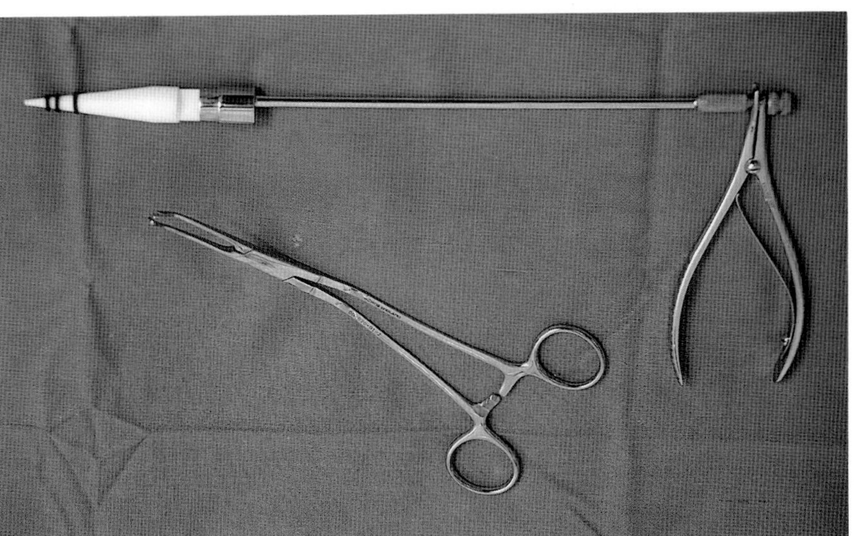

Fig. 36.5 The McGivney neoprene band ligator with St George's haemorrhoid-grasping forceps.

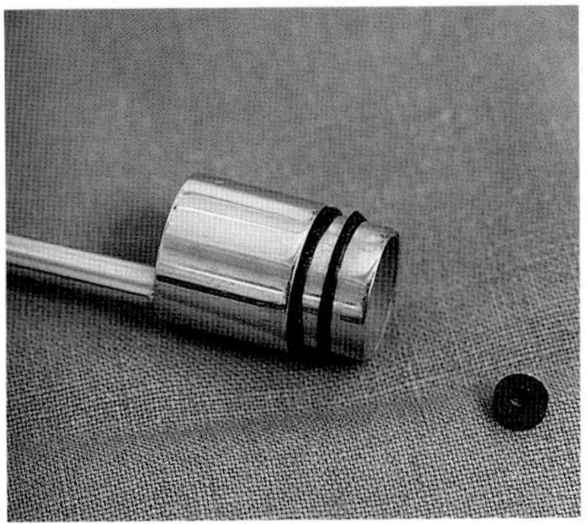

Fig. 36.6 Close-up of band applicator and neoprene bands.

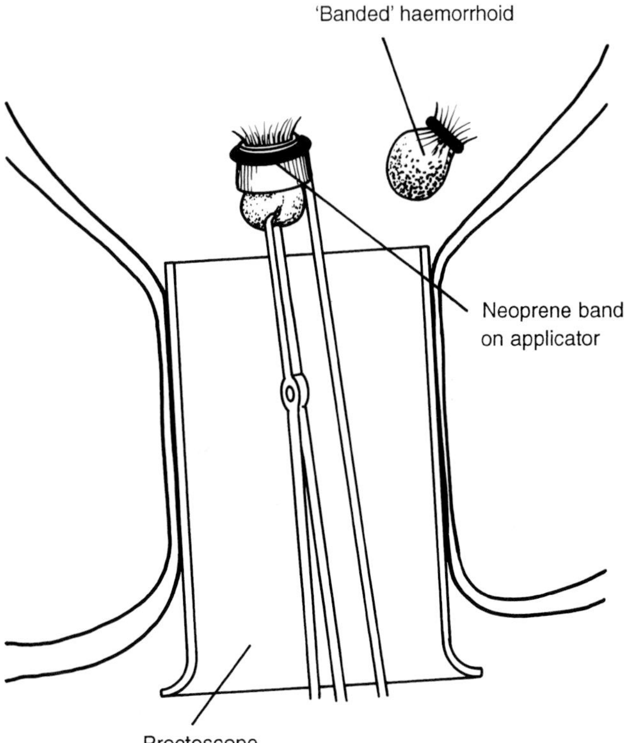

Fig. 36.7 Diagrammatic view of McGivney neoprene band ligator and siting of banding. (Redrawn from G.J. Hill, *Outpatient Surgery,* by permission of WB Saunders & Co.)

36.6 MANUAL DILATATION OF THE ANUS

This treatment for haemorrhoids was known in ancient Greece, practised in the Middle Ages, and recently revived by Peter Lord [42]. Normally done under a general anaesthetic, nevertheless it can be performed under local infiltration or caudal anaesthesia. Young patients with much anal spasm, and haemorrhoids associated with anal fissure seem to achieve most relief from this procedure; contraindicated are the elderly and those with a lax anal canal, who fare particularly badly, with a risk of permanent incontinence of faeces.

37

Varicose veins

Marius, Roman Consul, having both his legs full of great tumours, and disliking the deformity, determined to put himself in the hands of an operator. When, after enduring a most excessive torment in the cutting, never flinching or complaining, the surgeon went to the other, he declined to have it done saying 'I see the cure is not worth the pain'.

Plutarch's Lives, 186–55 BC

Varicose veins are one of the commonest problems encountered in general practice, it has been estimated that one person in five in the population either has, or will develop varicose veins of the legs. Women are affected more than men, and the most frequent reasons for seeking advice and treatment are discomfort, fear of ulceration, and appearance.

As far as minor surgery is concerned, there are three successful treatments – sclerotherapy, stab avulsions and multiple ligations. However, not all varicose veins are suitable for treatment – indeed in some, treatment might even be contraindicated or give very poor results.

37.1 ANATOMY

There are two sets of veins in the leg: deep and superficial, being separated from each other by the fascia, and being connected to each other by perforating veins. The perforating veins have valves which allow blood to pass from the superficial veins to the deep veins, but not the reverse.

The long saphenous vein is the longest vein in the body – it starts at the medial dorsal end of the venous arch on the dorsum of the foot, lying 2 cm in front of the medial malleolus, and passing up the leg to join the femoral vein about 3 cm below the inguinal ligament.

The short saphenous vein starts behind the lateral malleolus as an extension of the dorsal venous arch, it passes up the back of the calf in the midline, to join the popliteal veins (Fig. 37.4). Valves are frequent throughout the course of the superficial veins, most notably at the junction of the long saphenous and femoral vein, and it is incompetence of these valves which results in varicosities.

By the action of the calf muscles, blood is actively pumped from the feet to the abdomen; and during exercise, pressures up to 250 mmHg have been recorded in these veins. If valvular breakdown occurs in the perforating veins, blood at this pressure is forced outwards into the superficial veins causing varicosities and eventual ulceration secondary to capillary stasis.

Varicose veins may conveniently be classified into three categories.

37.1.1 Type I varicose veins (Fig. 37.1)

These veins are dilated, but have competent valves; there is no oedema, but the patient may be troubled with attacks of superficial thrombophlebitis; they are common in men.

37.1.2 Type II varicose veins (Fig. 37.2)

These veins are dilated; the valves in the superficial veins are incompetent, but the valves in the deep and perforating veins are still intact. These veins are therefore ideal for treatment.

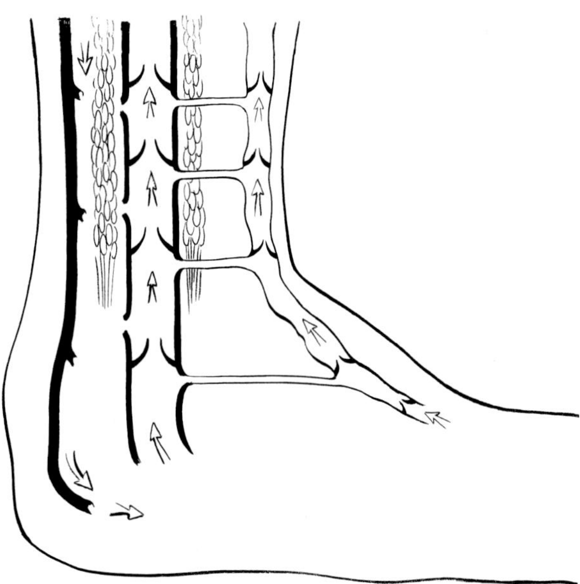

Fig. 37.1 Type I varicose veins. Dilated veins with competent valves.

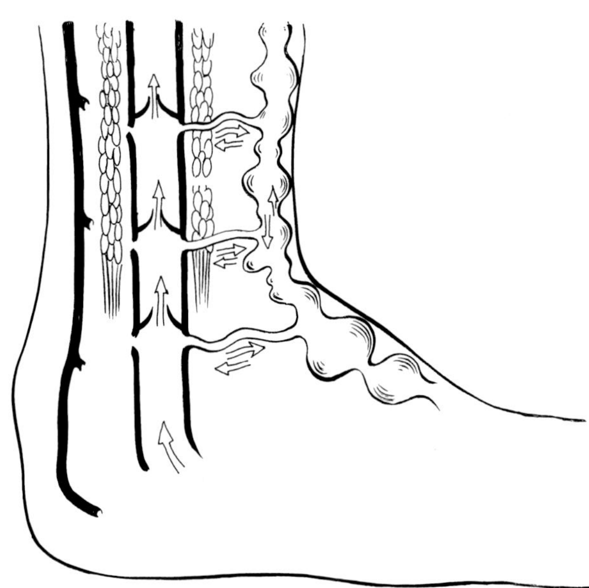

Fig. 37.2 Type II varicose veins. Dilated veins, valves in the superficial veins are incompetent, but valves in the deep and perforating veins are intact. These are ideal for injections.

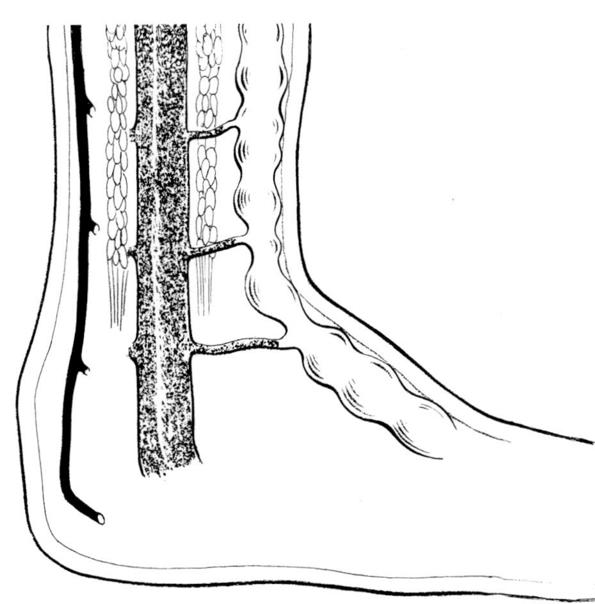

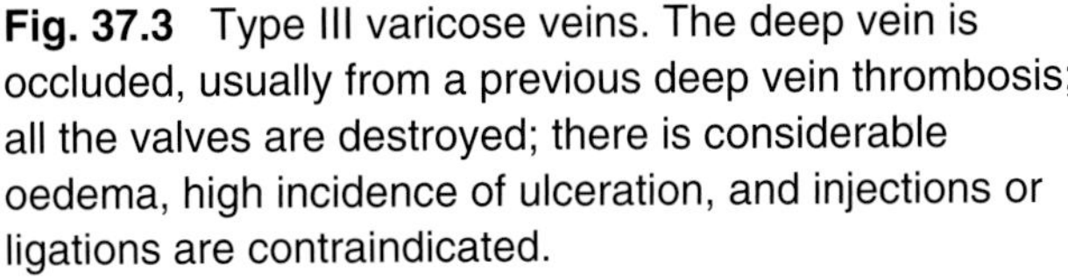

Fig. 37.3 Type III varicose veins. The deep vein is occluded, usually from a previous deep vein thrombosis; all the valves are destroyed; there is considerable oedema, high incidence of ulceration, and injections or ligations are contraindicated.

37.1.3 Type III varicose veins (Fig. 37.3)

In type III varicose veins, the deep vein is occluded, usually from a previous deep-vein thrombosis, all the valves are destroyed, there is considerable oedema, distension of the superficial veins, and a high incidence of venous ulceration. As the limb is now relying on the superficial veins to maintain a venous circulation, treatment by ligation or sclerotherapy is contraindicated and will make the situation worse. In many instances, the patient only seeks help when varicose ulceration has occurred; this is still not too late to commence treatment of the veins, as by reducing the superficial venous pressure, healing of the ulcer will be facilitated.

37.2 SELECTION OF PATIENTS

A simple selective procedure will improve results and avoid unnecessary treatment for unsuitable cases.

1. A careful history should be obtained to exclude any serious systemic disease.
2. A past history of deep-vein thrombosis in the affected leg is an absolute contraindication to sclerotherapy.
3. Veins which are confined to below the knee are most suitable for sclerotherapy. Those above the knee are difficult to bandage effectively and are better ligated.
4. Current medication is noted; patients taking the combined contraceptive pill or oestrogens for any other reasons should be asked to stop medication for 1 month before treatment if this is practicable.
5. If ulceration is present, check the arterial system and test the urine for sugar.
6. A test of saphenofemoral incompetence is made as follows. The patient lies down and the leg is raised to 30° to empty the superficial veins. A narrow tube is applied as a tourniquet around the upper thigh, the leg is lowered, and the patient asked to stand up. If just the saphenofemoral valve is incompetent, the superficial veins will fill slowly over 30 seconds from below upwards. If the perforating veins at a lower level are leaking, the superficial veins will fill rapidly, in which case other tourniquets may be applied progressively at lower levels until the site of leakage is identified. A second simple test is to apply a tourniquet around the leg at the level of the tibial tubercle and ask the patient to walk around for 1 min. If the perforating vein valves are competent, the superficial veins empty.
7. As the recommended treatment involves daily periods of walking by the patient, it is not advisable to offer injections if for any reason the patient cannot walk at least 3 miles each day.
8. Patients with obese legs should be advised to lose weight before offering a course of injections.
9. Any known allergic reaction to STD (sodium tetradecyl sulphate) is a contraindication to sclerotherapy.

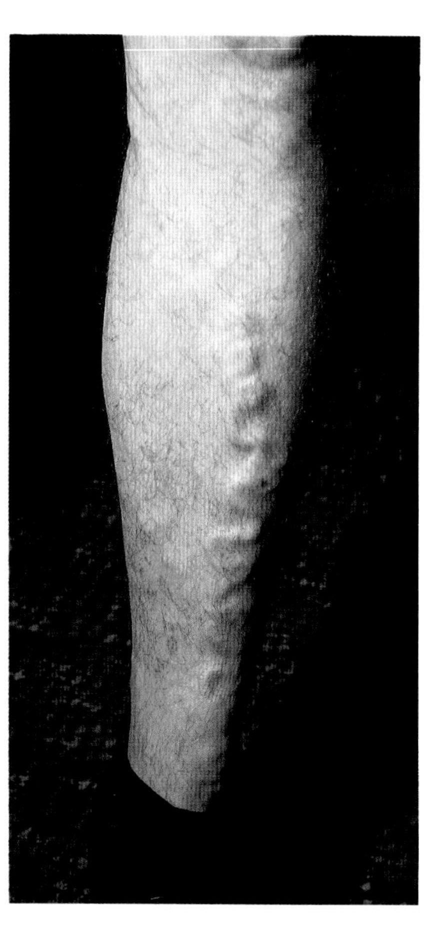

Fig. 37.4 Varicose veins affecting the short saphenous vein below the knee ideal for sclerotherapy.

37.3 SCLEROTHERAPY

The object of sclerotherapy is to obliterate the lumen of the vein by injecting an irritant solution directly inside it, and compressing the inflamed surfaces together. Current interest in the technique was revived by Professor Fegan in Dublin [43, 44, 45] and, provided suitable patients are selected carefully i.e. Type I or II veins below the knee, the results of treatment are very good.

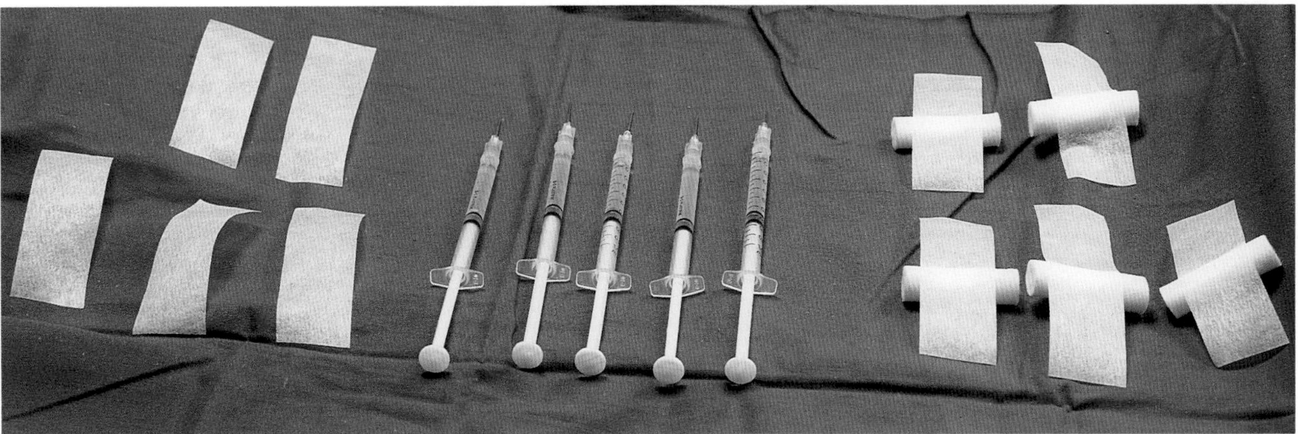

Fig. 37.5 Syringes with 3% STD adhesive tapes and cotton-wool rolls in readiness for sclerotherapy.

Instruments required (Fig. 37.5):

6 × 1 ml sterile syringes
6 × 25 swg × 5/8 in. (0.5 mm × 16 mm) needles
vial 5 ml of 3% STD solution (sodium tetradecyl sulphate) or
  ampoules of ethanolamine oleate
elastic web bandage 3 in. (7.6 cm) × 5 m
tubular elastic stockinette (Tubigrip)
size E 8.75 cm × 1 m or
size F 10 cm × 1 m
Sorbo rubber pads or large cotton dental rolls
adhesive tape (Micropore) 1 in. (2.5 cm).

Good illumination is essential. The number of injections likely to be given is noted, and the same number of syringes filled with 3% STD or ethanolamine oleate solution; usually 0.7 ml per syringe is sufficient. One strip of adhesive tape, 1 in. × 4 in. (2.5 cm × 10 cm) per syringe is stuck to the glass shelf of the instrument trolley in readiness, and a second strip 1 in. × 4 in. with a large cotton dental roll, per syringe, also attached to the shelf.

With the patient standing on a low stool the veins to be injected are identified using a felt-tip marker (Fig. 37.6). Still with the patient standing, and the doctor kneeling, the needle of the preloaded syringe is inserted in the vein and the plunger very slightly withdrawn (Fig. 37.7). Dark blood enters the syringe, confirming that the needle is in the correct place.

Without moving the syringe or needle at all, they are carefully taped in position using the first strip of adhesive (Micropore) tape. The second

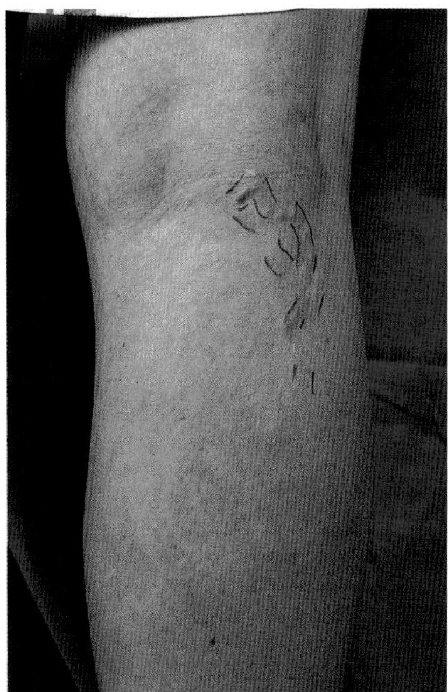

Fig. 37.6 The veins to be injected are first marked with a felt-tip pen, with the patient standing.

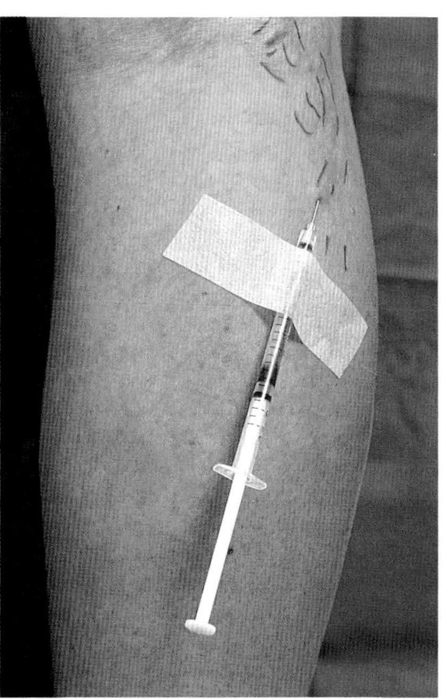

Fig. 37.7 With the patient standing, the first syringe is taped in position with the needle inside the vein.

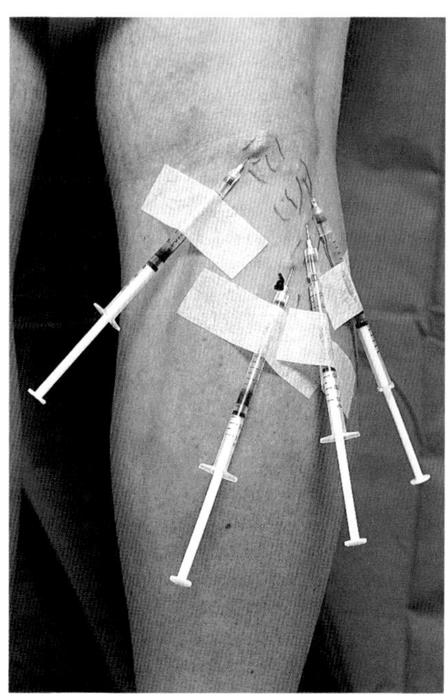

Fig. 37.8 Other syringes are now taped in position after placing the needle inside the vein.

injection is performed in exactly the same way, taping the syringe in place as before. Several injections may be given at one session (Fig. 37.8), but the total volume of sclerosant should not exceed 4 ml.

With all syringes taped in position, the operator carefully helps the patient to lie down on the couch or operating table and elevates the leg to about 30° above the horizontal. With an assistant holding the leg, the doctor now applies finger and thumb over the segment of vein to be injected, thus isolating this short strip of vein. With the other hand the contents of the syringe are injected into this segment, and a compression pad applied before removing the needle (Figs 37.9, 37.10). It is important to keep the sclerosant in the empty and isolated segment for at least 30 seconds. If possible, an assistant maintains pressure over the injected site while the operator proceeds to inject the remaining sites.

When all sites have been injected, an elastic web bandage is applied from the toes to the knee and this is then covered with an elasticated tubular bandage (Tubigrip E or F) doubled back on itself to produce two layers of compression (Figs 37.11 and 37.12). The patient is given an instruction sheet, advised to walk at least 3 miles every day for the next 3 weeks when the bandages and pads are removed. It is wise to warn the patient that they may experience severe pain in the leg during the first 48 hours, but that this will subside. They may reapply the bandages themselves if too tight, but should not disturb the compression pads.

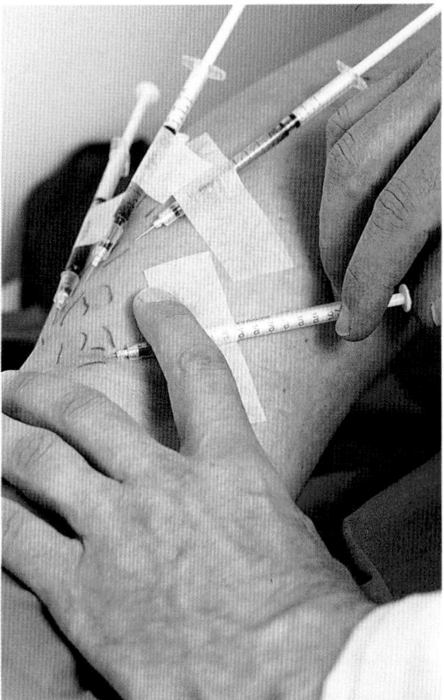

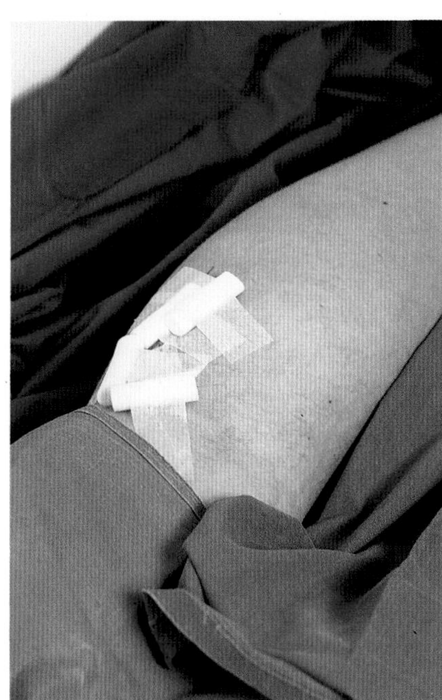

Fig. 37.9 With pressure on either side of the injection site, 0.5 ml 3% STD or ethanolamine oleate is injected into isolated segment of vein. (Gloves should be worn!)

Fig. 37.10 Cotton-wool rolls or Sorbo-rubber pads are now placed over each injection site.

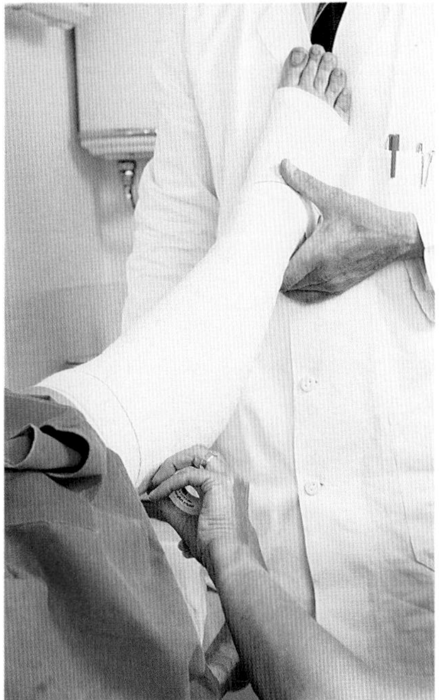

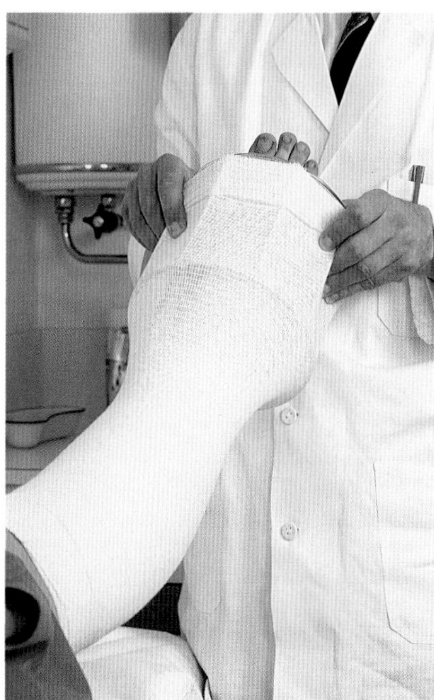

Fig. 37.11 An elastic web bandage (3 in.) is now applied from the toes to the knee.

Fig. 37.12 An elasticated tubular bandage (Tubigrip) is now applied over the bandage, folding itself back to give two layers.

37.3.1 Complications of sclerotherapy

Pain is a common accompaniment of injection treatment and this generally settles in a few days. Occasionally, extravasation of the STD solution results in severe pain, followed by an area of necrosis that may slough and produce an ulcer. A dry dressing is all that is required, and healing may take very many months, leaving a permanent depressed scar, and a depressed patient! Under these circumstances it may be prudent to excise the ulcer and close the wound by primary suture.

Accidental intra-arterial injection would result in immediate, severe, burning pain over the distal distribution. Should this occur, the needle should be left in the artery and heparin and lignocaine slowly injected; this is obviously the most potentially serious complication in a technique which is otherwise remarkably free of complications.

37.4 STAB AVULSION FOR VARICOSE VEINS (For full details see Chapter 47)

As an alternative to sclerotherapy, or as an adjunct therapy, stab avulsion offers a good treatment for many superficial varicosities.

37.4.1 Technique

Stab incisions of not more than 3 mm are made over the sites of previously marked varicosities. The underlying vein may then be picked up with a single skin hook, and by grasping with mosquito forceps, as much of the vein gradually teased out and then avulsed. Closure is with skin closure strips, covered with a compression bandage for 3 days followed by graduated compression stockings (Class II) for the next 3 weeks (Fig. 37. 13).

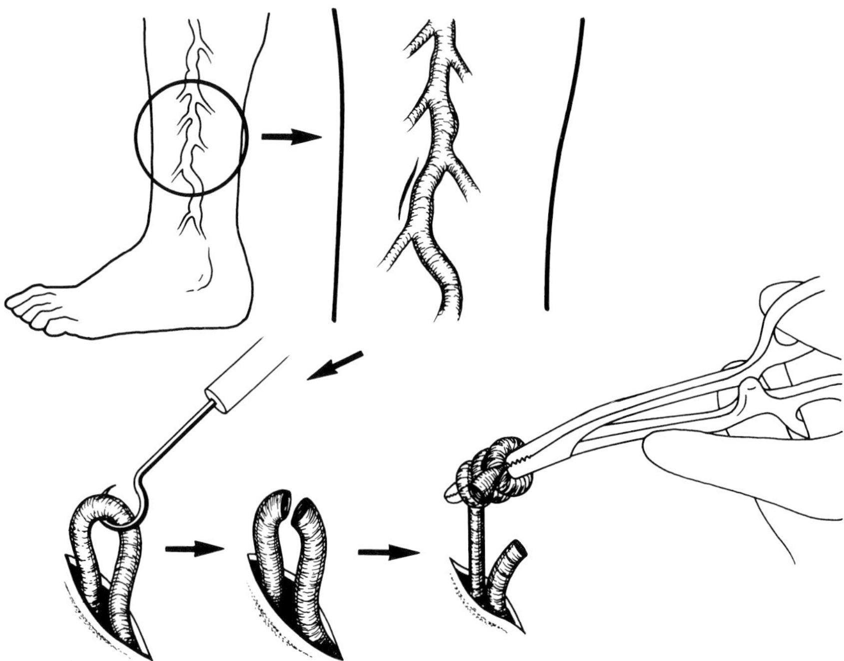

Fig. 37.13 Stab avulsion for varicose veins.

38

Minor surgical procedures in gynaecology

If thou examinest a woman suffering in her abdomen so that the menstrual discharge cannot come away from her ... apply Frankincense and incense between her two loins and cause the smoke thereof to enter her flesh

Edwin Smith, Surgical Papyrus, 3000–2500 BC

As well as all the usual intradermal lesions which can effect the skin over the perineum and vulva, several lesions of the cervix, vagina, and labia can be effectively treated with the minimum of instruments and equipment. Also included is cervical cytology and the insertion of intrauterine contraceptive devices, together with repair of episiotomy following delivery.

38.1 CERVICAL CYTOLOGY

During the last decade most general practitioners have learned to take routine cervical smears for cytology. The procedure itself is quite straightforward, using a vaginal speculum (preferably not lubricated with jelly) the cervix is visualized. Good illumination is essential, whether external spotlight, integral fibreoptic illumination, or tungsten-filament bulbs. The cervix is first inspected, and any unusual features such as excessive discharge, bleeding, erosions, polypi, etc. noted. The purpose-designed wooden cervical spatula is placed at the entrance to the external cervical os, and rotated through 360 degrees, thus obtaining cells from the whole area. These are then transferred to a microscope slide by wiping the spatula on the glass in one direction only, followed by immediate fixation with suitable preservative. The slide is then labelled with the patient's name and the appropriate request form completed. Bacterial swabs may also be taken at the same time if necessary (Fig. 38.1).

38.2 ENDOMETRIAL CELL SAMPLERS

These are now also available, by means of which the secretions inside the uterine cavity can be aspirated by gentle suction and sent for cytology examination; this will often obviate the need for a diagnostic D and C.

38.3 BRUSH CYTOLOGY

As a means of obtaining endometrial cells for cytological examination, small brushes similar to a 'bottle brush' are available. By visualizing the

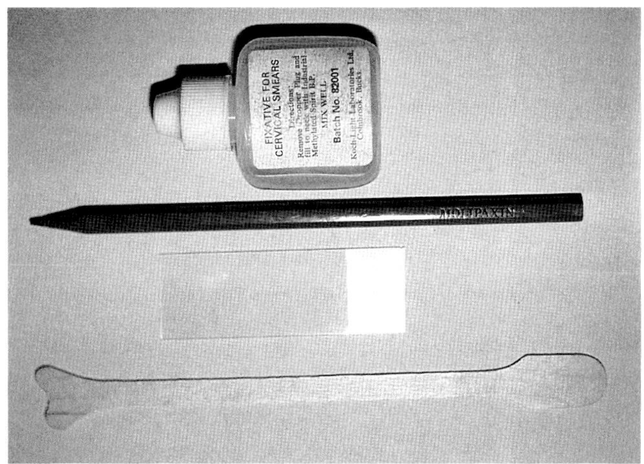

Fig. 38.1 All that is needed to take a cervical smear.

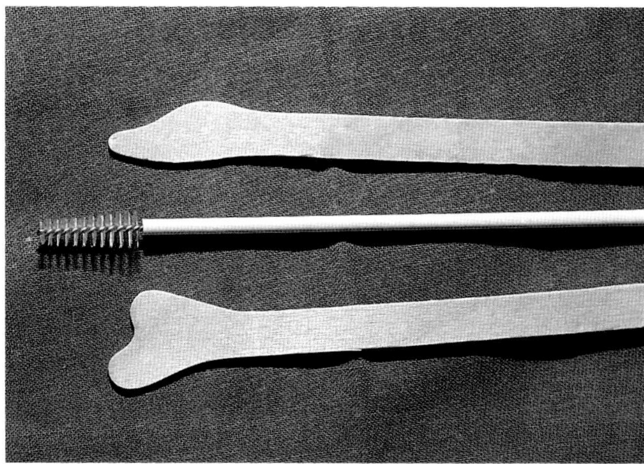

Fig. 38.2 Cervical smear spatulae and cyto-brush.

cervical os, the brush is gently inserted as far as possible without causing pain and rotated once and withdrawn. The microscope slide is then prepared in the same way as when using a spatula (Fig. 38.2).

38.4 CAUTERIZATION OF CERVICAL EROSIONS

The popularity of cauterizing every cervical 'erosion' has waned in recent years with the realization that many so-called erosions were not causing any symptoms and were not a sign of disease. Where an erosion is giving symptoms such as a heavy discharge, repeated infections, and discomfort, it may be effectively treated with any one of these methods of cautery: silver nitrate, cryotherapy, electrocautery, and diathermy. Silver nitrate is still the simplest, cheapest, and quickest means of treating a moderate erosion and disposable applicators with a silver nitrate bead are readily available (Chapter 15).

38.4.1 Technique of silver nitrate application

The cervix is visualized, and any cervical smears or bacterial swabs taken. The silver nitrate is now applied to the cervix, including the external cervical os; the area treated immediately turns white. The patient should be warned to expect an increased watery, sometimes blood-stained discharge for several weeks. A topical antiseptic or antibiotic cream may be given during this time to reduce risks of secondary infection.

38.5 CRYOSURGERY FOR CERVICAL EROSIONS

A nitrous oxide or liquid nitrogen cryoprobe is ideal for cauterizing troublesome cervical erosions. Treatment is quick, simple to apply, and has a high success rate and patient acceptability (Chapter 18).

38.5.1 Technique

Good visualization of the cervix is essential; one hazard of using the cryoprobe is that it can adhere to adjacent vaginal walls if they accidentally touch the probe tip or side and result in a small 'burn'. The cone-shaped applicator is placed on the cervix before starting to freeze; this enables it to be accurately positioned. Once in position the nitrous oxide or liquid nitrogen is switched on and freezing commences. The probe will become adherent to the cervix at this stage, generally 1–2 min is sufficient treatment time, and the probe either allowed to thaw out spontaneously or be 'de-frosted' with the built-in de-froster attachment. One treatment is normally all that is required, but a greater depth of penetration is obtained by giving a second freeze immediately following thawing if this is felt necessary. Follow-up is exactly as for silver nitrate.

38.6 ELECTROCAUTERY OF CERVICAL EROSIONS

As the cervical nerve endings are not sensitive to heat, any erosion may be cauterized using the electrocautery. Care must be taken if cauterizing the cervical os or cervical canal not to cause fibrosis, scarring and stenosis; likewise during treatment, if steam is produced which passes inside the uterus, pain is caused. To avoid the risk of stenosis, linear radial cauterization should be employed, using the standard V-shaped platinum wire electrode.

38.7 DIATHERMY OF CERVICAL EROSIONS

The use of standard bipolar diathermy requires a general anaesthetic; unipolar high-frequency diathermy may be used successfully without any anaesthetic. The Hyfrecator electrode is held a short distance away from the cervix, the current switched on, and a stream of sparks drawn from the electrode to the cervix (Chapter 17). This fulgurization effectively cauterizes the cervix. As with all other methods of cautery, the patient should be warned to expect an increased watery, blood-stained discharge for several weeks following treatment. An antiseptic or antibiotic cream may be applied during this time to reduce secondary infection.

38.8 VAGINAL VAULT GRANULATIONS FOLLOWING HYSTERECTOMY

Granulations in the vault of the vagina are relatively common following hysterectomy; they may cause a blood-stained discharge or even frank bleeding, both of which can cause anxiety to the patient.

Examination with a vaginal speculum reveals typical messy granulations, easily friable, and which bleed on the slightest touch. Treatment is simple, using silver nitrate to each granulation. Normally one application is sufficient to cure the condition.

38.9 GENITAL WARTS

These warts tend to develop in large clusters, affecting the penile and vulvar skin as well as mucous membranes, and the perianal skin. Examination with the electron-microscope shows clearly the human wart virus as the causative agent.

Genital warts can be confused with condylomata lata of syphilis, and as both conditions are sexually transmitted, both could coexist; it is therefore essential to examine the sexual partner as well, and screen both serologically for venereal diseases.

Treatment can be difficult and requires much patience. Vaginal and rectal examinations should be performed using a speculum to identify the extent of visible lesions.

Cryotherapy is probably the treatment of choice, applied once or twice weekly until cured. Alternatively podophyllin 25% in soft paraffin applied daily for 3 days is effective but more uncomfortable. Podophyllotoxin 0.5% solution applied twice daily for 3 days is effective for penile warts. In pregnancy podophyllin should not be used because of possible teratogenic effects.

The immunosuppressed patient, and also some pregnant patients develop warts at an alarming rate, ending up with huge fungating cauliflower-like lesions. The earlier treatment can be offered the better.

38.10 REPAIR OF EPISIOTOMY

A good repair of an episiotomy or second-degree tear following delivery can occasionally be quite difficult; however, time taken identifying each layer is well spent, makes the repair easier, and results in better, more comfortable healing. As with any surgical procedure, good illumination is paramount; the patient should be supported in the lithotomy position and a small swab on a cord inserted to the top of the vagina; this helps to control oozing from the uterus as well as helping to identify the extent of the laceration in the posterior vaginal wall. The top of this laceration must be identified, and the first suture inserted in the posterior vaginal wall just above the laceration. Chromic catgut 2/0 (metric 3.5) is suitable for this stitch (Ref. Ethicon W 565). Using a continuous stitch, the posterior vaginal wall is closed. Next, one or two interrupted catgut sutures are placed in the muscle layer between the posterior vaginal wall and skin. Finally, the perineal skin is approximated using either interrupted braided silk suture Ethicon W 667 (metric 3, 2/0) on a curved reverse cutting needle, interrupted chromic catgut stitches, a subcuticular catgut, or Dexon suture, depending on the preference of the operator (Figs 38.3 and 38.4).

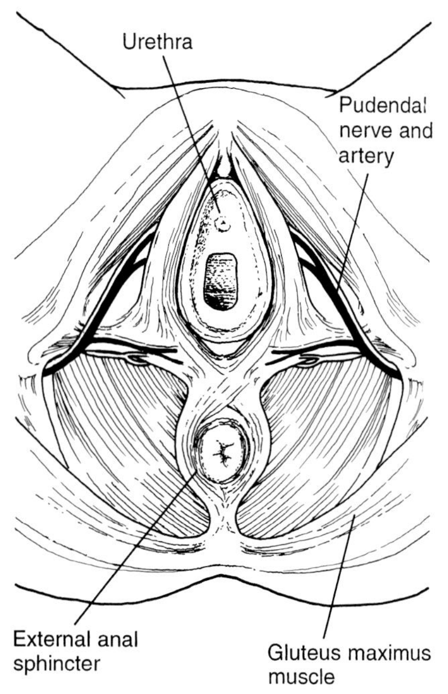

Fig. 38.3 Episiotomy: surgical anatomy.

38.11 BARTHOLIN'S CYSTS AND ABSCESSES

These can be extremely painful, some rupture spontaneously; those that do not may be treated either by aspiration, aspiration and injection of fucidic acid gel, or marsupialization.

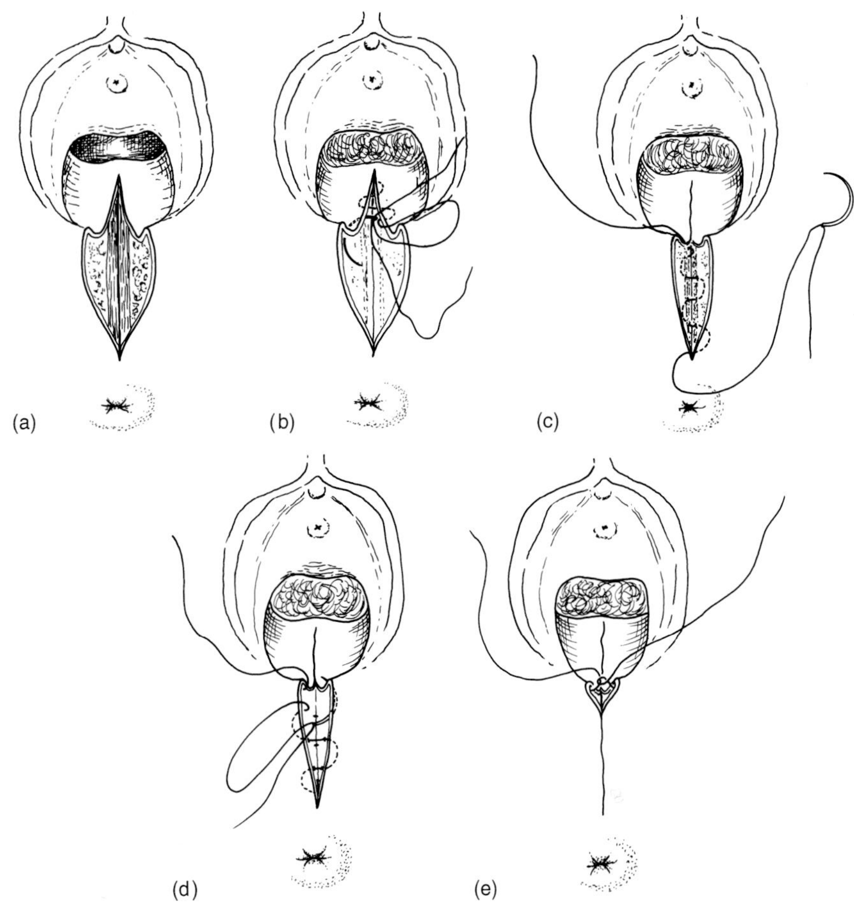

Fig. 38.4 a Episiotomy or second-degree tear. (**b**) Posterior vaginal wall sutured with a continuous 2/0 catgut suture. (**c**) Interrupted catgut sutures to skin and perineal muscles with buried knots. (**d**) The final result.

38.11.1 Aspiration

Although one would not expect aspiration alone to cure an abscess, nevertheless, it is found that many Bartholin's abscesses respond to a single aspiration using a wide-bore needle and syringe. As an added safeguard, injection of fucidic acid gel following aspiration seems to give improved results.

38.11.2 Marsupialization

Recurrent Bartholin's abscesses are best treated by marsupialization. This consists in creating a permanent sinus by incision, followed by suturing the lining of the cyst to the outside skin; it is very effective and normally results in a permanent cure (Fig. 38.5).

38.12 URETHRAL CARUNCLE

This is a relatively common condition, particularly in postmenopausal women, resulting in prolapse of the urethral mucosa which then causes bleeding, frequency, and dysuria. Mild cases may be treated with topical oestrogen-containing creams, possibly supplemented with systemic

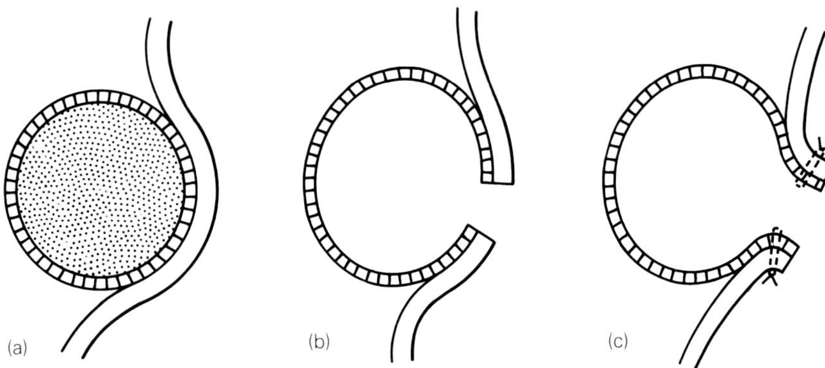

Fig. 38.5 Marsupialization of Bartholin's abscess. (**a**) Abscess; (**b**) incised; (**c**) inside capsule sutured to outside skin creating permanent sinus.

hormone replacement therapy. Where this fails, the mucosa may be treated with the diathermy or electrocautery, or cryocautery under local anaesthesia, inserting an indwelling Foley catheter afterwards until the oedema has subsided.

38.13 IUCD INSERTION

As a method of contraception, intrauterine devices have become popular in the last 30 years. There are now many different sizes, shapes and materials to choose from, and the practitioner will need to refer to the instruction leaflets provided with each device to determine the method of insertion.

38.13.1 Counselling

The patient and her partner should discuss with the doctor the pros and cons of this method of contraception; they should realize that no coil is 100% effective, that the periods following insertion may be much heavier and longer than previously, that occasionally the coil is expelled spontaneously, and that she should report for regular check-ups and cervical cytology. Although it has been shown to be a far safer procedure than was originally forecast, nevertheless, resuscitation facilities should be available for the unexpected vasovagal attacks. Similarly the risks of introducing infection are very much less than was anticipated – however, a rigid no-touch technique should be used throughout.

38.13.2 Technique

Whether the patient is lying on her left side or on her back depends on the preference of the doctor; whichever position is used, it is essential to visualize the cervix clearly. Using vulsellum forceps, the anterior lip of the cervix is grasped, and downward traction applied; this has the effect of straightening the longitudinal axis of the uterus and makes insertion easier. A uterine sound may be used to ascertain the dimensions and shape of the uterus – however, it is not always necessary as the coil and introducer may serve as a sound during insertion and give just as much information (Figs 38.6 and 38.7).

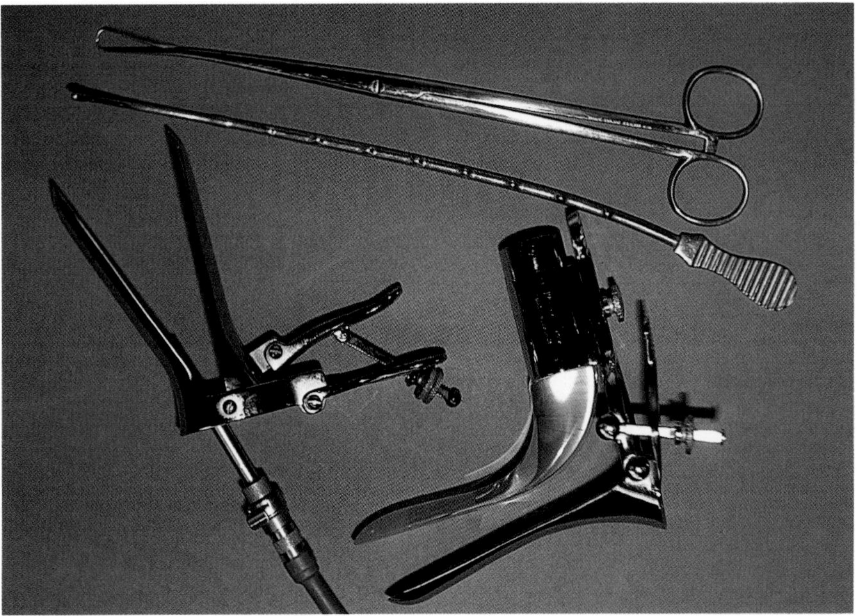

Fig. 38.6 Instruments required for IUCD insertion.

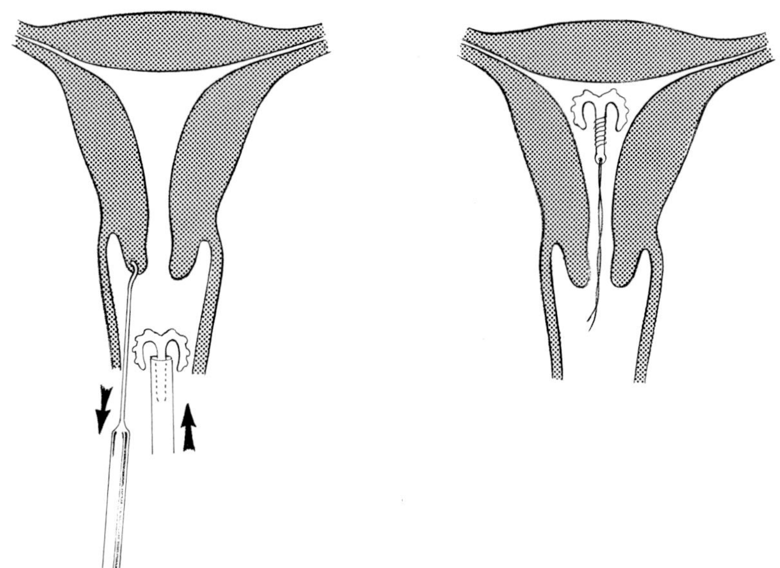

Fig. 38.7 IUCD insertion; the cervix is steadied by the application of a pair of vulsellum forceps, and slight traction applied. The IUCD is then inserted inside the uterine cavity.

The coil is loaded into the introducer, which may be given a very slight bend at the tip using the fingers and thumb of the left gloved hand; this simple manoeuvre makes sounding and insertion much easier and is to be recommended. Using gentle pressure, and if necessary slight rotation to 'feel' the direction of the cervical canal, the coil is introduced into the uterine cavity until it is felt to touch the fundus. The introducer is then withdrawn leaving the coil in position. The threads are then cut using McIndoe curved 7 in. (17.8 cm) scissors, and the vaginal speculum removed. The patient is requested to return for a coil check in 4 weeks and if all is well, annually thereafter. Copper-containing coils have a limited life of 2–5 years and need to be changed after this interval. Generally the optimum time to insert a coil is at a 6-week postnatal examination, or at the end of a menstrual period. Nulliparous patients tend to have more abdominal cramps and side-effects.

38.14 REMOVAL OF THE 'LOST' COIL

Occasionally the threads of an intrauterine coil are drawn up inside the uterine cavity, so that when the patient reports for a routine check they are not visible. At this point it is not possible to tell whether the coil has been extruded, or the threads are inside the uterus. Ultrasound examination will confirm the presence and situation of the coil, but if subsequently it is necessary to remove the coil, the threads need to be retrieved.

Gentle exploration with an Emmett thread retriever or a very fine single skin hook may bring down the threads, as may the introduction of a cervical cytology brush in the hope of engaging the threads. If all these measures fail, the patient may need to be referred to a gynaecologist.

38.15 HORMONE IMPLANTS

The discovery that hormone replacement therapy (HRT) can significantly reduce the incidence of osteoporosis and consequent fractures, as well as reducing the death rate from cardiovascular disease, menopausal symptoms, and carcinoma of the ovary, has resulted in renewed interest in the form of therapy.

Earlier attempts at oestrogen replacement alone, whilst abolishing menopausal symptoms, were found to cause endometrial hyperplasia and an increased incidence of carcinoma of the body of the uterus.

By adding cyclical progestogens and therefore a withdrawal bleed, the risk of endometrial disease was abolished, but the resumption of menstruation was not always acceptable to many women.

Further research then showed that oestradiol gave better protection against osteoporosis than did synthetic oestrogens [46]. Oestradiol can be given as tablets, injection, vaginal cream or pessary, transdermal patches, or subcutaneous implants. Low-dose continuous regimes are now available whereby both oestrogens and progestogens are given continuously. This offers all the advantages of HRT without the withdrawal bleed.

To give adequate protection against osteoporosis it seems necessary to give hormone replacement therapy for at least 5 years following the menopause. Obviously in patients who have had a hysterectomy, progestogens, whether cyclical or continuous, need not be given, and simple oestrogen therapy is all that is required.

Oestradiol is manufactured as crystalline slow-release pellets in three strengths 25 mg, 50 mg and 100 mg. For the average woman 50 mg seems to be adequate, and should last up to 6 months. It is administered as a subcutaneous implant through a trocar and cannula, usually in the abdominal wall.

38.15.1 Technique

The correct size of trocar and cannula should be chosen to match the size of the implant (Fig. 38.8). The point of insertion is chosen: usually this lies

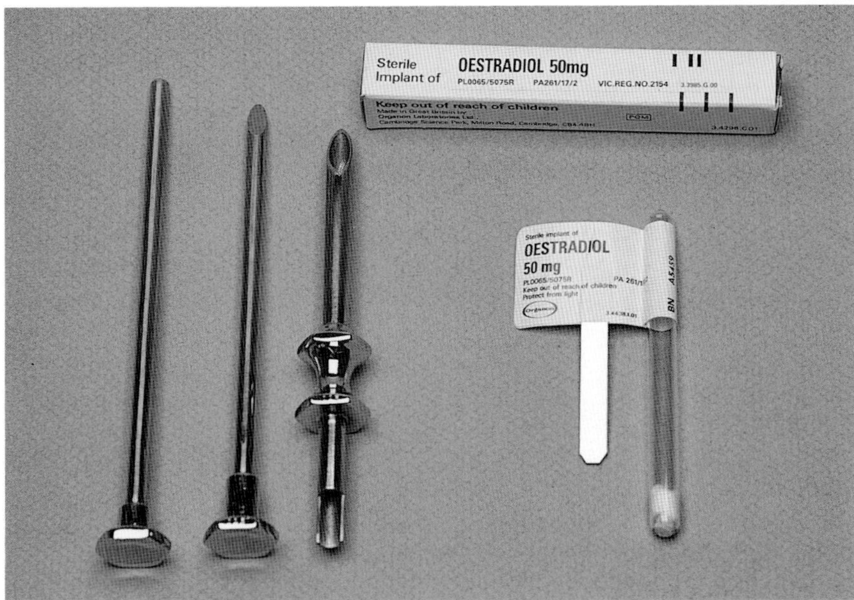

Fig. 38.8 Instruments required for hormone implant.

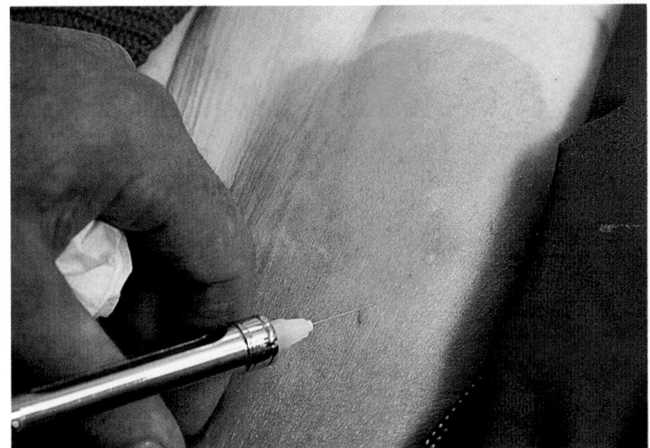

Fig. 38.9 Local anaesthetic infiltrated at site of implant.

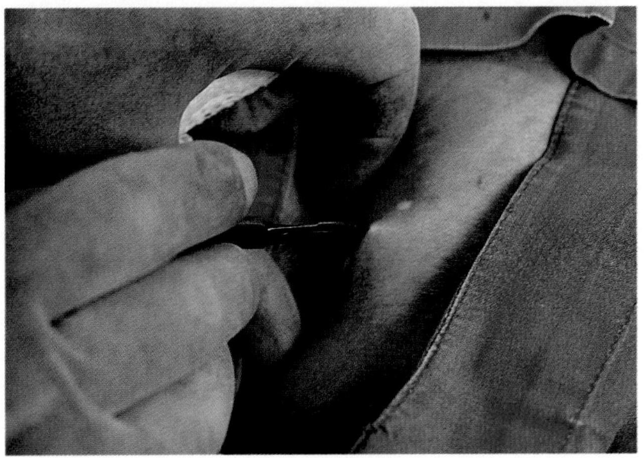

Fig. 38.10 Small incision using no. 11 scalpel blade on no. 3 handle.

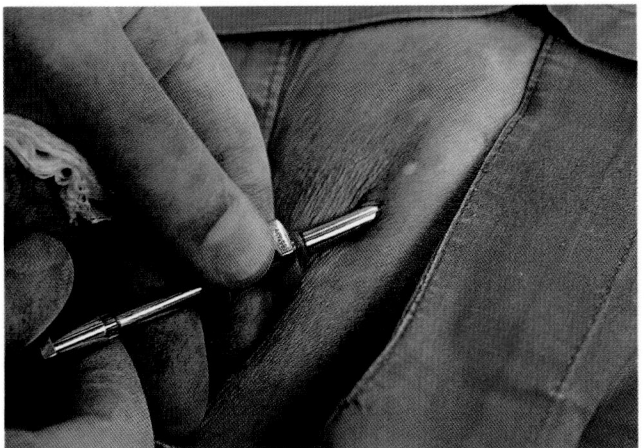

Fig. 38.11 Trocar and cannula pushed through incision.

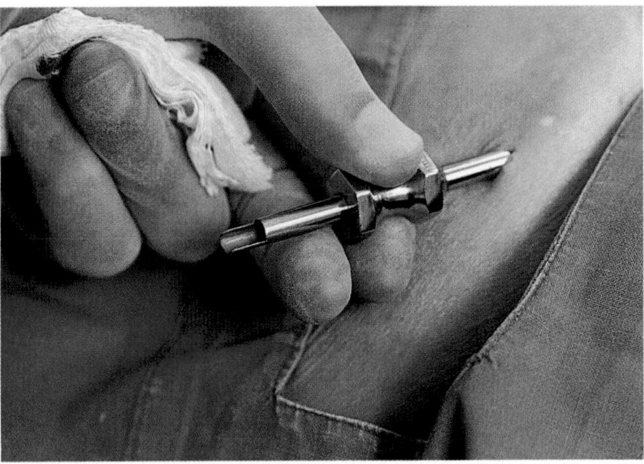

Fig. 38.12 Obturator withdrawn.

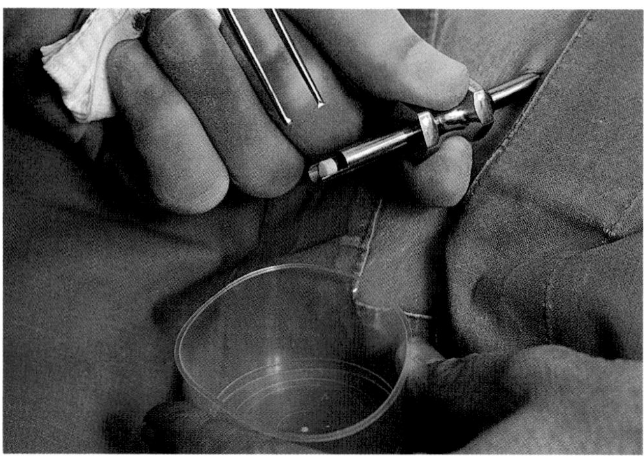

Fig. 38.13 Pellet of oestradiol inserted in cannula.

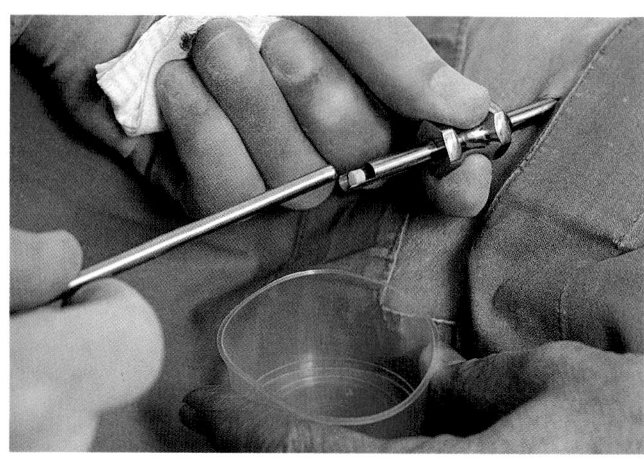

Fig. 38.14 Obturator ready to insert pellet through cannula.

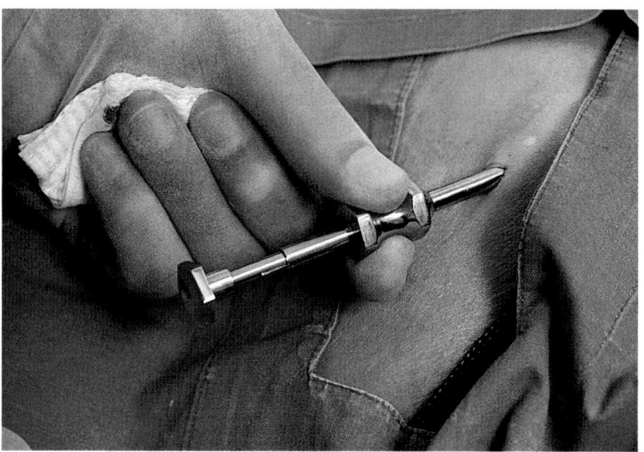

Fig. 38.15 Pellet inserted subcutaneously.

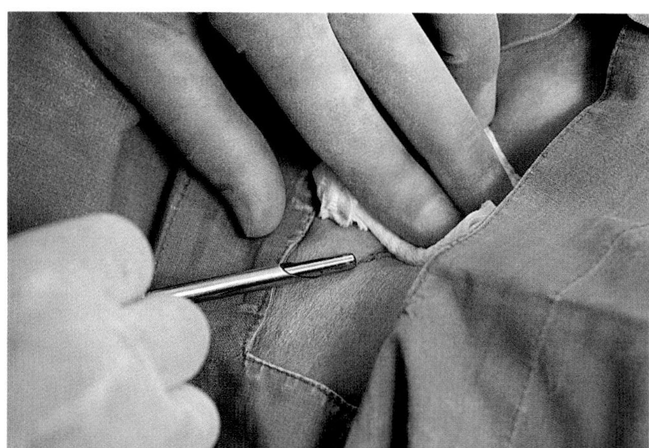

Fig. 38.16 Trocar and obturator removed. Pressure applied to reduce bleeding.

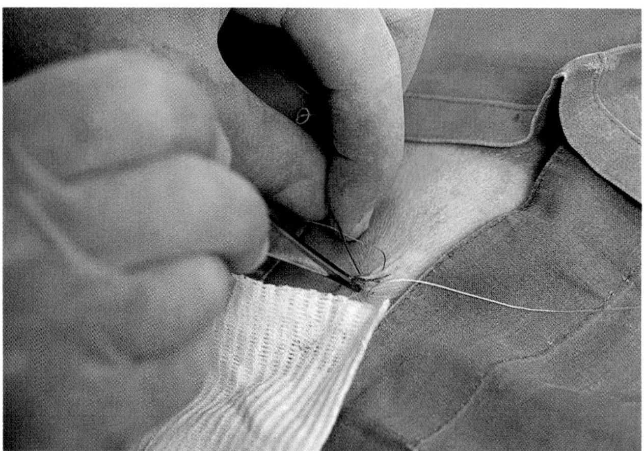

Fig. 38.17 One stitch or skin-closure strip to close incision.

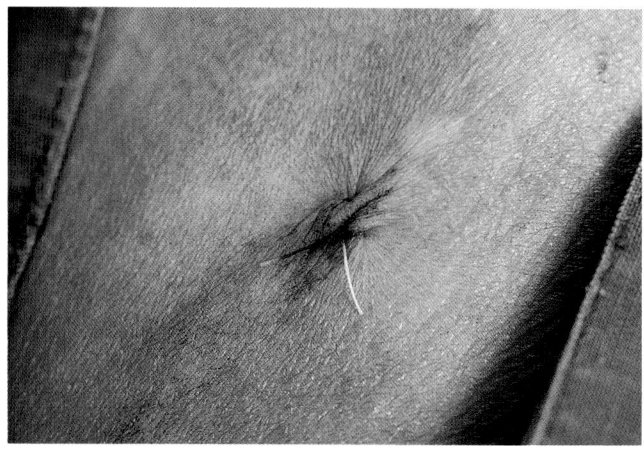

Fig. 38.18 Stitch may be absorbable, depending on preference.

on a line 2 in. above the inguinal ligament. A mark is made on the skin, which is then painted with povidone-iodine in spirit.

Using a 30 swg needle and dental syringe (or equivalent) a small quantity of local anaesthetic is infiltrated into the overlying skin and an incision 5mm long made with a sharp-pointed scalpel blade (size 11) on a no. 3 handle (Figs 38.9 and 38.10).

Whilst this is being done, the assistant opens the sterile tube containing the oestradiol pellet and places it in a sterile gallipot or container. The trocar with obturator is next pushed through the small skin incision into the subcutaneous fat layer (Fig. 38.11), and the obturator removed (Fig. 38.12).

With extreme care the hormone implant is next picked up with sterile forceps and placed in the cannula. It is helpful if the nurse or assistant keeps the sterile gallipot or container under the cannula while placing it in position, to avoid dropping it on the floor! (Fig. 38.13).

Using the blunt, longer obturator, the implant is pushed through the cannula to lie in the subcutaneous fatty layer (Figs 38.14 and 38.15). The cannula is now removed, and at the same time firm pressure is applied over the track of the cannula to reduce any bleeding (Fig. 38.16). Closure is by means of one single suture or Steri-strip (Figs 38.17 and 38.18).

Normally most patients feel the benefits within a few days, and can usually tell when it is wearing off. An interesting phenomenon of tachyphylaxis has been observed, where the patient is sure the implant needs replacing at steadily shorter intervals, whereas if serum oestradiol levels are measured, more than adequate levels are still circulating. Thus requests for further implants at closer intervals should be resisted, and where possible a 6-monthly schedule adhered to.

Where there is a loss of libido, a simultaneous implant of testosterone 100 mg together with oestradiol 50 mg seems to be helpful.

38.16 INSERTION OF PROGESTOGEN IMPLANTS (NORPLANT) (Figs 38.19–38.24)

Levonorgestrel has been manufactured as a set of six subdermal implants for long-term reversible contraception. The protection lasts up to 5 years, after which time the six rods should be removed.

Insertion is by means of a thin trocar and cannula similar to oestradiol implants but, unlike the latter, they need to be placed subdermally rather than in the subcutaneous fat.

A template is provided to mark the skin for insertion, usually in the upper inner arm, and the procedure is done under local infiltration anaesthesia.

The manufacturers recommend individual tuition in the insertion and removal of these implants.

Comprehensive counselling is necessary before insertion, as some patients experience irregularities of their menstrual cycle which require earlier removal.

Problems can be encountered with removal of the six rods – these are usually due to faulty insertion but the doctor should be aware that the

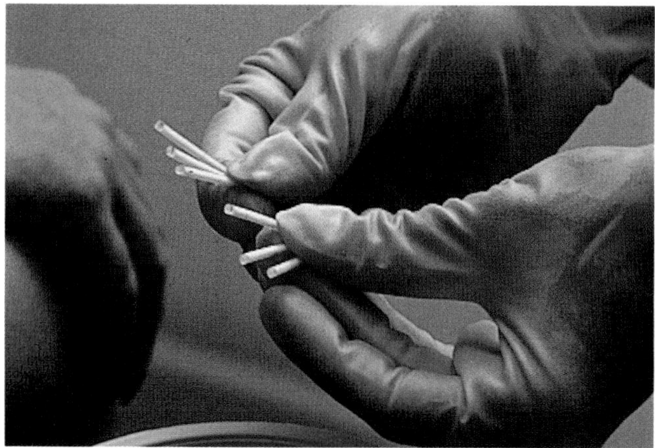

Fig. 38.19 The six Norplant implants (photograph by courtesy of Hoechst Roussel).

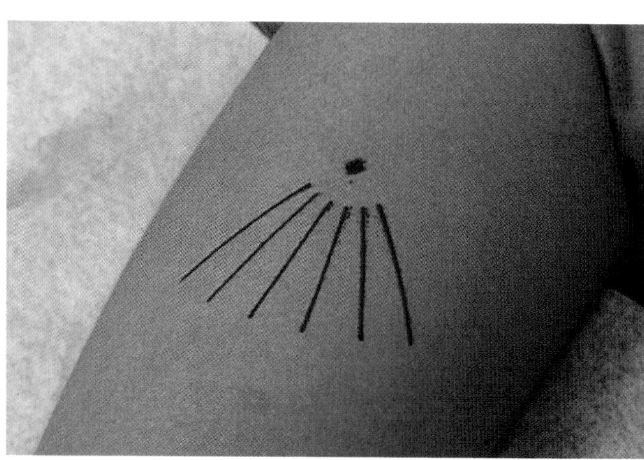

Fig. 38.20 Using the template, the sites for the implants are marked on the skin (photograph by courtesy of Hoechst Roussel).

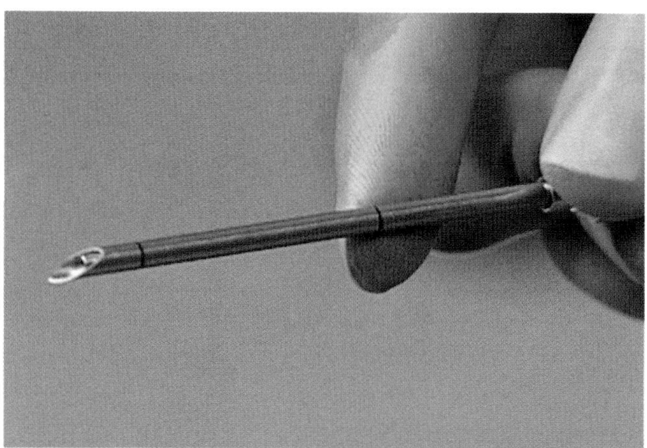

Fig. 38.21 The special trocar and cannula for introducing the Norplant implants (photograph by courtesy of Hoechst Roussel).

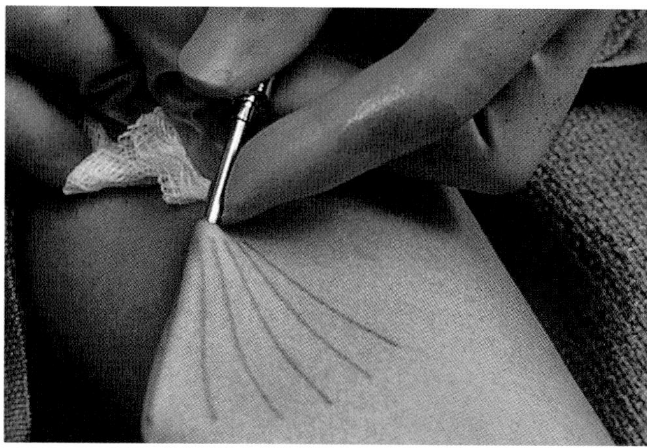

Fig. 38.22 After infiltration with lignocaine, the trocar is inserted subdermally, lifting up the skin as shown (photograph by courtesy of Hoechst Roussel).

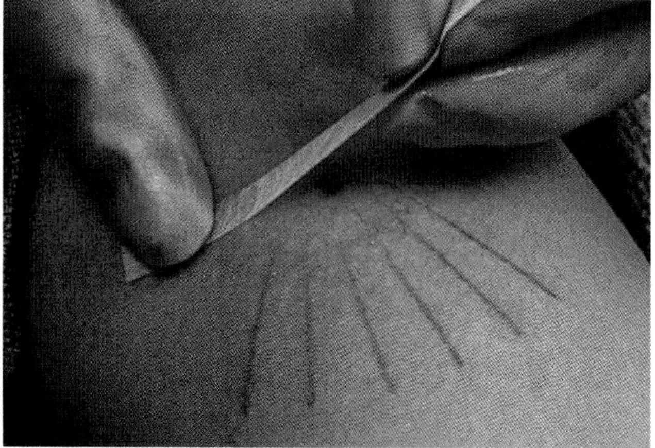

Fig. 38.23 After inserting the six rods, the wound is closed with skin closure strips (photograph by courtesy of Hoechst Roussel).

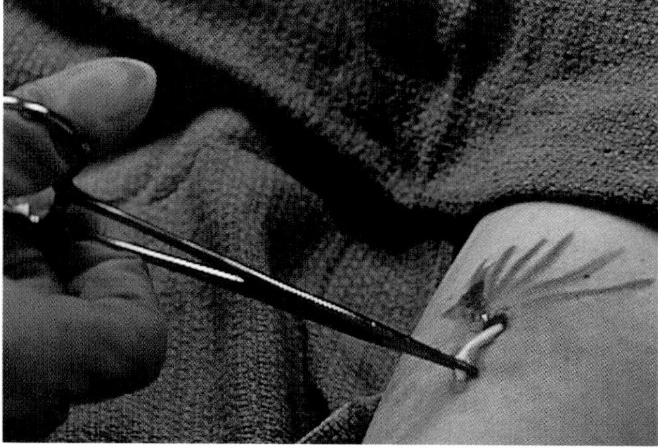

Fig. 38.24 Using forceps to remove the implant (photograph by courtesy of Hoechst Roussel).

procedure may not be as straightforward as anticipated so that tuition is essential.

A consent form, signed by the patient and doctor, should be completed prior to insertion (Fig. 38.25).

Fig. 38.25 Consent form for fitting progestogen implant.

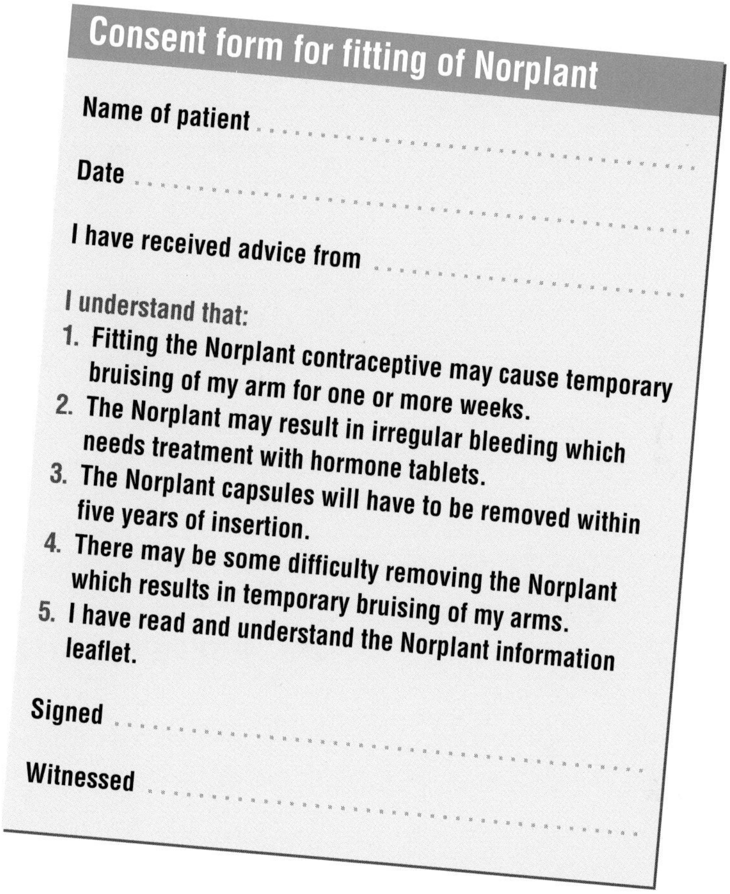

Consent form for fitting of Norplant

Name of patient ....

Date ....

I have received advice from ....

I understand that:

1. **Fitting the Norplant contraceptive may cause temporary bruising of my arm for one or more weeks.**
2. **The Norplant may result in irregular bleeding which needs treatment with hormone tablets.**
3. **The Norplant capsules will have to be removed within five years of insertion.**
4. **There may be some difficulty removing the Norplant which results in temporary bruising of my arms.**
5. **I have read and understand the Norplant information leaflet.**

Signed ....

Witnessed ....

39

Vasectomy

But amongst other causes of barreness in men, this also is one that maketh them barren ... the incision, or cutting of their veins behind their ears

De Morbis Foemineis, 1686

Vasectomy as a method of contraception has become increasingly popular in the last decade; it is an operation which can be performed by the general practitioner surgeon under local anaesthesia, but because of the medicolegal implications, extra attention must be given to counselling, record-keeping, technique, histology, and follow-up. It involves resecting a small portion of the vas deferens on either side of the scrotum. Although the operation should be considered irreversible, due to increasing divorce rates patients change their minds, so a technique of vasectomy which will allow reversal should be performed if possible [47].

39.1 PREOPERATIVE COUNSELLING

Where there is a stable relationship, it is obviously preferable to see both patient and wife or partner together although the consent of the spouse is not legally necessary.

The details of the operation need to be carefully explained to the patient, together with the possible risks of failure and the difficulty of reversal should the patient subsequently change his mind. The importance of follow-up is explained, and the patient is warned not to relax any contraception until at least two negative sperm tests have been performed.

A consent form (Fig. 39.1) needs to be signed by the patient. The Department of Health has produced a recommended form (HC(90) – Appendix A(2) which can be used for vasectomy.

Instruments required:

- Warm, aqueous povidone-iodine (Betadine solution)
- 10 ml syringe
- two 25 swg × 5/8 in. (0.5 mm × 16 mm) needles
- scalpel handle size 3
- scalpel blade size 15
- pair fine pointed, straight iris scissors 4 1/2 in. (11.4 cm)
- pair toothed dissecting forceps 5 in. (12.7 cm)
- two pairs fine, curved,
- Halstead mosquito artery forceps
- pair 'vasectomy' forceps or fine Allis forceps

CONSENT FORM

For sterilisation or vasectomy

APPENDIX A (2)

Health Authority ....
Hospital ....
Unit Number..............................

Patient's Surname ....
Other Names ....
Date of Birth ....
Sex: *(please tick)* Male ☐ Female ☐

DOCTORS *(This part to be completed by doctor. See notes on the reverse)*

TYPE OF OPERATION: STERILISATION OR VASECTOMY

Complete this part of the form

I confirm that I have explained the procedure and any anaesthetic (general/regional) required, to the patient in terms which in my judgement are suited to his/her understanding.

Signature.............................. Date..../..../.....

Name of doctor..............................

PATIENT

1. Please read this form very carefully.

2. If there is anything that you don't understand about the explanation, or if you want more information, you should ask the doctor.

3. Please check that all the information on the form is correct. If it is, and you understand the explanation, then sign the form.

I am the patient

I agree
- to have this operation, which has been explained to me by the doctor named on this form.
- to have the type of anaesthetic that I have been told about.

I understand
- that the operation may not be done by the doctor who has been treating me so far.
- that the aim of the operation is to stop me having any children and it might not be possible to reverse the effects of the operation.
- that sterilisation/vasectomy can sometimes fail, and that there is a very small chance that I may become fertile again after some time.
- that any procedure in addition to the investigation or treatment described on this form will only be carried out if it is necessary and in my best interests and can be justified for medical reasons.

I have told
- the doctor about any additional procedures I would not wish to be carried out straightaway without my having the opportunity to consider them first.

For vasectomy
I understand
- that I may remain fertile or become fertile again after some time.
- that I will have to use some other contraceptive method until 2 tests in a row show that I am not producing sperm, if I do not want to father any children.

Signature ....

NHS Management Executive

Fig. 39.1 Form of consent for vasectomy

Kilner needle holder
Hyfrecator (optional).

Surgical sutures:
catgut metric gauge 2 (4/0) curved cutting needle. Ref. Ethicon W 480 (chromic) or W 470 (plain)
braided polyester (Mersilene) metric gauge 1.5 (4/0) curved cutting needle. Ref. Ethicon W 316

39.2 TECHNIQUE (Figs 39.2–39.24)

All instruments should be sterilized by autoclaving or using a hot-air oven, and an absolutely aseptic technique employed throughout; an infected postoperative scrotal haematoma is disastrous. The patient should shave the scrotal skin on both sides, and follow this with a bath.

A right-handed surgeon should stand on the left of the patient; this allows gentle traction to be applied to each vas with the left hand. Each vas is identified by careful palpation and the presence of any abnormality such as a varicocele excluded.

The skin is painted with warmed povidone-iodine aqueous solution (Betadine), the vas identified, and isolated to the lateral side of the cord. A small intradermal weal of lignocaine is raised and a 1 cm incision made in the skin, down to the outer sheath of the vas, which is then further anaesthetized with a second injection of lignocaine into the sheath surrounding the vas. Using special vasectomy forceps or fine Allis forceps, the vas in its sheath is picked up, and the sheath separated using fine-pointed iris scissors. The vasectomy forceps are now reapplied, this time around the vas inside the sheath, and a short section of vas freed from its sheath posteriorly. The sheath is mobilized from the front of the vas distally for about 1 cm to prepare a pocket for burying the vas later. It is now possible to apply a pair of fine Halstead mosquito artery forceps at either end of the isolated portion of vas and excise the middle piece, which is sent for histology. A 1 cm portion of 'mesentery' is separated from the proximal portion of vas, and then ligated with 4/0 (metric gauge 2) catgut, as is the vas itself.

The distal end of the vas is ligated with non-absorbable braided polyester 4/0 (metric gauge 1.5). Each end of the divided vas is now coagulated with the unipolar diathermy (Hyfrecator). To prevent any chances of re-anastamosis, the proximal and distal ends of the vas are enclosed in different fascial planes as follows: the lower end is buried in the pocket of the sheath previously prepared, while the upper end of the vas is secured outside the sheath.

Skin closure is achieved by inserting one blade of a small pair of Allis forceps inside the incision deep to the dartos muscle, the other in the skin and suturing through both with 4/0 (metric gauge 2) plain catgut. The same procedure is then performed on the opposite side and both skin incisions painted with Whitehead's varnish, Nobecutane or collodion.

A scrotal support or close-fitting pants are applied and the patient allowed to return home after 15 minutes rest.

It is essential to warn the patient that he will continue to produce viable spermatozoa for 3 months or more following vasectomy, and thus must continue with alternative forms of contraception until two consecutive sperm tests are returned showing no motile spermatozoa in fresh (less than 2 hours old) specimens. Failure to take notice of this advice has resulted in more than one unplanned pregnancy.

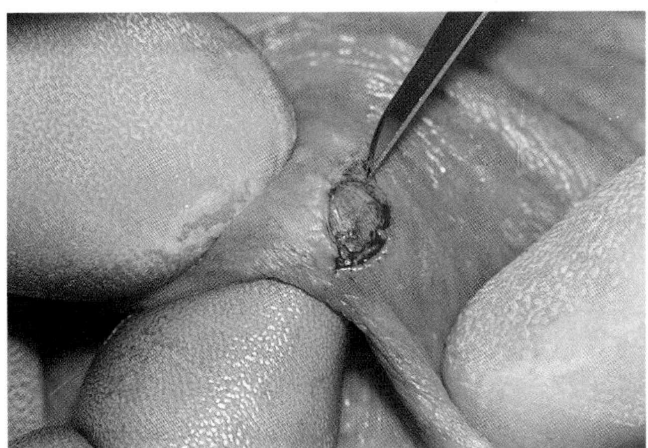

Fig. 39.2 The vas is isolated always lateral to the cord, and held between the finger and the thumb of the left hand. After raising a small intradermal weal with the lignocaine, a 1 cm incision is made through it down to the outer surface of the sheath of the vas. (Figures 39.2–39.24 by kind permission of the late Mr W. Keith Yeates.)

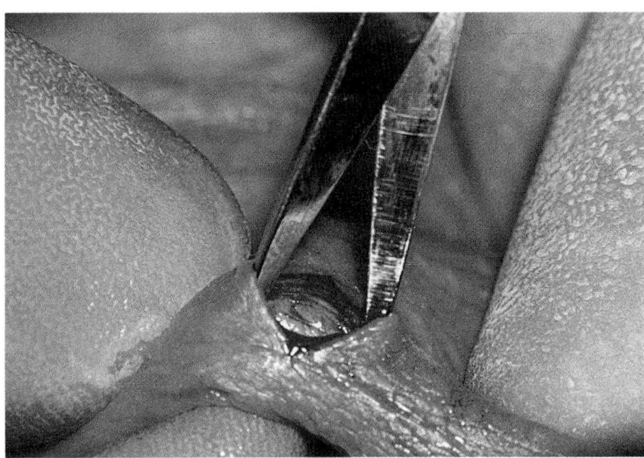

Fig. 39.3 After another very small amount of lignocaine has been injected in each side of the vas and into its sheath, the sheath is delineated by introducing and opening the blades of fine-pointed scissors.

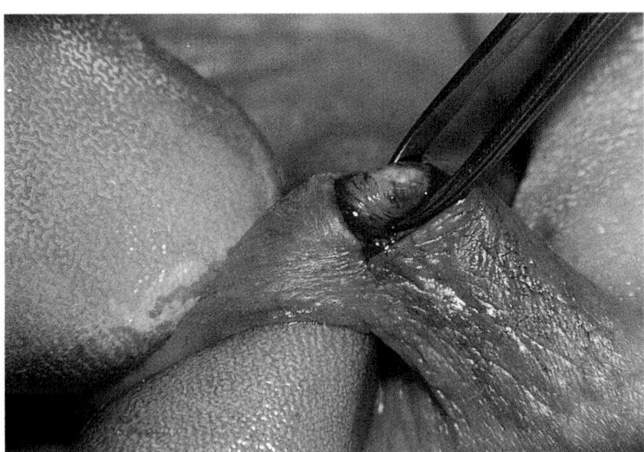

Fig. 39.4 The vas in its sheath is then picked up with a fine pair of Allis forceps.

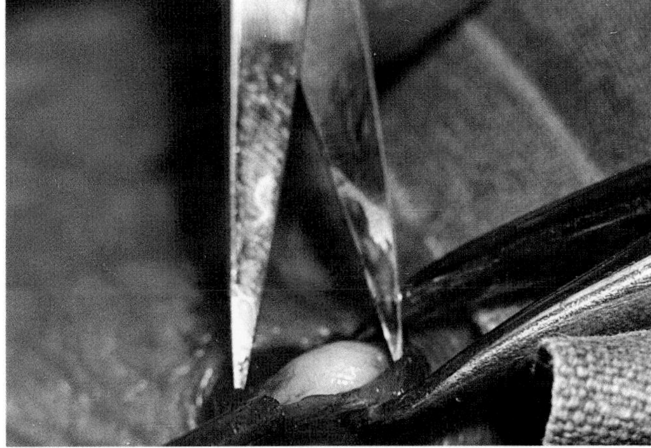

Fig. 39.5 A blunted towel clip is applied round the vas in its sheath; the latter is then opened with the fine pointed scissors, exposing the bare vas.

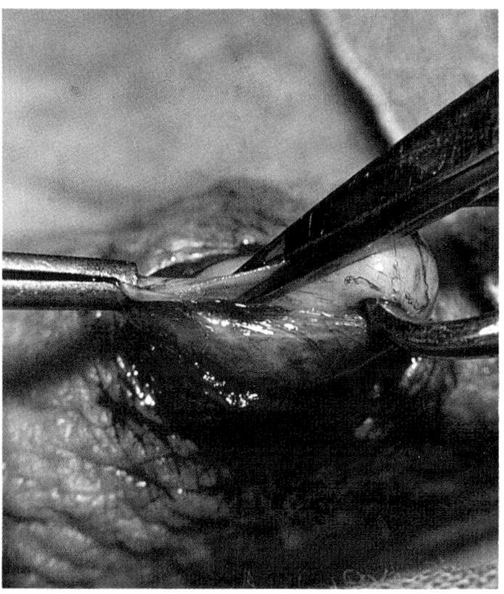

Fig. 39.6 The exposed vas is held with toothed dissecting forceps while the towel clip is opened and then reapplied inside the sheath under the vas itself. The lower part of the sheath of the vas is then picked up with small, toothed dissecting forceps, and the fine adhesions between it and the vas divided with the scissors.

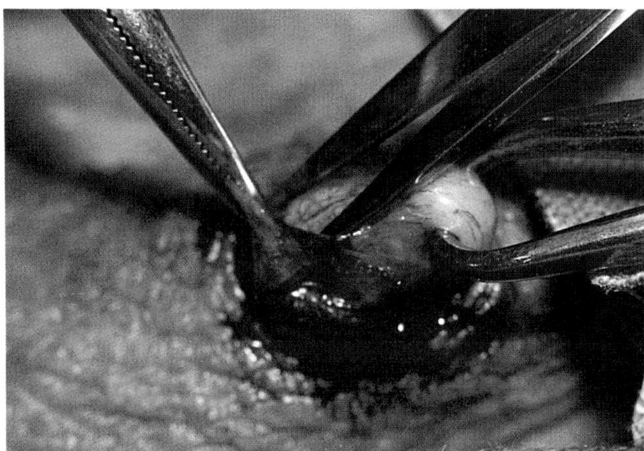

Fig. 39.7 The lower edge of the pocket created is held with haemostatic forceps, which are then left on.

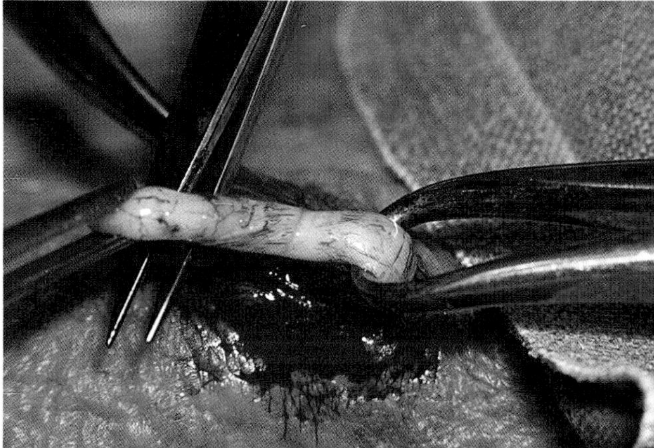

Fig. 39.8 A short section of vas is picked up with the toothed dissecting forceps, and isolated from the posterior part of its sheath.

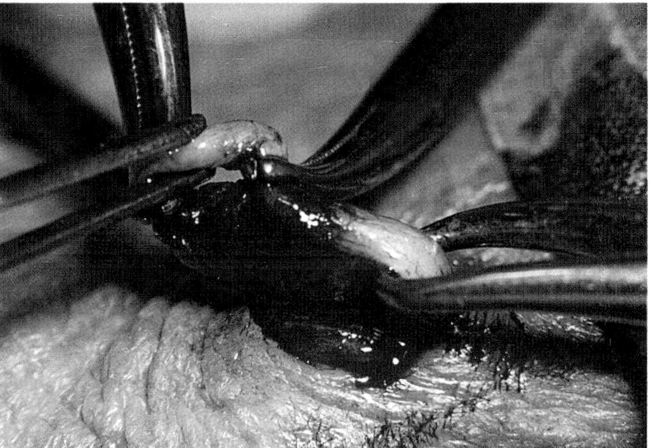

Fig. 39.9 A pair of haemostatic forceps is applied at each end of the isolated vas.

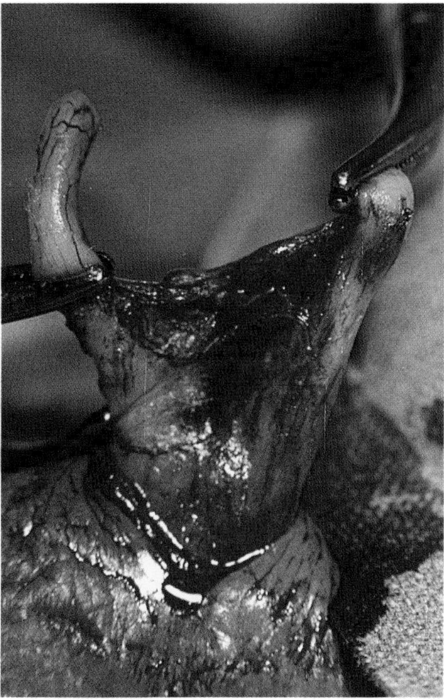

Fig. 39.10 The vas is now divided.

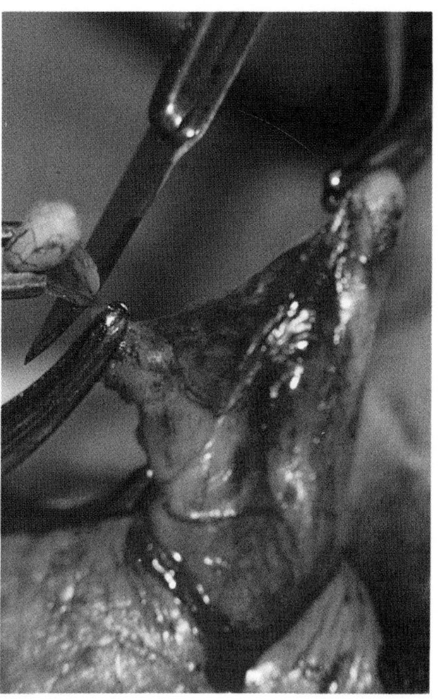

Fig. 39.11 A portion of the vas is excised and sent for histological examination.

Fig. 39.12 The 'mesentery' attached to the upper end of the vas is then held with haemostatic forceps, which are used to strip off the mesentery from the upper end for about 1 cm.

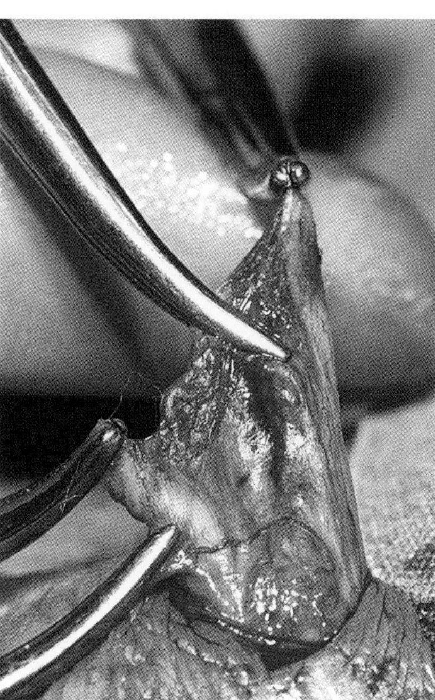

Fig. 39.13 Proximal end of vas freed from mesentery.

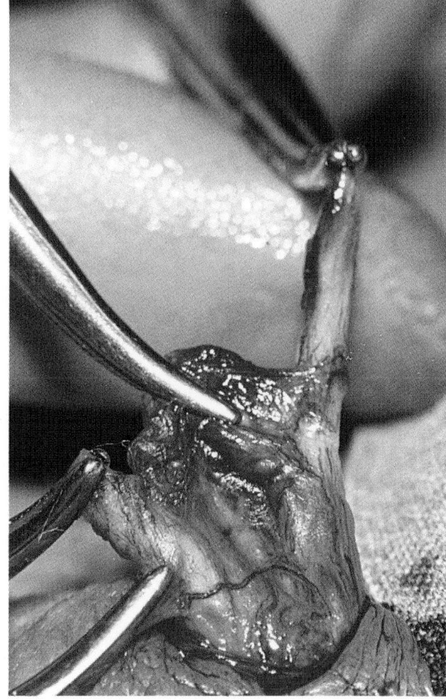

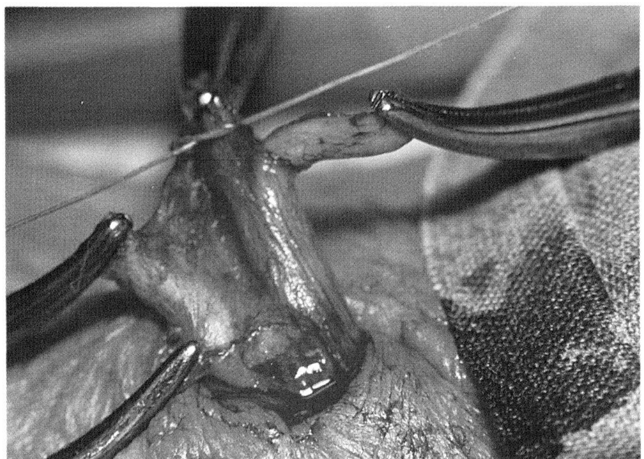

Fig. 39.14 The mesentery is ligated with 4/0 catgut.

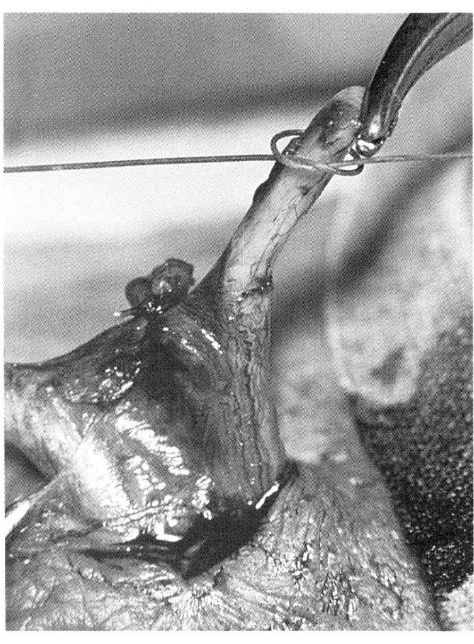

Fig. 39.15 The upper end of the vas is ligated with 4/0 catgut.

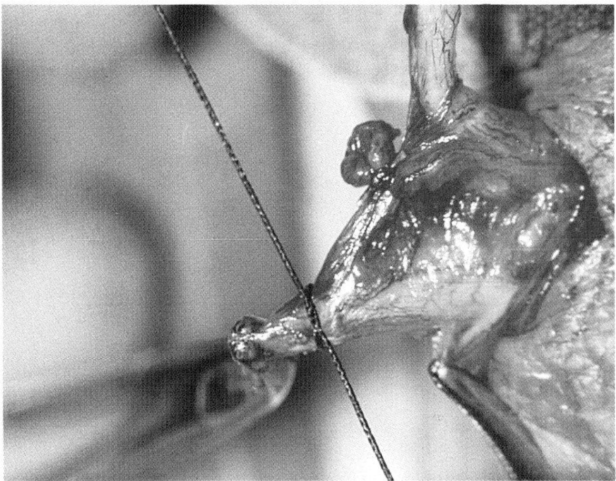

Fig. 39.16 The lower end is ligated with non-absorbable material (silk or braided nylon).

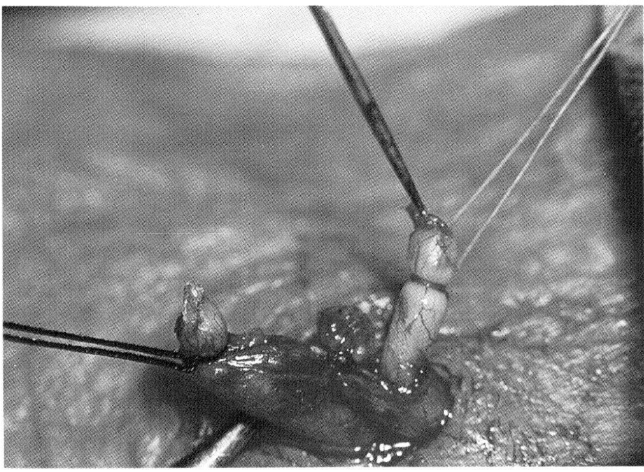

Fig. 39.17 The ligatures round each end of the vas are left long and held in haemostatic forceps, which keeps the field on full view throughout the procedure. Diathermy is applied to both cut ends.

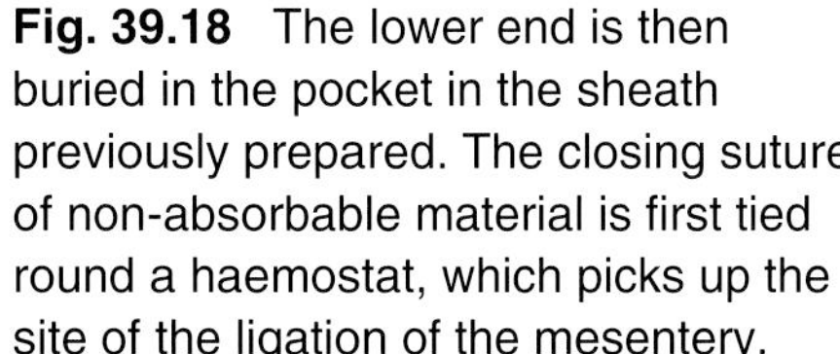

Fig. 39.18 The lower end is then buried in the pocket in the sheath previously prepared. The closing suture of non-absorbable material is first tied round a haemostat, which picks up the site of the ligation of the mesentery.

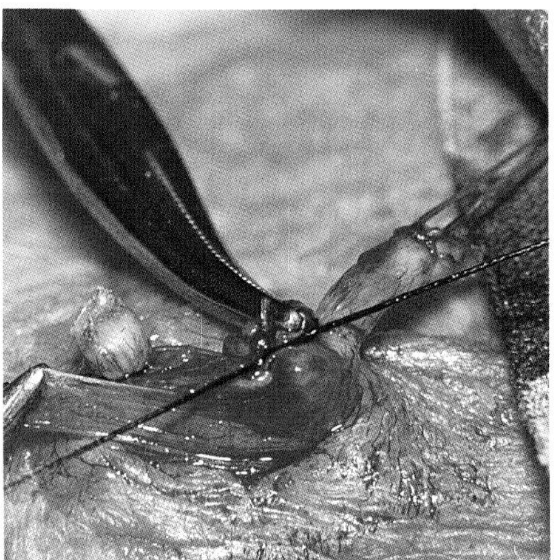

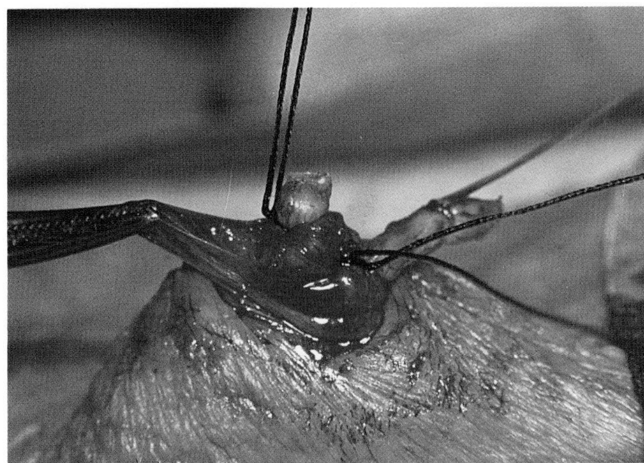

Fig. 39.19 The lower edge of the pocket is opened by traction on the haemostat previously applied.

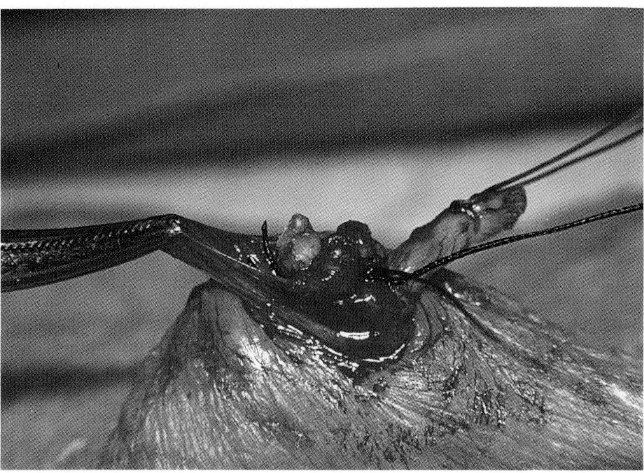

Fig. 39.20 The ligature round the lower end of the sectioned vas is cut.

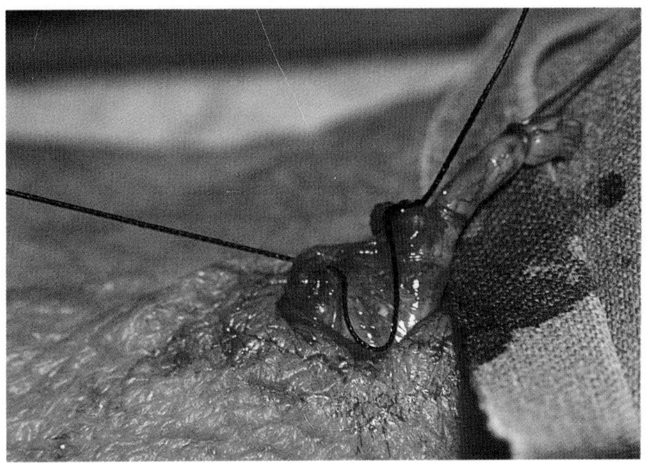

Fig. 39.21 The suture is passed through the margins of the sheath.

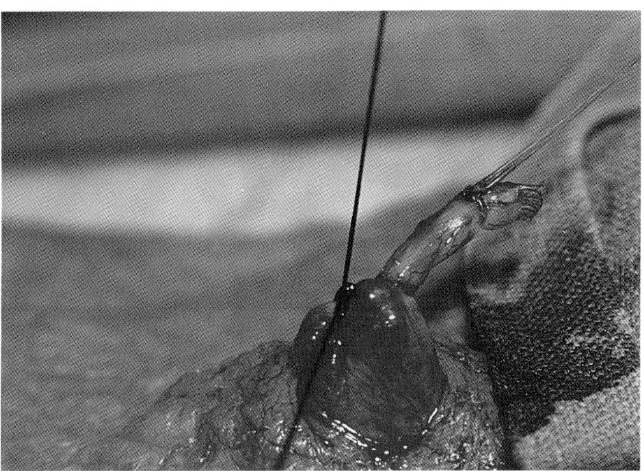

Fig. 39.22 The sheath is then closed over the lower end of the vas.

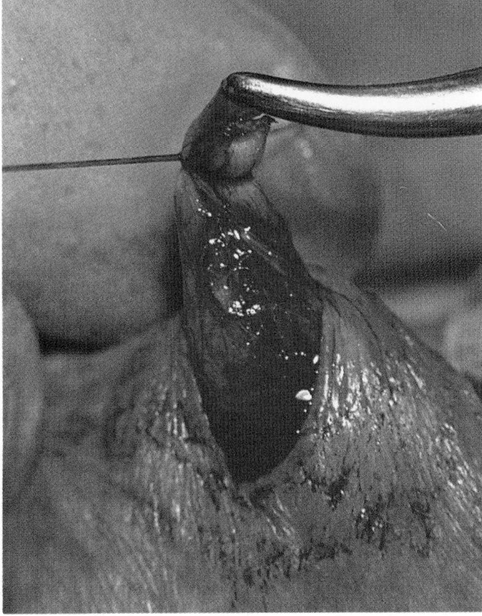

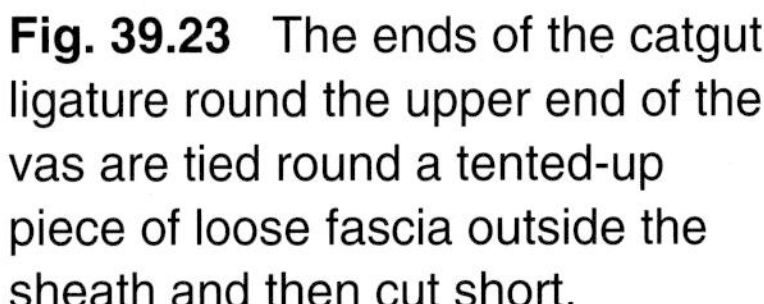

Fig. 39.23 The ends of the catgut ligature round the upper end of the vas are tied round a tented-up piece of loose fascia outside the sheath and then cut short.

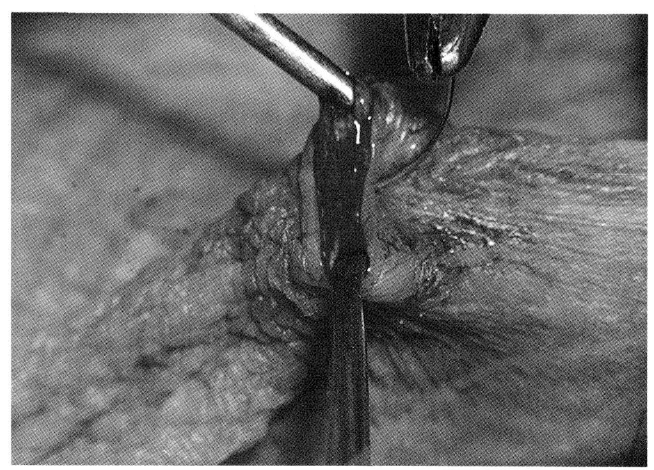

Fig. 39.24 The skin is closed by inserting the blade of a small pair of Allis forceps inside the incision deep to the dartos, the other end being held in a similar fashion with fine-toothed dissecting forceps. The effect of this is to ensure that the suture of 4/0 plain catgut will include the dartos layer. This is very important for haemostasis. A similar procedure is then performed on the opposite side. At the end of the operation, both incisions are painted with Whitehead's varnish, and the scrotum powdered to remove the stickiness of the povidone-iodine. A scrotal support is applied.

For medicolegal reasons, it is important to record the following in writing:

1. That the patient and his wife have had the operation carefully explained to them.
2. That the exceptionally rare possibility of failure has been explained and is understood.
3. A histology report confirming that a portion of vas has been excised on either side.
4. Two negative sperm tests following operation.

Photocopies of duplicate forms of each should be given to the patient, with the originals being kept permanently by the doctor.

39.3 POSTOPERATIVE CARE

The patient may experience discomfort, but not usually pain, which can be controlled with mild analgesics. He should be advised to keep the skin dry for 4 days; no restrictions need be imposed on intercourse, provided contraception is practised until azoospermia is achieved. Mild bruising is common and of no significance; very rarely, a large haematoma occurs, which can look alarming, but which normally settles on conservative treatment alone. Given careful selection, adequate counselling, and the doctor's personal knowledge of the patient, vasectomy is an excellent method of contraception once a couple feel their family is complete.

40

Lymph gland biopsy

A Scrofula is an indurated gland, mostly forming in the neck, armpits and groins. ... When the base of the scrofulous tumour runs out into a narrow point, we may cut it away readily

Paul of Aegina, 7th Century AD

Excision of an enlarged lymph node for histological examination may give valuable information and help to establish a definite diagnosis, but it can be a difficult operation and the doctor should be aware of certain possible problems:

1. Many lymph nodes give the appearance of being quite superficial, but are found at operation to be situated much deeper than anticipated.
2. Bleeding may be more brisk than with other excision procedures.
3. The lymph nodes need very careful handling to preserve their histology, as they tend to be somewhat friable.
4. Avoid the inguinal area and axilla if possible because of the risk to underlying structures.

Given these constraints, however, excision biopsy of suitably accessible lymph glands is a useful procedure which on occasions gives important information in establishing a diagnosis.

40.1 SELECTION OF PATIENTS

Certain preliminary investigations will help to establish a diagnosis and may make the need for lymph node biopsy unnecessary. These include a full blood count, haemoglobin, differential white cell count and platelets, ESR, or plasma viscosity, serum proteins and electrophoresis, liver function tests, LE cells, autoantibody screening, chest X-ray, and possibly blood culture, if pyrexial, and bone marrow.

These tests, together with a careful clinical examination will establish a diagnosis in the majority of patients; those remaining will then be helped by excision of a gland for histological examination. Before embarking on surgery, a representative gland should be chosen and excision should be undertaken.

40.2 TECHNIQUE FOR EXCISION OF GLAND

Instruments required:

scalpel size 3
scalpel blade size 10

toothed dissecting forceps 5 in. (12.7 cm)
McIndoe's scissors, curved 7 in. (17.8 cm)
Kilner needle holder 5¼ in. (13.3 cm)
two pairs Halstead mosquito artery forceps curved 5 in. (12.7 cm)
surgical suture 4/0 (1.5 metric) monofilament Ethilon (Ref. Ethicon W319) with curved, reverse cutting needle
povidone-iodine in spirit (Betadine alcoholic solution)
10 ml 1% lignocaine with adrenaline 1:200 000
syringes and needles.

The overlying skin is painted with povidone-iodine in spirit and the area anaesthetized by infiltration using 1% lignocaine and adrenaline 1:200 000. An incision is now made down to the gland, which may be dissected free using the curved McIndoe's scissors and scalpel, holding the gland with the toothed dissecting forceps. Bleeding can be troublesome, but normally responds to firm pressure; should any small bleeding points not be controlled by pressure, they may be clipped and ligated (Figs 40.1, 40.2).

Closure is by interrupted 4/0 sutures to the skin, with coated Vicryl sutures to the deeper layers if a dead space has been left. The excised gland should be placed in 10% formol saline, immediately labelled and sent for histological examination.

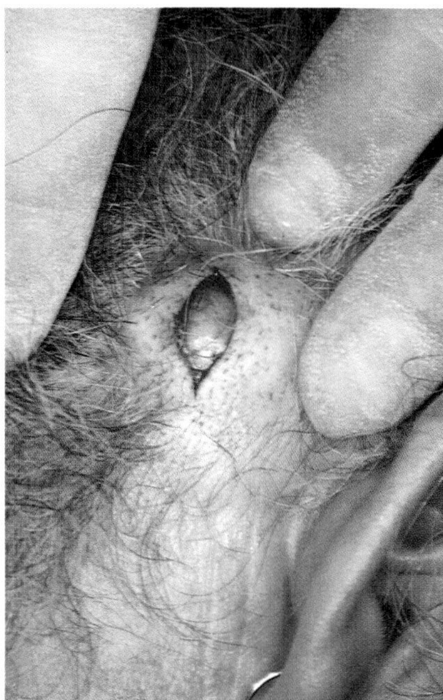

Fig. 40.1 Lymph gland biopsy; technique similar to removal of sebaceous cyst.

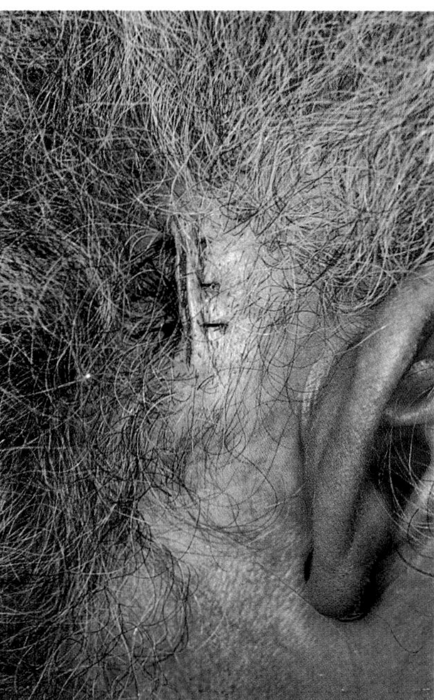

Fig. 40.2 Lymph gland biopsy; closure with interrupted braided silk sutures.

41.2.2 Incision with tenotomy knife

This is done under a local anaesthetic. As with rupture of the ganglion, recurrence rates are high, but the treatment is quick, simple, and generally leaves no scar (Figs 41.2, 41.3).

41.2.3 Catgut suture transfixing the ganglion

Described in the 18th century, the treatment consisted in drawing a thread through the ganglion. This may most conveniently be done by inserting a chromic catgut suture through the skin and through the ganglion. The

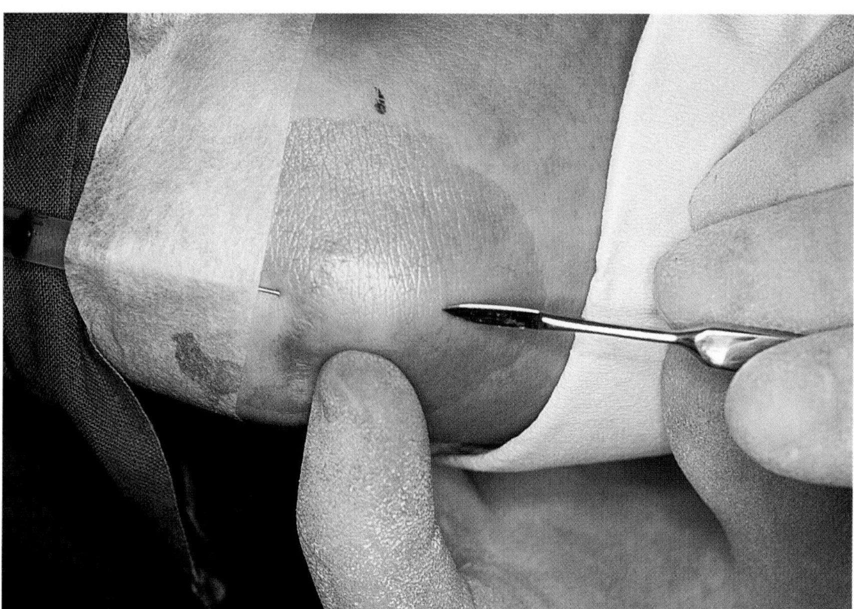

Fig. 41.2 Ganglion on dorsum of wrist.

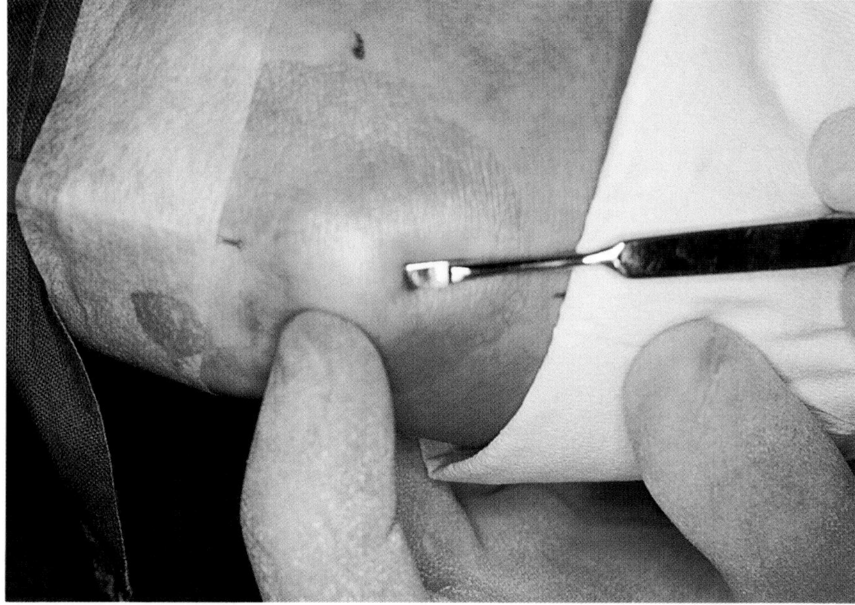

Fig. 41.3 Incision with tenotomy knife. Contents expressed by pressure. Recurrence likely.

action of the suture is to pierce the wall of the ganglion, allowing the contents to leak away under the skin, and secondly to produce an irritant inflammatory reaction within the ganglion in the hope of causing fibrosis and cure.

41.2.4 Aspiration and sclerosant injection

In recent years good results have been obtained by aspirating the gelatinous contents, and reinjecting a sclerosing solution. This simple treatment offers an 80% cure rate, the same as excision, but does not leave a scar, and is considerably quicker and easier to perform.

41.2.5 Excision

If all other treatments fail excision under a bloodless field may be performed, but even this treatment has a failure rate, and it is wise to warn the patient of this possibility at the initial consultation. It is a time-consuming operation which needs to be done meticulously, and if general anaesthesia is unavailable, an intravenous regional block needs to be performed, which demands a qualified assistant.

41.3 TECHNIQUE FOR ASPIRATION AND SCLEROSANT INJECTION

Instruments required:

Two 2 ml syringes
19 swg needle (White)
25 swg needle (Orange)
3% STD injection
Two dental rolls
Micropore tape 1 in.
Elastocrepe bandage 3 in.
Betadine alcoholic solution (povidone-iodine in spirit)
2% lignocaine.

The skin overlying the ganglion is liberally painted with povidone-iodine in spirit (Fig. 41.4).

Lignocaine 2% is now infiltrated from a point on the skin, through to the ganglion itself, injecting 0.5–1 ml local anaesthetic into the cyst. This has the effect of thinning the gelatinous contents, which will make aspiration easier as well as anaesthetizing the area (Fig. 41.5).

One millilitre of 3% STD (sodium tetradecyl sulphate) is now drawn up in a 2 ml syringe, and the needle discarded. Using the 19 swg needle attached to an empty sterile 2 ml syringe, the ganglion is entered and the contents aspirated. This may be assisted by simultaneous pressure over the ganglion with the thumb or finger of the opposite hand (Figs 41.6, 41.7).

With patience, all the gelatinous contents of the ganglion can be aspirated through the 19 swg needle.

Having emptied the ganglion, the syringe is disconnected from the

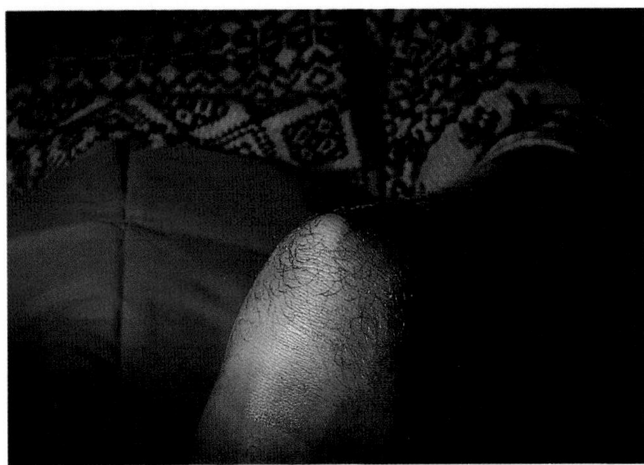

Fig. 41.4 Skin overlying the ganglion is painted with povidone-iodine in spirit.

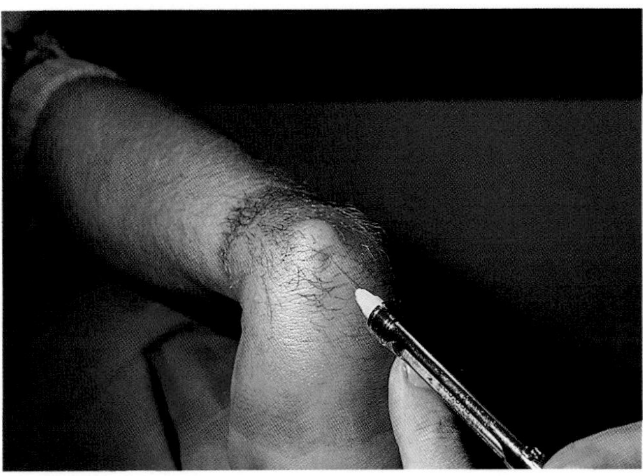

Fig. 41.5 One per cent lignocaine is infiltrated into the overlying skin and into the ganglion itself.

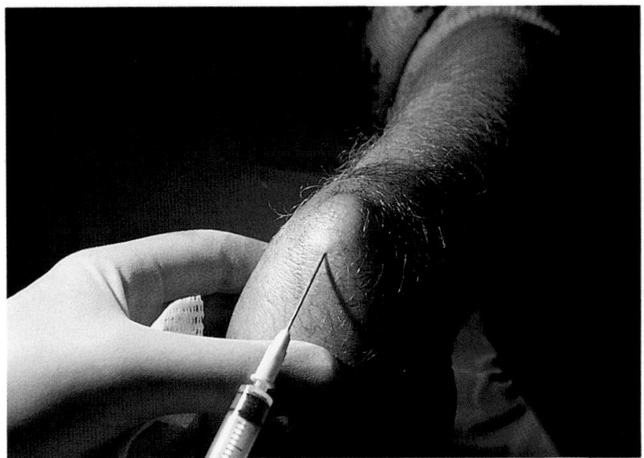

Fig. 41.6 Using a 19 swg needle the contents of the ganglion are aspirated.

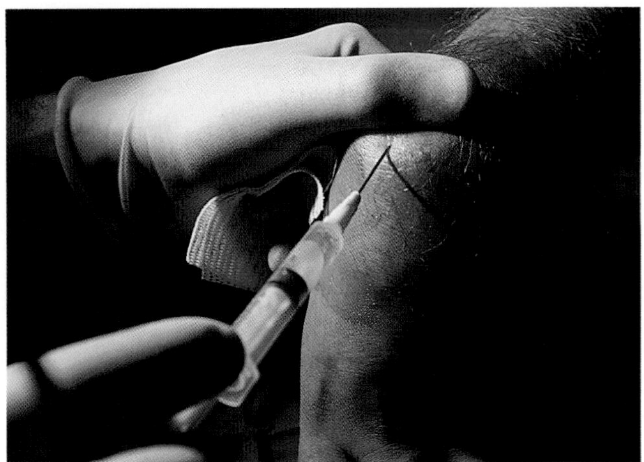

Fig. 41.7 Pressure applied whilst aspirating helps to empty the cyst.

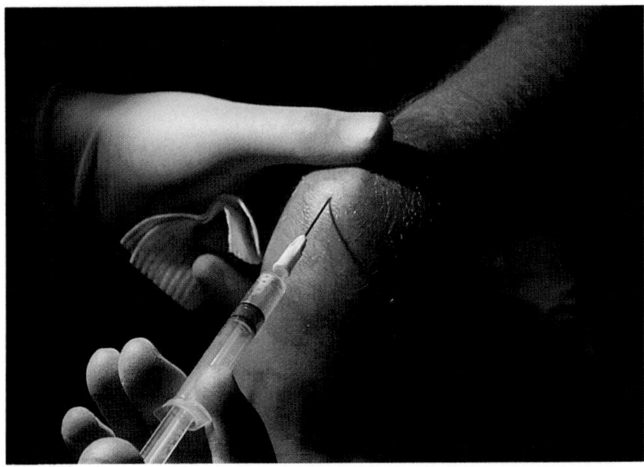

Fig. 41.8 Sclerosant injected into empty ganglion cyst.

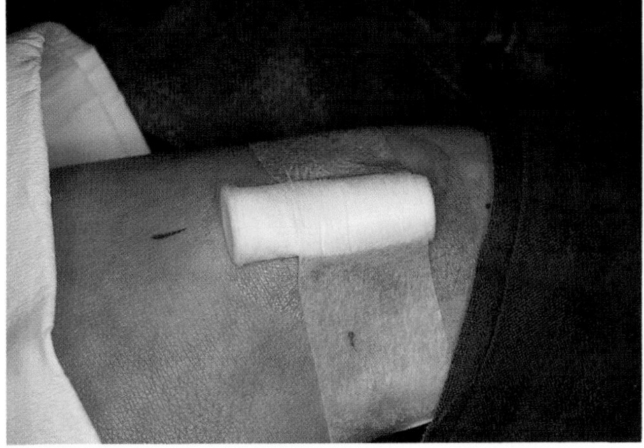

Fig. 41.9 A dental roll is applied over the site of the ganglion.

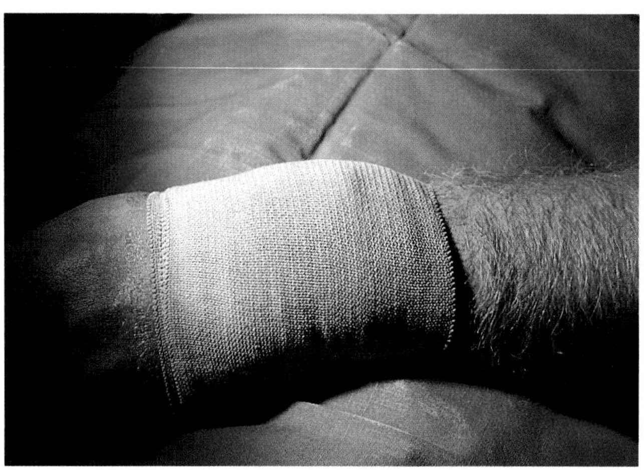

Fig. 41.10 Firm bandage is applied over the dental roll and left undisturbed for 2 weeks.

needle, which is left inside the empty ganglion sac, the volume of aspirate noted, and STD, exactly half the volume aspirated, is now injected through the needle (Fig. 41.8).

Pressure is now applied over the ganglion with a gauze swab while the needle and syringe are withdrawn. A dental roll is taped over the site of the ganglion and this is covered by a firm elastocrepe bandage (Figs 41.9, 41.10).

This is now left undisturbed for 2 weeks, after which time it is removed. No further follow-up is needed. This simple treatment offers an 80% cure rate, similar to that for excision, and is now the treatment of choice for ganglion.

Three per cent sodium tetradecyl sulphate is known to cause marked inflammation when injected in leg veins; it is interesting to note that such reactions are rare when the sclerosant is injected into ganglia – the reason for this is not fully understood.

41.4 THE MUCOUS CYST (GANGLION) ON THE FINGER

Mucous cysts are commonly seen over the terminal interphalangeal joints of the fingers. They frequently occur over the lateral edge and interfere with writing and knitting. Some disappear spontaneously but many recur. They may be excised, sclerosed, cauterized chemically or electrically, treated with cryotherapy or radio-surgery, but a very simple treatment which patients can undertake themselves once shown is to prick with a sterile needle, express the clear jelly, and apply a firm tape dressing daily for 6 weeks. Micropore tape (1/2 in.) is ideal. It should be applied around three quarters of the finger and replaced whenever it becomes loose. If the patient is given a supply of sterile needles they can be instructed to repeat the procedure should the cyst recur (Figs 41.11, 41.12 and 41.13).

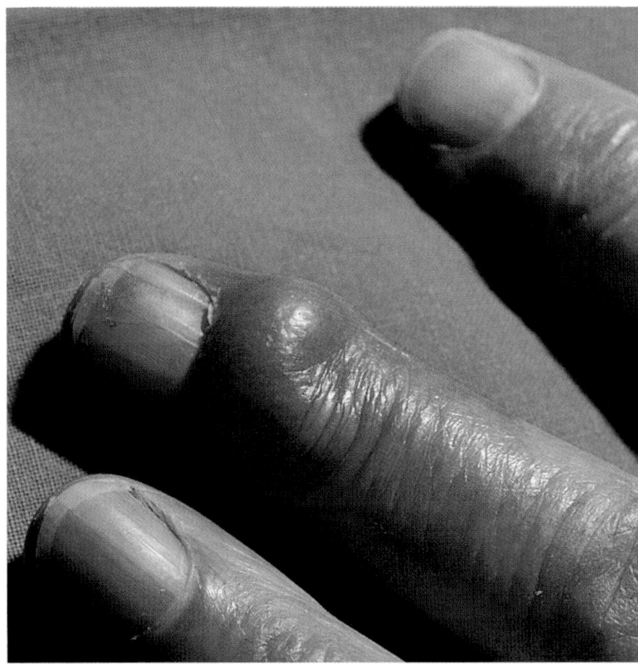

Fig. 41.12 After pricking with a sterile needle, jelly may be expressed and the cyst emptied.

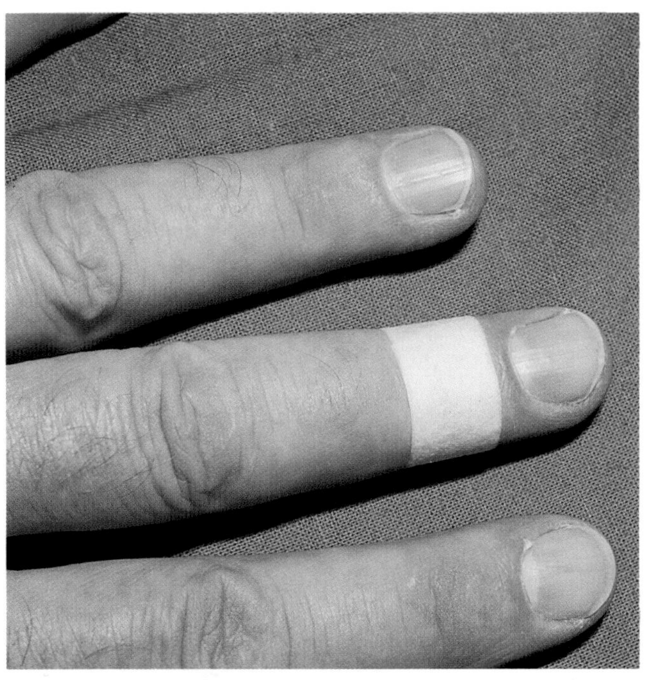

Fig. 41.12 After pricking with a sterile needle, jelly may be expressed and the cyst emptied.

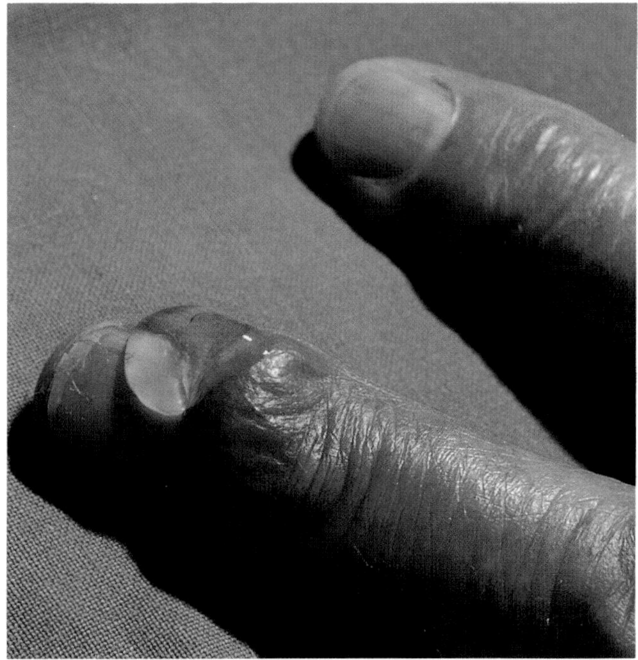

Fig. 41.13 The finger should be taped daily for 6 weeks to prevent recurrence.

42

Radio-surgery

Apply the cautery to the artery itself after having quickly removed the finger, and keep it there until bleeding is arrested.

Albucasis, AD *936*

Radio-surgery now has an established place throughout the world in dermatology, gynaecology, facial and cosmetic surgery, vascular and podiatric practice. Its use in minor surgery is increasing rapidly and it can now achieve far more superior results than other more conventional surgical techniques.

Radio-surgery is a procedure in which tissue is removed or destroyed by electrical energy. This energy is converted to heat as a result of tissue resistance but, unlike electrocautery, the heat is generated in the tissues themselves and the actual electrode remains cold.

42.1 BACKGROUND

The control of bleeding by the application of heat was probably first used by the Ancient Egyptians and there are numerous accounts of heated metal instruments being used to destroy tissues and control haemorrhage.

Electric current has been used in medical equipment for over a century. The traditional electrocautery consists of a platinum wire which could be heated to red heat by the application of an electric current – this had the ability to both cut and coagulate tissues.

Later, with the advent of alternating current and transformer circuitry, high-frequency electric currents were used in medicine to coagulate, cut and destroy tissues, and today diathermy equipment is found in every operating theatre in the world.

In standard diathermy, a high-frequency electric current is passed through the patient. Two electrodes are used – a large plate electrode which is moistened and strapped to the patient's leg, and an 'active' electrode which is used to touch tissues. The heating effect is dependent on the electrical 'density', i.e. where the current is spread over a large surface area there is minimal generation of heat, but where it is concentrated at a small point, enough heat is generated to cut, coagulate or destroy tissue (Fig. 42.1).

Low-frequency alternating current caused muscle contractions (the Faradic effect as used in physiotherapy); high-frequency (>10 000 Hz) currents did not have this effect, but resulted mainly in heating of the tissues.

The invention of the vacuum tube, as used in radios and televisions, allowed the production of amplified electric currents which would cut

Fig. 42.1 Diagrammatic illustration of radio-surgery showing the distribution of energy.

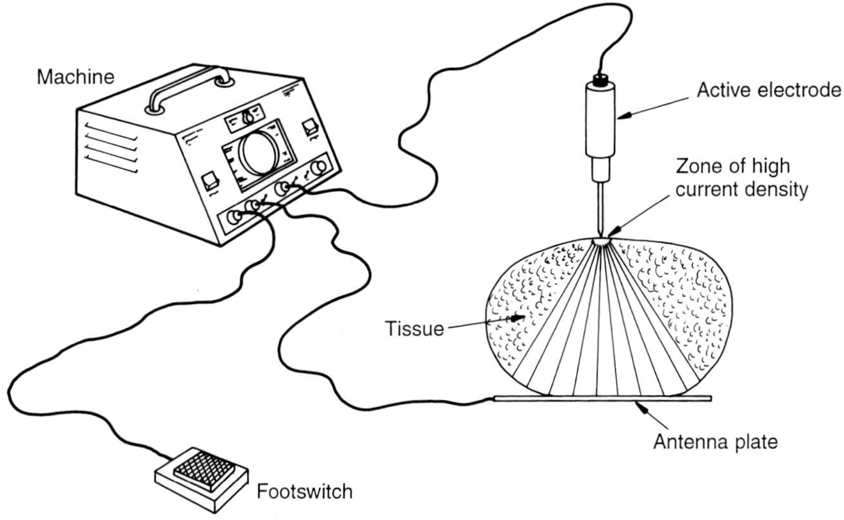

Fig. 42.2 Comparison of different electrical frequencies and their respective uses.

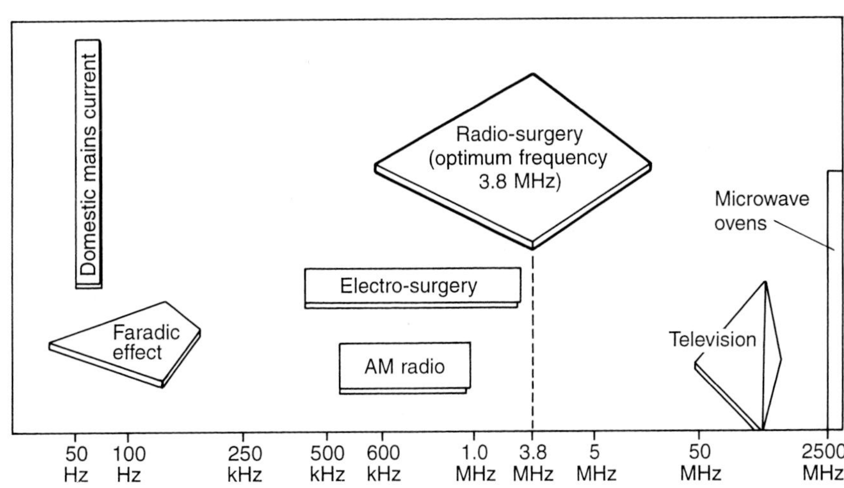

Fig. 42.3 Different waveforms and modes of action.

	Waveform	Use	Oscilloscope confirguration
I	Fully filtered and fully rectified	Cutting	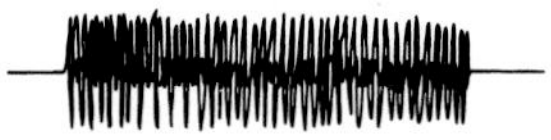
II	Fullt rectified	Cut and coagulate	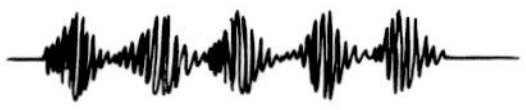
III	Partially rectified	Haemostasis	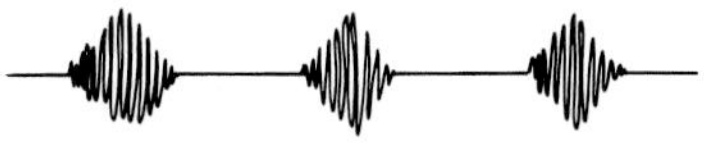
IV	Markedly damped (spark gap)	Fulguration and electra desiccation	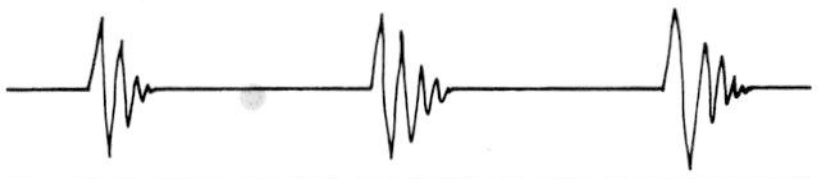

tissues, and in 1978 Maness showed that 3.8 million cycles per second (mega-hertz) was the optimal frequency for cutting soft tissues. This frequency is still used in modern radio-surgery units (Fig. 42.2).

Furthermore, in modern radio-surgical instruments several different waveforms can be generated, each having different characteristic effects on tissues, viz. incision, excision, coagulation (Fig. 42.3).

Radio-surgery is an atraumatic method of cutting and coagulating soft tissues. No pressure is needed and the cells are vaporized in the path of the radiowaves causing them to split apart much like a hot wire through polystyrene. This results in less trauma to the cells, less fibrous scarring, and less postoperative discomfort; the other advantage is that the electrodes are also self-sterilizing in use.

42.2 DIFFERENT WAVEFORMS

The five different waveforms commonly used are as follows:

1. A pure filtered waveform (pure micro-smooth cutting) (Fig. 42.4). This is used for skin incisions and wire loop excisions where

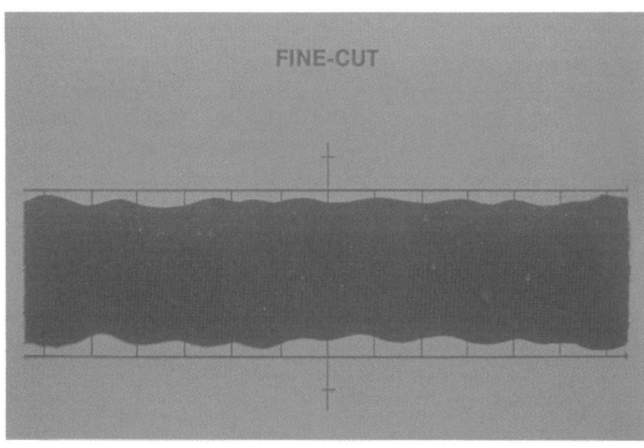

Fig. 42.4 Fully filtered waveform (cutting).

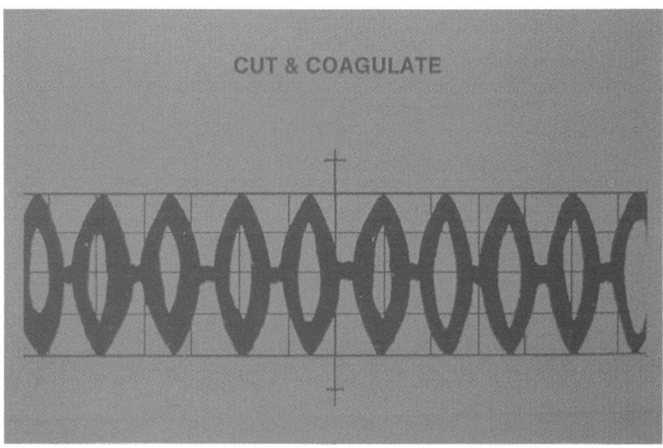

Fig. 42.5 Fully rectified waveform (cutting and coagulation).

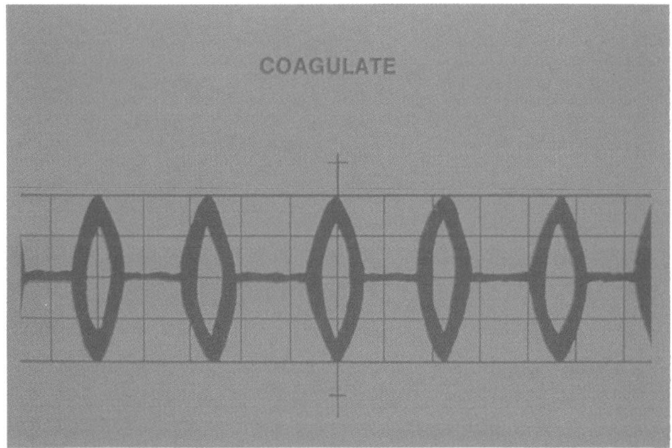

Fig. 42.6 Partially rectified waveform coagulation).

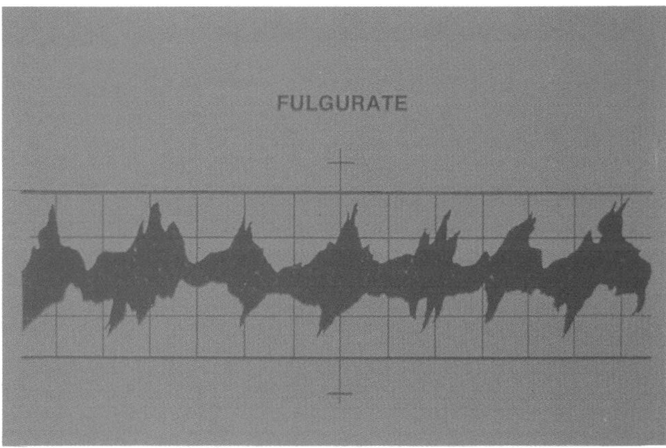

Fig. 42.7 Marked damped (spark-gap) waveform (fulguration).

haemostasis is not expected to be a problem. This waveform gives the least lateral heat, and therefore the least tissue damage.

2. A fully rectified waveform (blended cutting and coagulation) (Fig. 42.5). This is used for skin tags, papillomata, keloids, keratoses and removal of naevi where slight bleeding might be expected. It cuts as well as coagulates small blood vessels and gives slight lateral heat to the tissues.
3. A partially rectified waveform (hospital-type control of bleeders) (Fig. 42.6). This is primarily for haemostasis – it cannot be used for cutting but is excellent for coagulation, telangectasia and spider veins.
4. A fulgurating current (spark-gap tissue destruction) (Fig. 42.7). This is very similar to the unipolar diathermy (Hyfrecator) and gives superficial tissue damage by holding the needle electrode close to the tissue and allowing a stream of sparks to burn the tissues. It is suitable for superficial haemostasis and destruction of small basal cell carcinomata and cysts.
5. Bipolar coagulation (Fig. 42.8). Very precise haemostasis may be obtained by using bipolar forceps. Each blade is connected to the radio-surgical unit so that the current passes between the points of the forceps. It is very useful for picking off individual bleeding vessels in micro-surgery.

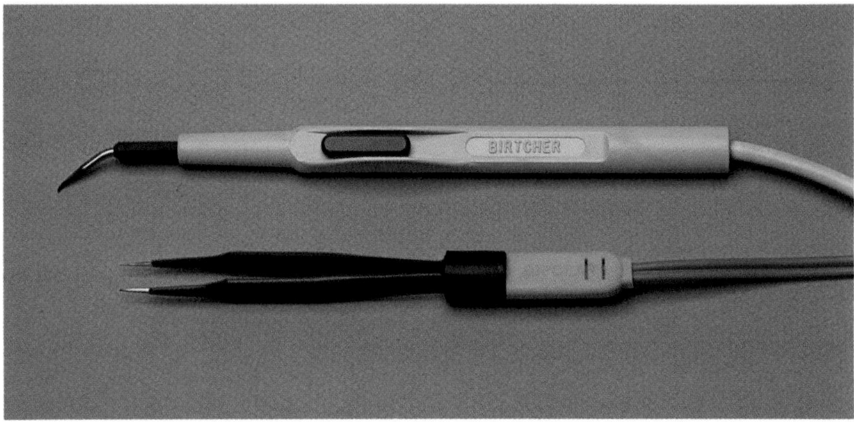

Fig. 42.8 Finger-switch and bipolar forceps.

The heat generated in the tissues as the electrode passes through them is described as lateral heat and can be calculated from the formula

$$H = T \times I \times W \times S \times F$$

where T = time during which the electrode is in contact with the tissues;
I = power intensity;
W = waveform (pure filtered gives least lateral heat and partially rectified gives the most lateral heat);
S = surface area of the electrode in contact with the tissues (the smaller, the less heat); and
F = frequency of application (allow time between successive treatments for the tissues to cool).

The more lateral heat produced, the more is the tissue damaged, so it follows that for the best results, the needle electrode should be of the finest diameter, the power setting should be the lowest compatible with smooth cutting, the appropriate waveform should be selected, and no pressure should be used.

There are several radio-surgical units on the market, each with different characteristics, waveforms and power outputs. The author uses an Ellman Surgitron FFPF unit (Figs 42.9, 42.10, 42.11), and all settings and waveforms refer to this machine. Where the doctor possesses an alternative instrument, reference should be made to the maker's handbook for power settings, etc.

Most radio-surgical units will comprise the following:

1. An electrical generator connected to the domestic electricity supply which converts the mains voltage (110 at 60 Hz or 240 volts at 50 Hz) to high-frequency current of 3.8 MHz. It has a switch which will select different waveforms.

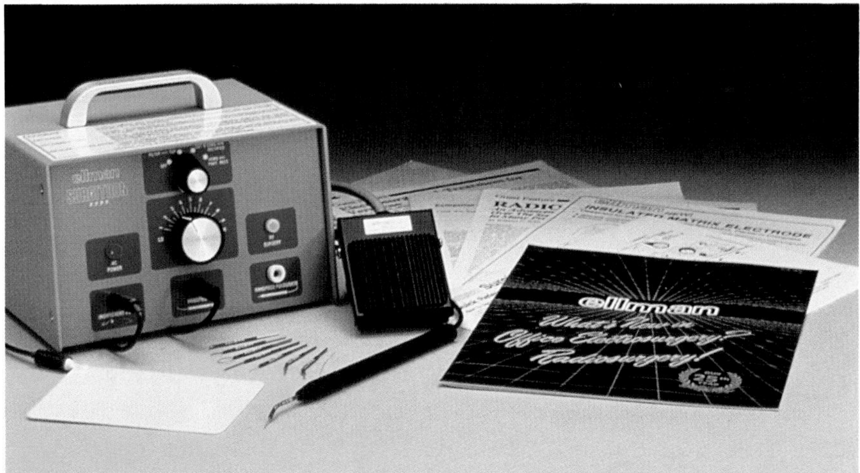

Fig. 42.9 The Ellman Surgitron FFPF radio-surgical unit.

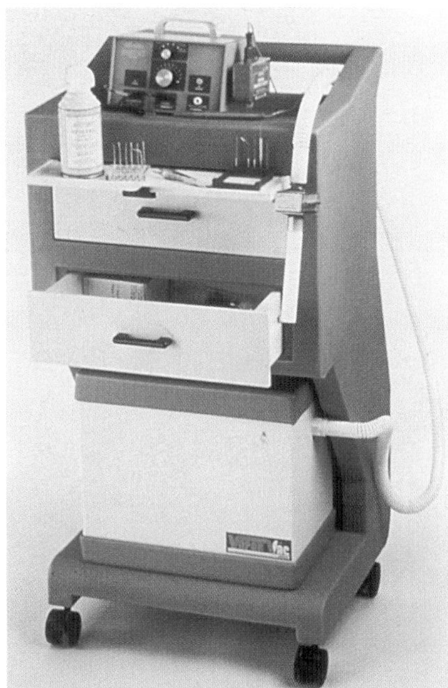

Fig. 42.10 The Ellman Surgitron on trolley with Vapor-Vac.

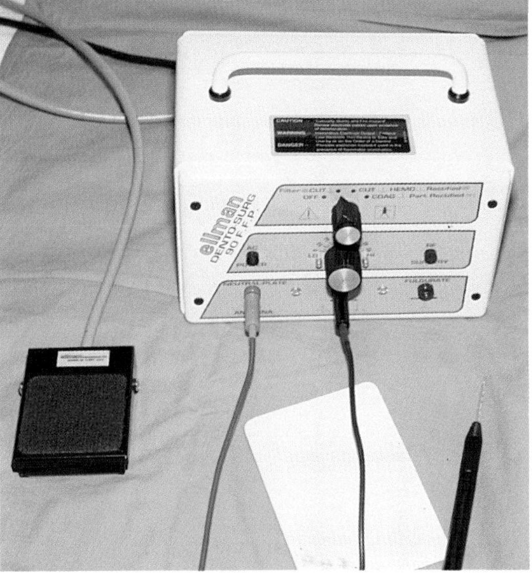

Fig. 42.11 The Ellman Dento-Surg 90 watt radio-surgical unit.

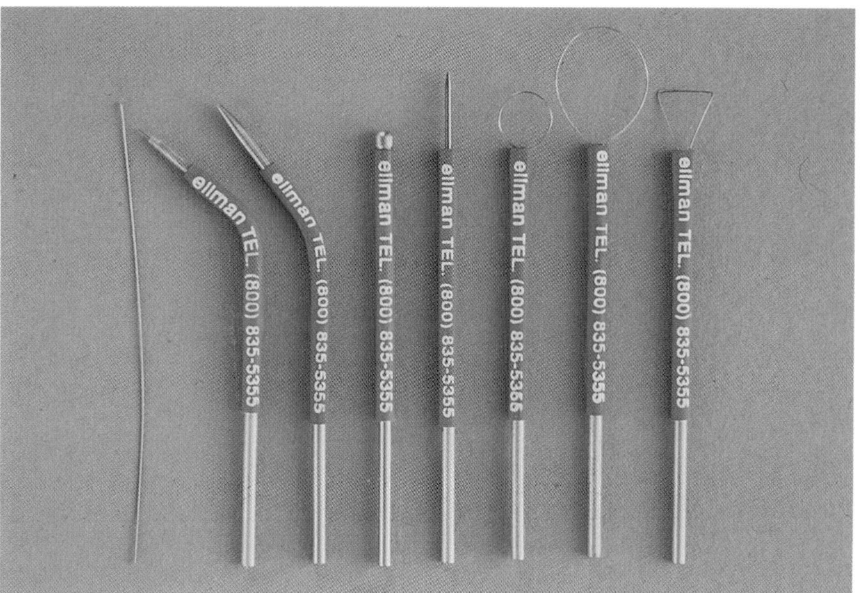

Fig. 42.12 Selection of electrodes for Ellman radiosurgery unit.

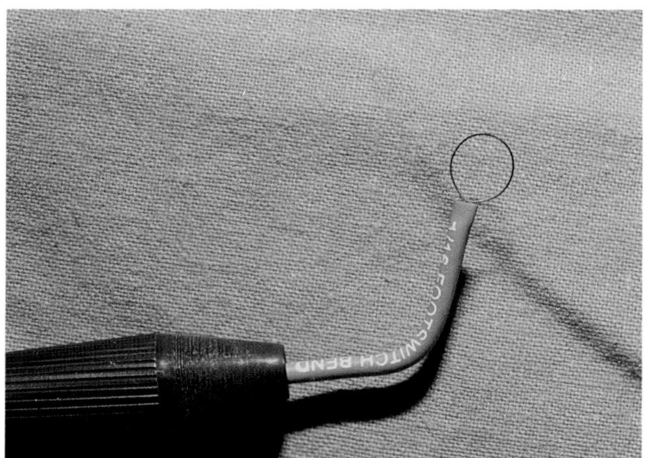

Fig. 42.13 The tungsten wire loop electrode.

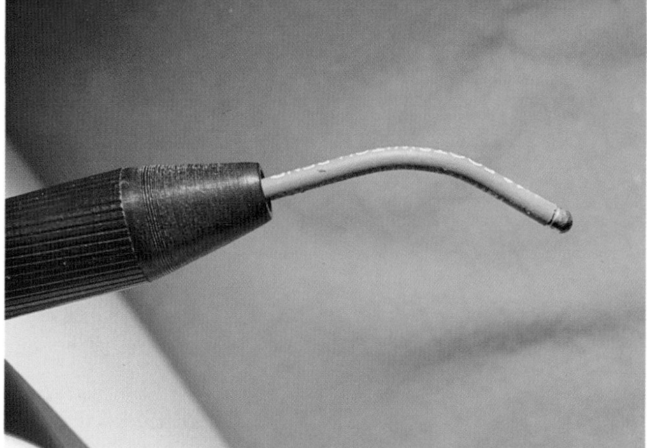

Fig. 42.14 The ball-ended 'coagulation' electrode.

2. A passive electrode or ground plate or dispersive electrode (Fig. 42.11). This is usually a small plastic covered plate which is placed in close proximity to the patient – it does not need to make electrical contact with the patient (unlike hospital diathermy) and acts like an antenna to concentrate the radio waves.
3. A treatment handle connected to the generator by a flexible wire. Different shaped electrodes are inserted into this handle and clamped in position. Electrodes, manufactured from surgical quality tungsten, may be single wire for incision or fulguration, loop electrodes for cutting (electro-section) (Fig. 42.12) or ball-ended for haemostasis (Fig. 42.13). Fine, bipolar forceps are also available for precise haemostasis.

   A handle which holds a standard scalpel blade is also available so that the surgeon can use both conventional cutting as well as radio-section (Figs 42.15, 42.16, 42.17).

4. A foot switch or finger-operated switch on the electrode handle (Figs 42.8 and 42.18).
5. A smoke evacuator (Figs 42.19, 42.20, 42.21). This is essential where any number of radio-surgical procedures are being performed, particularly in wire loop excision of the cervix in gynaecology. Viral filters and activated charcoal filters can be incorporated in the extraction circuit making the radio-surgery operation almost odourless! A room ventilator is also a very good idea.

Other equipment needed includes:

1. Latex gloves. These should be worn at all times; for the majority of superficial skin lesions they need not be sterile, but for deeper procedures sterile gloves should be worn.
2. Masks. Where viral lesions are being removed it is a sensible precaution to wear a surgical mask. There has been documented evidence that the wart virus DNA is liberated during carbon dioxide laser surgery, and it is possible that this can occur with the plume of smoke released during radio-surgery.
3. Appropriate sterile instruments to handle tissues, e.g. fine forceps and skin hooks.
4. Autoclave to sterilize the electrodes and instruments.

42.3 LEARNING THE TECHNIQUE OF RADIO-SURGERY

Radio-surgical instruments are powerful, and a totally different technique from that of conventional scalpel surgery has to be learned. Most of the poor results are entirely due to inexperience and faulty technique.

The first major difference is that **no pressure must be used**. This is hard to learn for a surgeon who has been trained to press the scalpel firmly through the tissues. In radio-surgery it is the radio wave which does the cutting.

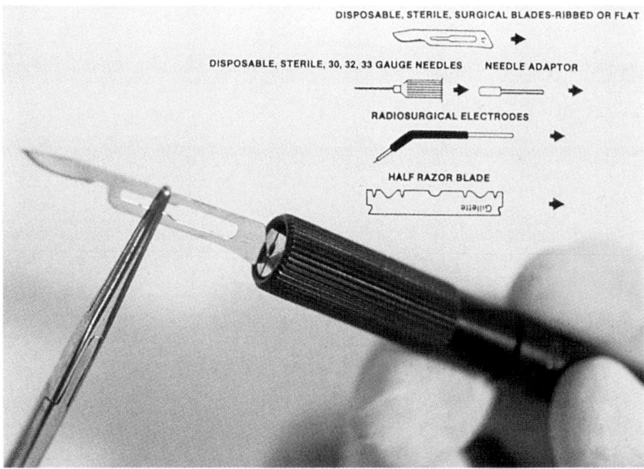

Fig. 42.15 Conventional scalpel blades may be used with a radio-surgical unit, combining both modes of cutting.

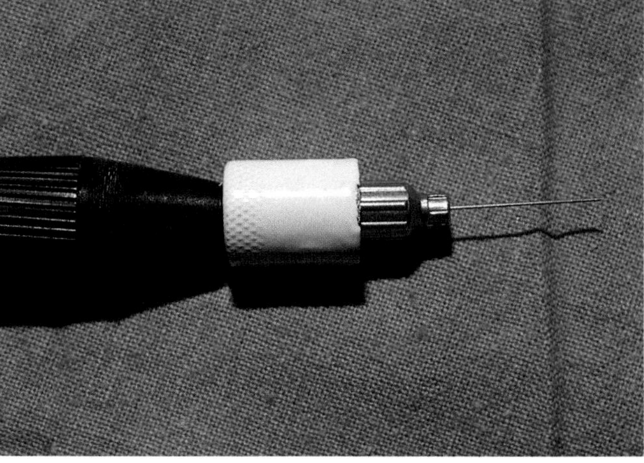

Fig. 42.16 Attachment which can take disposable 30 swg needles to use as a scalpel.

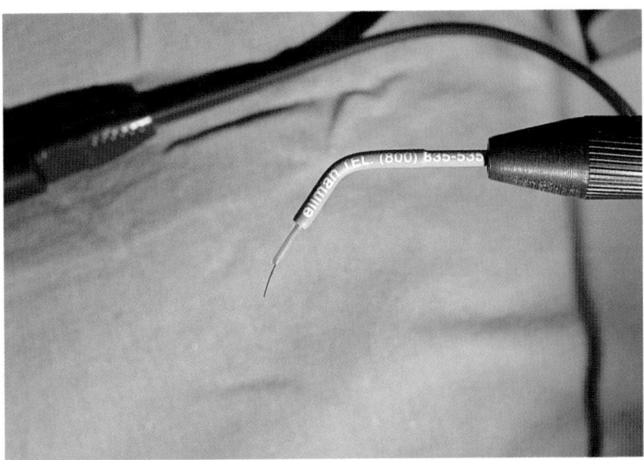

Fig. 42.17 Needle electrode.

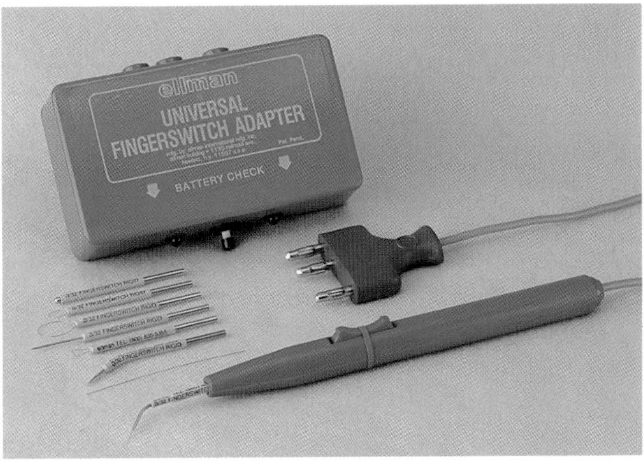

Fig. 42.18 Hand-piece with finger switch and switching unit which plugs into the side of the Surgitron FFPF.

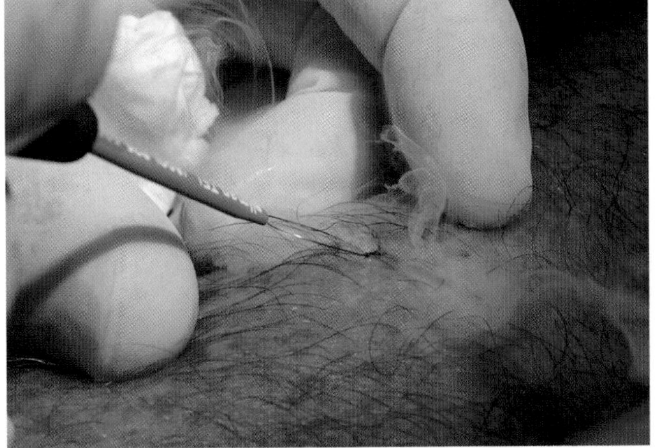

Fig. 42.19 Considerable smoke is produced with radio-surgery.

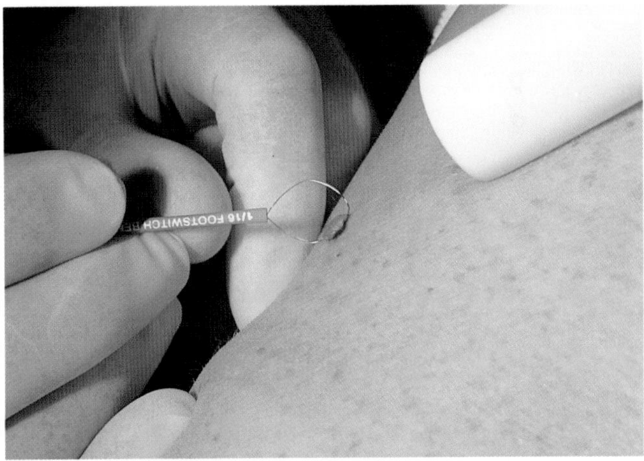

Fig. 42.20 The use of a vacuum extraction unit is strongly recommended both for visibility and patient comfort.

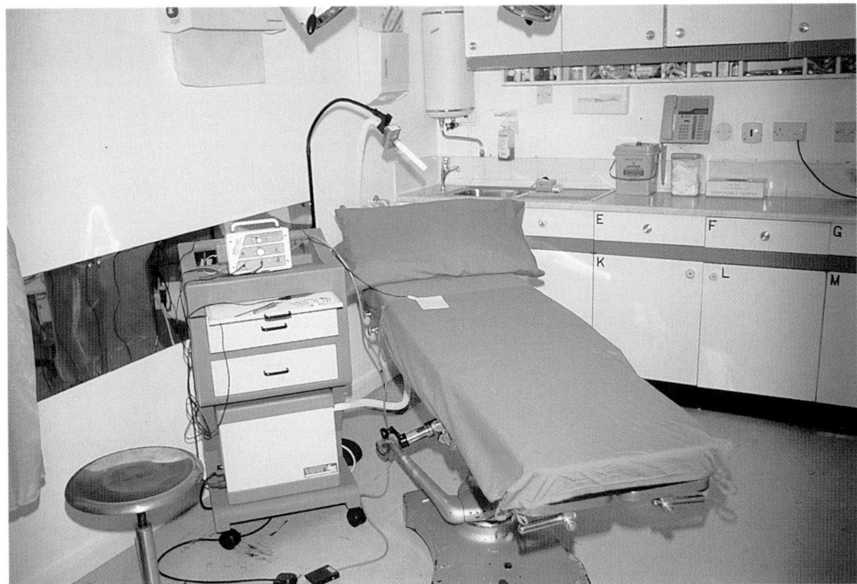

Fig. 42.21 Radio-surgical unit and trolley with vacuum extraction along-side treatment couch.

Secondly, there are no absolute power settings on the machine – these need to be learned by trial and error and experience. For example, a small moist lesion will require much less power to remove than a larger fibrous keratinized lesion.

Thirdly, if repeated incisions are to be made on the same lesion time should be allowed to let the edges cool between cuts – usually up to 10 seconds.

Fourthly, rather than removing the whole lesion at the first attempt, better cosmetic results are obtained by first removing a representative sample for histological examination and then gradually 'planing' off the remainder of the lesion until it is flush with the surrounding skin (Figs 42.22, 42.23, 42.24).

One of the simplest teaching aids is a piece of raw steak placed on the passive base electrode. Starting with high power, different techniques of cutting and coagulation may be tried, and then, by reducing the power, the effects of too low or too high current are discovered (Figs 42.25, 42.26, 42.27).

Many videotapes have now been produced demonstrating radio-surgery, and these can be highly recommended for teaching.

Tuition by a colleague familiar with the technique of radio-surgery is well worth the time and effort, followed by treating several patients under supervision.

42.4 WARNINGS

1. Cardiac pacemakers. No patient with a cardiac pacemaker should be treated with radio-surgery without prior consultation with their cardiologist. Fixed-rate pacemakers are least likely to experience problems, but demand-led pacemakers may well be affected and result in arrhythmias. It is, therefore, essential to enquire from every patient in advance whether they have a pacemaker.
2. No spirit-based or inflammable skin antiseptic should be used. In fact, it is probably unnecessary to use any form of skin preparation.
3. Any allergic history of the patient to local anaesthetics (very rare), skin preparations, and postoperative skin applications and tapes should be noted.
4. Delayed bleeding can occur. This is usually light but can cause alarm to the patient. It can be minimized by not using adrenaline with the local anaesthetic, and by applying a solution of 20% aluminium chloride or Monsell's solution on a cotton-wool applicator at the end of the procedure. It is also helpful to advise the patient about applying finger pressure for 10 minutes should any oozing occur.
5. Explosion risks exist in the presence of bowel gases and/or oxygen, as they do with diathermy and electrocautery.
6. Electrical shocks and burns. These can be minimized by not allowing any part of the patient to touch any metal and by the operator wearing rubber gloves.
7. Finally – inexperience.

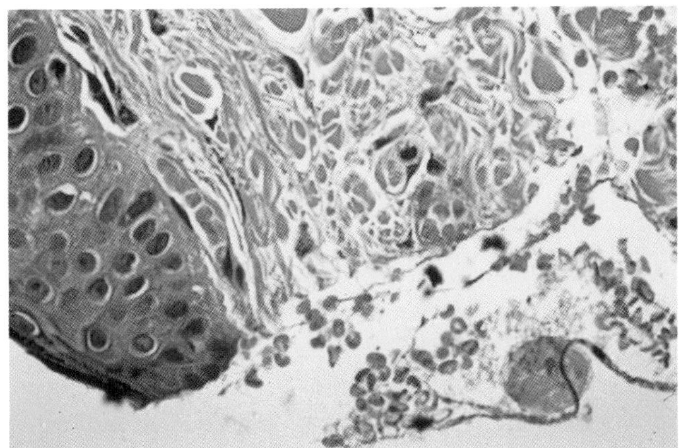

Fig. 42.22 Histological appearance of tissue cut with scalpel.

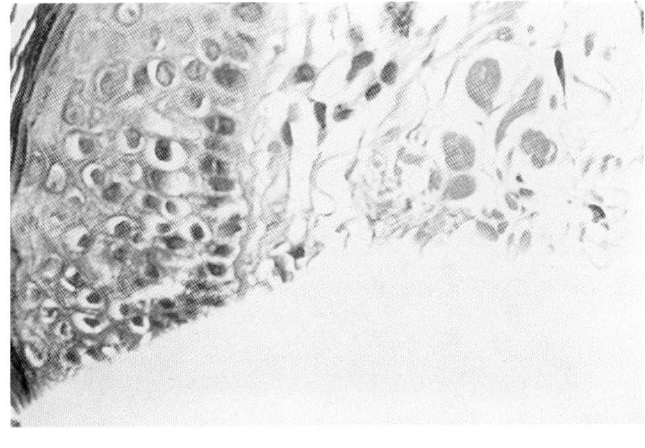

Fig. 42.23 Histological appearance of tissue cut with radio-surgery. Note less cellular damage.

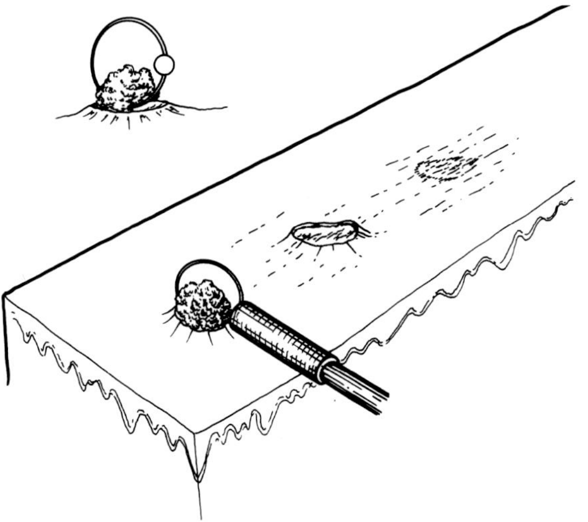

Fig. 42.24 Diagram showing removal of top of naevus for histological examination and then 'planing' down with a wire loop electrode.

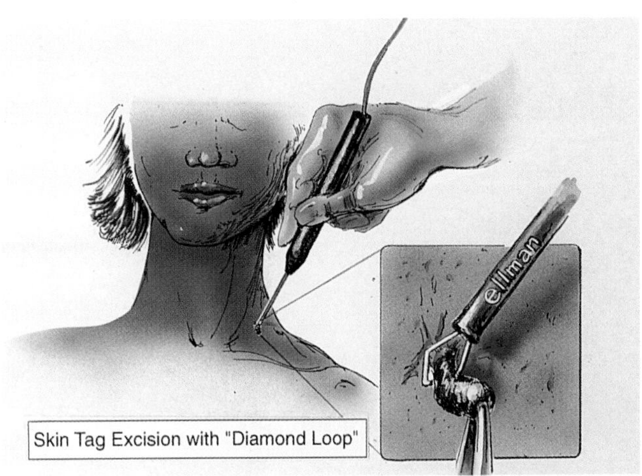

Fig. 42.25 Use of wire loop electrode.

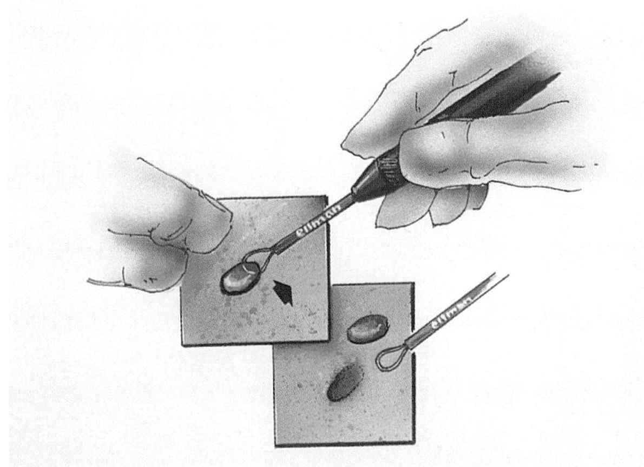

Fig. 42.26 Removing lesion with wire loop.

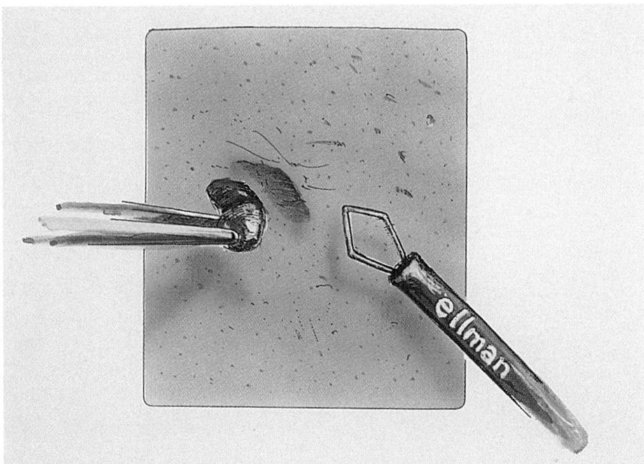

Fig. 42.27 Removing lesion with forceps and wire loop.

42.5 AVOIDANCE OF COMPLICATIONS

As with all medical and surgical treatments, complications can occur, but the majority are avoidable – careful preoperative assessment of both patient and equipment will prevent many mishaps.

1. Check all wires and replace any which are frayed or where there is a break in the insulation.
2. Check all electrodes. Broken wires will cause lacerations. Discard any worn tips.
3. Too deep an excision will result in unnecessary scarring.
4. Watch the foot switch or finger switch. Don't let an assistant accidentally tread on the foot switch, and don't tread on it yourself inadvertently as accidental burns can occur to the patient.
5. Check hand-piece is inserted in correct socket.
6. Check power control has not been increased at the end of a previous procedure, e.g. to steam-clean electrodes.
7. Too much tissue destruction making histology impossible. This may be due to incorrect power or waveform setting, or a lesion which is too shallow. In this case cut off the top with a conventional scalpel and then treat the base with the radio-surgical unit.
8. Check that the patient does not have a cardiac pacemaker.
9. Check the patient is not on aspirin or anticoagulants.
10. Beware lower limbs in diabetic patients.

42.6 CLEANING ELECTRODES

All electrodes can be steam sterilized in an autoclave, as can the wires, plugs and antenna baseplate. Furthermore, in use the electrodes are self-sterilizing. However, during use, carbon particles and debris can become adherent to the tungsten wire, reducing the efficiency and causing 'drag'. A very simple way of removing this and also for sterilizing the electrode is 'steam cleaning'.
To steam clean electrodes (Fig. 42.28):

1. Gloves should be worn.
2. Set the unit to cutting waveform (pure filtered).
3. Set power dial to 5.
4. Place two gauze pads together and fold in half.
5. Saturate with water.
6. With the electrode in the hand-piece, place it between the folds of the gauze.
7. Activate for 2 seconds while moving the electrode back and forth within the gauze, with almost no finger pressure. Repeat. (A sizzling sound can be heard as steam is generated. Be careful not to burn fingers holding the swab.)

Certain electrodes are bendable to make for easier access, but the tungsten wire should always be treated with great respect as it is very fragile.

Fig. 42.28 Care of electrodes (Ellman International Inc

Care of electrodes

Preventing electrode breakage

Electrodes are made of surgical grade tungsten wire and will eventually volatize and break. If misused, they will carbonize and rapidly wear out. To increase their efficiency and prolong their life follow these recommendations.

1. Plug handpiece into the correct terminal.
2. The correct waveform should be used. **Never** try to cut on partially rectified.
3. The antenna plate should be in close proximity to the operative site. (i.e. in face surgery, place behind the head). The antenna may be placed behind cloth or under a pad. **It does not need** to have skin contact.
4. Have your assistants handle the electrodes by the **insulated shafts only**. The wires are surgical grade tungsten with very thin diameters.

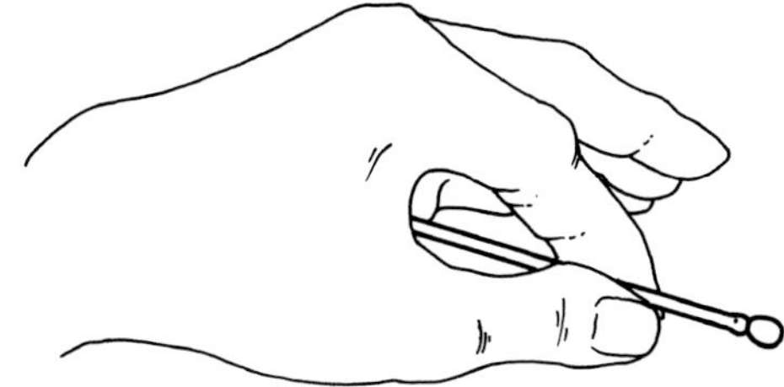

5. If using bendable electrodes, **only bend** the electrodes at their insulated shaft.

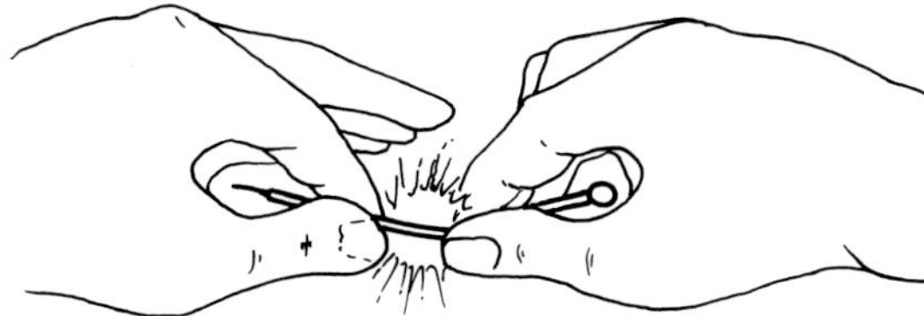

6. Tissue should be moist.
7. Always activate the unit **before** making contact with the tissue.
8. **Never apply pressure**. Always remember that the radiowaves are doing the cutting.
9. If there is resistance, drag, or tissue sticking to the electrode, the power setting is **too low**. This will cause bending and breakage. Adjust accordingly by raising power gradually.
10. If there is sparking (which causes carbonization), the power is **too high**. Adjust accordingly by lowering power gradually.
11. Electrode loops need slightly **higher power** than straight wires (adjust up gradually) and are more fragile.
12. If you get stuck in the tissue, **do not force** the electrode. De-activate the unit and carefully remove the electrode from the tissue.

Cleaning electrodes during surgery

1. Set radiosurgical instrument at cut or cut/coag waveform.
2. Set power dial between 3 and 5.
3. Place two gauze pads together and fold in half.
4. Saturate the gauze with tap water.

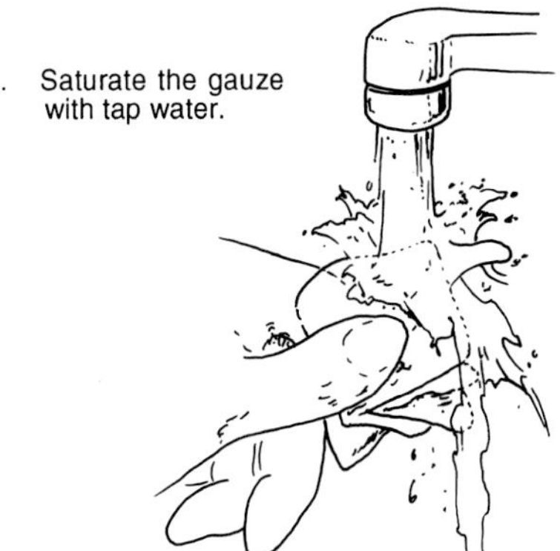

5. With electrode in the handpiece, place it between the folds of the gauze.
6. Activate unit for 1–2 seconds while moving electrode back and forth within the gauze with little or no finger pressure. Repeat procedure (you should hear a 'sizzling' sound). This volatizes the water molecules and 'steam cleans' your electrodes.

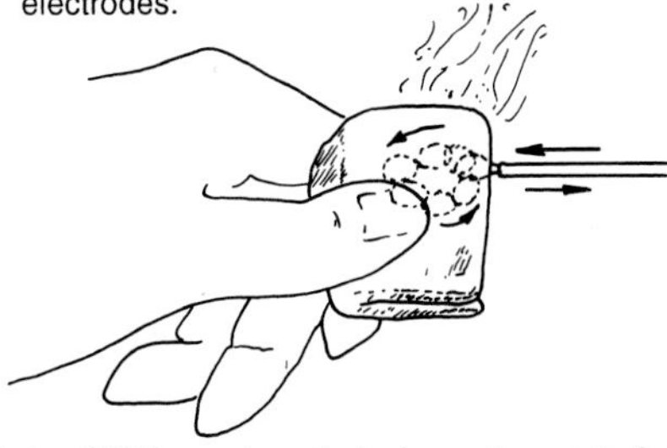

****Note:** OSHA requires that gloves be worn during all clinical procedures and during cleaning, disinfecting, and sterilizing of instruments including electrodes.

Care and cleaning of electrodes after use

1. **Do not scrub** electrodes with a brush or an abrasive.
2. To remove blood or tissue, place the electrode in hydrogen peroxide or in an ultrasonic cleaner for 3–5 minutes.
3. Place electrodes in an autoclave bag, being sure that electrodes lay side by side and **not** on top of each other.
4. Place electrode autoclave bag on top of other surgical instrument bags to prevent breakage.

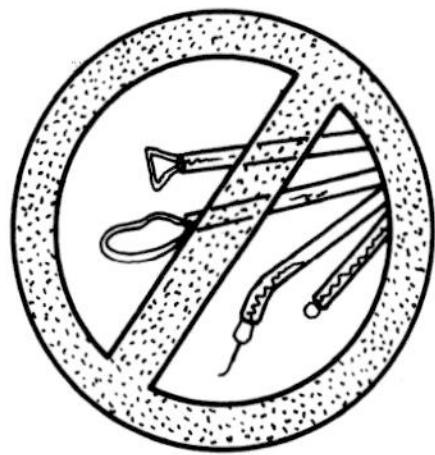

Important: A periodic visual inspection of your electrodes is strongly recommended. If the tungsten wire is broken or if the insulated coating is 'nicked', torn, cracked, or damaged in any way, replace the electrode.

42.7 GENERAL GUIDELINES FOR RADIO-SURGERY

1. Always select the correct waveform.
2. Never try to cut on partially rectified waveform (coagulation).
3. The antenna plate should be as near as possible to the operative site – it does not need to have skin contact with the patient.
4. Tissues should be moist.
5. Always activate the unit before making contact with the tissues.
6. Never apply pressure – let the radiowave do the cutting.
7. If there is resistance or 'drag' or tissue sticking to the electrode, the power setting is too low.
8. If there is sparking the power setting is too high.

42.8 CARE OF ELECTRODES AFTER USE

1. Do not scrub with a brush or abrasive.
2. Blood and secretions may be removed by soaking in a solution of hydrogen peroxide, or by using an ultrasonic bath for 5 minutes.
3. Autoclave electrodes in a separate container to avoid damage from other larger instruments.

42.9 PREPARATION OF THE PATIENT

1. It is essential to explain to the patient in advance the technique of radio-surgery, and what to expect both during the procedure and also the postoperative management.
2. Where a vacuum extractor unit is used it is helpful to explain to the patient that most of the noise will be coming from that, and that the operative electrode and unit is silent.
3. Ensure any rings and jewellery are removed, particularly if situated near the operation site.
4. Make the patient comfortable, and ask them not to make any jerky or unexpected movements if at all possible.
5. Warn the patient about the smell of burning and also to expect to see some smoke, even if the vacuum extractor is used.
6. Pre-printed preoperative and postoperative information sheets are invaluable and usually answer most of the patient's questions.

42.10 ANAESTHESIA

With few exceptions, local infiltration anaesthesia is required, exactly as with conventional surgery or electrocautery. This should be with plain lignocaine rather than with added adrenaline as there is a slightly increased risk of postoperative oozing where adrenaline has been used. The finest gauge needle should be used to administer the anaesthetic (30 swg or finer).

Because infiltration of the tissues might distort the size and shape of skin lesions, it is helpful to mark the boundaries of the 'mole' or 'naevus' with a skin marking pen before injecting the local anaesthetic.

42.11 APPLICATIONS OF RADIO-SURGERY

A chart showing the applications of radio-surgery, lesions which may be treated, choice of waveform and which electrode to use is shown in Fig. 42.29.

The following conditions may be treated with radio-surgery:

Actinic keratoses
Basal cell carcinoma
Blepharoplasty
Bowen's disease
Cauterisation of bleeding vessels
Cervical biopsies
Cervical conization (LLETZ)

Fig. 42.29 Quick reference chart showing applications of radio-surgery, lesions which may be treated, choice of waveform and which electrode to use (Ellman International Inc.).

Procedure	Waveform	Electrode
Abscessess	I, II	A8, B and C series
Anal fissure	II	A2
Basal cell carcinoma	II, IV	A3, A8, B and C series
Biopsy	I	A8, B and C series
Carbuncles	II	A8, B and C series
Caruncles	II	A8, B and C series
Cervical erosion	II	B series, W1–5 series
Condyloma	II	B series
Cysts	I, II, IV	A8, B and C series
Development of skin flaps	I, II	H15, A8, E series
Ear-piercing	I	A3
Epilation	III	D7, A1
Epistaxis (nose bleeds)	III	H8, H9, D2
Fistulas	II	A2
Furuncles	II	A8, B and C series
Haemorrhoids	II, III	B and D series
Haemostasis	III	D, J series. H40
Keloids	II, III	A3, J series
Keratosis	I, II	B and C series
LLETZ/LEEP	I, III	W1–5 series
Matrixectomy	III	H10
Nasal polyps	II	H7, B series
Naevi	I, II	A8, B and C series
Rectal polyps	II	H7, B series
Rectal skin tags	II	B and C series
Rhinitis (inflammation of the nasal mucous membrane)	II	B and C series
Skin incisions	I, II	A8, H15
Skin tags	I, II	A8, B and C series
Telangiectasia	III	A1, D7, H17
Tumours	I, II, IV	A8, B and C series
Verrucae	II	B and C series
Xanthoma	I, II	A8, B and C series

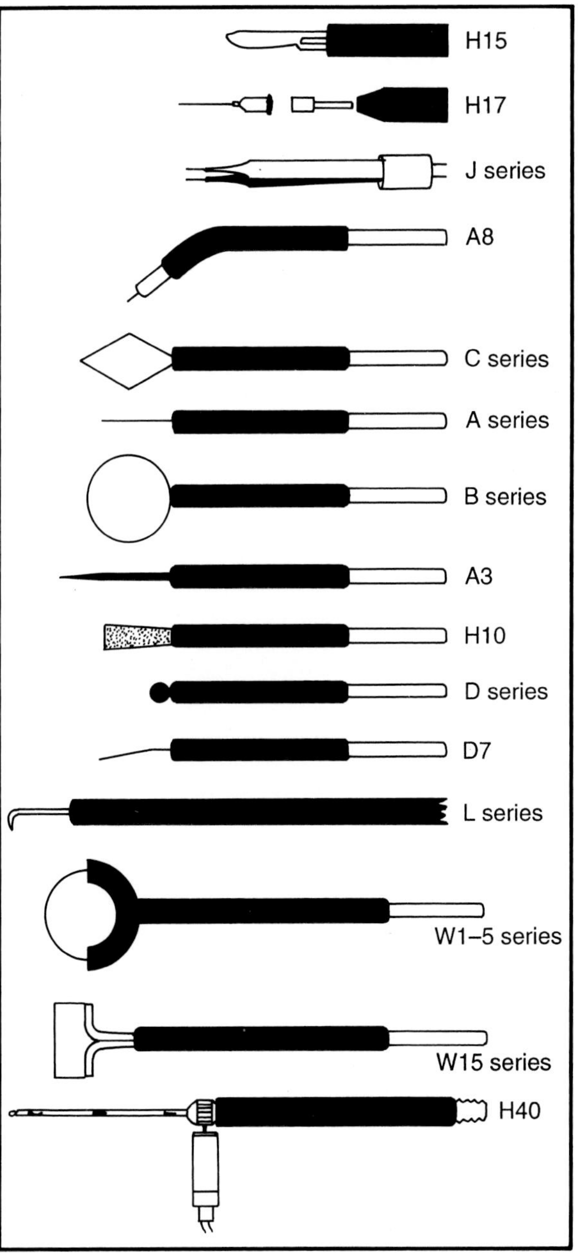

Chalazion
Condylomata accuminata
Cosmetic surgery
Epilation
Excision of skin lesions
Fibro-epithelial polyps
Hair transplants
Haemorrhoids
Ingrowing toe-nails
Keloids
Mucosal lesions inside the mouth
Naevi
Palato-uvuloplasty
Pyogenic granuloma
Rhinophyma
Sebaceous cysts
Seborrhoiec warts
Skin tags
Syringoma
Tattoo removal
Telangectasia
Xanthelasmata

Some of these procedures are obviously beyond the scope of this book, but those which can be considered minor surgical procedures are included under the following headings:

1. Removal of skin lesions (Figs 42.30–42.61).
2. Treatment of ingrowing toe-nail (Figs 42.62–42.67).
3. Telangectasia and thread veins (Figs 42.68 and 42.69).

42.12 RADIO-SURGERY IN CONJUNCTION WITH CRYOSURGERY

Excellent cosmetic results can be achieved with radio-surgery alone, but even better results may sometimes be obtained if the area treated by radio-surgery is sprayed with liquid nitrogen immediately postoperatively.

The rationale behind this is, first, to blend the edges of the wound and make for a smoother junction between healthy and treated skin and, secondly, when treating lesions such as basal cell carcinoma, squamous cell carcinoma and intra-epithelial carcinoma (Bowen's disease) any microscopic spread by neoplastic cells may be destroyed.

In practice, the lesion is marked with a skin pen, removed or destroyed using the radio-surgical electrode, any bleeding vessels are coagulated using the ball-ended electrode, and the base is then frozen using liquid nitrogen cryospray, extending the freezing to 1 or 2 mm beyond the edge of the wound.

Healing will then be a combination of the effects of radio-surgery and freezing.

42.13 INTRADERMAL NAEVI

Some of the most impressive results of radio-surgery are with the removal of intradermal naevi and other similar lesions. Because the amount of thermal damage is so slight, remarkable cosmetic results can be obtained (Figs 42.30–42.61).

A wire loop electrode is used, and this should be held at right-angles to the skin. A smooth, light action is required with no pressure.

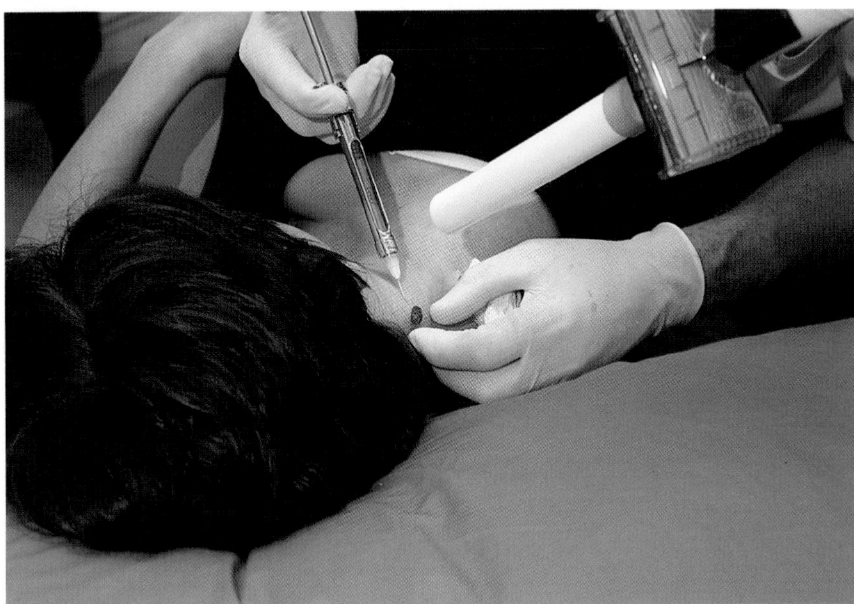

Fig. 42.30 Removal of pigmented naevus on neck. Stage 1: injection of the base with local anaesthetic.

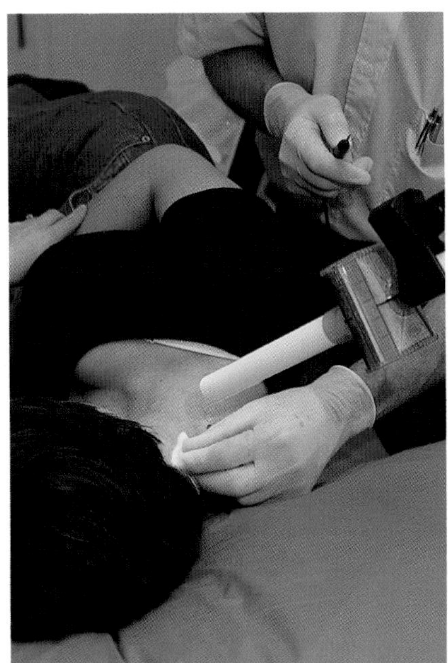

Fig. 42.31 Removal of pigmented naevus on neck. Stage 2: moistening the lesion with water or saline.

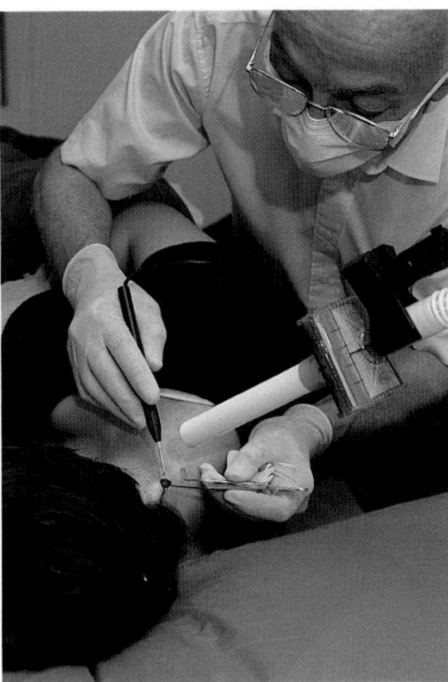

Fig. 42.32 Removal of pigmented naevus on neck. Stage 3: removing the lesion using a wire loop and forceps.

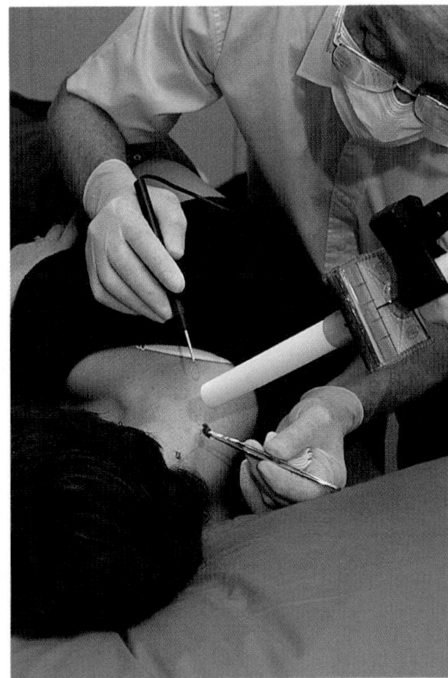

Fig. 42.33 Removal of pigmented naevus on neck. Stage 4: planing down the base flush with surrounding skin.

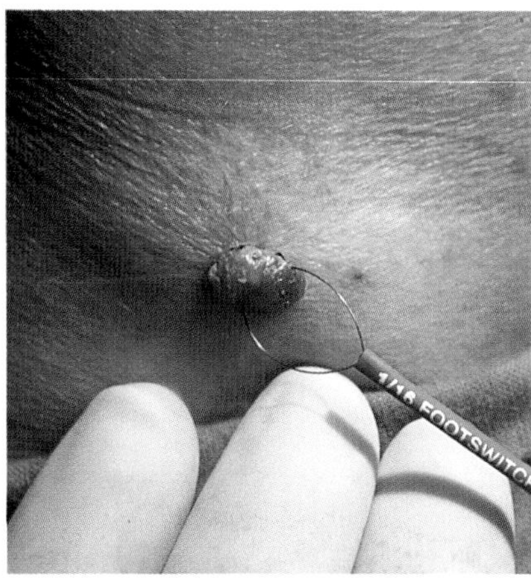

Fig. 42.34 Removal of pigmented naevus on neck. Stage 5: specimen ready to put in histology pot.

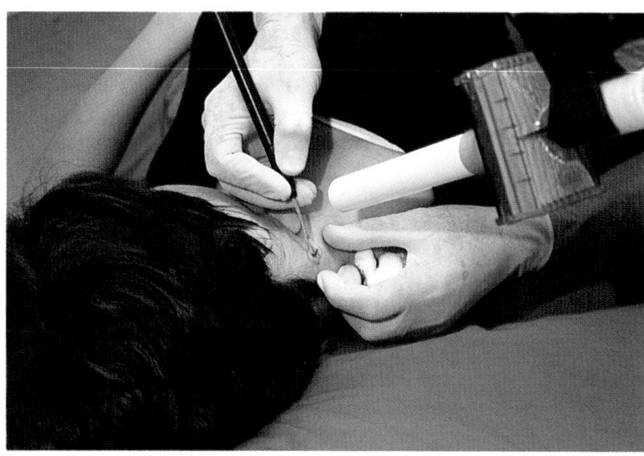

Fig. 42.35 Removal of intradermal naevus with the tungsten wire loop electrode.

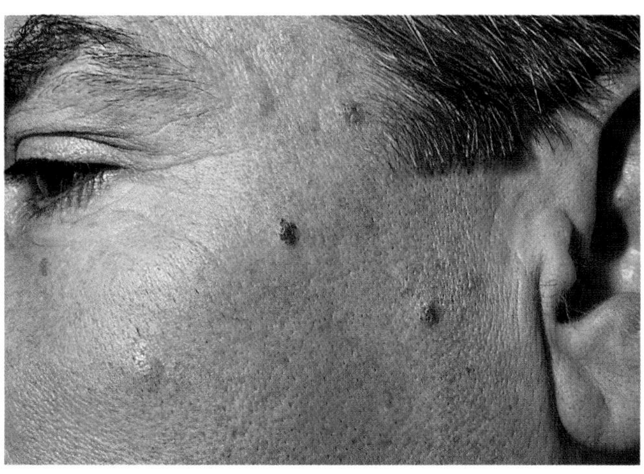

Fig. 42.36 Patient with multiple pigmented intradermal melanocytic naevi on face.

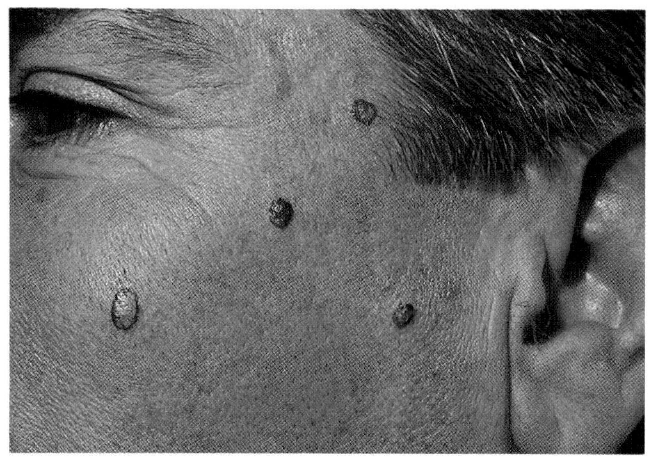

Fig. 42.37 Each naevus is marked with a pen.

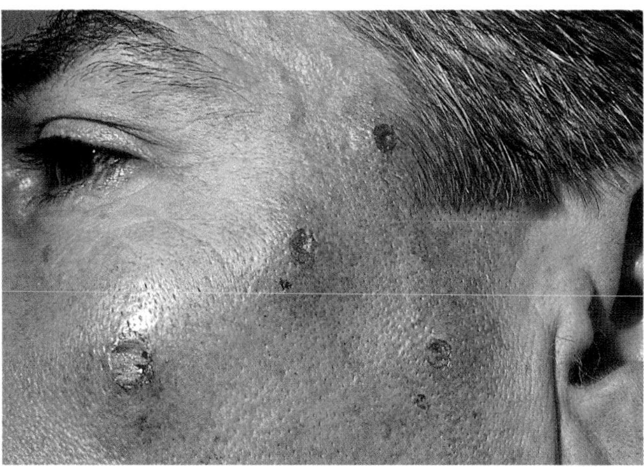

Fig. 42.38 Immediately after removal with the wire loop electrode.

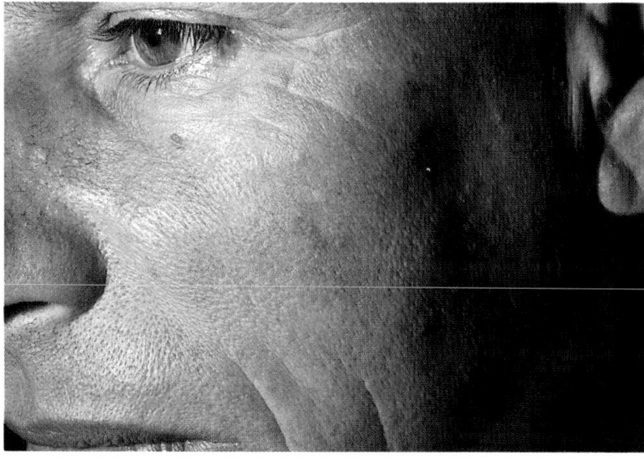

Fig. 42.39 Same patient 6 weeks later.

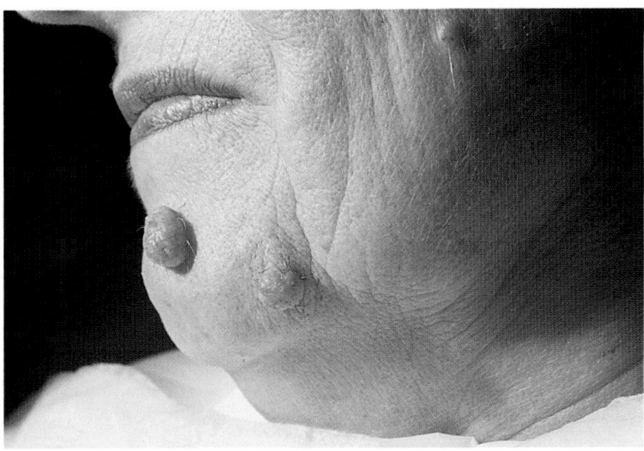

Fig. 42.40 Patient with fibroepithelial polyp on chin and two intradermal naevi on face.

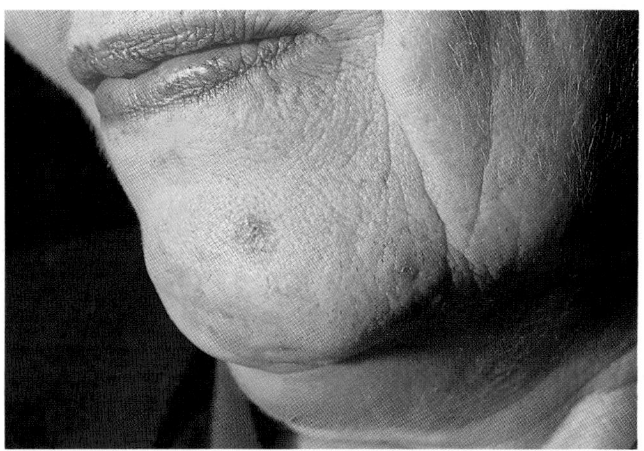

Fig. 42.41 Same patient 6 weeks later.

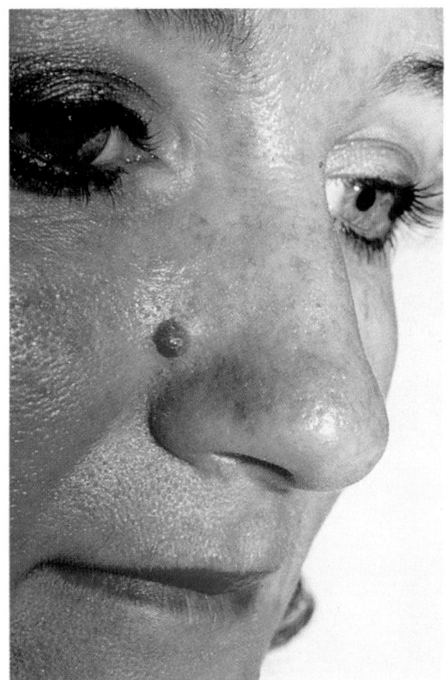

Fig. 42.42 A common site for intradermal naevus (photograph by courtesy of Dr Sheldon Pollack).

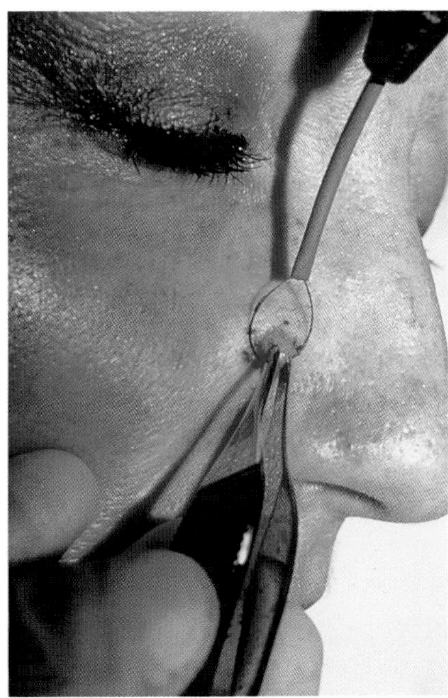

Fig. 42.43 Removal with the wire loop electrode (photo-graph by courtesy of Dr Sheldon Pollack).

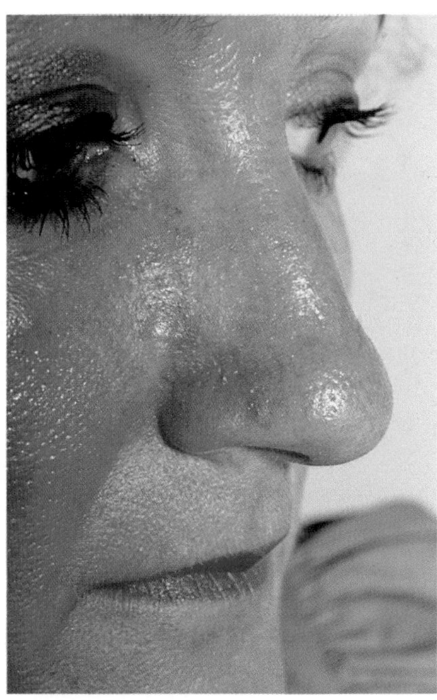

Fig. 42.44 Same patient 3 months later (photograph by courtesy of Dr Sheldon Pollack).

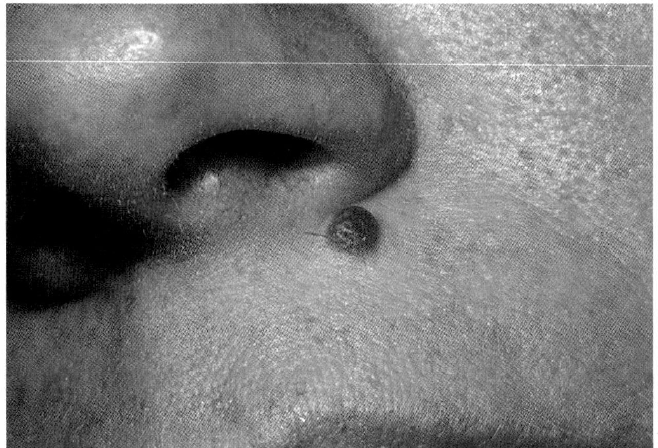

Fig. 42.45 Pigmented melanocytic naevus on upper lip (photograph by courtesy of Dr Randolph Waldman).

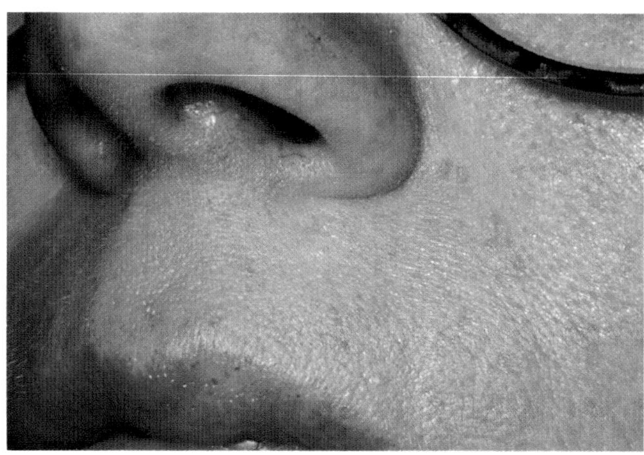

Fig. 42.46 Same patient 3 months later (photograph by courtesy of Dr Randolph Waldman).

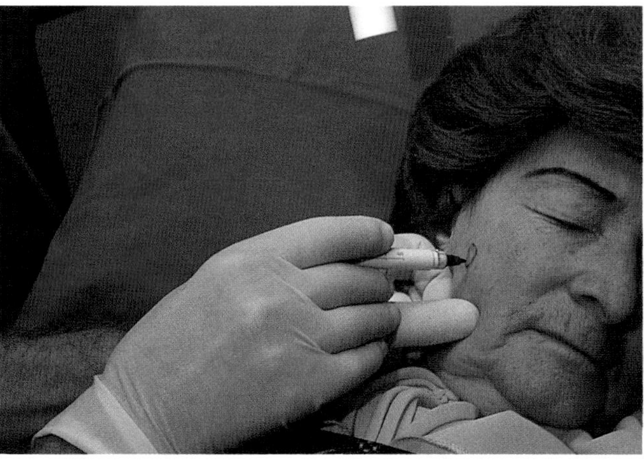

Fig. 42.47 Patient with actinic keratosis on right of face; marking with a skin pen.

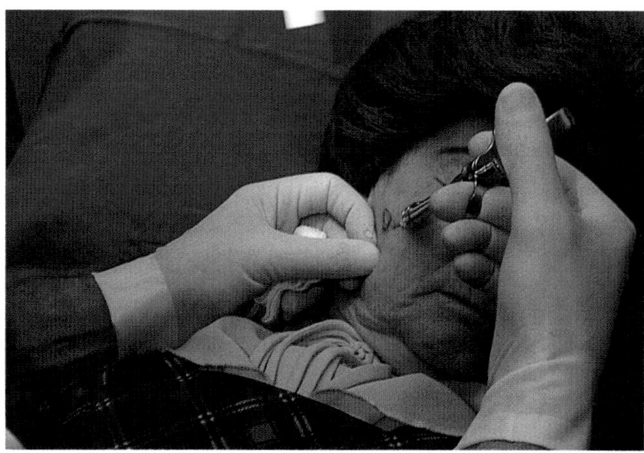

Fig. 42.48 Same patient – infiltrating the base with local anaesthetic.

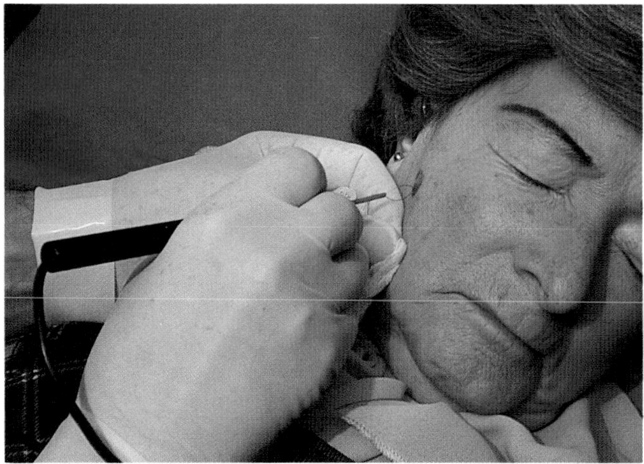

Fig. 42.49 Removal of keratosis with wire loop electrode.

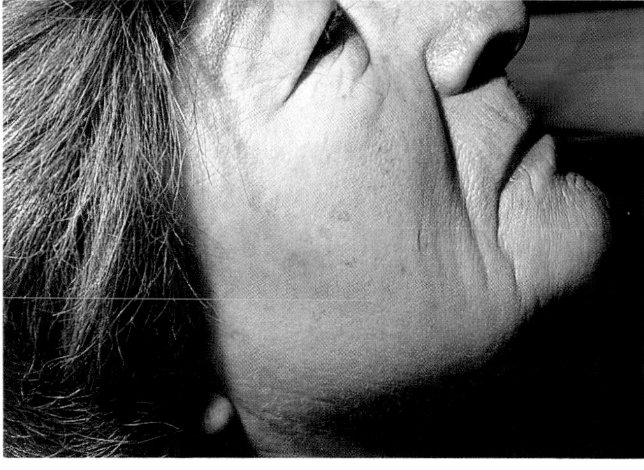

Fig. 42.50 Same patient 4 weeks later.

Fig. 42.51 Two darkly pigmented seborrhoeic warts on abdomen.

Fig. 42.52 Same patient immediately after removal with wire loop electrode.

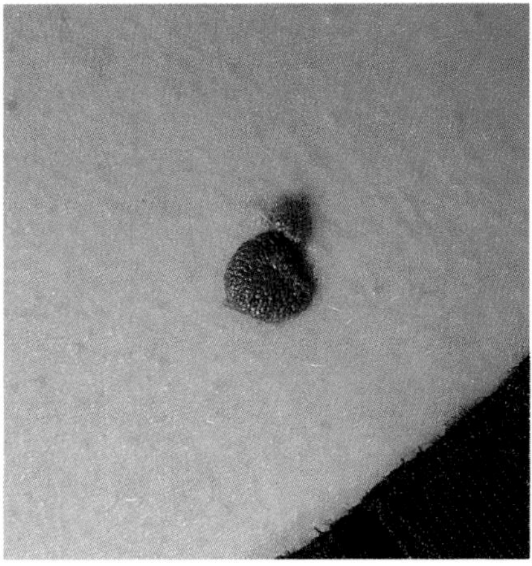

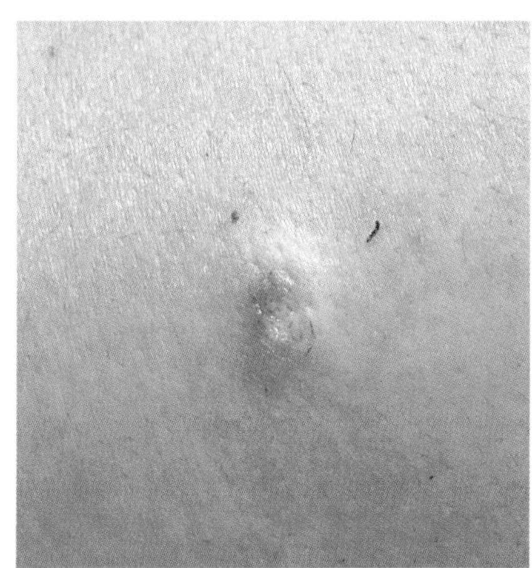

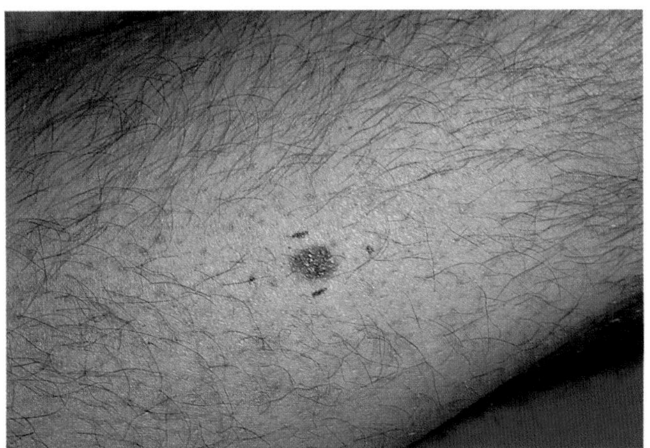

Fig. 42.53 Dysplastic naevus on right thigh – preliminary marking of margin to be excised.

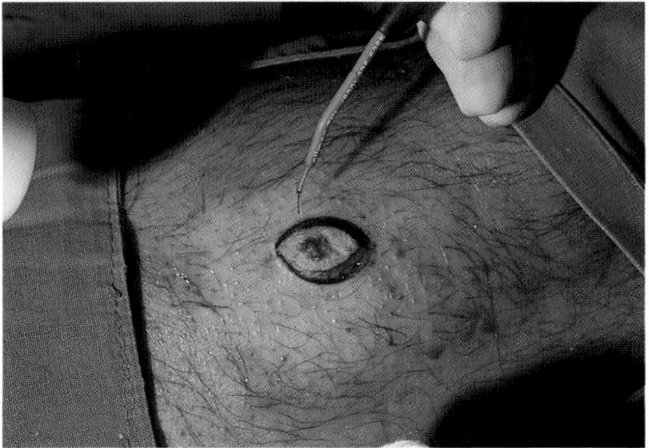

Fig. 42.54 Excising the lesion using the needle electrode – note absence of bleeding.

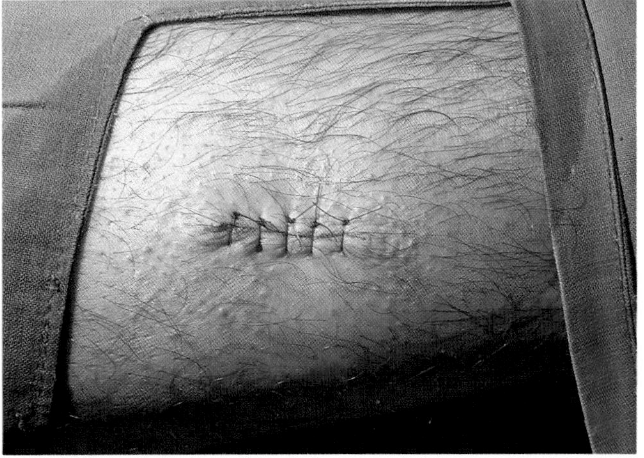

Fig. 42.55 Conventional suturing of wound after excision.

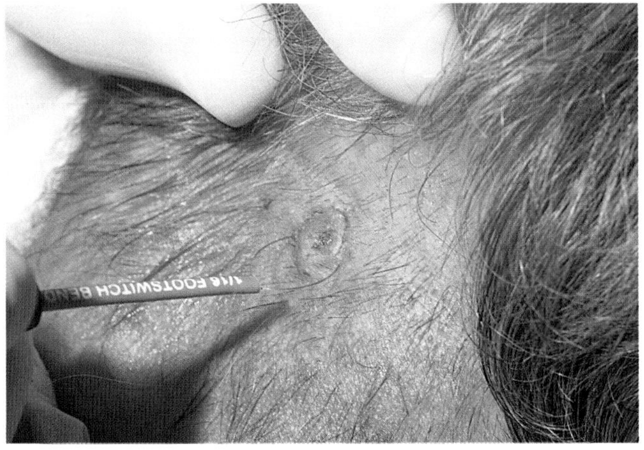

Fig. 42.56 Wire loop excision of seborrhoeic keratosis at back of neck – too much pressure being applied resulting in too deep a cut.

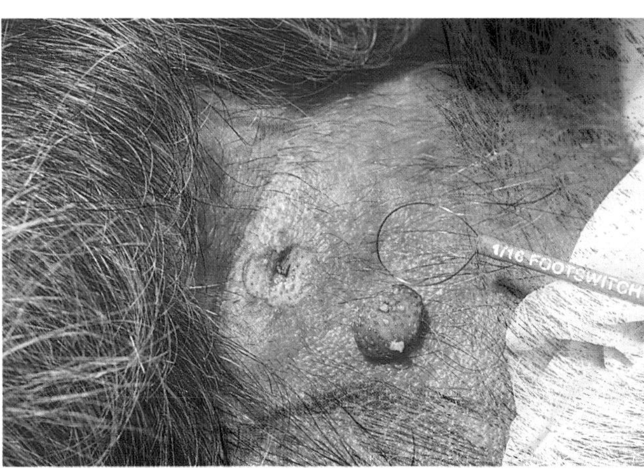

Fig. 42.57 Cut is too deep in this case – these lesions are very superficial and only need 'planing' off.

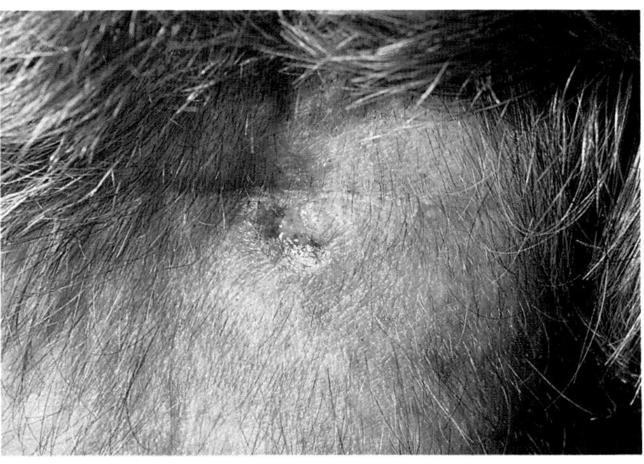

Fig. 42.58 Same patient 3 weeks later – the wound will heal eventually and be acceptable, but better results would have been obtained with a shallower cut.

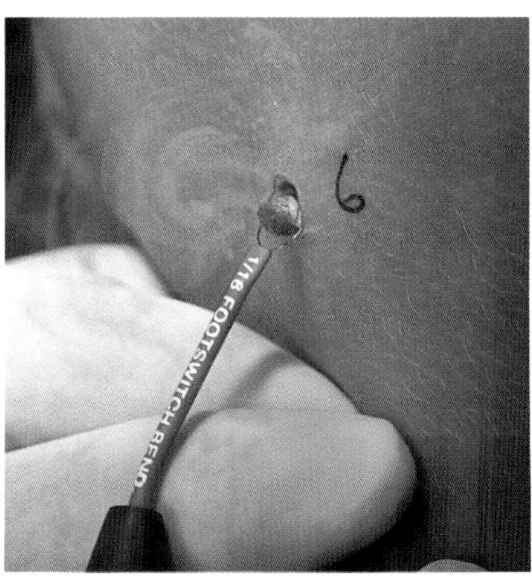

Fig. 42.59 Wire loop too small and cut too deep.

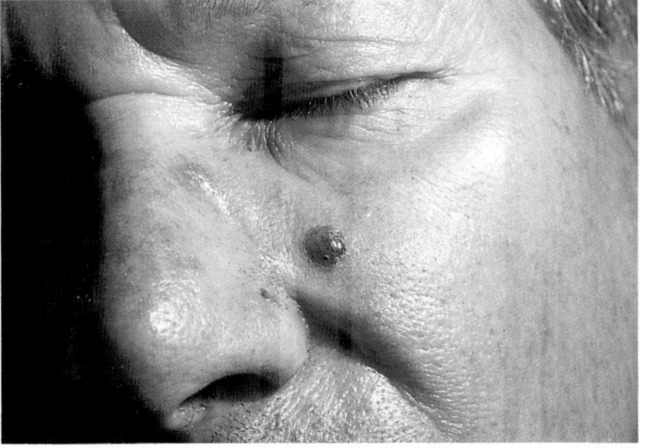

Fig. 42.60 Intradermal naevus on side of nose.

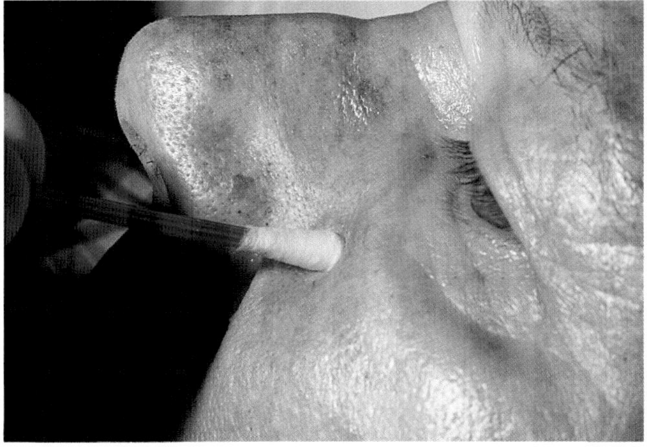

Fig. 42.61 Minor bleeding may be controlled by pressure from a swab soaked in 20% aluminium chloride or Monsell's solution.

42.13.1 Technique

1. Mark the edges of the naevus with a skin marker pen (Fig. 42.37).
2. Infiltrate beneath and around the base of the naevus with lignocaine using a 30 swg needle and dental syringe.
3. Position the antenna plate electrode near the lesion – skin contact is not necessary.
4. Switch on the unit and allow it to warm up.
5. Turn the power setting to '2' on 'cut' or 'cut and coagulate'.
6. Ensure your assistant has a histology pot available, with 10% formol saline in which to preserve the specimen, and also has the vacuum extractor ready for use.
7. Moisten the naevus with a small gauze swab soaked in water.
8. Holding the wire loop electrode at right-angles to the lesion, practise one or two strokes to ensure accuracy and avoidance of shakes or unwanted movements (Fig. 42.35).
9. Switch on the power using the foot switch or finger-tip control.
10. Pass the wire loop smoothly through the lesion (Fig. 42.35). If sticking occurs, increase the power; if sparking occurs, reduce the power.
11. Place the specimen in the histology pot and label.
12. Trim the remainder of the lesion using small smooth strokes, wiping any charred debris away from the base of the lesion with a moist gauze swab. Finally, 'feather' the edges to blend with adjacent skin (Fig. 42.24).
13. If any bleeding vessels are noticed, seal with the ball-ended electrode at setting 3 on 'coagulation' (partially rectified).
14. If mild oozing occurs, apply a cotton bud swab soaked in 20% aluminium chloride in spirit (Fig. 42.61). (Remember, this is inflammable so do not re-apply the electrode.)
15. Apply a small 'spot' plaster or leave exposed to the air.

42.13.2 Postoperative Care

Various regimes have been advocated for the postoperative management of lesions treated with radio-surgery. The aim is to prevent infection and to keep the area relatively moist to accelerate healing. Small lesions are probably best left exposed to the air and frequently washed with warm soapy water using cotton wool, taking care not to rub the surface too vigorously in case it causes bleeding from capillaries. Larger or deeper wounds are probably best covered with non-adherent dressing and antibiotic ointment, changing every other day or more frequently if there is much discharge. Any signs of spreading infection should be promptly treated with systemic antibiotics as well as topical antibiotics. A patient information sheet given at the end of the operation helps to remind the patient how to look after the wound (Chapter 50).

42.14 INGROWING TOE-NAILS (Figs 42.62–42.65)

Excellent results have been reported using radio-surgery to ablate the germinal epithelium, and cure rates in excess of 98% have been reported.

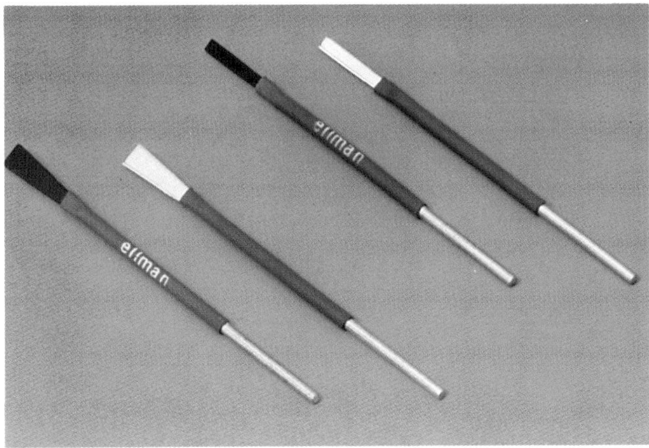

Fig. 42.62 Selection of electrodes for ingrowing toe-nails.

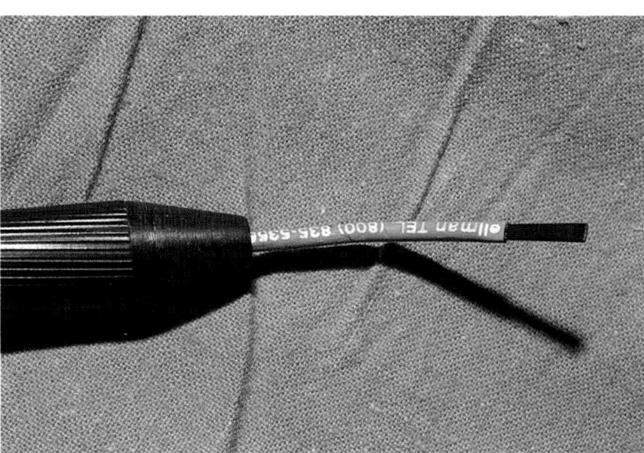

Fig. 42.63 The nail matrixectomy electrode.

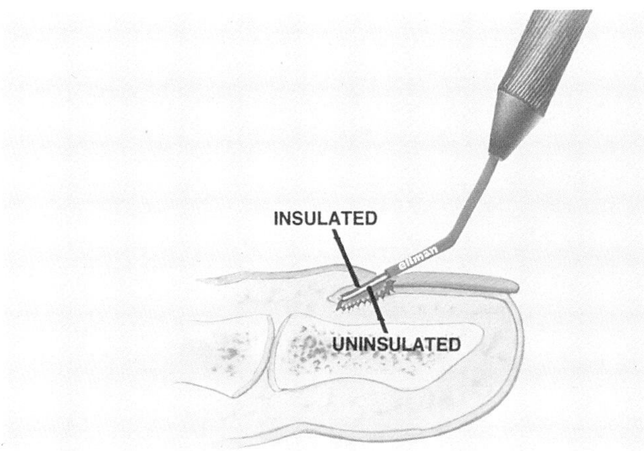

Fig. 42. 64 Diagram showing placement of electrode with insulated side uppermost beneath eponychium and metal side face downwards, in proximity but not pressing against the germinal epithelium.

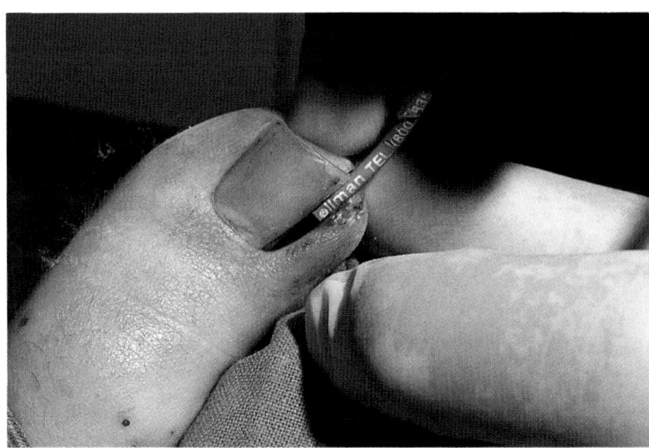

Fig. 42.65 The nail matrixectomy electrode in use.

The technique is basically identical to nail matrix phenolization (Chapter 30), but instead of destroying the germinal epithelium with phenol the matrix is destroyed electrically. This is achieved by using a specially designed matrixectomy electrode which is insulated on one side to protect the overlying eponychium (Fig. 42.62).

42.14.1 Technique

1. Some doctors prefer to use a tourniquet and a bloodless field, others prefer not to use a tourniquet. As the radio wave will coagulate any bleeding vessels, a tourniquet is certainly not essential.
2. A ring block of local anaesthetic is performed and the antenna plate is placed under the leg.
3. Using a pair of Thwaites nail nippers, stitch scissors, or a scalpel

blade, a thin strip of nail including the nail base on the affected side is removed.

4. Any granulations are removed with a sharp-spoon Volkmann curette.
5. The nail matrixectomy electrode is now inserted its full length so that the exposed part lies next to the germinal epithelium and the insulated part lies under the eponychium (Figs 42.63, 42.64, 42.65).
6. The power dial is set at '3' on 'partially rectified' (coagulation).
7. The current is applied for 2–4 seconds and the electrode is then slowly withdrawn over the next 5 seconds. Better results are obtained if the metal side of the electrode is raised slightly away from the nail matrix rather than pressing firmly against it.
8. Normally bleeding is not a problem.
9. A dressing of Bactigras or similar non-adherent material is applied, with or without triple antibiotic cream, depending on the degree of preoperative infection.
10. Where there is any significant preoperative infection, it is advisable to give the patient systemic antibiotics as well as topical applications.
11. The first postoperative dressing is done on the third day, and thereafter at approximately weekly intervals until fully healed.
12. The patient is seen again at 3 months to ensure that there has been no regrowth of nail.
13. Where there have been granulations and infection alongside the nail, some doctors spray these with liquid nitrogen followed by a strong steroid and antibiotic ointment and a final dressing.

42.15 RECURRENT 'SPICULES' OF NAIL

1. Occasionally a small 'spicule' of nail regrows despite what appeared to be a matrixectomy (Fig. 42.66). These can occur whatever the original method of matrix destruction.
2. A specially designed 'spicule' electrode is available to deal with this situation. It comprises a Teflon-insulated shaft and a small pointed

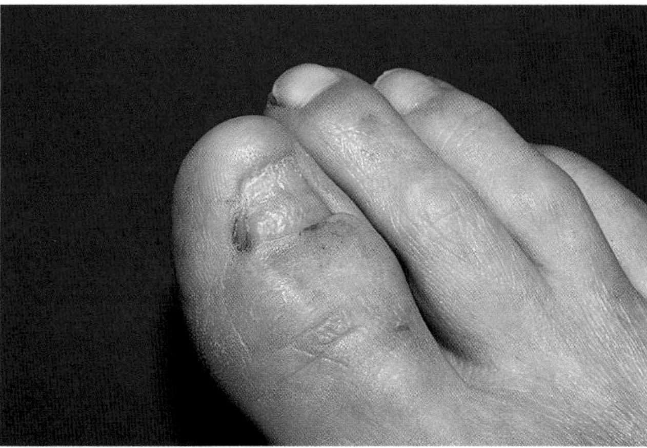

Fig. 42.66 Total nail-bed ablation with phenol 3 months previously – note a small spicule of nail regrowing at the edge.

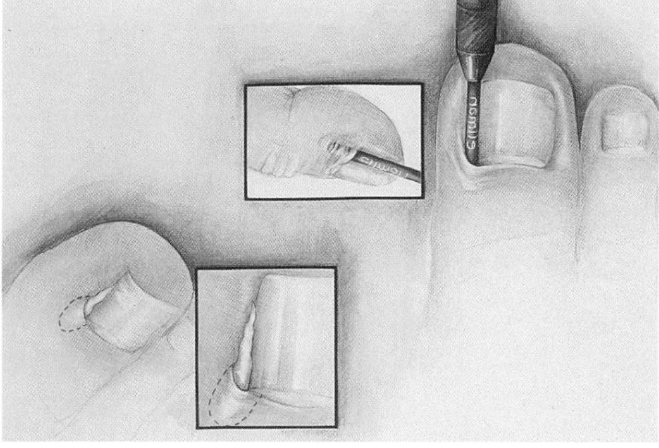

Fig. 42.67 Diagram showing use of nail spicule electrode.

metal electrode at the end (Fig. 42.67). After removing the spicule under local anaesthesia, the 'spicule' electrode is inserted under the eponychium down to the germinal epithelium, and the offending matrix destroyed using the partially rectified (coagulation) current waveform at setting '2' for 5 seconds. To be absolutely sure of success, it is helpful to wait 15 seconds for the tissues to cool and then repeat the treatment.

3. Postoperative dressings are the same as for matrixectomy.

42.16 TELANGIECTASIA AND THREAD VEINS (Figs 42.68 and 42.69)

Spider naevi and thread veins can be obliterated very successfully using radio-surgery. The technique is both quick, simple and easy to learn, and gives excellent results.

42.16.1 Materials and method

1. The radio-surgical unit is set to partially rectified (coagulation).
2. The power setting is between 'low' and '1'.
3. A fine 30 swg needle is attached to the hand-piece and, if necessary, bent to an angle of 45 degrees. Alternatively, the specially designed insulated shaft needles may be used.
4. With the patient in a comfortable position, the foot switch is continuously depressed and each telangectasis is lightly touched or 'tapped' along its course (Fig. 42.69).
5. Any bleeding points can be treated with a cotton-wool bud soaked in 20% aluminium chloride in spirit (remember, this is inflammable) or Monsell's solution.
6. More than one treatment session may be required.
7. Thread veins are dealt with in the same manner.
8. Generally, facial telangiectasia respond better to radio-surgery than the thread veins found on the lower limbs.

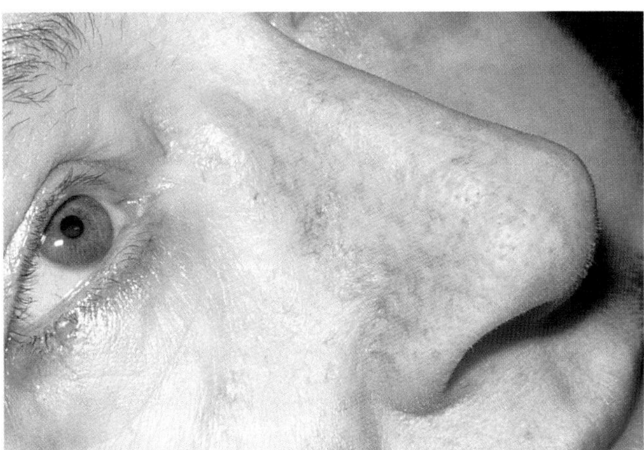

Fig. 42.68 Telangiectasis on side of nose (photograph courtesy of Dr Randolph Waldman).

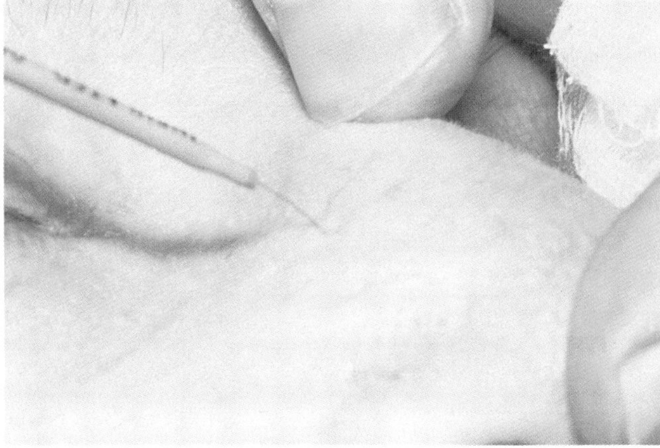

Fig. 42.69 Needle electrode being used to treat telangiectasis (photograph courtesy of Dr Randolph Waldman).

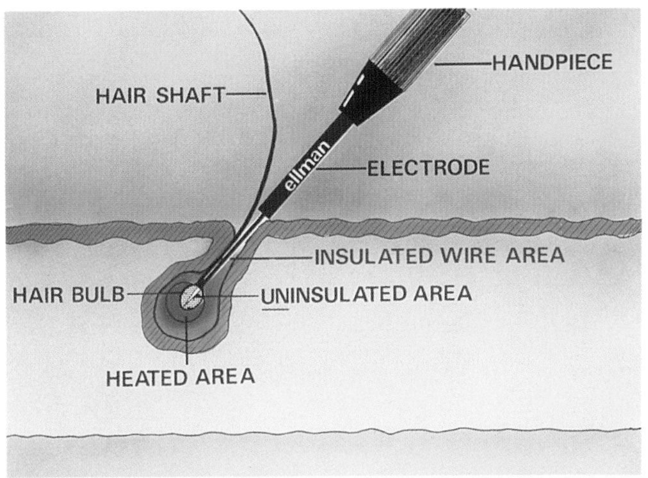

Fig. 42.70 Diagram showing insulated needle electrode for epilation.

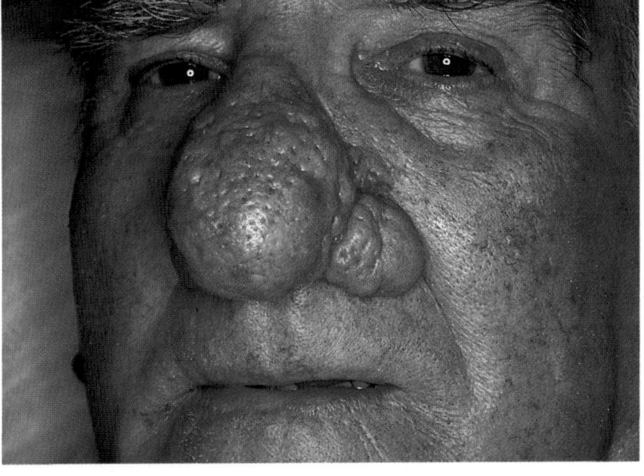

Fig. 42.71 Patient with rhinophyma suitable for treatment with radio-surgery.

42.17 EPILATION

Radio-surgery is very effective for epilation. Fine, insulated needle electrodes are best (Fig. 42.70). The needle is inserted to the hair root, parallel to the hair, and the waveform set to partially rectified (coagulation) lowest setting 0–1. Gentle traction on the hair will free it.

42.18 RHINOPHYMA

This distressing condition (Fig. 42.71) can now be very effectively treated using radio-surgery and the large wire loop electrode. Local infiltration anaesthesia may be employed, and successive layers of excess tissue planed off. Any troublesome bleeding vessels can be coagulated using the ball-ended electrode and partially rectified waveform. Following planing and coagulation, the raw area and adjacent margins may be treated with liquid nitrogen cryospray for 15–20 seconds.

42.19 XANTHELASMATA

These can be treated either by fulguration using a very fine spark, or by coagulation using the ball-ended electrode. Larger lesions can be planed off using the fully rectified (cut and coagulation) waveform and a wire loop. As they are very superficial, only minimal treatment is needed.

42.20 SEBORRHOEIC KERATOSES

These are generally very superficial and only light 'planing' is needed. The wire loop electrode at power setting 2–3 on fully rectified (cut and coagulation) gives very good results. It is important to keep the keratosis moistened during treatment. Some dermatologists also give the base a freeze with liquid nitrogen cryospray immediately after radio-surgery.

42.21 CERVICAL DYSPLASIA

For those doctors trained in colposcopy and the treatment of cervical intra-epithelial neoplasia (CIN), radio-surgery using the specially designed wire loop electrodes offers a very quick and efficient method of removing suspicious areas of cervix – the LLETZ technique (large loop excision of the transformation zone) or LEEP (loop electrosurgical excision procedure). A good vacuum extraction system is needed. Any troublesome bleeding can be controlled using the ball-ended electrode and partially rectified (coagulation) waveform. For full details of this technique the reader should refer to a textbook of gynaecology.

42.22 MISCELLANEOUS OTHER USES FOR RADIO-SURGERY

Radio-surgery is also widely used in dentistry, plastic and reconstructive surgery, ENT and ophthalmology, and is not covered in this book. The reader who wishes to learn these techniques is advised to refer to the relevant papers or textbooks.

43

Miscellaneous minor surgical procedures

To draw out splinters
Incence, Dough, Sea-salt, Wasp's Dung, Fat, Red-lead and Wax, Apply thereto: it draws the matter out

Ebers Papyrus, 1500 BC

43.1 SUBUNGUAL HAEMATOMA

This is extremely painful due to the pressure of trapped blood underneath the nail. Release of the blood results in an immediate relief of pain. One of the simplest methods is to rest the electrocautery V tip against the nail, switch on the current, and allow the wire to burn a small hole through the nail. As the nail itself is devoid of any nerve endings, the procedure is totally painless, provided undue pressure is not applied to the nail by the cautery. Once all the blood is released, the hole may be sealed with collodion or clear nail varnish, and allowed to grow out (Figs 43.1–43.5).

An even neater hole may be produced by using the cold-point electrocautery burner.

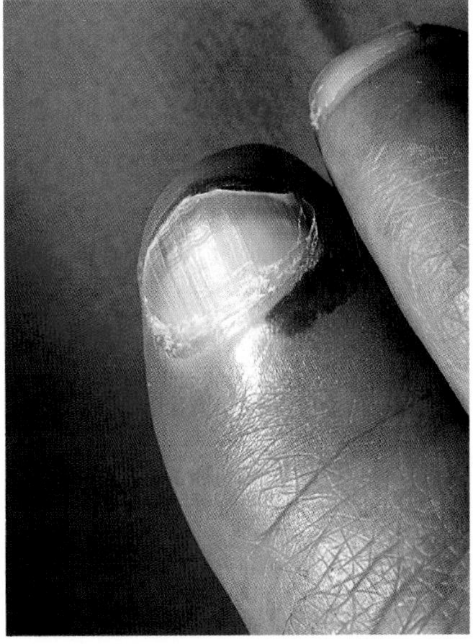

Fig. 43.1 Subungual haematoma.

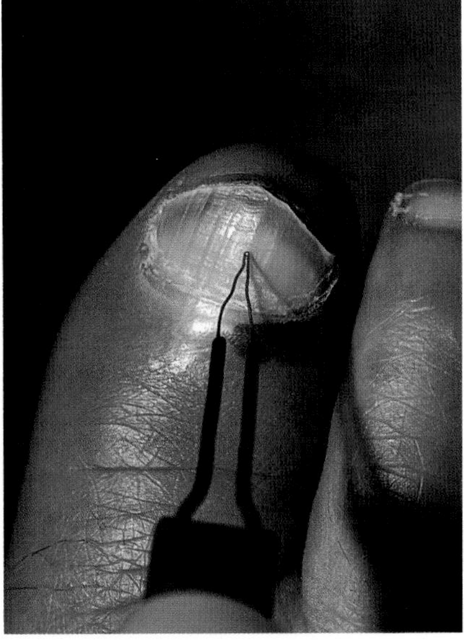

Fig. 43.2 Fine-point electrocautery burner is rested against the nail.

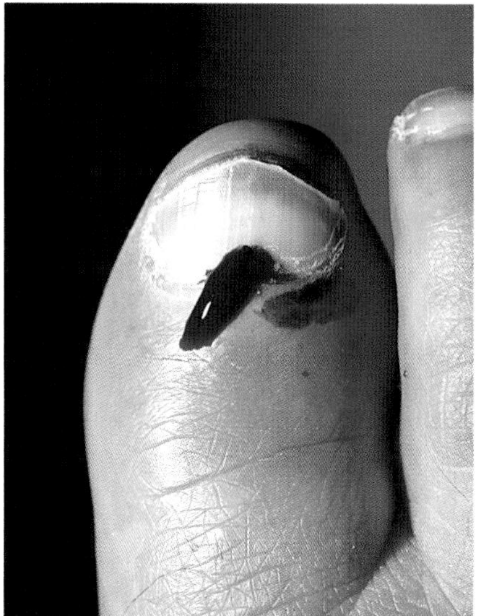

Fig. 43.3 No anaesthetic is required, and blood is released.

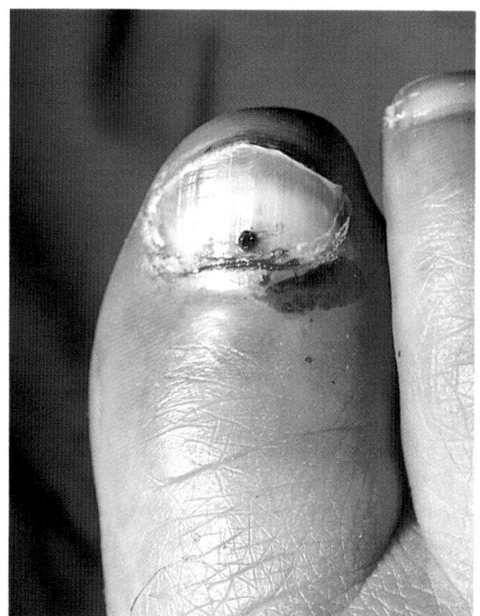

Fig. 43.4 Residual hole in nail is allowed to grow out. When dry, it may be sealed with clear nail varnish.

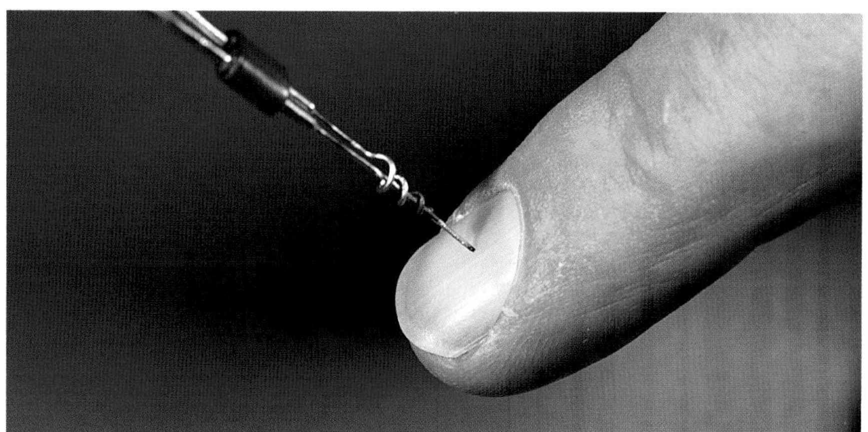

Fig. 43.5 An even neater hole may be made using a cold-point electrocautery burner.

43.2 REMOVAL OF SUBUNGUAL SPLINTERS

These can be extremely painful, as can any attempts at removal.

It may help to leave the splinter for 2 days, during which slight suppuration will occur, loosening the splinter and making subsequent removal easier.

Many splinters may be removed under Entonox analgesia: the patient takes 20 deep breaths of the gas, and most splinters may then be removed painlessly.

Alternatively the digit may be anaesthetized by performing a digital nerve or ring block with or without a rubber strip tourniquet. The splinter is then grasped with a pair of splinter forceps or straight Halstead's mosquito forceps and removed. Very deep embedded splinters may sometimes be removed by using a 21 swg (0.8 mm) needle which has had the point bent backwards to form a hooked barb.

43.3 SMALL SCALP LESIONS

Where a suture is judged inappropriate, small scalp lacerations can be closed by twisting a few hairs on either side of the wound and knotting them together over the centre of the laceration. To prevent the knots slipping undone, they should be sprayed with Tinct. Benz. Co., Whitehead's varnish, collodion, or Nobecutane. Thereafter the knot is left to grow out, or is cut out after 10 days. Alternatively the wound may be closed using a cyanoacrylic tissue adhesive (Histoacryl) (Chapter 11).

43.4 XANTHELASMATA

These may be treated with topical applications of monochloroacetic acid or pure liquefied phenol BPC. Great care is needed to avoid accidental burns to the eye or surrounding skin, and repeated small applications are preferred (Figs 43.6 and 43.7).

Other treatments include cauterization using the unipolar diathermy (Hyfrecator) electrocautery, or freezing with the cryoprobe, or infrared coagulation with a sapphire interface.

43.5 REMOVAL OF FOREIGN BODIES IN EARS AND NOSES

Young children frequently insert small pieces of rubber, paper, plastic, peas and nuts etc. in nostrils and ears. If not noticed at the time, the first symptom may be a unilateral, offensive, blood-stained discharge. Examination of the nose or ear with an auriscope reveals the cause, and the offending object may usually be removed with a pair of Tilley's aural forceps. Foreign bodies in ears may be difficult to grasp, and may be more conveniently syringed out using an ear-syringe and warm water. Steel ball-bearings may need a powerful ophthalmic electromagnet for removal.

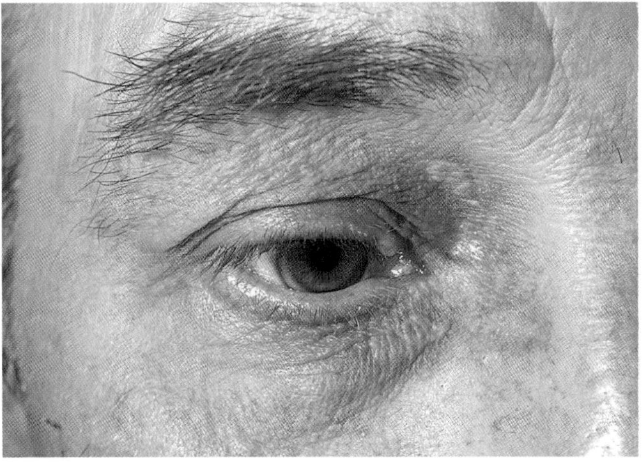

Fig. 43.6 Typical shallow xanthelasmata, suitable for careful treatment with monochloroacetic acid.

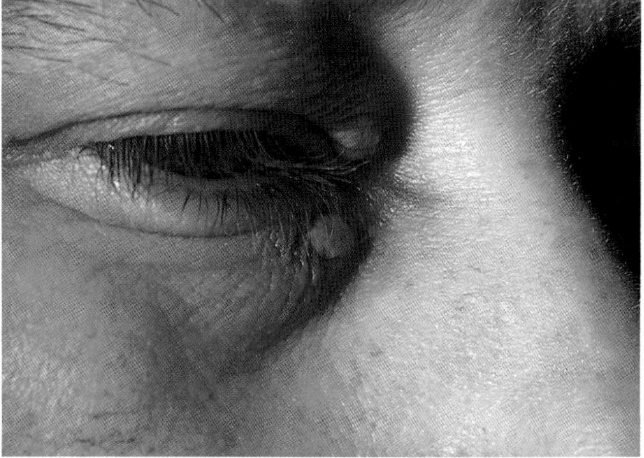

Fig. 43.7 More prominent xanthelasmata, also very near inner canthus of eye. Great care is needed if treatment is judged to be necessary.

43.6 STONE IN THE SALIVARY DUCT

Obstruction to a salivary gland by a calculus in the duct gives a classical picture of intermittent swelling of the gland whenever the patient attempts to eat. If the calculus can be felt with the examining finger, a small bleb of local anaesthetic is injected, and a suture placed deeply behind the stone, which serves to steady the duct and also prevents the stone slipping into the hilum of the gland. An incision in the long axis of the duct is made over the stone, which may then be easily lifted out. The suture is removed, and no further treatment is needed.

43.7 EAR-LOBE CYSTS

These are particularly common and troublesome, occurring more frequently in young male patients. Many of the cysts become infected and discharge spontaneously. Treatment consists of either dissecting the cyst free after infiltrating the area with local anaesthetic, or incising the cyst, expressing the contents, and cauterizing the lining of the cyst with a small cotton wool swab applicator soaked in pure liquefied phenol.

If the doctor possesses a pair of chalazion ring forceps, these are ideal for holding the ear-lobe and fixing the cyst. The introduction of fucidic acid gel into the cavity before closure enables healing by primary intention to occur.

43.8 HAEMANGIOMA OF THE LIP

These lesions are relatively common, and may be readily treated by electrocautery, diathermy, cryotherapy or photocoagulation. After preliminary infiltration with local anaesthetic, the needle of the Hyfrecator or electrocautery is inserted into the centre of the haemangioma; more than one treatment may be necessary to obtain a good cosmetic result (Figs 43.8–43.10).

43.9 SKIN GRAFTING

Small skin grafts may be performed in the general practitioner's surgery, usually to treat skin loss following accidents. Tips of fingers are the commonest site; if only a small piece of skin has been lost, grafting is unnecessary, but if the complete tip of the digit has been removed, a pinch-skin graft may be attempted.

A donor site is chosen, usually the thigh or arm, and after preliminary infiltration, the chosen piece of skin excised. This is then carefully sutured in place over the injured digit, a tulle-gras dressing applied, and a firm, dry sterile gauze dressing applied and left in place for at least a week.

43.10 NASAL POLYPI

These may be removed with a wire snare; often they are multiple, and are situated in inaccessible sites, but if the doctor is fortunate enough to see a solitary nasal polyp situated near the entrance, it can be snared off after

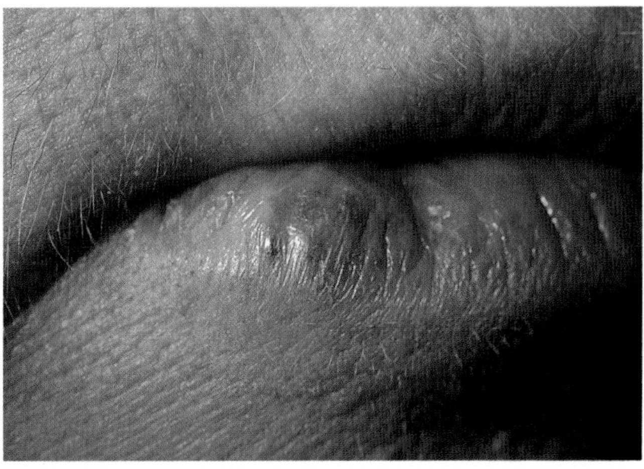

Fig. 43.8a Haemangioma on lower lip. Easily treated with electrocautery or Hyfrecator.

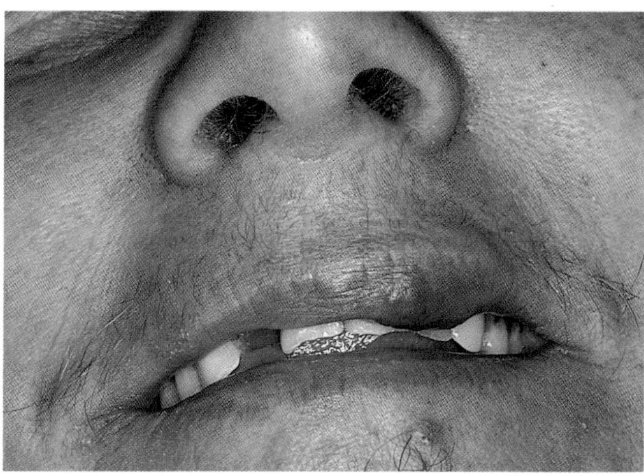

Fig. 43.8b Haemangioma on upper lip.

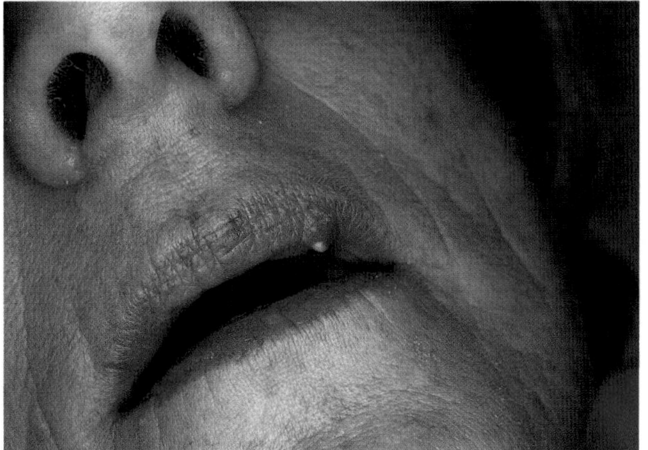

Fig. 43.9 Needle of Hyfrecator inserted in centre of haemangioma.

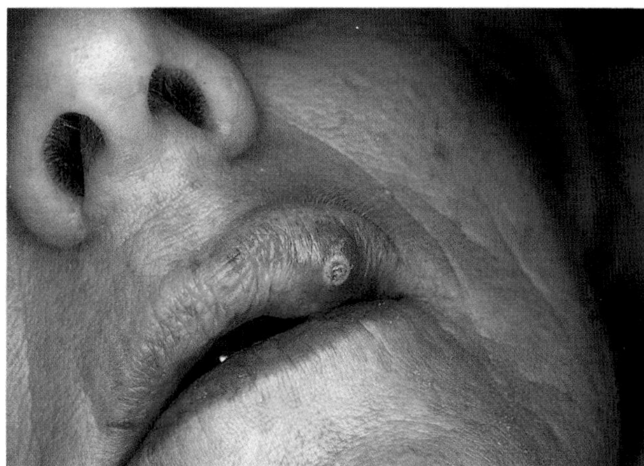

Fig. 43.10 Appearance immediately following fulguration with Hyfrecator.

preliminary topical local anaesthesia. Bleeding can be brisk, but usually stops spontaneously. Good illumination, preferably a spotlight and a head-mirror, is essential.

43.11 CONGENITAL EXTRA DIGITS

The majority of extra digits are inherited, and may be removed easily at birth either by tying a braided silk suture around the base, or preferably using the electrocautery (Figs 43.11–43.14).

43.12 ACCESSORY AURICLES

Accessory auricles or preauricular skin tags or polypi may be removed either by tying a braided silk suture around the base, or by excision and suturing, occasionally by the use of the electrocautery (Figs 43.15–43.18).

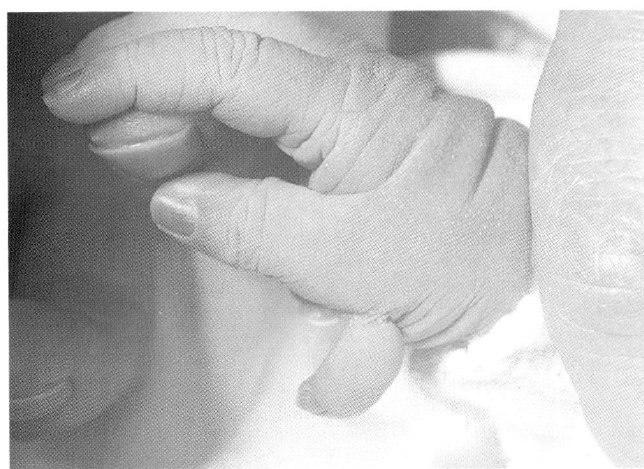

Fig. 43.11 Baby with extra 'thumb'.

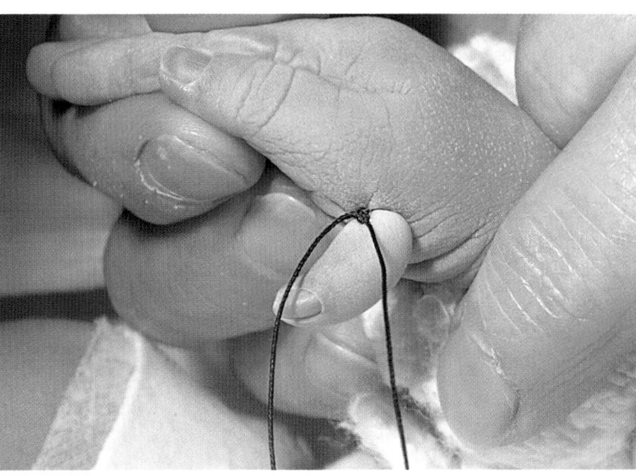

Fig. 43.12 Thread may be tied around the base, or alternatively the digit may be removed immediately with the electrocautery.

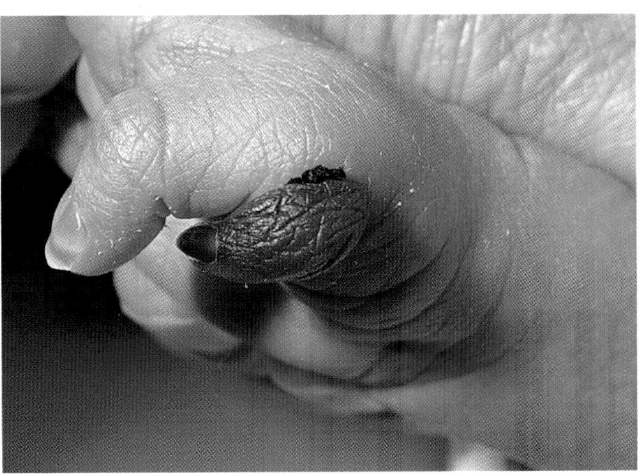

Fig. 43.13 After 2 weeks, the extra digit begins to separate.

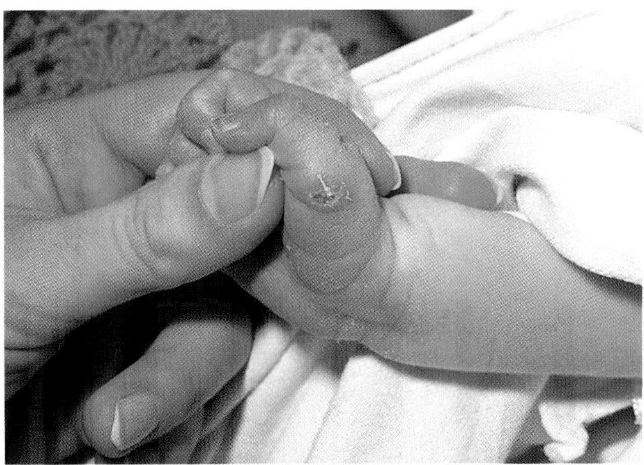

Fig. 43.14 The end result, 4 weeks later.

43.13 SUPERNUMERARY NIPPLES

Many patients suffer considerable embarrassment by the presence of supernumerary nipples but feel their problem is too trivial to consider treatment. Excision is simple, effective and quick, and may be performed under local infiltration anaesthesia (see Intradermal lesions, Chapter 22, and Incisions, Chapter 10), paying particular attention to the direction of the ultimate scar.

43.14 REMOVAL OF PACEMAKER

One prerequisite before cremation can be authorized is the removal of any cardiac pacemakers or implants, and the general practitioner may be asked to do this by the undertaker or relatives (Fig. 43.19).

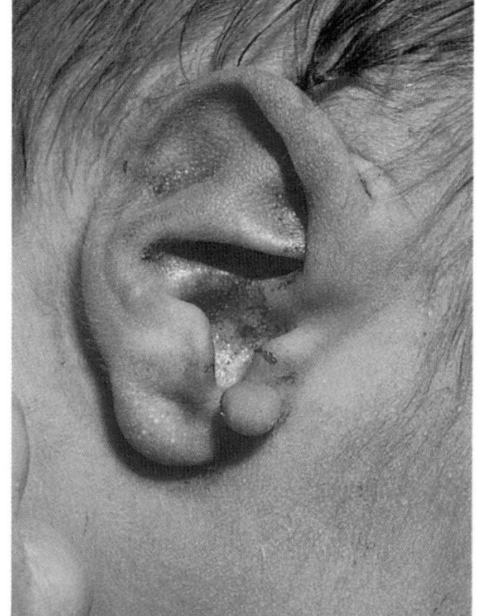

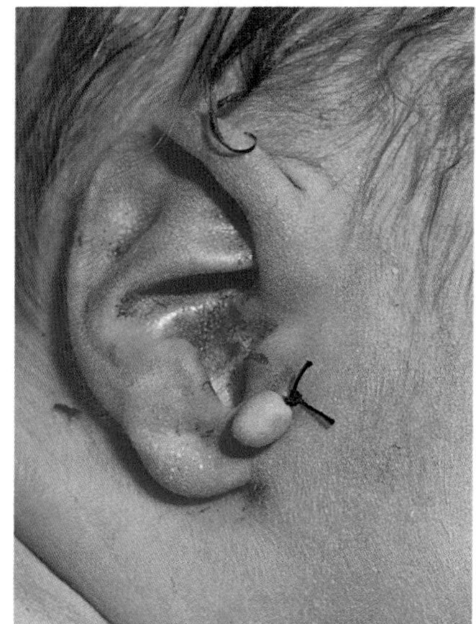

Fig. 43.15 An accessory auricle.

Fig. 43.16 Thread may be tied around the base, or alternatively the papilloma may be removed immediately with the electrocautery.

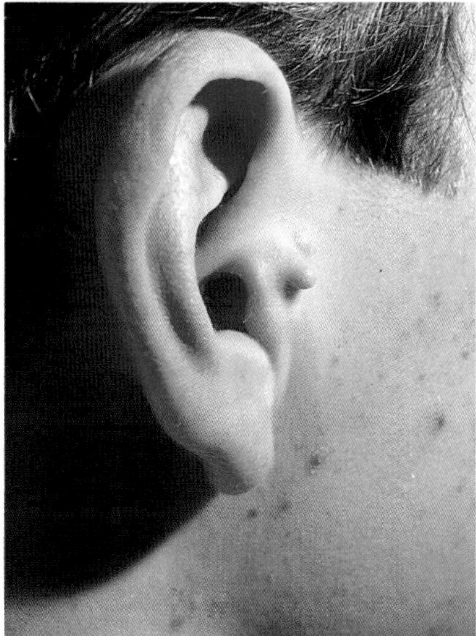

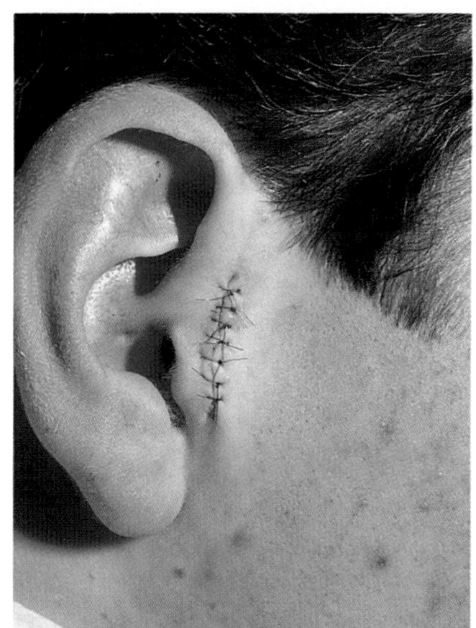

Fig. 43.17 Accessory auricle too broad to tie off.

Fig. 43.18 Accessory auricle excised under local anaesthetic.

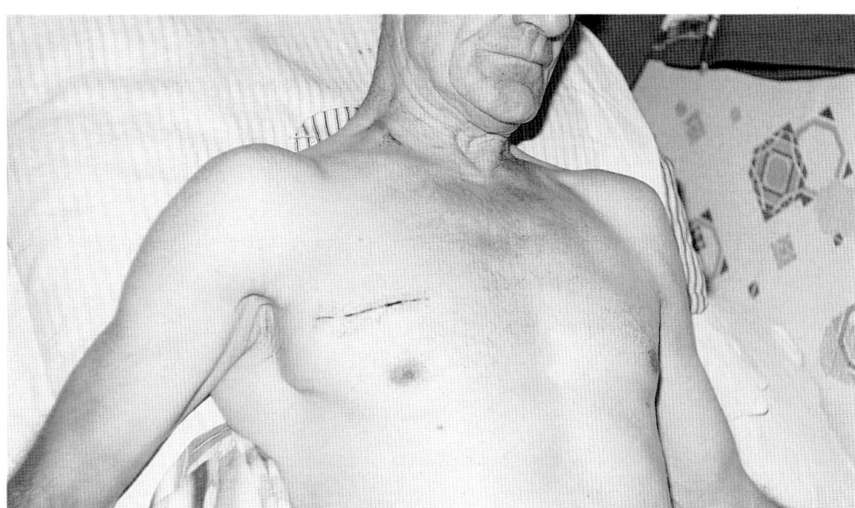

Fig. 43.19 Typical site for cardiac pacemaker.

A simple suture pack is all that is required (Chapter 2), an incision is made over the pacemaker which may be easily removed, together with the flexible wire electrode. The skin is then closed with interrupted sutures or adhesive tape.

43.15 FOREIGN BODY REMOVAL UTILIZING A BLOODLESS FIELD

The removal of small pieces of glass or metal can be extremely difficult if the operating field is covered with blood. Attempts to locate or remove such objects usually provoke further bleeding. It tends to be forgotten that a bloodless operating area can be obtained in any limb or digit by the use of a rubber tourniquet.

Any injection of local anaesthetic, either infiltration, digital nerve block or ring block should be given first and the injured site then covered with a dry dressing or small ring pad if fragments of glass are likely to be embedded. A rubber strip or Esmarch bandage may then be applied to exsanguinate the part, and a tourniquet applied. In the case of digits, this can be a thin rubber tube and artery forceps; limbs should have a pneumatic tourniquet applied. The absence of bleeding then enables the doctor to locate and remove any fragments of glass or metal more easily.

43.16 CIRCUMCISION

The majority of boys should have fully retractile foreskins by the age of 4 years. Where recurrent attacks of balanitis have occurred, or where there is a marked phimosis or paraphimosis, circumcision may be considered.

General anaesthesia is normally used, but where this is unavailable or contraindicated, local infiltration using 1% plain lignocaine may be used, forming a ring block around the base of the penis.

Having produced anaesthesia, the foreskin should be retracted fully if possible and the glans cleaned with a moist swab. Using fine, straight

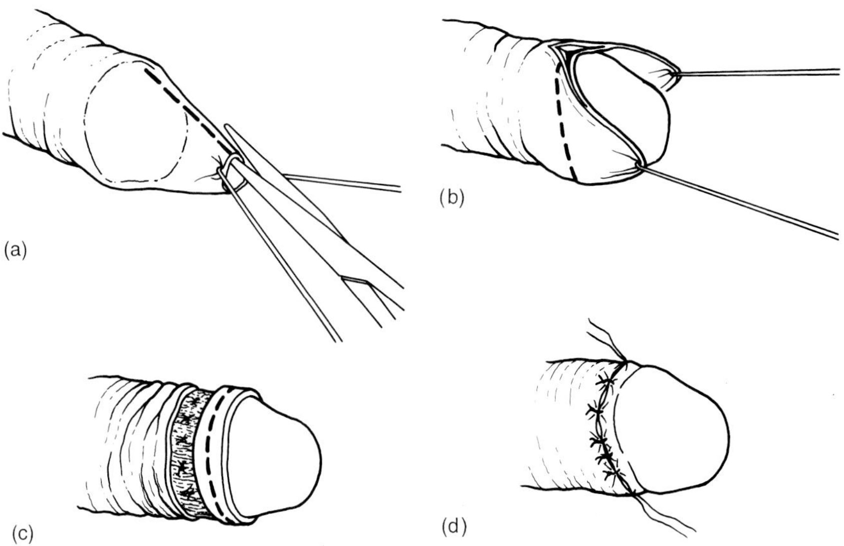

Fig. 43.20 Circumcision. Dissection method. (**a**) Dorsal slit. (**b**) The prepuce is trimmed parallel with the coronal sulcus. (**c**) All bleeding points are ligated, and the deep skin layer is trimmed. (**d**) Skin closure.

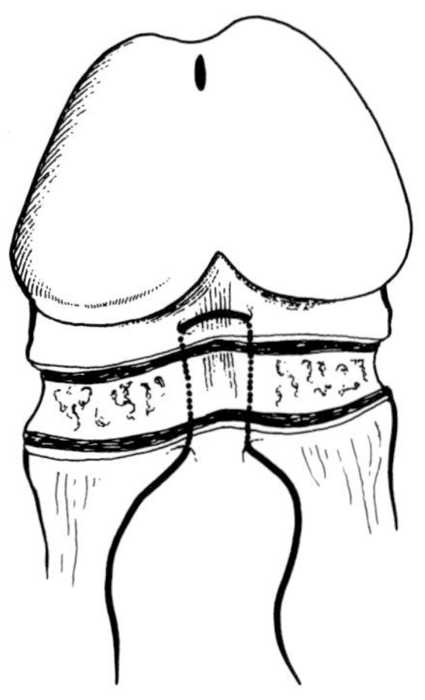

Fig. 43.21 The 'three-in-one' fraenal stitch.

mosquito forceps the tip of the foreskin is grasped, and dorsal and ventral midline cuts are made using straight scissors up to within 5mm of the coronal sulcus. Next, using curved scissors, the foreskin is trimmed parallel to the sulcus, also leaving a margin of 5 mm.

Any bleeding points can be secured using 4/0 catgut or Dexon, and the skin edges sutured using interrupted 4/0 Dexon or similar absorbable suture. Finally the stitch line is sprayed with Nobecutane spray or painted with tinct. benz. co. and a dry gauze swab applied (Fig. 43.20).

It is important not to damage the urethra, and unipolar diathermy is not recommended to control bleeding because of the risk of vascular thrombosis. It is also important to arrange postoperative supervision, to check regularly for any postoperative bleeding. This can arise from the fraenal artery, and may be picked up in a special three-in-one stitch (Fig. 43.21).

43.17 REMOVAL OF FISH-HOOKS

During the fishing season, a number of patients are always seen with fish-hooks embedded in various parts of their anatomy. Attempts by the patient to remove the hook usually fail due to the barb. If a pair of strong wire-cutters are available, the eye of the hook should be cut off, and then with a needle holder or artery forceps, the hook pushed through the skin and removed (Figs 43.22–43.24).

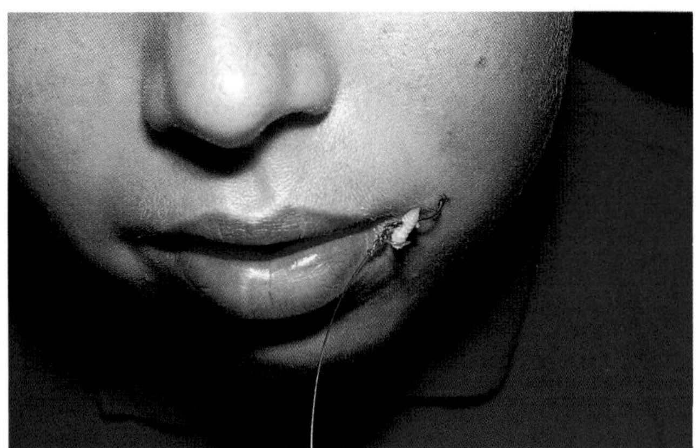

Fig. 43.22 A fish-hook embedded in the cheek, complete with maggot!

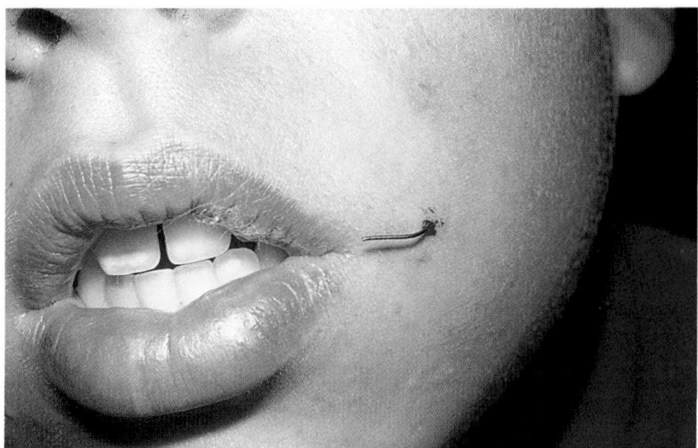

Fig. 43.23 One end of the hook is cut off with wire-cutters.

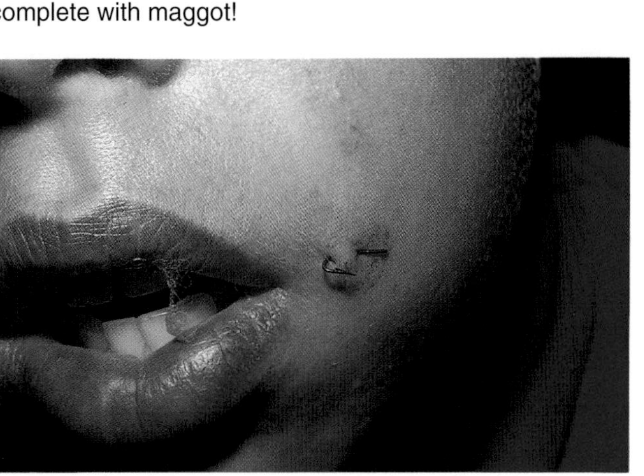

Fig. 43.24 The hook may now be pushed through, and removed.

43.18 PINCH-GRAFTS TO VARICOSE ULCERS

Every doctor and every nurse has one or two 'Heart-sink' patients with varicose ulcers which stubbornly fail to heal! Occasionally, in suitable patients, pinch-grafts will heal such ulcers and are well worth trying.

Before attempting grafting, the base of the ulcer should be clean, granulating, free from infection as much as possible, and fairly shallow. To this end Inadine non-stick dressing applied directly to the ulcer under gauze and pressure bandages, changed frequently if necessary, will ensure optimum grafting conditions.

The donor site is normally the upper outer thigh. An area is chosen and anaesthetized. This may be by infiltration, but a simple method of anaesthetizing the skin is by the use of Emla cream under waterproof occlusion. This is applied 2 hours before the grafting.

Pinch skin grafts are taken as follows. Using a 21 swg needle, a small

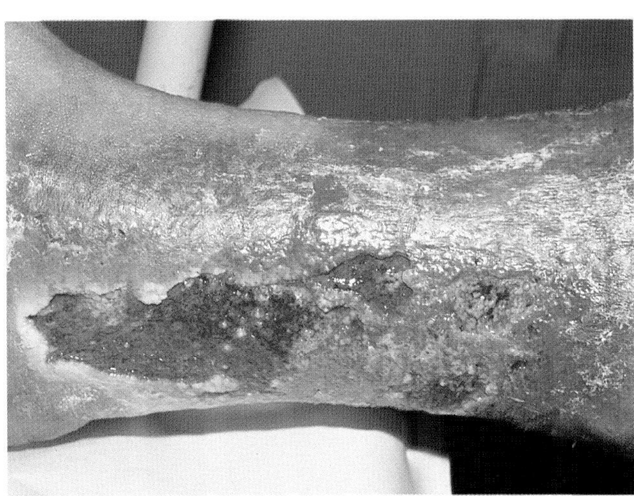

Fig. 43.25 Chronic, painful varicose ulcer defying attempts to heal it.

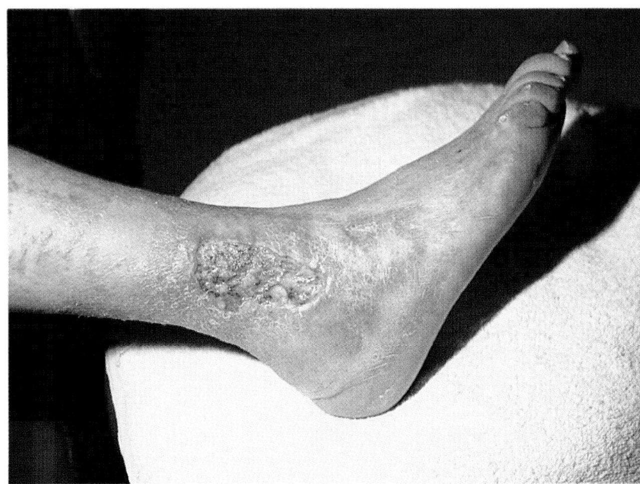

Fig. 43.26 Aim to clean the ulcer and encourage granulations in the base.

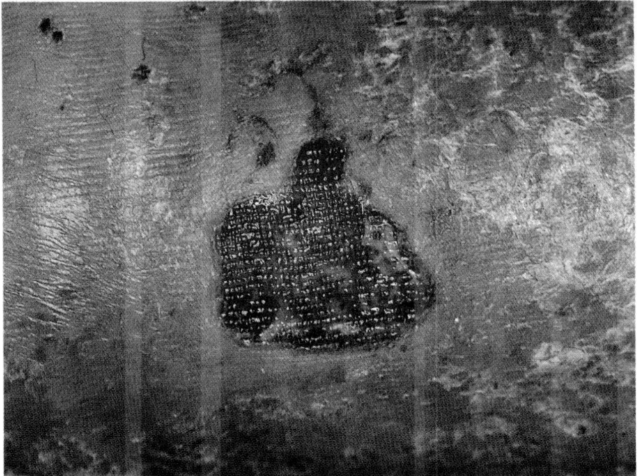

Fig. 43.27 The ulcer, treated with Inadine dressings, ready for pinch-skin grafting.

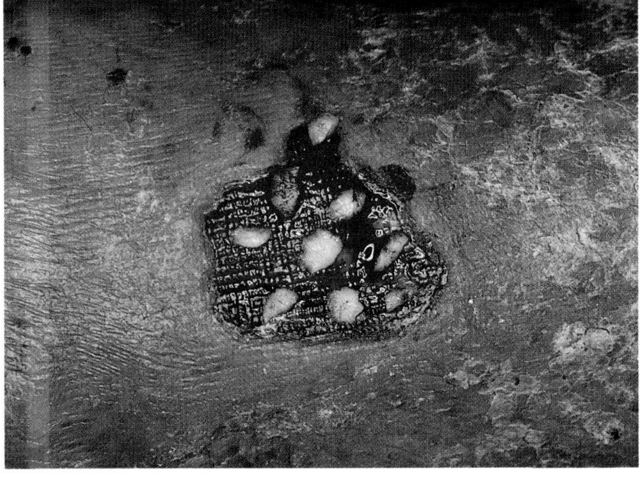

Fig. 43.28 Islands of skin taken from the thigh are laid evenly over the ulcer.

piece of skin is picked up and cut off using a scalpel. This is then laid on the ulcer. Similar 'islands' of skin are prepared, until the ulcer is covered with small pieces of skin, spaced about 5 mm apart or less (Figs 43.25–43.28).

A dressing of Inadine (povidone-iodine in non-stick base) is carefully placed over the grafted area, taking care not to dislodge the grafts (Fig. 43.29).

A layer of sterile gamgee or multiple layers of gauze are then applied, covered by an elastocrepe bandage, which in turn is covered by an elasticated tubular bandage (Tubigrip E or F). The donor site (Fig. 43.30) is covered with a similar dressing.

The grafted area is now left undisturbed for up to 2 weeks: the absence of pain is a promising sign that epithelialization is occurring. After 2 weeks the dressing is changed, and another applied. When successful, the ulcer is found to be healed after 6 weeks (Fig. 43.31).

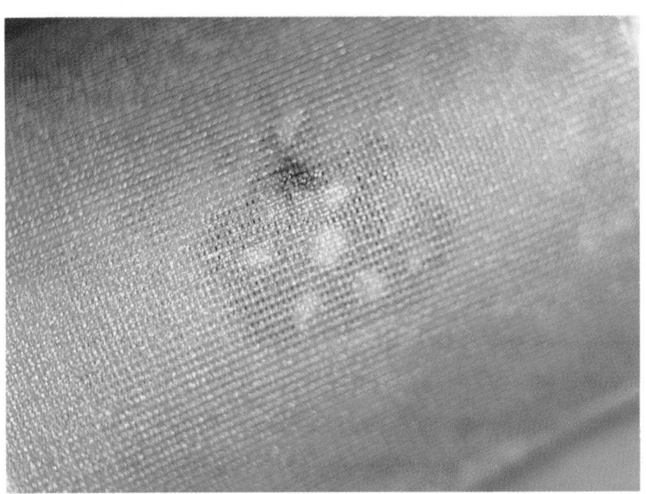

Fig. 43.29 These are covered with Inadine dressing and bandaged firmly in place.

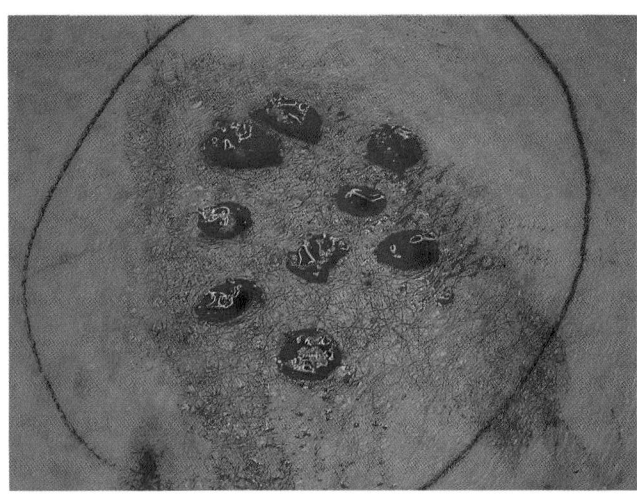

Fig. 43.30 The donor sites on the thigh. These are covered with a non-stick dressing.

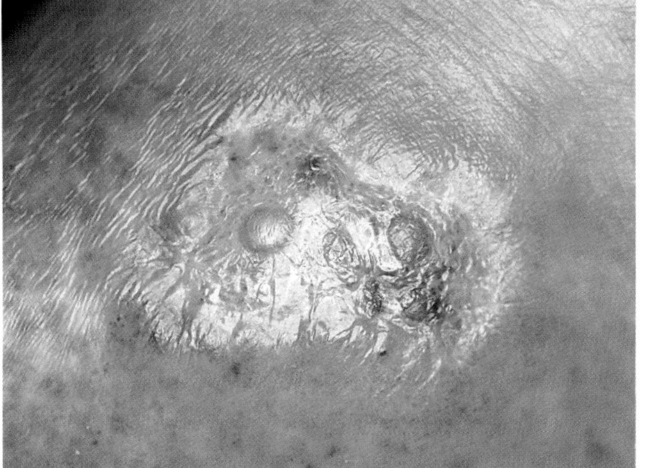

Fig. 43.31 The healed ulcer, 6 weeks later. (Remained healed for 2 years, then small recurrence.)

43.19 SPIDER NAEVI

These vascular lesions are quite common in children and young adults. They may be solitary or multiple and are due to a cutaneous arteriole feeding a leash of fine blood vessels radiating from the centre.

Treatment consists of sealing the feeding arteriole. This may most conveniently be done by the use of the cold-point electrocautery.

The needle of the cold-point burner is rested against the centre of the spider naevus, and gentle pressure applied. If correctly positioned, the naevus will blanch and disappear. By resting the needle against this arteriole and switching on the current, a localized burn in the skin occurs.

No anaesthetic is used, the procedure takes less than 1 second, and is extremely successful (Fig. 43.32, and Chapter 16). Radio-surgery ablation of the feeding arteriole is also very successful using a needle electrode and a low setting (Chapter 42).

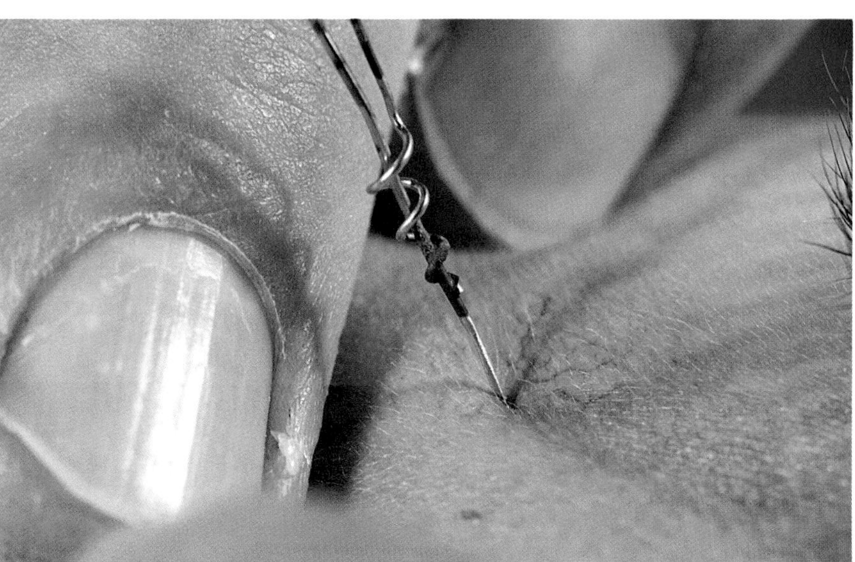

Fig. 43.32 Spider naevus being treated with cold-point electrocautery burner – no anaesthetic is used – the central arteriole blanches when pressure is gently applied.

In the absence of a cold-point burner, a conventional A-shaped platinum wire burner may be used, or the needle electrode of the Hyfrecator diathermy, or even by touching the centre with a sharpened wooden applicator dipped in monochloroacetic acid.

43.20 BIOPSY OF THE TEMPORAL ARTERY (Figs 43.33 and 43.34)

Polymyalgia rheumatica and temporal arteritis are relatively common in the elderly. Untreated, temporal arteritis may be followed by sudden loss of vision, which is permanent and occurs without warning. Systemic steroids give dramatic results, and prevent the onset of blindness.

The diagnosis is usually made on clinical findings plus a markedly raised sedimentation rate (ESR), but occasionally the diagnosis is not straightforward and it may be helpful to biopsy a branch of the superficial temporal artery. As these vessels lie above the deep fascia on the temporalis muscle, they are easily palpated.

Fig. 43.33 Temporal artery: anatomy.

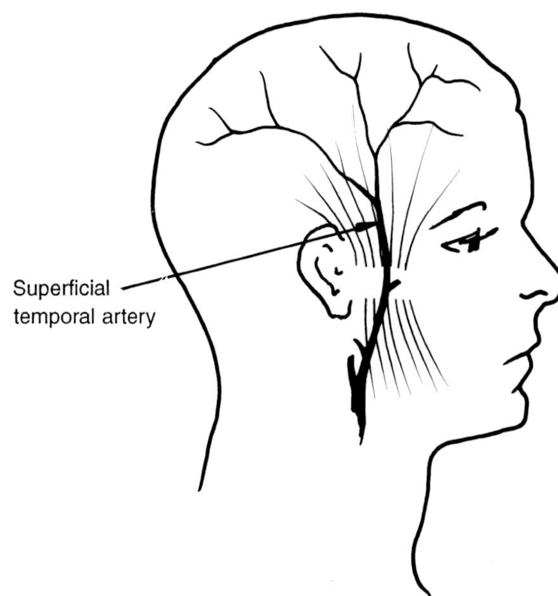

Fig. 43.34 Temporal artery: biopsy.

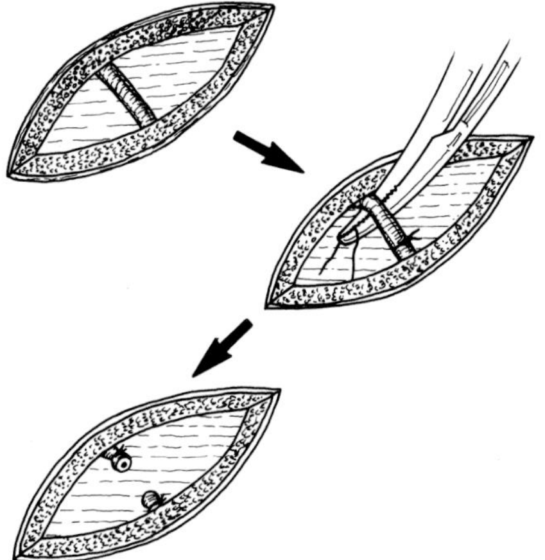

43.20.1 The operation

Any overlying hair is shaved, the area painted with povidone-iodine in spirit and infiltrated with 1% or 2% lignocaine with added adrenaline 1:80 000.

An incision is made over the artery, in a skin crease line. If possible the edge of the wound is retracted, either by an assistant or by using a small self-retaining retractor.

By blunt dissection using a pair of curved Halstead's mosquito forceps, the artery is freed, and two ligatures of 3/0 coated Vicryl applied, spaced 1.5 cm apart. The isolated segment of artery is carefully excised and placed immediately in a histology pot with 10% formol-saline.

The wound is then closed with interrupted 4/0 monofilament nylon sutures and sprayed with Nobecutane spray. No other dressing is required.

43.21 DIVISION OF TONGUE-TIE

Where a very tight fraenum is preventing the tongue from protruding to its full length, and particularly if it is thought to be interfering with the development of speech, it may be easily divided using the electrocautery or radio-surgical unit. Any bleeding points can normally be sealed with the cautery or coagulation tip of the radio-surgical electrode, and it is not normally necessary to suture the divided edges.

43.21.1 The operation

Fifteen minutes before the operation, the patient (usually a child) is asked to apply 4% topical lignocaine on a cotton-wool swab to the underneath part of the tongue, and to keep repeating the application to anaesthetize

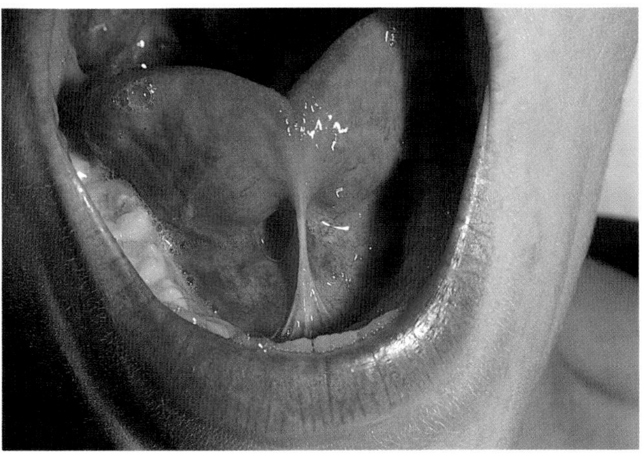

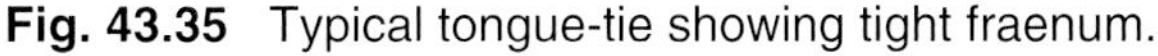

Fig. 43.35 Typical tongue-tie showing tight fraenum.

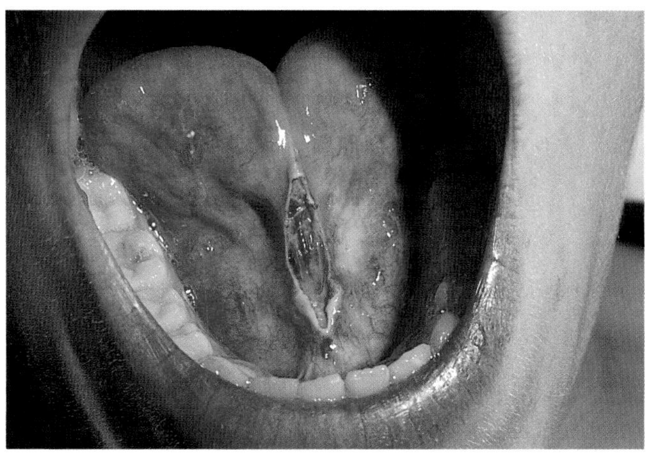

Fig. 43.36 Fraenum divided using either electrocautery or radiowave surgery.

the fraenum. Using a dental syringe and 30 swg needle, a small quantity (1 ml) of lignocaine is infiltrated into the area at either end of the fraenum to supplement the topical anaesthesia. Using a gauze swab, the tongue is held with the operator's left hand and drawn upwards to stretch the fraenum.

With the C28 cordless electrocautery and ring cutter electrode or radiosurgical unit and diamond wire loop electrode and cutting and coagulation waveform, the fraenum is now carefully divided. Any bleeding vessels are sealed using the ball-ended electrode (Figs 43.35 and 43.36).

Postoperatively, the patient is instructed to keep the mouth clean with frequent mouth rinses, and healing occurs rapidly over the next few days.

43.22 CHONDRODERMATITIS HELICIS CHRONICUS (Figs 43.37 and 43.38)

This is a common, painful nodule arising on the edge of the ear. The patient finds it is painful to lie on it when in bed.

Intralesional injection of triamcinolone using a dental syringe and a 30 swg needle sometimes effects a cure, as does careful use of liquid nitrogen cryosurgery.

Where these two methods fail, wedge excision and suture is the treatment of choice. Closure is with the finest monofilament Prolene sutures 6/0 or finer) which are removed after 7 days and the edges held together with skin adhesive strips for another 7 days.

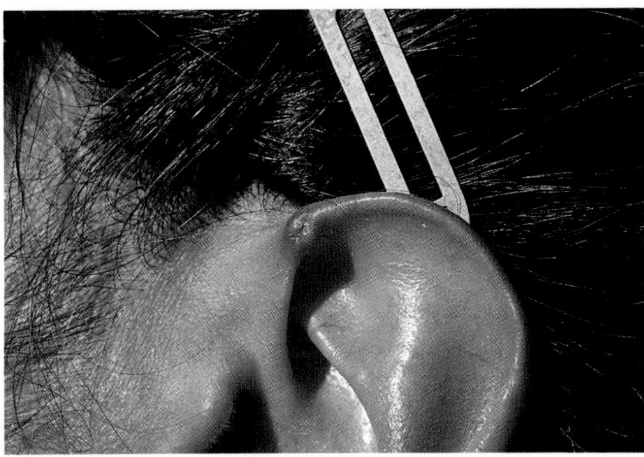

Fig. 43.37 A typical lesion of chondrodermatitis helicis chronicus.

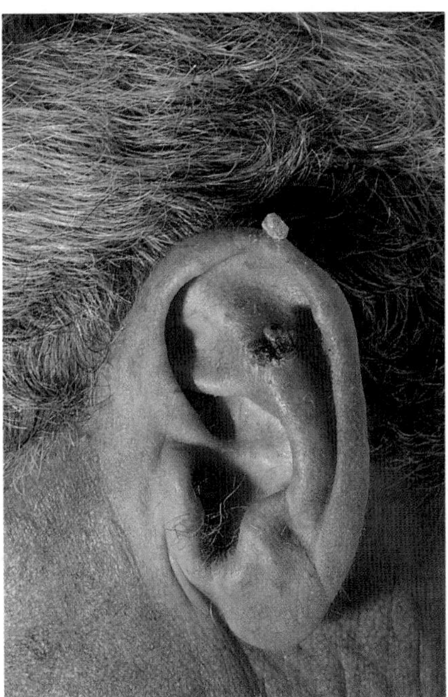

Fig. 43.38 This looks similar to chondrodermatitis helicis chronicus but turned out to be two areas of actinic keratosis, both of which cleared with liquid nitrogen spray.

44

Resuscitation

How is the surgeon transported, to discover motion returning to the lips and eyelids of a man apparently dead and when he perceives that the heart palpates and respiration is restored!

Dominique-Jean Larrey, 1766–1842

Every hospital and doctor's surgery should have facilities for giving emergency resuscitation for the 'collapsed' patient, and a basic knowledge of first aid and cardiopulmonary resuscitation is essential for members of the staff working in these premises.

The combined manual of first aid produced by the St John Ambulance Association, the St Andrew's Ambulance Association, and British Red Cross Society is excellent. A patient who has collapsed at the surgery may be suffering from any of the following:

1. A vasovagal attack (faint)
2. Profound vasovagal attack leading to a convulsion
3. Epileptic attack
4. Myocardial infarction
5. Allergic reaction to drugs administered
6. Anaphylactic reaction to drugs administered
7. Pulmonary embolism
8. Concealed haemorrhage
9. Cerebrovascular attack (stroke)
10. Acute psychiatric crisis
11. Cardiac arrest.

It is helpful to keep all resuscitation equipment together in one place, known to all members of the staff. The exact contents of any 'resuscitation kit' will vary depending on the preference of the doctors, but the following will provide a nucleus which can be supplemented with additional equipment if needed:

1. A selection of plastic airways
2. Endotracheal tubes
3. Laryngoscope
4. Intravenous cannulae
5. Giving sets for intravenous fluids
6. Oxygen cylinders and giving sets
7. Suction apparatus
8. Positive-pressure inflator (Ambu)
9. Sphygmomanometer
10. Electrocardiogram machine or monitor

11. Cardiac defibrillator
12. Large selection syringes and needles
13. Emergency drugs, intravenous fluids and plasma expanders.

44.1 THE VASOVAGAL ATTACK

This is undoubtedly the commonest cause of 'collapse' seen by the doctor. The patient may complain of not feeling well, becomes pale, sweaty, anxious, with cold, clammy skin and a slow imperceptible pulse. The patient is usually sitting or standing at the time, and if left in this position, will lose consciousness due to cerebral ischaemia secondary to hypotension. It is a common accompaniment to injections or painful or unpleasant experiences and is usually self-limiting as consciousness returns as soon as the patient falls to the ground.

First aid treatment consists of laying the patient on the floor and elevating the lower limbs to increase the venous return to the heart, watching the airway at the same time. Recovery is normally rapid. Because vasovagal attacks can occur in the most unexpected patients it is a good rule always to insist that the patient lies on the couch or operating theatre table rather than be seated in a chair for any minor surgical procedure.

44.2 PROFOUND VASOVAGAL ATTACK LEADING TO CONVULSION

In this, the patient appears to faint, but then has a short epileptiform convulsion. Unlike a major epileptic fit, the patient recovers consciousness quickly and is able to resume his or her activities without any impairment. Treatment consists of laying the patient down and placing him or her in the recovery position. If the airway can be guarded, the patient may be placed on his or her back and the lower limbs elevated to hasten recovery of consciousness.

44.3 MAJOR EPILEPTIC CONVULSION

This may arise in a patient known to suffer from epilepsy, or may occur without any previous history of attacks. If a solitary fit occurs, the patient should be placed in the recovery position and the airway guarded. Should multiple fits occur (status epilepticus) intravenous diazepam should be given, and oxygen administered via a high-concentration mask.

44.4 MYOCARDIAL INFARCTION

A patient may suffer a myocardial infarction while in the doctor's surgery; immediate resuscitation may be life-saving. Nitrites and aspirin given immediately may reduce the severity of the infarction, oxygen should be given via a high-concentration face-mask, pain relieved by diamorphine or morphine, nausea by cyclizine, bradycardia by intravenous atropine. The early insertion of an intravenous cannula is valuable as it gives access to the circulation should subsequent collapse occur or should thrombolytic therapy be considered. Arrangements to transfer the patient to hospital should be made, and if possible electrocardiographic monitoring done, with cardiac defibrillation available should cardiac arrest occur.

44.5 ALLERGIC REACTION TO DRUGS ADMINISTERED

It is always wise to enquire from the patient whether he or she has any allergies or drug sensitivities, and beware of any interractions with drugs to be administered. Should a reaction occur, intravenous antihistamines and steroids should be administered; an intravenous cannula inserted, regular blood-pressure checks made, and any shock corrected.

44.6 ANAPHYLACTIC REACTION

These are extremely rare, but very frightening when they occur. Sudden circulatory collapse occurs. The patient should be immediately placed on the floor or a couch; legs elevated and adrenaline administered, together with intravenous steroids, antihistamines, and fluid replacement. Oxygen and ventilation may be necessary. Check the expiry date for adrenaline regularly.

44.7 PULMONARY EMBOLISM

This may be very difficult to diagnose outside hospital. First aid treatment consists of maintaining an airway, the administration of oxygen, the introduction of an intravenous cannula, and urgent admission to hospital.

44.8 CONCEALED HAEMORRHAGE

This may arise from a bleeding duodenal ulcer, ruptured ectopic pregnancy, or following trauma from a ruptured liver, kidneys, or spleen. The patient will be shocked, with a rising, rapid, feeble pulse, and falling blood pressure. First aid treatment aims to restore the blood volume by the insertion of an intravenous cannula and administration of plasma expanders after first taking blood for grouping and cross-matching.

44.9 CEREBROVASCULAR ATTACK

As with a myocardial infarction, any patient may suddenly develop a cerebrovascular attack while attending the doctor. The patient with a cerebral haemorrhage suddenly loses consciousness, may have localizing signs, and may die within 48 hours. The only first aid treatment is the maintenance of an adequate airway and oxygen if necessary, with transfer to hospital. Occlusion of a cerebral artery from thrombosis or embolus may respond initially to rebreathing via a polythene bag. In this, a large polythene bag is placed over the nose and mouth and the patient requested to rebreathe until they find it uncomfortable. This allows the carbon dioxide levels in the lung to rise – giving cerebral vasodilatation. Additionally, intravenous dexamethasone has been used to reduce intracranial oedema.

44.10 THE ACUTE PSYCHIATRIC CRISIS

This may manifest itself as hypomania, excitability, confusion, delusions, or violence. There is usually a preceding history of psychiatric disturbance. First aid treatment consists of reassurance, and if necessary intravenous chlorpromazine or diazepam.

44.11 CARDIAC ARREST (Figs 44.1–44.7)

This is the most serious of all 'collapses'. It may arise following a myocardial infarction, following fright, or spontaneously with no obvious cause. It is diagnosed by an unconscious patient with absent pulses, and irregular, infrequent respirations which eventually stop. Following this, the pupils become widely dilated and fixed.

44.11.1 First-aid treatment

If an ECG monitor is immediately available, and the cause is shown to be ventricular fibrillation, immediate cardiac defibrillation should be performed, giving a DC shock of up to 400 joules, repeating if necessary. Oxygen and endotracheal intubation should be instituted, together with the insertion of an intravenous cannula. Following successful defibrillation, intravenous lignocaine 100 mg and dexamethasone 5 mg should be given.

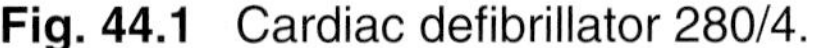

Fig. 44.1 Cardiac defibrillator 280/4.

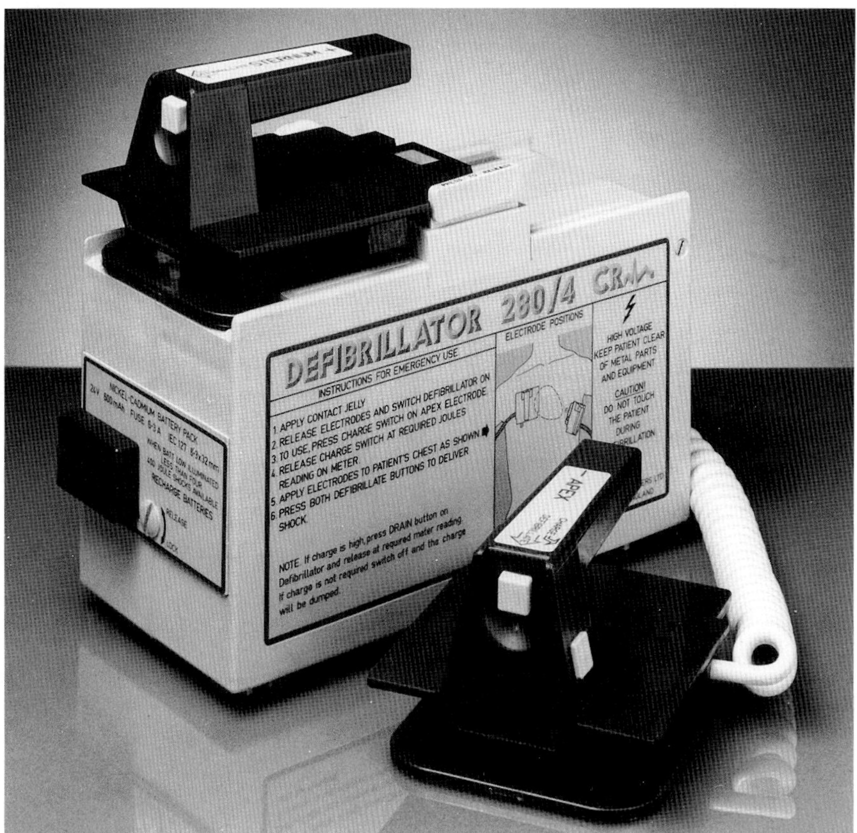

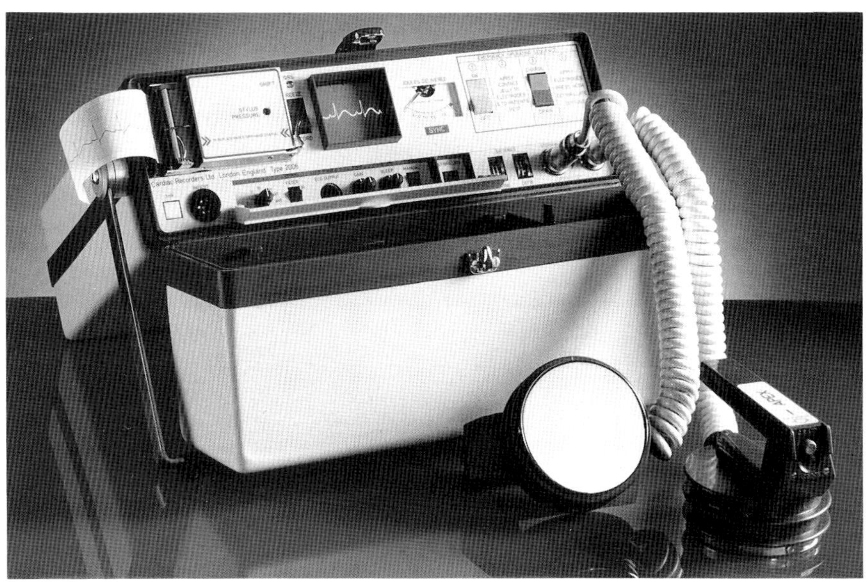

Fig. 44.2 Cardiac defibrillator monitor and ECG machine (Cardiac Recorders Type 2006).

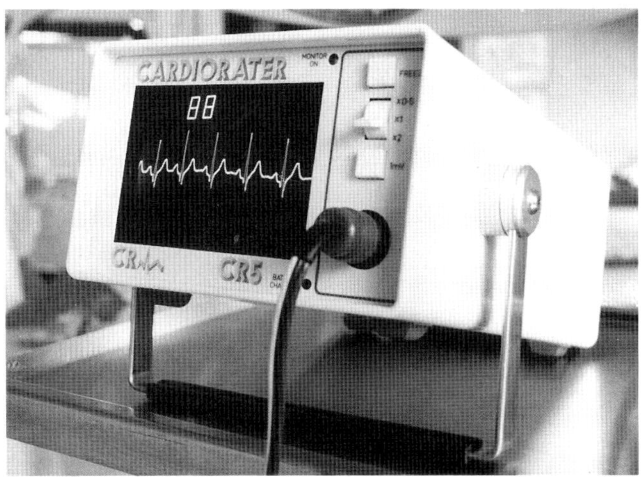

Fig. 44.3 The CR5 Cardiorater (Cardiac Recorders Ltd).

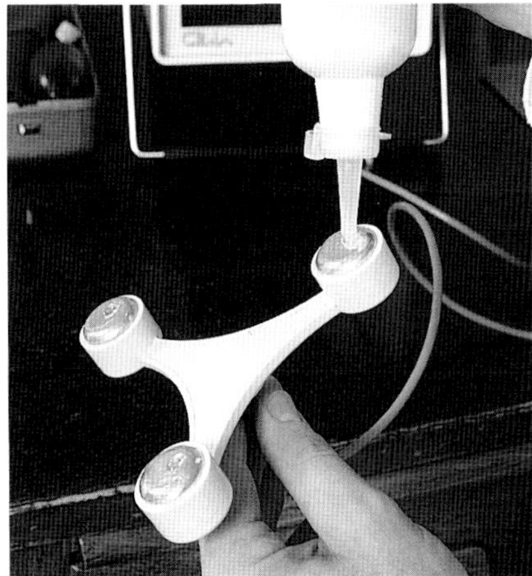

Fig. 44.4 A tripod chest electrode gives immediate tracings (Cardiac Recorders Ltd).

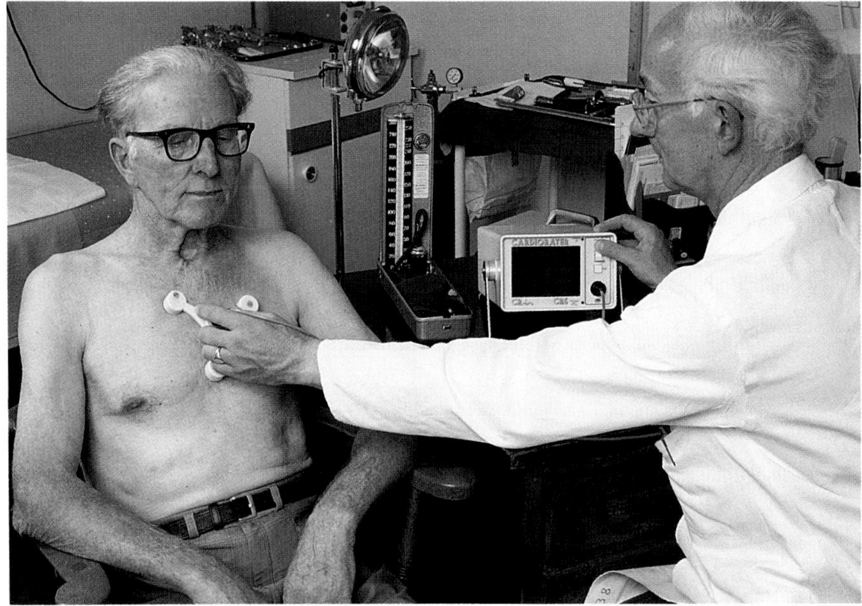

Fig. 44.5 The use of the tripod electrode with the CR5 cardiac monitor (Cardiac Recorders Ltd).

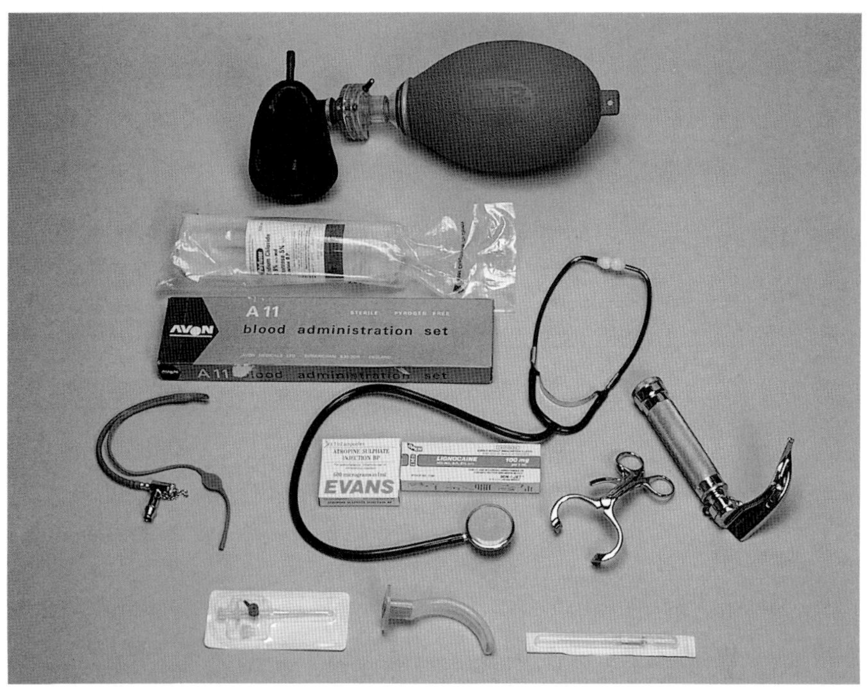

Fig. 44.6 Contents of a simple 'cardiac arrest' box.

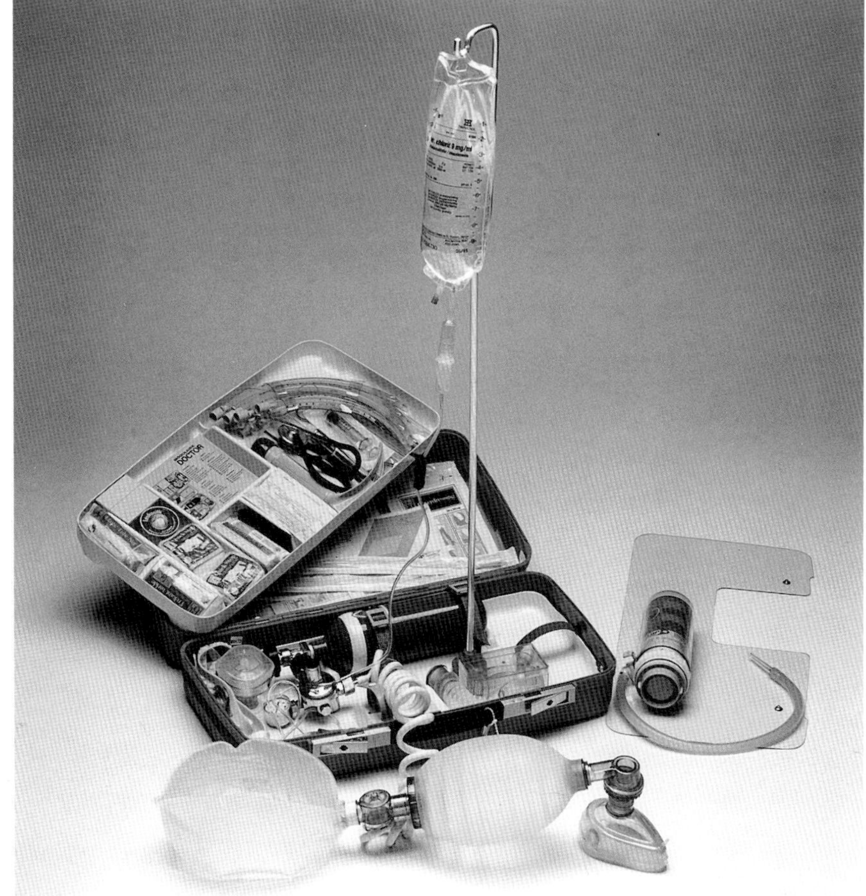

Fig. 44.7 A comprehensive resuscitation kit which may be kept in the treatment room, or in the boot of the doctor's car for immediate use both at road-traffic accidents and in the patient's home. Laerdal Modulated 'Doctor' complete (Laerdal Medical Ltd).

Severe bradycardia should be treated with intravenous atropine 300–600 μg while asystole should be treated with intravenous adrenaline 1:100 1 ml to induce ventricular fibrillation, which can be converted to sinus rhythm by DC defibrillation.

Acidosis is treated by intravenous sodium bicarbonate 8.4% 50–150 ml and cardiac failure by intravenous frusemide 20–40 mg.

Throughout all these procedures, cardiopulmonary resuscitation by mouth-to-mouth artificial respiration and external cardiac compression should be maintained (Fig. 44.8).

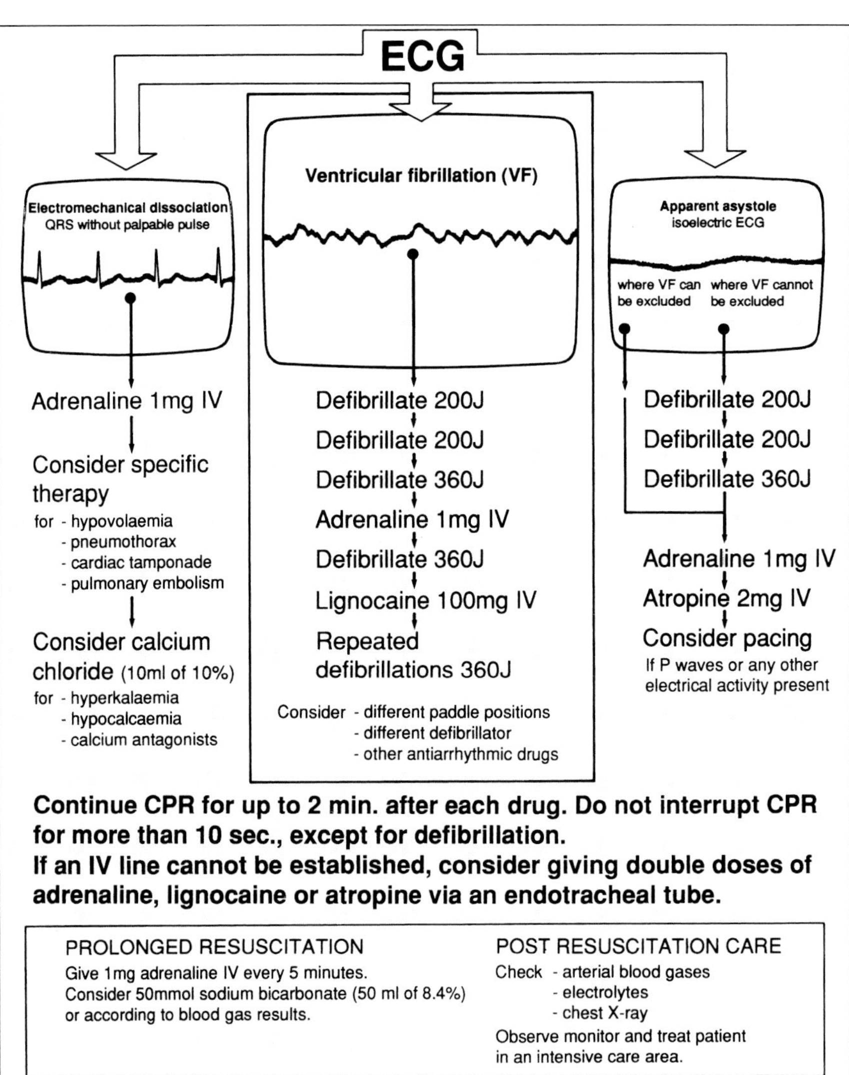

Fig. 44.8 Protocol for resuscitation produced by the Resuscitation Council of the UK 1984.

Part Three :

Advanced minor surgery

In the following five chapters are described four additional operations – decompression of the carpal tunnel, release of trigger finger, excision of ganglion and stab avulsion of varicose veins – which are well within the capability of the experienced general practitioner surgeon but carry additional risks. These should therefore only be undertaken after the doctor has had personal tuition from a colleague and has done several under supervision before embarking on his own.

Chapter 49 concludes with two more complex anaesthetic techniques – caudal epidural and intravenous regional anaesthesia (Bier's block). There are few occasions when the average doctor will use either of these methods of anaesthesia, particularly intravenous regional blocks which carry considerable risks should the cuffs fail. However, if the practitioner is faced with a situation where either would be appropriate, and the risks are fully understood, and the necessary back-up and resuscitation facilities exist, then it is helpful to know the procedures.

In the first edition of *Minor Surgery* decompression of the carpal tunnel, excision of ganglion and release of trigger finger were all described using intravenous regional anaesthesia (Bier's block) which in itself carries a significant risk, and this was the reason why it was decided not to include these procedures in the second edition. However, it is perfectly possible to produce a bloodless anaesthetic area without resorting to intravenous regional blocks, so it has been decided to reintroduce them in this edition.

Stab avulsion of varicose veins is a relatively new technique which lends itself admirably to minor surgery provided, again, that the doctor has had personal tuition and has performed several under supervision.

All four operations are supplemented with a small intravenous 'premedication' injection of fentanyl and midazolam to reduce the awareness of the orthopaedic tourniquet in operations on the hand, and to reduce awareness of avulsing segments of veins in the leg. It is therefore essential that an assistant is present throughout the whole of the operation and that suitable resuscitation facilities are available, a benzodiazepine reverser is available, and ideally blood-oxygen monitoring should be carried out.

Given all these restraints, these operations are nevertheless some of the more rewarding to do, giving excellent results.

45

Decompression of the carpal tunnel

She is woke up nightly by pains in the fingers, hands and up the fore-arms. The hands seem to become stiff and useless, and when she gets up – look, she says, as if they were dead. The pain is severe and prevents sleep. She connects her complaint with the use of water for scrubbing floors – she gave up her place as a servant on this account and her hands improved afterwards.

J. A. Ormerod, *On a peculiar numbness and paresis of the hands, 1883*

Decompression of the median nerve in the carpal tunnel is now one of the commonest operations on the hand, yet the first recorded carpal tunnel decompression was only carried out in 1941. The presenting symptoms are paraesthesia affecting the middle three fingers, with pain up the forearm; the patient is commonly a woman, and the right hand is affected more than the left; typically the pain and 'pins and needles' wake the patient at night, and relief is obtained by shaking the arm and hanging it out of bed.

Confirmation of the diagnosis may be obtained by applying pressure over the carpal tunnel to reproduce the symptoms, by tapping the carpal tunnel, or by acutely flexing the wrist for a minute (Chapter 22).

If early warning symptoms are ignored, wasting of the thenar muscles occurs and, even if the nerve is subsequently decompressed, recovery of wasted muscle seldom occurs (Fig. 45.1). It should also be remembered

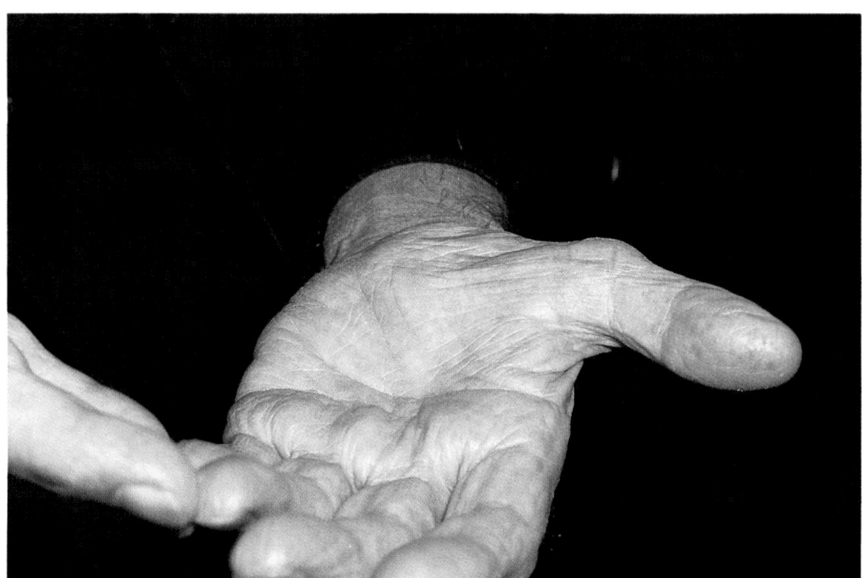

Fig. 45.1 Untreated, compression of the median nerve may result in severe wasting of the thenar muscles.

that cervical nerve root entrapment at C7 level will also give pain in the hand and numbness of the middle finger, so it is important to check the neck at the time of the initial examination.

Non-surgical treatment consisting of splinting, diuretics and steroid injection is worth trying (Chapter 22). If a steroid injection relieves the symptoms which later recur, at least the doctor knows decompression will work and can thus confidently recommend it.

Surgical decompression is a much simpler operation than is generally realized. A bloodless operating field is essential, so an orthopaedic tourniquet and Esmarch bandage are required. Likewise, complete aseptic operation conditions are mandatory – this means CSSD packs or autoclaving, gowns, masks and sterile surgical gloves.

45.1 INSTRUMENTS

The following instruments are required:

Povidone-iodine in spirit (Betadine alcoholic solution)
1 dental syringe and 30 swg needle
1 cartridge local anaesthetic (without added adrenaline)
1 orthopaedic tourniquet
1 Esmarch bandage
Sterile pads, bandages and gauze
1 scalpel handle size 3
1 scalpel blade size 15
1 self-retaining retractor (West Weitlander or similar)
1 double-ended McDonald's dissector
1 stitch scissors
1 Kilner needle-holder 5¼in. (13.3 cm)
1 pair fine-toothed Adson's dissecting forceps 4¾in. (12 cm)
1 surgical suture 3/0 monofilament nylon or Prolene on curved cutting needle.
Skin closure strips 3M Ref. R1547 12 mm × 100 mm (½in. × 4 in.)

Where the doctor requires a bloodless field and anaesthesia in a limb, a safer alternative to a Bier's block is to infiltrate the area with local anaesthesia and then to apply an orthopaedic tourniquet and Esmarch bandage. This is particularly effective for decompression of the carpal tunnel and release of trigger finger, and exploration for foreign bodies.

45.2 TECHNIQUE FOR PRODUCING ANAESTHETIC BLOODLESS FIELD

1. Remove any rings from fingers on the affected hand.
2. Explain procedure in detail to the patient.
3. Give intravenous 'premedication injection' of fentanyl 100 μg and midazolam 2–4 mg. This is given slowly over 1–2 minutes into a vein in the opposite arm. If an intravenous cannula is inserted at this stage and taped in position, the doctor then has access to the circulation for the remainder of the operation. This would be valuable if the midazolam needed to be reversed.

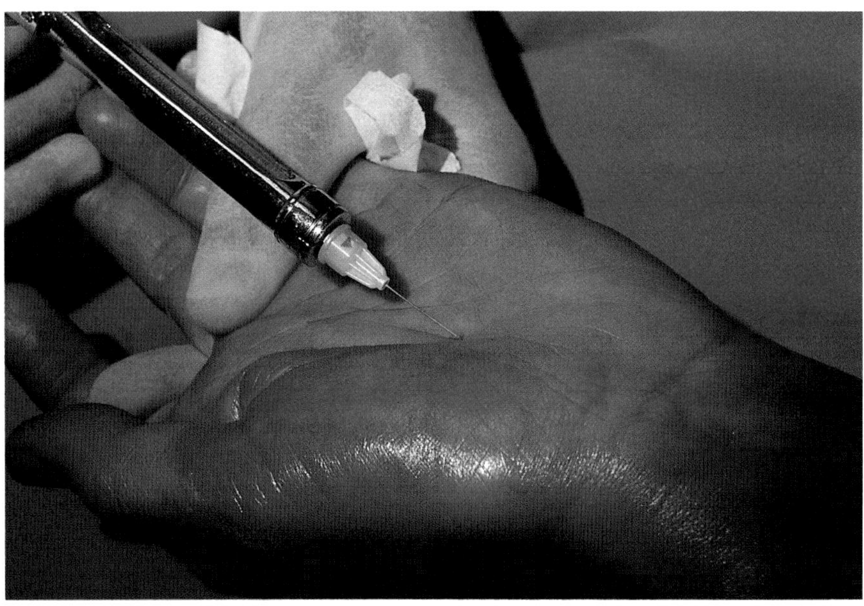

Fig. 45.2 Infiltrating the line of the incision with local anaesthetic.

4. Paint the palmar surface of the hand and wrist with povidone-iodine in spirit.
5. Infiltrate the line of the thenar crease with local anaesthetic (without added adrenaline) using a dental syringe and 30 swg needle (Fig. 45.2).
6. Paint the skin a second time with povidone-iodine in spirit and cover with a sterile pad.
7. Apply the orthopaedic tourniquet over a layer of cotton-wool over the upper arm and bandage in position.
8. Raise the arm, keeping the sterile pad in position over the palm, and apply the Esmarch bandage tightly from the finger-tips to the lower edge of the orthopaedic tourniquet.
9. Pump the tourniquet to above arterial pressure (approx. 300 mmHg)
10. Unwind the Esmarch bandage and remove the sterile pad.

45.3 THE OPERATION

The overlying skin is again painted with povidone-iodine in spirit (Betadine alcoholic solution) and a sterile drape placed over the area. As with excision of ganglion and release of trigger finger, full aseptic technique is employed – this means wearing sterile surgical gown, mask and gloves.

A skin incision is made in the thenar crease as shown (Fig. 45.3); correctly placed it will be exactly between the thenar and hypothenar muscles, exactly over the median nerve. Self-retaining or individual hand-held retractors are now placed in the wound and opened to expose the underlying fatty tissues and dense fibrous transverse ligament (Fig. 45.4). The incision is cautiously deepened until the glistening median nerve is seen. At this stage, the McDonald's dissector (Fig. 45.5) is gently introduced below the transverse ligament and in front of the median nerve, and the ligament is divided by cutting down on the blade of the dissector

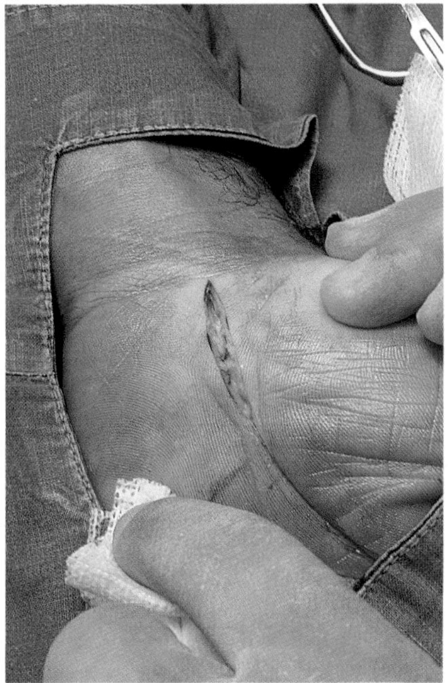

Fig. 45.3 The incision is made in the proximal palmar crease as shown.

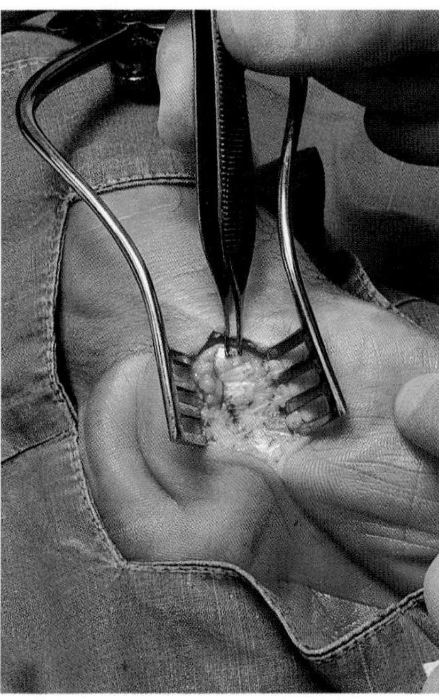

Fig. 45.4 A self-retaining retractor makes the operation much easier.

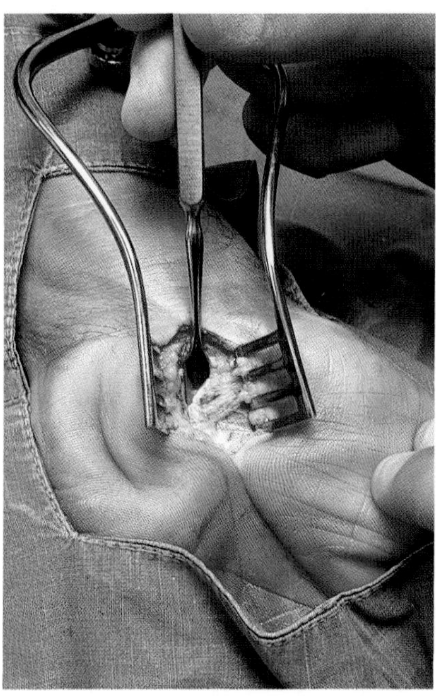

Fig. 45.5 The McDonald's dissector is slipped under the retinaculum, in front of the nerve.

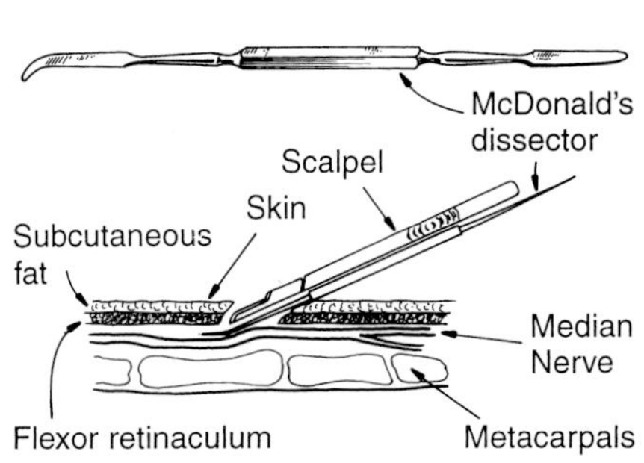

Fig. 45.6 The McDonald's dissector is inserted in front of the median nerve to protect it, and the deep transverse ligament is divided using the Number 15 scalpel blade with the back of the blade resting against the McDonald's dissector.

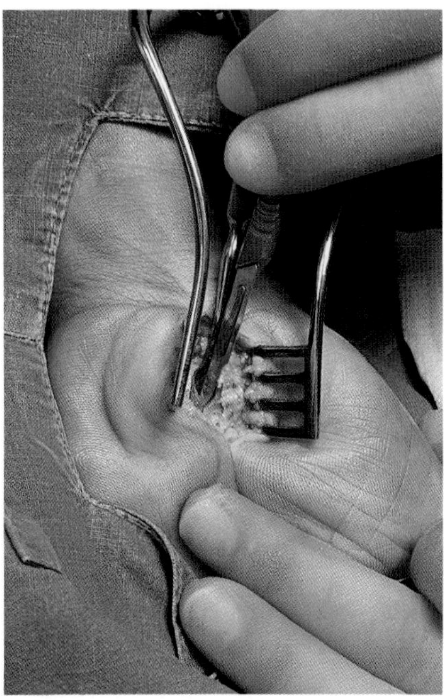

Fig. 45.7 With the McDonald's dissector protecting the nerve, the retinaculum is split with a small scalpel blade.

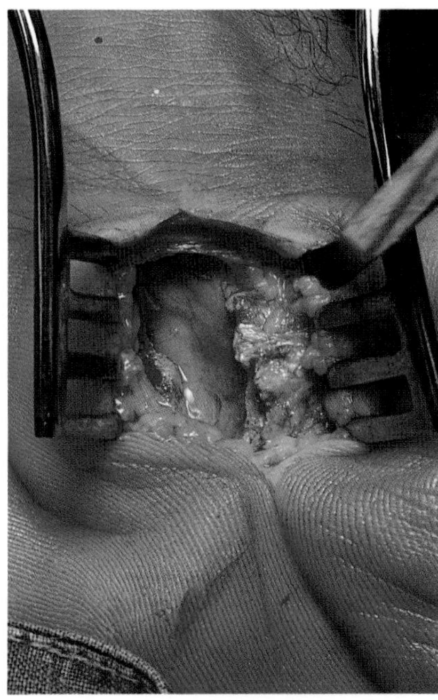

Fig. 45.8 The median nerve is now exposed. (Note what a large structure it is.)

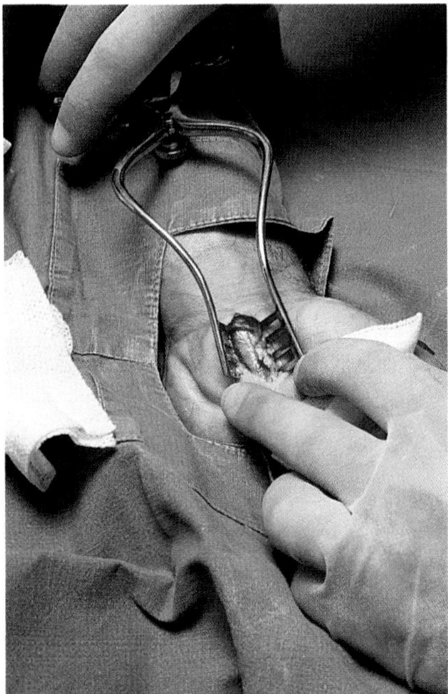

Fig. 45.9 The retractor may now be removed.

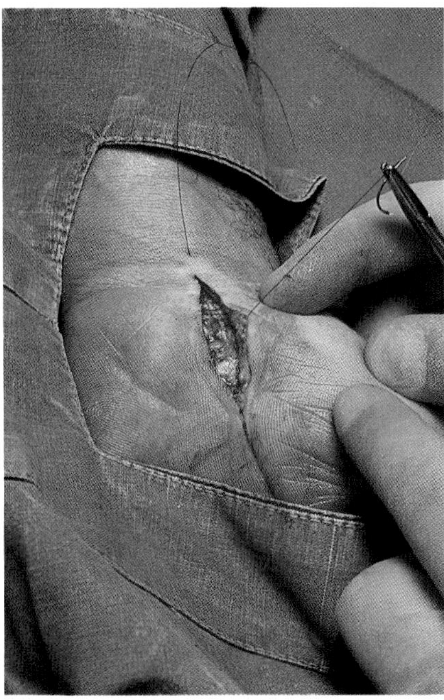

Fig. 45.10 Skin closure is with a subcuticular monofilament nylon suture alone.

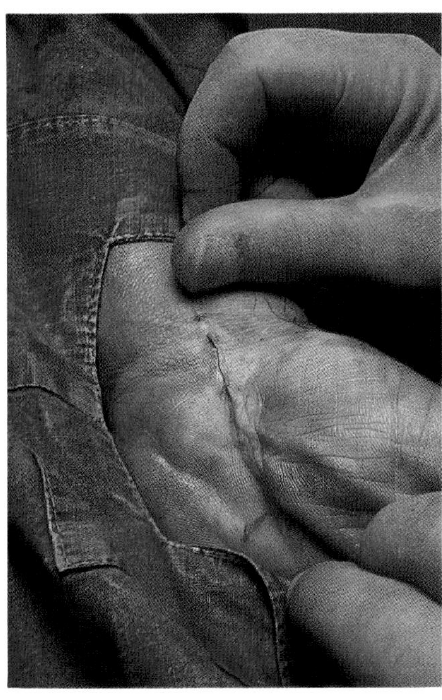

Fig. 45.11 A subcuticular stitch gives a neat scar, and it is quick to insert and is easy to remove.

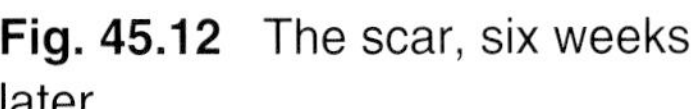

Fig. 45.12 The scar, six weeks later.

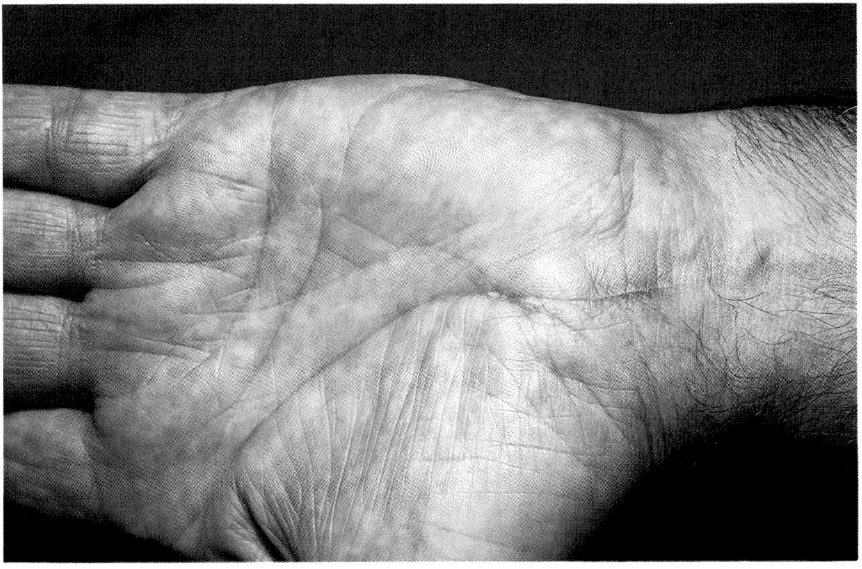

which is protecting the nerve (Fig. 45.6). The median nerve may now be freed both proximally and distally with the aid of the McDonald's dissector, and particular note made of any branches to the thenar muscles or skin, which should be preserved (Figs 45.7 and 45.8).

When the operator is satisfied that the median nerve is no longer compressed within the carpal tunnel, the retractors may be removed (Fig. 45.9) and the wound closed. Just the skin is sutured; either with interrupted braided silk 3/0 (metric gauge 2) or a neater scar may be obtained by using a subcuticular monofilament polyamide 63/0 (metric gauge 2) suture, strengthened with adhesive skin closure strips Ref. 3M R1547 ½in. × 4in. (12mm × 100mm) (Figs 45.10 and 45.11). Sterile gauze swabs are now folded in half and taped in position over the incision to act as a mild pressure dressing – these are then covered with cotton wool and a firm elasto-crepe bandage. When applying the cotton wool, it is important to place it between all the fingers.

The arm is now elevated, and the assistant applies pressure over the incision while the doctor releases both tourniquets. Pressure is maintained for at least 5 minutes; following this the arm is placed in a triangular sling with the palm of the operated hand on the opposite shoulder.

Assuming all is well, the dressing is left undisturbed until the 10th post-operative day when the sutures are removed, leaving the Steri-strips. A sterile dry dressing is reapplied over the strips and lightly bandaged and left in place for a further 4 days, by which time healing is complete.

The patient usually obtains immediate relief of all symptoms – occasionally it may take several months to recover, and frequently there is a tender area underneath the scar which arises from the exposed nerve – this likewise recovers gradually over several months; however, if any significant degree of muscle wasting has occurred, this does not usually recover.

Carpal tunnel syndrome, diagnosed before irreversible damage to the nerve has occurred, is one of the most satisfactory conditions to treat surgically.

46

Release of trigger finger

It seemed most likely that it was a thickening of the tendon sheath at a specific point. On March 7th 1894, I excised the common tunnel of extensor pollicis brevis over a length of one centimetre

Fritz de Quervain, Concerning a Form of Chronic Tenovaginitis, 1868–1940

Trigger finger and trigger thumb (tenovaginitis stenosans and de Quervain's syndrome) are cause by a constriction of the flexor tendon sheath combined with a secondary localized thickening of the tendon. This results in difficulty in extending the joint, which often straightens suddenly with a palpable 'click'. Commonly the constriction occurs in front of the metacarpophalangeal joint under the annular ligament. Relief may be obtained by injecting corticosteroid (methylprednisolone acetate) into the sheath but, if the condition recurs, surgery is indicated.

A bloodless operating field is essential, therefore an orthopaedic tourniquet and Esmarch bandage are required. Likewise, complete aseptic operation conditions are mandatory – this means CSSD packs or autoclaving, gowns, masks and sterile surgical gloves.

46.1 INSTRUMENTS

The following instruments are required:

Povidone-iodine in spirit (betadine alcoholic solution)
1 dental syringe and 30 swg needle
1 cartridge local anaesthetic (without added adrenaline)
1 orthopaedic tourniquet
1 Esmarch bandage
Sterile pads, bandages and gauze
1 scalpel handle size 3
1 scalpel blade size 15
1 self-retaining retractor (West Weitlander or similar)
  or 2 Kilner double-ended retractors (cat's paw retractors)
2 pair Halstead's mosquito artery forceps, curved 5 in. (12.7 cm)
1 double-ended McDonald's dissector
1 stitch scissors
1 Kilner needle-holder 5 1/4 in. (13.3 cm)
1 pair fine-toothed Adson's dissecting forceps 4 3/4 in. (12 cm)
1 surgical suture 4/0 monofilament nylon or Prolene on curved cutting needle
Skin closure strips 3M Ref. GP 41 6 mm × 75 mm

Where the doctor requires a bloodless field and anaesthesia in a limb, a safer alternative to a Bier's block is to infiltrate the area with local anaesthesia and then to apply an orthopaedic tourniquet and Esmarch bandage. This is particularly effective for decompression of the carpal tunnel and release of trigger finger, and exploration for foreign bodies.

46.2 TECHNIQUE FOR PRODUCING ANAESTHETIC BLOODLESS FIELD

1. Remove any rings from fingers on affected hand.
2. Explain procedure in detail to the patient.
3. Give intravenous 'premedication injection' of fentanyl 100 µg and midazolam 2–4 mg. This is given slowly over 1–2 minutes into a vein in the opposite arm. If an intravenous cannula is inserted at this stage and taped in position for the duration of the operation, the doctor then has access to the circulation. This is valuable should the midazolam need to be reversed.
4. Paint the palmar surface of the hand and wrist with povidone-iodine in spirit.
5. Infiltrate the line of the distal palmar crease with local anaesthetic (without added adrenaline) using a dental syringe and 30 swg needle (Fig. 46.1).
6. Paint the skin a second time with povidone-iodine in spirit and cover with a sterile pad.
7. Apply the orthopaedic tourniquet over a layer of cotton wool over the upper arm, and bandage in position.
8. Raise the arm, keeping the sterile pad in position over the palm, and apply the Esmarch bandage tightly from the finger-tips to the lower edge of the orthopaedic tourniquet.
9. Pump the tourniquet to above arterial pressure (approx. 300 mmHg).
10. Unwind the Esmarch bandage and remove the sterile pad.

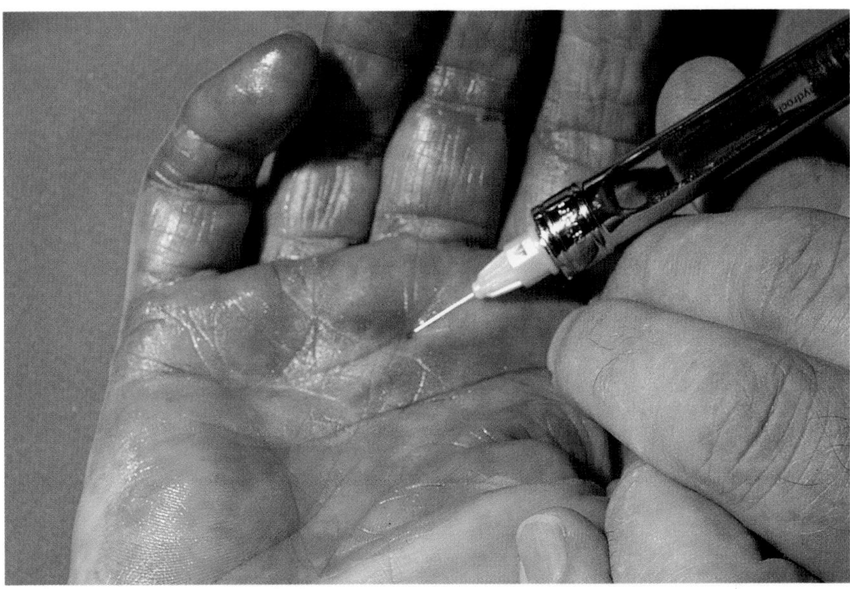

Fig. 46.1 The line of the distal palmar crease is infiltrated with local anaesthetic (without added adrenaline) using a dental syringe and 30 swg needle.

46.3 THE OPERATION

The overlying skin is liberally painted with povidone-iodine in spirit (Betadine alcoholic solution), a sterile drape is placed over the area, and full aseptic precautions observed. A surgical gown, mask and gloves should be worn.

A small transverse incision is made in the distal palmar crease for trigger fingers, and the proximal thumb crease for trigger thumb (Fig. 46.2).

The incision is deepened until the flexor sheath is exposed, taking care to avoid the digital nerves and blood vessels on either side. For this stage of the operation it is easier and safer to use curved fine artery forceps for dissection rather than scissors or scalpel (Fig. 46.3).

The proximal part of the annular ligament and tendon sheath is divided, and the patient is asked to move the fingers to demonstrate that any triggering has been released. It is preferable to leave the distal portion of the

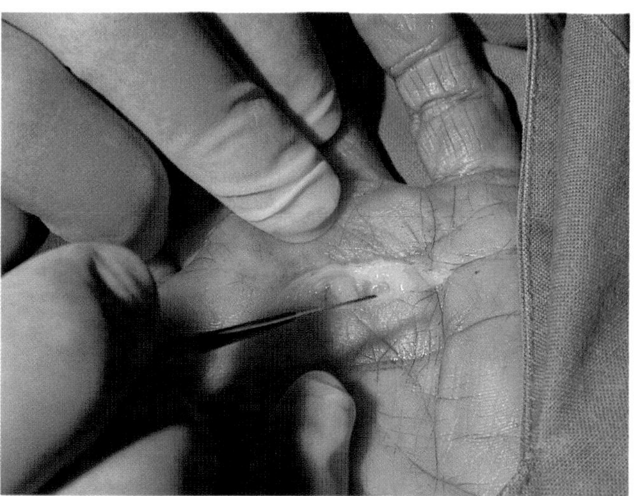

Fig. 46.2 Small transverse incision in distal palmar crease.

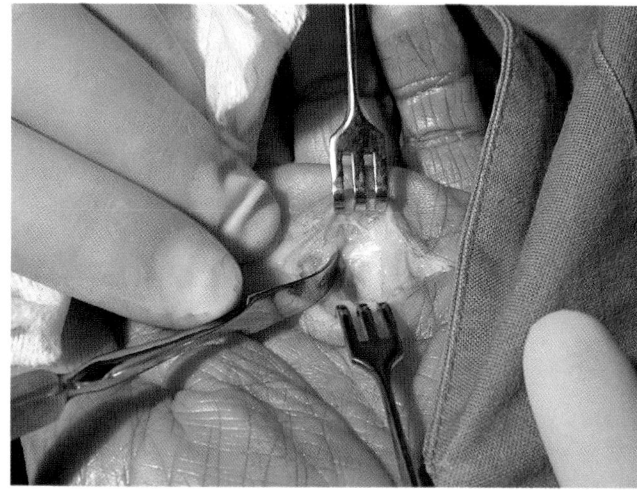

Fig. 46.3 The incision is deepened using curved fine artery forceps.

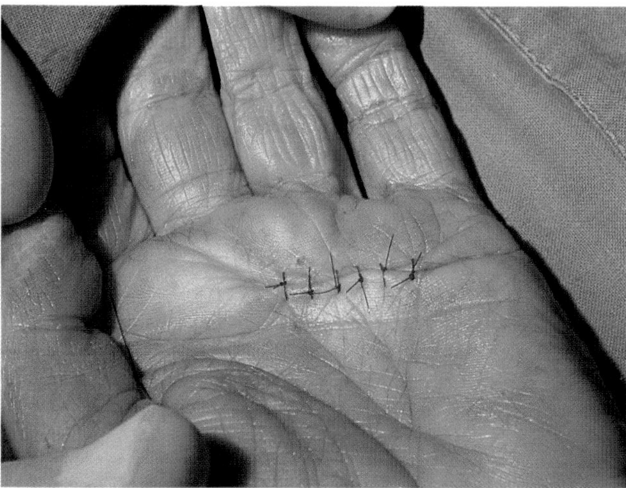

Fig. 46.4 Closure of the wound.

annular ligament, as troublesome bowing of the tendon can occur if this is divided. It is not necessary, nor desirable, to remove any thickening of the tendon itself for fear of subsequent weakening and spontaneous rupture.

Closure is by one subcuticular monofilament suture or interrupted sutures (Fig. 46.4) supplemented by skin closure strips.

A sterile dressing is applied over the incision, covered with cotton wool and an elastocrepe bandage, and the arm placed in a triangular sling with the affected hand on the opposite shoulder.

The dressing is left completely undisturbed until the suture is removed on the 10th postoperative day. The skin closure strips are left in place, and the hand lightly bandaged for two more days, after which no restrictions need be imposed, and the patient is encouraged to use the fingers as much as possible.

47

Stab avulsion varicose veins

Marius, Roman Consul, having both his legs full of great tumours, and disliking the deformity, determined to put himself in the hands of an operator. When, after enduring a most excessive torment in the cutting, never flinching or complaining, the surgeon went to the other, he declined to have it done saying 'I see the cure is not worth the pain'

Plutarch's Lives, 186–55 BC

Anatomy, types of varicose veins and sclerotherapy have been covered in Chapter 37 and, for the majority of veins below the knee, sclerotherapy still gives very good results. However, even better results can be achieved by the multiple stab avulsion technique by the purchase of just one additional instrument, namely, vein forceps (Fig. 47.5a).

The principle of treatment is to make numerous small stab incisions along the course of the vein, and then to tease out segments of vein through these incisions. By grasping this vein with strong artery forceps it may be forcibly avulsed.

In effect one is 'stripping' the vein, but in small sections. The advantage over stripping is that irregular tributaries may be treated, and both long and short saphenous veins treated.

As with sclerotherapy, if there is any evidence of saphenofemoral incompetence, these patients should be referred for ligation in the groin. Failure to recognize this will result in a high recurrence rate and disappointed patients.

Normally, stab avulsions are done under general anaesthesia, but it is perfectly possible to perform them under local anaesthesia. Because the actual avulsion of the vein can be uncomfortable, an intravenous premedication injection of midazolam and fentanyl is given. This enables the patient to remain relaxed and pain-free, and it also has an amnesic effect.

It is important to warn the patient in advance not to drive for at least 24 hours following the injection and to arrange transport home.

A scrubbed assistant is needed for this operation.

47.1 INSTRUMENTS

The following instruments are required:

- 1 pair of vein forceps (Fig. 47.5a)
- 1 pair of strong, straight, artery forceps
- 1 scalpel handle size 3 with size 15 blade
- 1 10 ml syringe with 25 swg needle
- 1 skin marker-pen

Steri-strips size $^{1}/_{2}$in. × 4in. (12mm × 100mm) Ref. 3M R1547
Micropore tape 1in.
Sterile gauze swabs
Elastocrepe bandages 4in.
Tubigrip size F2 × 1 metre
Elastic web bandage 3in. × 5 metres
Ampoules, midazolam and fentanyl
5ml syringe and 23swg needle
10ml ampoule 1% lignocaine, plain
1 aerosol spray skin adhesive (Dow Corning Medical Adhesive 'B')

47.2 OPERATIVE TECHNIQUE (Figs 47.1–47.12)

1. With the patient standing, all varicose veins are marked using the skin marker-pen and the proposed sites of incisions are marked (Fig. 47.1).
2. With the patient lying down an intravenous premedication injection of midazolam (2–4mg) and fentanyl (100μg) is given slowly. (If 'sleep-doses' of midazolam are given it is advisable to use a pulse oximeter to monitor oxygen saturation).
3. Sterile drapes are placed under the leg and injections of 1% lignocaine given where marked along the course of the veins (Fig. 47.3).
4. Starting distally, a small stab incision is now made adjacent and parallel to the segment of vein to be removed (Fig. 47.4).
5. Using the vein forceps, the vein is brought out through the incision (Fig. 47.5b), and grasped with artery forceps (Fig. 47.6).
6. Using a twisting action much like a windlass, more vein may be pulled out (Fig. 47.7) until it eventually tears free.
7. The assistant now places a folded gauze swab over the incision and applies firm pressure to prevent bleeding.
8. The operator moves along the course of the vein and repeats the procedure at the next point which has been marked. If a good

Fig. 47.1 With the patient standing, the veins are marked out.

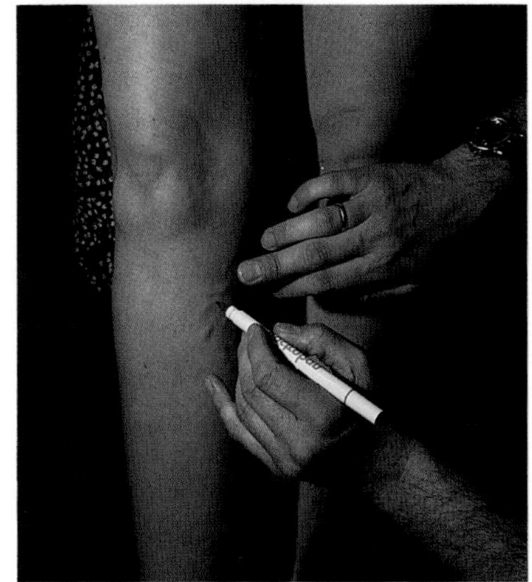

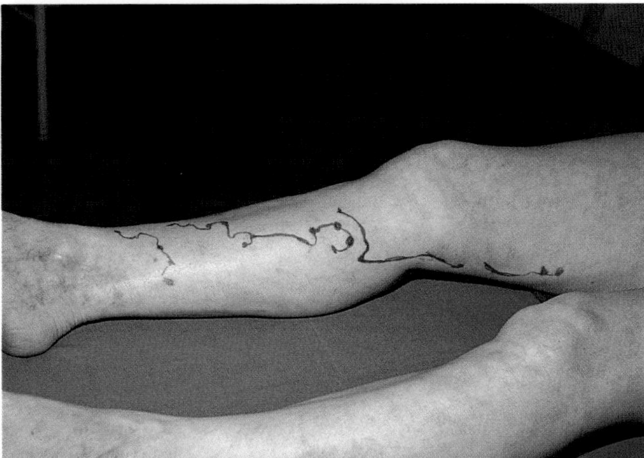

Fig. 47.2 Marked branches of the long saphenous vein.

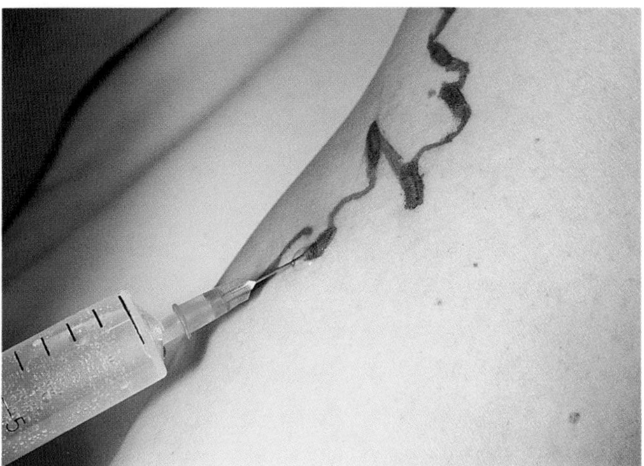

Fig. 47.3 1% lignocaine is injected at the sites along the vein.

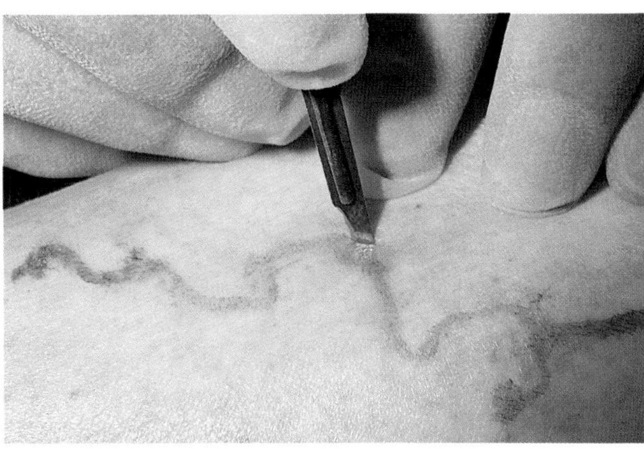

Fig. 47.4 Using a No. 15 blade a small stab incision is made alongside the vein.

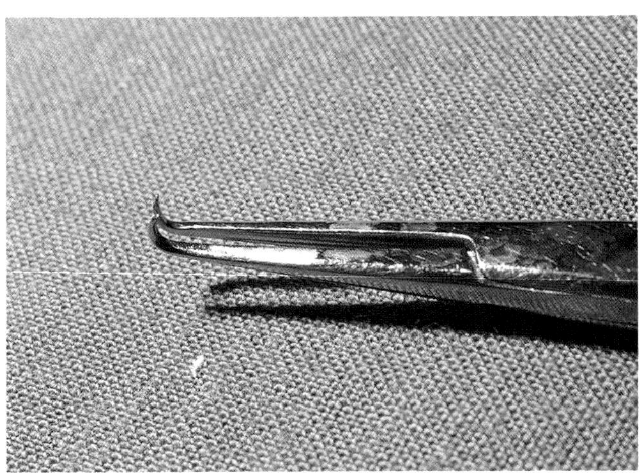

Fig. 47.5a The vein forceps look like a pair of very fine mosquito artery forceps with the tips turned back to form two very small hooks (Caterham Surgical Supplies Ltd).

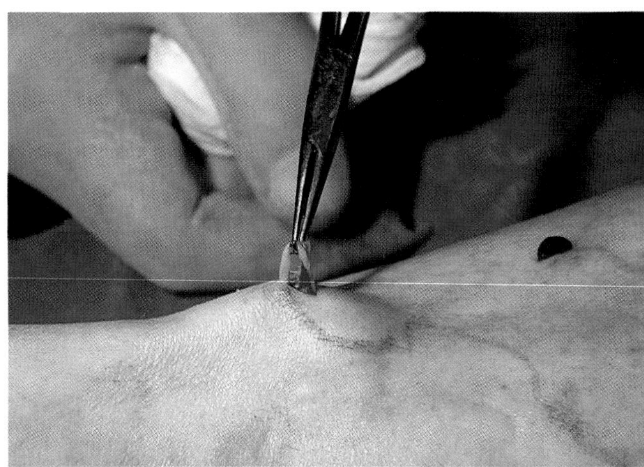

Fig. 47.5b The vein forceps are inserted through the stab incision and the vein is pulled through the skin.

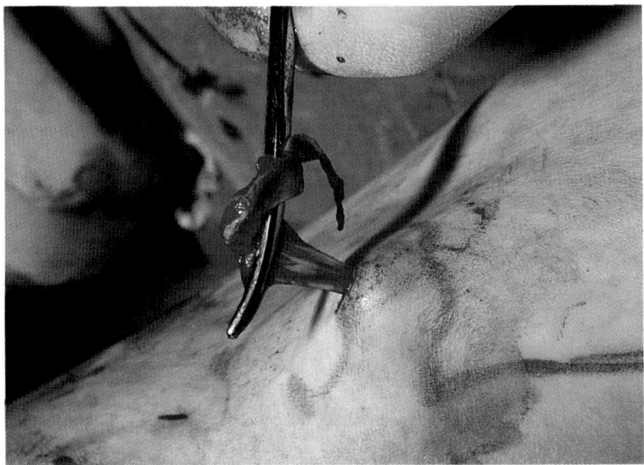

Fig. 47.6 Using artery forceps, the vein is gradually 'teased' out of the wound.

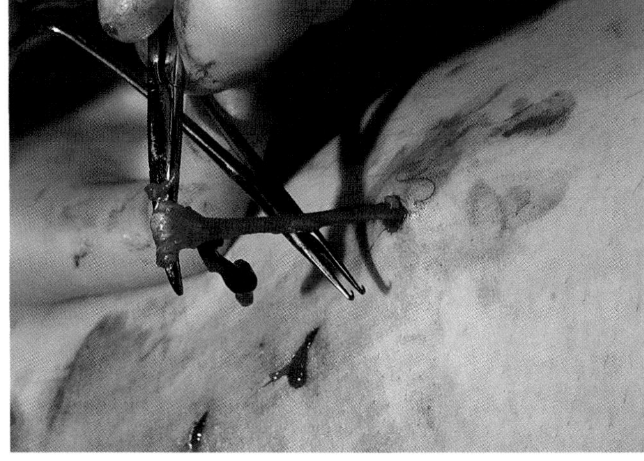

Fig. 47.7 By twisting the forceps a longer section of vein may be avulsed.

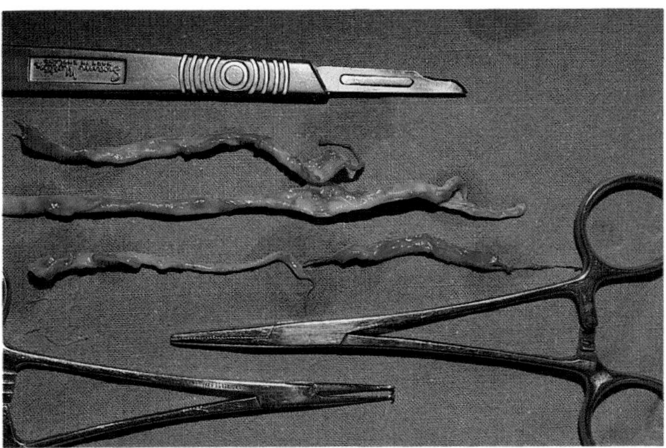

Fig. 47.8 Instruments needed, together with typical sections of avulsed vein.

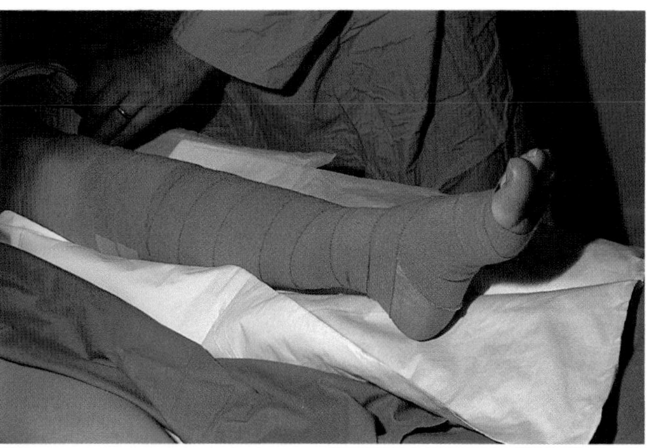

Fig. 47.9 The leg is bandaged with 4 in. Elastocrepe from the toes to above the top incision.

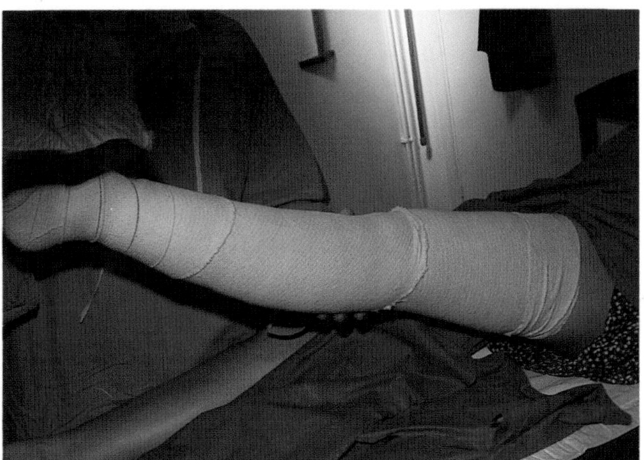

Fig. 47.10 Two layers of elasticated tubular bandage (Tubigrip) size F are applied.

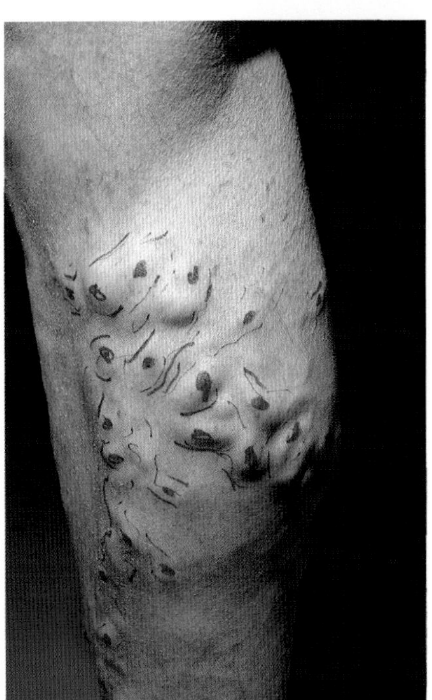

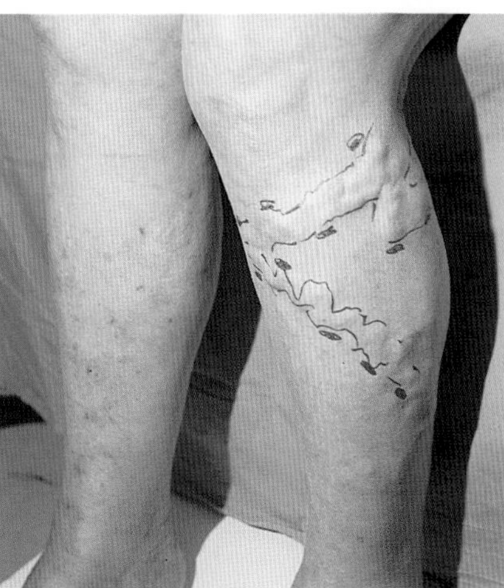

Fig. 47.11 Typical varicosities before operation.

Fig. 47.12 'Before and after'. The leg on the left was treated 6 months previously. The scars of the stab avulsions can still be seen. The leg on the right has been marked and is ready for treatment.

segment of vein was obtained it may be possible to miss out the next marked spot and move on to the next.

9. It is not always possible to obtain good segments of vein, usually because they are friable and tear easily. This does not seem to make a significant difference to the outcome as there has been an interruption of the vein itself.
10. When all segments of veins have been avulsed, the incisions are closed with Steri-strips. To ensure good adhesion, the skin is sprayed liberally with a medical adhesive prior to the application of each Steri-strip.
11. Folded gauze swabs are now placed over each incision and taped in position with 1 in. micropore tape.
12. A 4 in Elastocrepe bandage is now applied from the toes to above the topmost incision (Fig. 47.9).
13. This is then covered with two layers of Tubigrip F (Fig. 47.10).
14. Finally, a 3 in elastic web bandage is applied firmly over the Tubigrip extending from the toes to above the previous bandages. This is primarily to prevent any bleeding on the way home.
15. The patient then remains on the premises for at least 2 hours during which the effects of the midazolam wears off.
16. Before going home the bandages are checked and a postoperative patient information sheet is given.
17. The patient is advised to go straight home and straight to bed, and to remain there for the next 12 hours.
18. Once the patient is in his or her own bed, the outermost elastic web bandage may be removed after 1 hour.
19. The patient is encouraged to be fully ambulant after the initial 12 hour rest and to remove all bandages and dressings after 10 days (this is best done in the bath where they can be soaked off.)
20. The Tubigrip bandage is reapplied for the next 4 days when the patient is seen for a check-up.
21. Some bruising is normal, but this disappears quickly over the next few weeks.
22. The patient is seen for a final check at 2 months.

It is helpful to give the patient both a preoperative and a postoperative information sheet.

48

Excision of ganglion

They are most frequently met with over the tendons upon the back of the wrist: the most certain method of treatment is to make a small puncture into the sac, and to draw a cord through it, or after the puncture is made, to press out the contents and then inject some gently stimulating fluid, as port wine and water heated blood warm

Encyclopaedia Britannica, 1797

Ganglia are extremely common; they are cystic swellings surrounded by a fibrous tissue wall, occurring in the vicinity of joint capsules and tendon sheaths. Most have crystal clear gelatinous contents, apart from some in which bleeding has occurred. The cause is not fully understood, but may be a degenerative process in the mesoblastic tissues surrounding the joint. The commonest site is the dorsum of the wrist (Fig. 48.1) (60–80%) followed by the flexor aspect of the wrist adjacent to the radial artery (15–20%). Smaller ganglia occur in the flexor sheaths of the fingers, dorsum of foot, ankle and head of fibula.

Untreated, many ganglia disappear spontaneously; many others appear not to trouble the patient and may be left alone. Treatment is indicated if the patient is complaining of unacceptable symptoms, usually pain or limitation of function. Many treatments have been advocated – all carry a recurrence rate, and the patient should be advised of this accordingly. Simple rupture of the cyst by pressure occasionally succeeds, as does incision with a tenotomy knife, aspiration and injection of sclerosants but

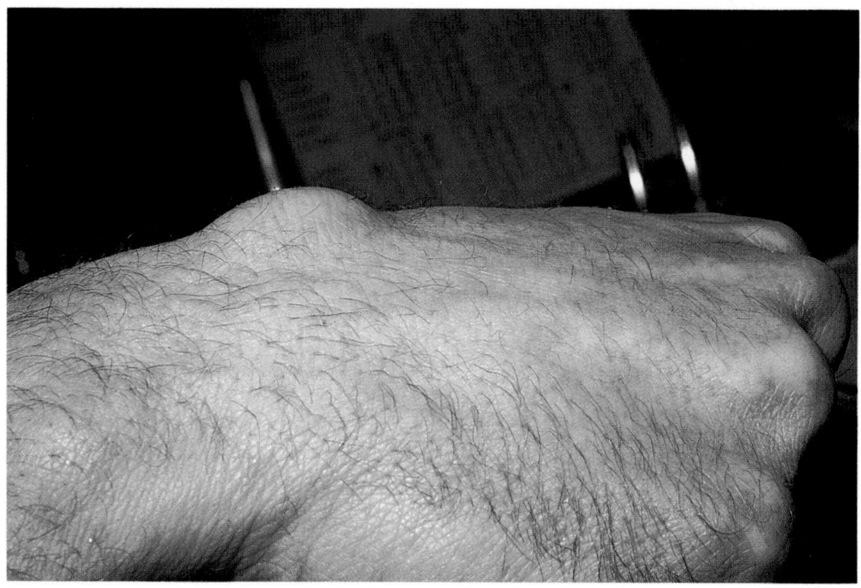

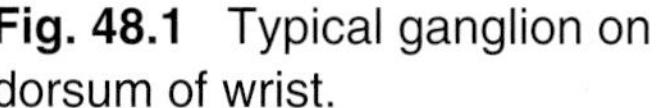

Fig. 48.1 Typical ganglion on dorsum of wrist.

many surgeons recommend excision as offering the best chance of cure.

It is essential to have a bloodless operating field, secured by a pneumatic tourniquet, as the dissection can be quite difficult and the ganglion extend deeper than anticipated. Thus a general anaesthetic or intravenous regional block or tourniquet and local infiltration is required; the latter being the method chosen for the average general practitioner.

Many patients will assume that excision of a ganglion will be no different from a small sebaceous cyst; it is therefore important to let them know that it is quite a complicated procedure, that they should not drive a car immediately following operation and that, despite a meticulous dissection, recurrence is still possible.

48.1 INSTRUMENTS

The following instruments are required:

Povidone-iodine in spirit (Betadine alcoholic solution)
1 dental syringe and 30 swg needle
1 cartridge local anaesthetic (without added adrenaline)
1 orthopaedic tourniquet
1 Esmarch bandage
Sterile pads, bandages and gauze
1 scalpel handle size 3
1 scalpel blade size 15
1 self-retaining retractor (West Weitlander or similar)
  or 2 Kilner double-ended retractors (cat's paw retractors)
2 pair Halstead's mosquito artery forceps, curved 5 in. (12.7 cm)
1 stitch scissors
1 Kilner needle-holder 5¼ in. (13.3 cm)
1 pair fine-toothed Adson's dissecting forceps 4¾ in. (12 cm)
1 surgical suture 4/0 monofilament nylon or Prolene on curved
  cutting needle.
Skin closure strips 3M Ref. GP 41 6 mm × 75 mm

Where the doctor requires a bloodless field and anaesthesia in a limb, a safer alternative to a Bier's block is to infiltrate the area with local anaesthesia and then to apply an orthopaedic tourniquet and Esmarch bandage. This is particularly effective for decompression of the carpal tunnel and release of trigger finger, and exploration for foreign bodies.

48.2 TECHNIQUE FOR PRODUCING ANAESTHETIC BLOODLESS FIELD

1. Remove any rings from fingers on affected hand.
2. Explain procedure in detail to the patient.
3. Give intravenous premedication injection of fentanyl 100 μg and midazolam 2–4 mg. This is given slowly over 1–2 minutes into a vein in the opposite arm. If an intravenous cannula is inserted at this stage and taped in position, the doctor then has access to the circulation for the remainder of the operation. This is valuable should the midazolam need to be reversed.

4. Paint the skin overlying the ganglion with povidone-iodine in spirit.
5. Infiltrate the skin over the ganglion with local anaesthetic (without added adrenaline) using a dental syringe and 30 swg needle.
6. Paint the skin a second time with povidone-iodine in spirit and cover with a sterile pad.
7. Apply the orthopaedic tourniquet over a layer of cotton-wool over the upper arm and bandage in position.
8. Raise the arm, keeping the sterile pad in position, and apply the Esmarch bandage tightly from the finger-tips to the lower edge of the orthopaedic tourniquet.
9. Pump the tourniquet to above arterial pressure (approx. 300 mmHg).
10. Unwind the Esmarch bandage and remove the sterile pad.

48.3 THE OPERATION

The overlying skin is liberally painted with povidone-iodine in spirit (Betadine alcoholic solution); a sterile drape is applied over the area, and full aseptic precautions observed. (A surgical gown, mask and gloves should be worn.)

The incision should follow a skin crease, normally transverse (Fig. 48.2), about 4 cm long, and any underlying nerves dissected free. The extensor retinaculum overlying the ganglion is incised, and a self-retaining retractor inserted. The bulk of the ganglion is seen superficial to the tendons, but when these are retracted, the deeper part of the ganglion may be seen (Figs 48.3 and 48.4) extending to the wrist joint or intercarpal joint. Gradually the main part of the ganglion is dissected free using a scalpel, applying traction with toothed dissecting forceps. Usually at this stage, the capsule is incised, liberating the typical clear jelly. This is often an advantage and makes the remaining dissection easier. The ganglion is now detached (Fig. 48.6) excising part of the joint capsule as well. It is quite in order to leave adjacent tendons without a synovial covering.

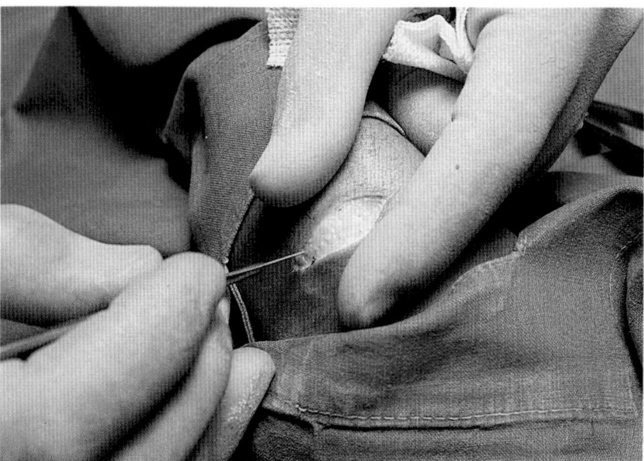

Fig. 48.2 A transverse incision is made over the ganglion in the line of a skin crease.

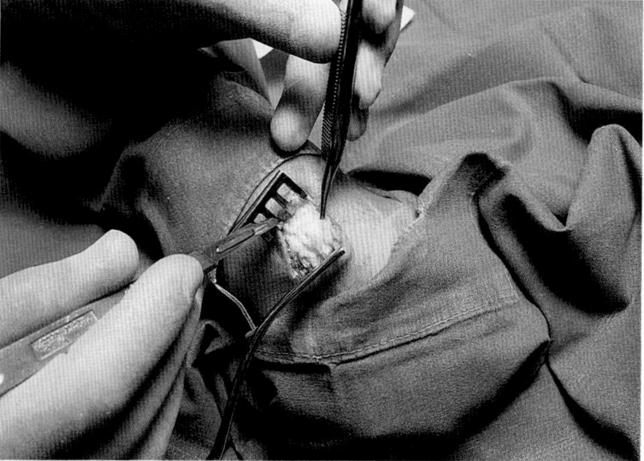

Fig. 48.3 A self-retaining retractor is inserted.

Closure is by one subcuticular monofilament polyamide suture, strengthened by skin closure strips (Figs 48.7, 48.8, 48.9, and 48.10). A sterile dry gauze dressing is applied covered with cotton wool and an elastocrepe bandage. The assistant now applies direct pressure over the site of the incision, and the doctor releases both tourniquets.

If all is well, the dressings are left undisturbed until the 10th postoperative day, when the suture is removed, leaving the Steri-strips in position. A light sterile dressing is reapplied over these for four more days and then removed.

48.4 EXCISION OF RHEUMATOID SYNOVIOMA (Figs 48.11 and 48.12)

This is performed using an identical approach to the excision of ganglion.

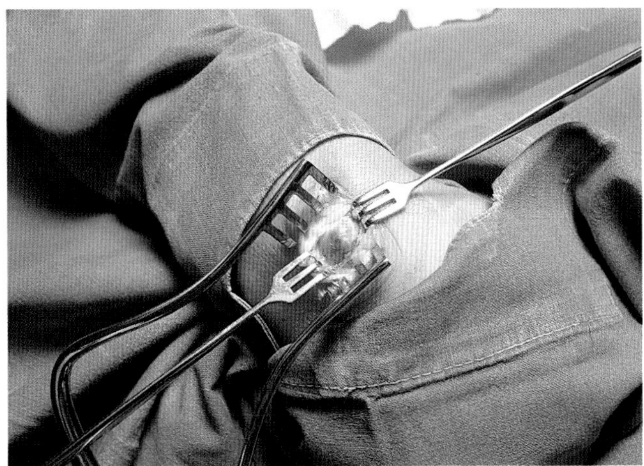

Fig. 48.4 If necessary, two cat's paw retractors may be used as well to improve access.

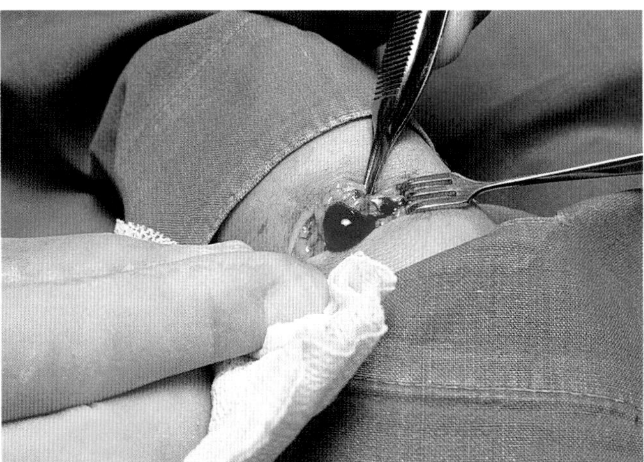

Fig. 48.5 The ganglion has been opened; blood-stained jelly is seen; this indicates possible previous trauma. Normally, the jelly is clear.

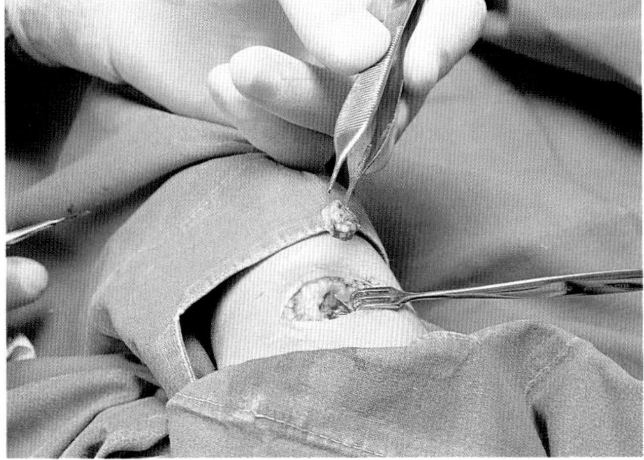

Fig. 48.6 The capsule of the ganglion has been excised.

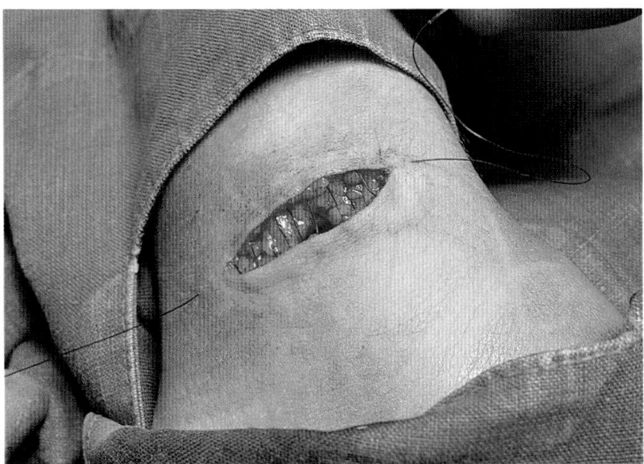

Fig. 48.7 A sub-cuticular monofilament nylon structure gives a neat scar.

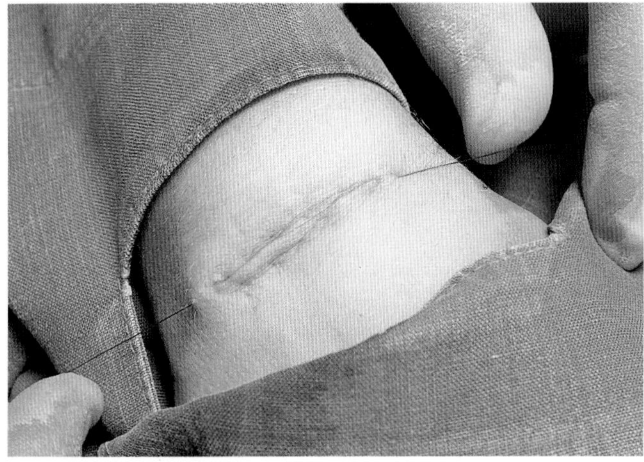

Fig. 48.8 Skin edges approximated with the subcuticular nylon stitch.

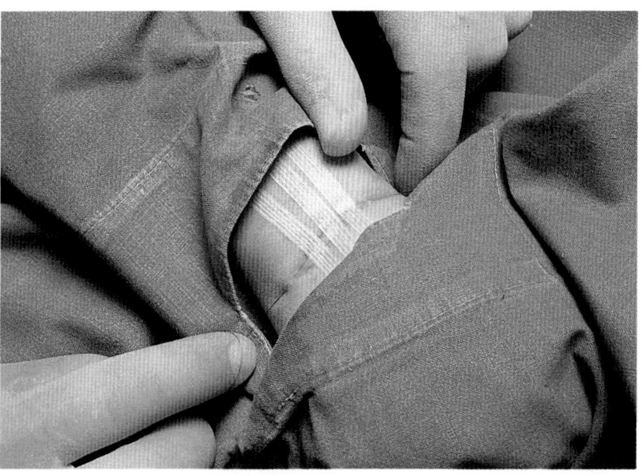

Fig. 48.9 Additional support may be given by the application of skin closure strips.

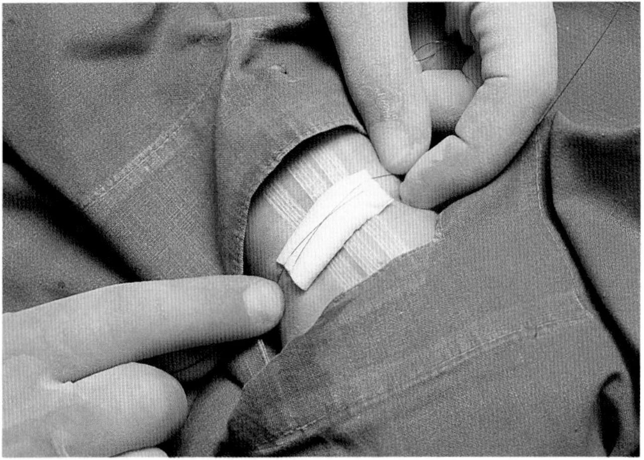

Fig. 48.10 The ends of the nylon suture are folded over a cotton wool roll, and taped in position.

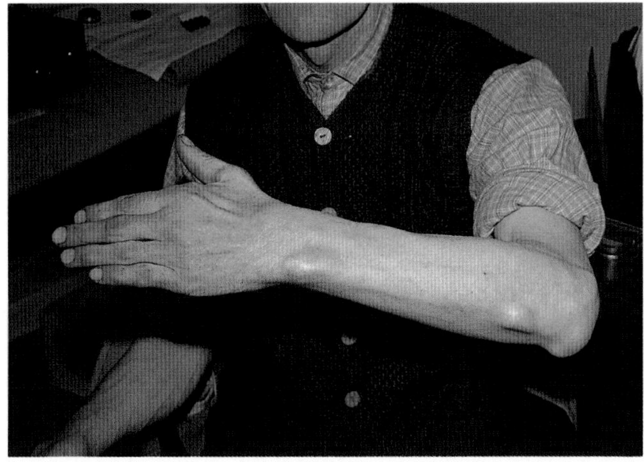

Fig. 48.11 Rheumatoid 'nodule' may be excised as for ganglion.

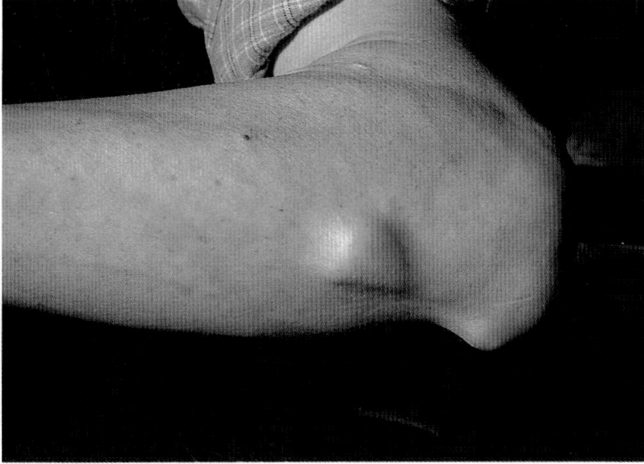

Fig. 48.12 Rheumatoid 'nodule'.

49

Caudal epidural and intravenous regional anaesthesia

Chapter 8 covers all the commonly used methods of anaesthesia suitable for minor surgery and, where possible, these are the techniques which can be recommended. However, there are rare situations where a caudal epidural anaesthetic or intravenous regional anaesthesia (Bier's block) might need to be given. Both carry risks but, provided the doctor is fully aware of these risks and takes appropriate action to minimize them, and has full facilities to deal with any complications, they are useful techniques and are included in this section of advanced minor surgical techniques.

49.1 EPIDURAL ANAESTHESIA

This method of anaesthesia has achieved great popularity, particularly in the obstetric and general surgery fields. Basically, a sterile solution of dilute local anaesthetic is introduced through a lumbar puncture-type needle into the extradural space, as opposed to a spinal anaesthetic where the solution is injected into the cerebrospinal fluid. The technique of high epidural anaesthesia is beyond the scope of this book, but caudal epidural anaesthesia is included as a valuable method of pain relief in patients with acute low back pain accompanied by muscle spasm, such as is found in prolapsed intervertebral disc lesions.

49.1.1 Technique of caudal epidural anaesthesia

Items required:

- 50 ml syringe filled with 40 ml 0.9% saline plus 10 ml 0.5% bupivacaine (Marcain)
- 2 ml syringe filled with methylprednisolone 80 mg (Depo-Medrone)
- 2 ml syringe with 1% lignocaine
- 20 swg spinal needle $3^1/_2$ in. (8.9 cm) long
- Sterile dressing pack.

The patient is placed prone on the operating theatre table or couch and a cushion placed under the pelvis to tilt the sacrum upwards.

Povidone-iodine (Betadine) alcoholic solution is painted over the overlying skin and 2 ml of 1% lignocaine is injected through to the sacral hiatus. The spinal needle is now inserted through the hiatus and just below the cornua. Some difficulty may be encountered in determining the exact

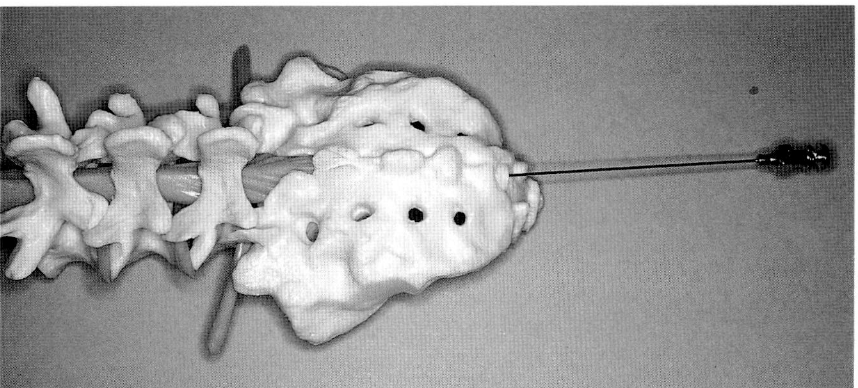

Fig. 49.1a Models to show caudal epidural injection.

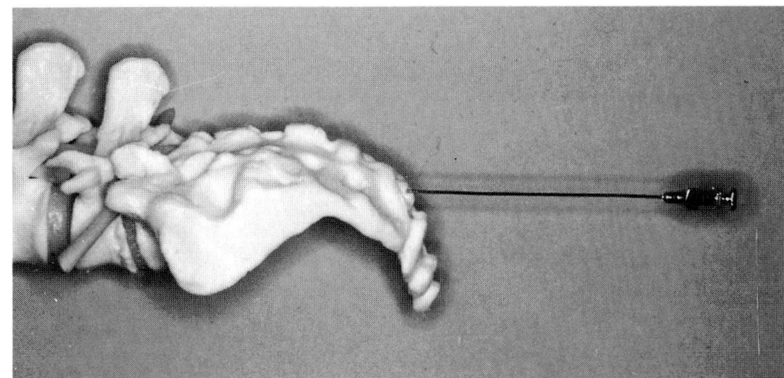

Fig. 49.1b Models to show caudal epidural injection.

angle, but it tends to be parallel to the surface of the 5th sacral segment (Fig. 49.1a, b).

After inserting the spinal needle to 5 cm the stylus is withdrawn and no fluid should be seen. If cerebrospinal fluid is seen, the procedure should be abandoned and repeated on another occasion. If blood is seen, the needle should be moved slightly until bleeding ceases.

The saline/Marcain mixture is now very slowly injected, taking 5–10 minutes.

After 40 ml has been injected, 2 ml of methylprednisolone is injected through the same needle, followed by the remaining 10 ml saline/Marcain solution. The needle is now withdrawn. After the injection the patient is left lying prone for 5–10 minutes before turning to the supine position. Half an hour later the patient may return home.

Provided an absolutely meticulous aseptic technique is employed, this is a valuable method of pain relief which can be used in general practice.

49.2 INTRAVENOUS REGIONAL ANAESTHESIA (BIER BLOCK)

The danger of intravenous regional block is that of cuff failure, whereby a large bolus of local anaesthetic is released into the circulation, resulting in major convulsions and even death.

Provided meticulous care is taken, two pneumatic tourniquets are used, and good resuscitation facilities are available, this is an extremely useful method of producing total anaesthesia, muscle relaxation, and a bloodless operating field in an arm or leg, and enables the general practitioner to increase the scope of minor surgery to include such operations as excision of ganglion, removal of foreign bodies, exploration, reduction of simple fractures, and even release of trigger finger and decompression of the carpal tunnel.

The technique was first described by August Bier in 1908 using procaine as the anaesthetic [50], but it was not until 1963 that the method achieved popularity using lignocaine [51]. As a result of the numerous side-effects of this drug, in 1965 the editorial of the Journal of the American Medical Association advised against the use of intravenous regional anaesthesia until safer agents were available.

By 1971 prilocaine had been recommended by Thorn-Alquist [52] and bupivacaine by Ware [53], who further reported favourably using bupivacaine in 1979 [54]. In 1983 serious side-effects were reported from various centres using bupivacaine for intravenous regional anaesthesia, and the drug of choice now appears to be prilocaine (Citanest). A review of the Bier's block technique by Pattison [55] in 1984 concluded that it is a safe, simple, effective, and well-tolerated method of regional anaesthesia. He could find no long-term complications attributable to the technique. The method consists of exsanguinating the limb and injecting a large volume of dilute anaesthetic intravenously through an indwelling needle; this passes retrogradely via the veins, venules, capillaries, arterioles and arteries, thence to skin, muscle and the whole limb, producing anaesthesia and muscle relaxation. Up to 1 hour operating time is obtained in a bloodless field with total anaesthesia and muscle relaxation. The following items are required for an intravenous regional block:

Orthopaedic pneumatic tourniquet
Standard sphygmomanometer and cuff
3 in. Esmarch bandage
Intravenous cannula size 18 swg (0.09 cm metric)
40 ml 0.5% prilocaine plain (Citanest).

49.2.1 Technique of Bier block for the arm

1. An intravenous cannula is inserted in a vein on the opposite limb. This is taped in position: it gives access to the circulation throughout the operation, and may be used to administer any premedication drugs intravenously (Fig. 49.2).
2. Cotton wool padding is applied around the upper arm, and an orthopaedic pneumatic tourniquet applied over it.
3. A sphygmomanometer cuff (or second orthopaedic tourniquet) is applied distal to the first tourniquet, covered with a non-stretch bandage, and inflated to just below arterial pressure. This distends the veins at the wrist. This second tourniquet acts as a safeguard should the first tourniquet fail (Fig. 49.3).
4. The 18 swg (0.09 cm) intravenous cannula is now inserted in a suitable vein, strapped in position with adhesive tape and the sphygmomanometer deflated (Fig. 49.4). A 1 ml syringe containing prilocaine is attached to the cannula and strapped in place (Fig. 49.5).

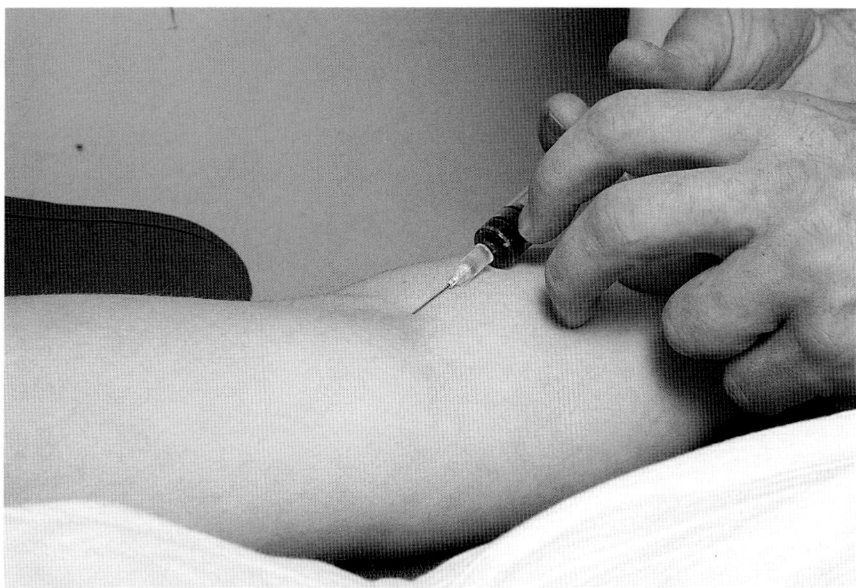

Fig. 49.2 An intravenous 'premedication' injection of midazolam and fentanyl is given.

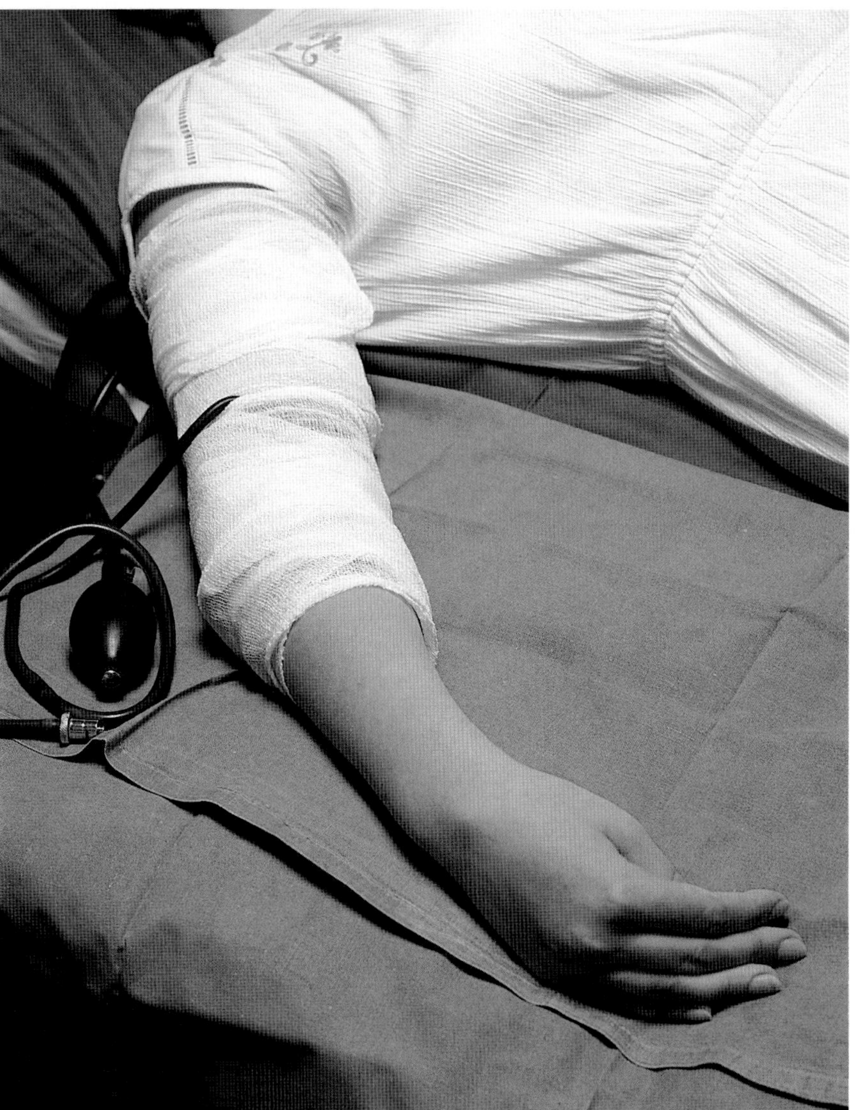

Fig. 49.3 An orthopaedic and sphygmomanometer cuff are applied to the upper arm and bandaged in place.

Fig. 49.4 After inflating one cuff to 80 mmHg, an intravenous cannula is inserted in a suitable vein.

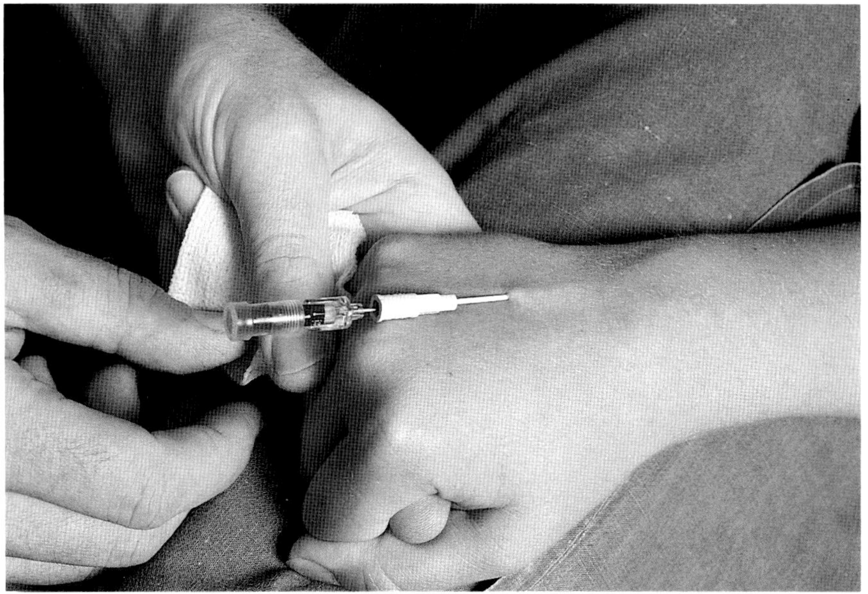

Fig. 49.5 The cuff is now deflated, the stylus withdrawn, leaving the cannula which is connected to a 1 ml syringe and prilocaine.

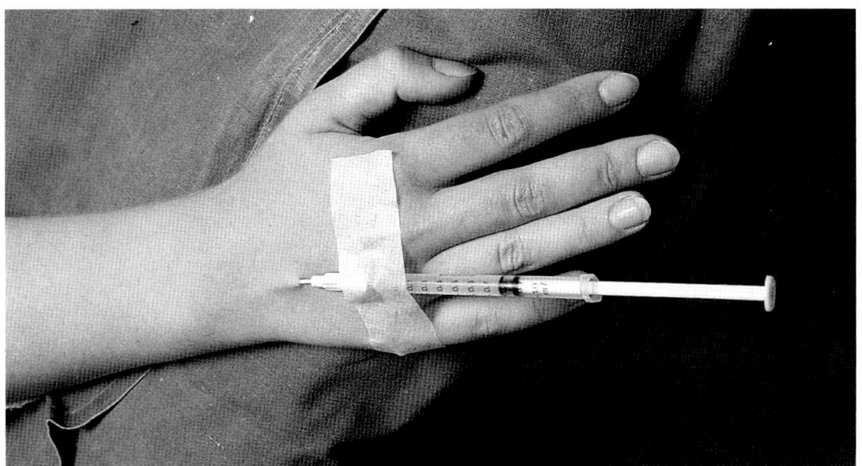

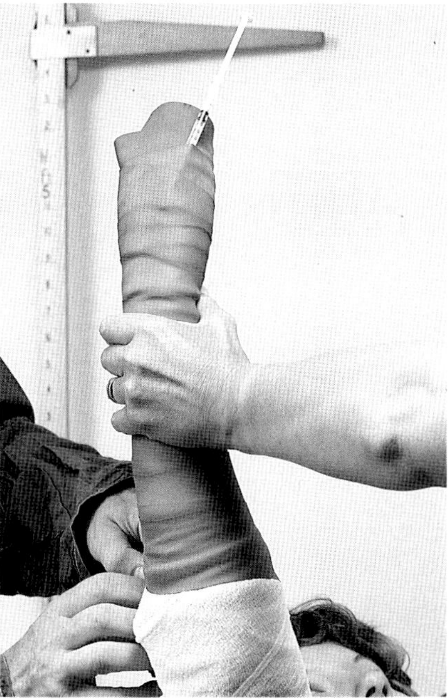

Fig. 49.6 The arm is elevated and an Esmarch bandage applied. The cuff is inflated to 300 mmHg and the bandage removed.

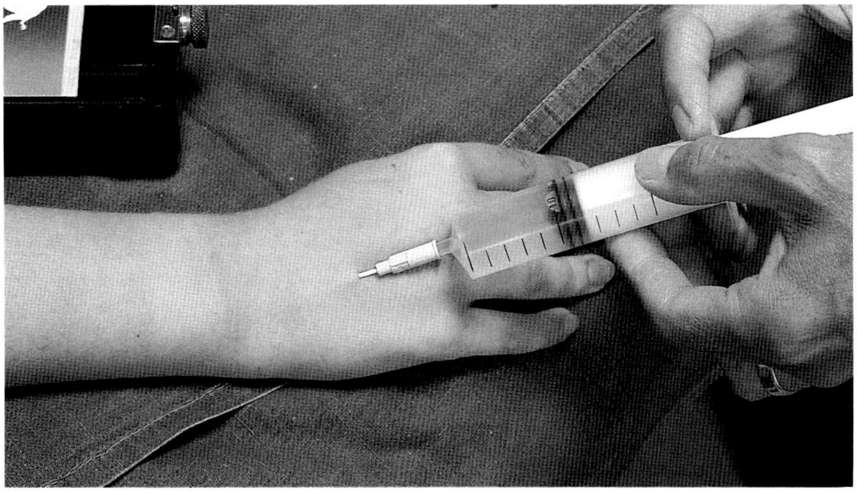

Fig. 49.7 After removing the Esmarch bandage, 30 ml 0.5% prilocaine is injected through the cannula, which is left in place for safety.

Part Four :

Administration

50

Providing information to the patient

Patients who are about to have an operation – whether major or minor – are anxious, and it is a common experience that, despite discussing the details of their forthcoming operation, most of the information is either not heard or is soon forgotten. This also applies after the operation is completed, when the doctor and nurse have spent a considerable amount of time and think that they have covered all the relevant points.

When an operation has been performed under an intravenous premedication injection of a benzodiazepine such as midazolam or diazepam, it is almost universal that the patient will remember nothing of what was said.

This can have profound psychological and even medicolegal implications, but can be prevented in almost all situations by the judicious use of pre-printed information leaflets which may be given to the patient both before and immediately after their operation. There can then be absolutely no doubt about what was intended, what to expect, when to seek further help, when to return for dressings or suture removal, and what sort of result can be anticipated.

If contact numbers are also included the patient will feel able to seek help both at an early stage, and also appropriately should there be any queries.

The following information sheets are some of those used by the author – each doctor can design his or her own sheets for their own particular situation; they can be kept in a loose-leaf folder for immediate use.

The Surgery

1 Carpal Tunnel: Preoperative information

1. The median nerve passes through a tight space at the wrist called the carpal tunnel – occasionally it becomes compressed in this tunnel causing pins and needles in the fingers, and pain which can extend up the forearm.
2. Some settle with splinting, others with tablets, and others following a steroid injection into the tunnel itself. However, when symptoms persist despite these medical measures, it is necessary to decompress the nerve surgically.
3. This will be done under a local anaesthetic supplemented by a premedication injection of a mild sedative and analgesic, and the operation will take about 30 minutes in all.
4. YOU SHOULD NOT DRIVE A CAR FOR AT LEAST 24 HOURS
5. Please make arrangements to be driven home 2 hours after the time of your operation.
6. Your hand will be bandaged and in a sling. The bandage needs to be left in place and not disturbed for 10 days when the stitch will be removed. The sling may be removed after 24 hours if comfortable.
7. It is advisable not to work for 2 weeks until after the stitch is removed.
8. If you have any questions, please do not hesitate to contact the surgery.

The Surgery

1A Carpal Tunnel Operation: Postoperative Instructions

1. The median nerve passes through a narrow tunnel at the wrist and your symptoms of pain and pins and needles have been due to pressure on this nerve.
2. The operation consisted of splitting the thick tissue which lies in front of the nerve, thus releasing the nerve and removing the pressure.
3. It may take several months before the symptoms disappear, depending on how long the nerve has been trapped; in some instances the pain and pins and needles disappear immediately, but the majority improve gradually. Where muscle wasting has occurred around the base of the thumb and little finger, release of the nerve will not improve this but will at least prevent it becoming any worse.
4. Keep the arm in a sling for 2 days, and do not disturb the bandage for 10 days.
5. There is only one single nylon suture holding the wound together; please make an appointment to have this stitch removed on

   ______________________________ at ______________________________

6. Please make an appointment to see the doctor in 6 weeks time to check that the scar is healing satisfactorily and that the symptoms are improving.
7. If you have any queries, please do not hesitate to telephone the surgery.

The Surgery

2 Ingrowing Toe-nails: Postoperative Instructions (Phenol)

1. A small strip of nail including the nail-bed has been removed, and the base treated with pure phenol to prevent this strip from regrowing.
2. When you arrive home, please rest on a settee with the feet elevated on a cushion for the remainder of the day – this reduces the discomfort and the tendency to bleeding.
3. Any simple analgesic tablet such as paracetamol may be taken for any postoperative discomfort.
4. Please make an appointment to see our nurse on

   ______________________ at ______________________

   and a second appointment to see our nurse on

   ______________________ at ______________________

5. If you have any queries, please do not hesitate to telephone the surgery.

The Surgery

2A Ingrowing Toe-nails: Postoperative Instructions (Wedge)

1. A small strip of nail on the infected side has been removed, including the nail-bed, to prevent this narrow strip from regrowing.
2. Sometimes, there is one stitch which needs to be removed on the 7th postoperative day.
3. When you arrive home, please rest on a settee with the feet elevated on a cushion for the remainder of the day – this reduces discomfort, minimizes bleeding, and helps healing.
4. Any simple analgesic tablet such as paracetamol may be taken for any postoperative discomfort.
5. Please make an appointment to see our Practice Nurse on

   ______________________ at ______________________

   and a second appointment to have the stitch removed on

   ______________________ at ______________________

6. If you have any queries, please do not hesitate to telephone the surgery.

The Surgery

2B Ingrowing Toe-nails: Postoperative Instructions (R.W.)

1. A small strip of nail on the infected side has been removed, together with any messy 'granulations'.
2. Using a radio-surgical unit, the nail-bed beneath this small strip of nail has been destroyed by passing a very high frequency electric current through it.
3. This means that the remaining nail will eventually be very slightly narrower, reducing the chances of an ingrowing nail happening again.
4. When you arrive home, please rest on a settee with the feet elevated on a cushion for the remainder of the day – this reduces any discomfort, minimizes bleeding and helps healing.
5. Any simple analgesic tablet such as paracetamol may be taken for any postoperative discomfort.
6. Please make an appointment to see our Practice Nurse on

   ______________________ at ______________________

7. If you have any queries, please do not hesitate to telephone the surgery.

The Surgery

3 Injection Treatment for Varicose Veins

Injection treatment for varicose veins consists of injecting an irritant fluid into the vein and applying a firm dressing over the injection site. The object of the treatment is to create a controlled inflammation inside the vein, and then by compressing the inflamed surfaces together, hope that they will adhere to each other, thus obliterating the lumen of the vein.

The following instructions should be followed:

1. The bandages should be left on (day and night) for 3 weeks. Some discomfort should be expected during the first few days; in a small number of patients it can be very painful, in which case you should take any simple analgesic tablet such as paracetamol, aspirin, codeine or ibuprofen at regular intervals until the pain subsides.
2. If the outer layers of the bandages work loose or begin to dig into the skin, it is helpful to remove the outer bandage carefully whilst lying down, and then to re-apply it firmly from the toes up to the knees, making sure not to disturb the pressure pads overlying the injection sites in the veins.
3. WALK AT LEAST THREE MILES EVERY DAY
4. If you wish to have a bath or shower, the bandaged leg may be kept dry by putting it inside a large waterproof polythene bag (e.g. bin liner) with two elastic bands around the top.
5. After 3 weeks please make an appointment to see the doctor to have the bandages removed.
6. If you have any queries, please do not hesitate to contact the surgery.

The Surgery

3A Stab Avulsion Varicose Veins: Information Sheet

Varicose veins may be treated by elastic support stockings, injections, stripping or, most recently, by stab avulsions.

In stab avulsion treatment, small 3 mm incisions are made in the skin overlying the vein, which is then gently pulled out. Multiple incisions are made, depending on the extent and severity of the veins. Normally no stitches are needed, and the incisions are closed just with Steri-strips with a small gauze dressing covering them. Elastic bandages are then applied over the dressings and remain in place for 2 weeks.

1. You may have a light meal before coming to the surgery if you wish.
2. If your leg is hairy, please shave it before you come – this will help with the application of the Steri-strips, and make it easier for you to remove them!
3. Ladies should wear a loose-fitting skirt.
4. Men should wear a pair of shorts under their trousers.
5. Please bring loose-fitting shoes or slippers to wear home as your foot will have several layers of bandages.
6. PLEASE ARRANGE TRANSPORT HOME 2 HOURS AFTER THE TIME OF YOUR OPERATION
7. Under NO circumstances must you drive yourself home or drive a car for at least 24 hours.
8. When you arrive home, go immediately to bed and remain there for at least 12 hours. Gentle walking is encouraged.
9. You will need to take one week off work, possibly two, depending on how comfortable the leg is, and what your job entails.
10. If your doctor has given you a prescription for special bandages or elastic stockings, collect them from the chemist and bring them with you on the day of the operation.
11. You will be given a postoperative instruction sheet on the day of the operation.
12. If you have any questions, please do not hesitate to telephone the surgery.

The Surgery

3B Stab Avulsion Varicose Veins: Postoperative Instructions

1. In this form of treatment, a small incision has been made in the skin adjacent to the varicose vein and a small segment of vein removed. Multiple incisions are made, depending on the extent and severity of the veins. Normally no stitches are used, and the incisions closed with just Steri-strips, covered by a small dressing, elastic bandages and Tubigrip.
2. To prevent any bleeding on the way home, an additional strong elastic bandage has been applied over all the above bandages, and this may be removed after you are in bed at home.
3. When you arrive home, **go immediately to bed and remain there for 12 hours**. This is essential, and is to allow the small blood vessels under the skin to seal off and let the bandages apply an even pressure over the leg.
4. Bleeding can occasionally occur under the bandages and some soak through. Should this occur, remain in bed, lie flat, and raise the foot; as the blood is coming from a vein and not an artery, raising the leg will stop the bleeding. If, however, you are concerned, please contact this surgery and speak to one of the doctors.
5. **Keep the bandages on for 10 days.**
6. If they feel uncomfortable or are working loose, it is permissible to re-apply them yourself – do this lying down rather than standing, and endeavour to keep an even pressure from the toes to the top of the dressing.
7. Gentle walking each day is helpful.
8. On the 10th day take off the Tubigrip and elastic bandage and have a bath. This will soak off the Steri-strips and dressings.
9. Bruising and discolouration is common at this stage and is harmless; it is due to blood collecting under the skin and disappears over the next few weeks.
10. Re-apply the Tubigrip for another 4 days.
11. Make an appointment to see one of our practice nurses 2 weeks after the date of your operation to check that everything is healing satisfactorily.
12. TWO MONTHS after your operation, would you make an appointment to see the doctor for a final check.
13. If you have any queries, please do not hesitate to contact the surgery.

The Surgery

4 Injection Treatment for Ganglion

A ganglion is a cyst filled with clear jelly; it is often situated near a joint, and may cause pain and slowly increase in size. Some eventually rupture spontaneously and disappear, but this may not happen for up to three years.

1. Injection treatment consists of drawing off the jelly from the ganglion and then injecting an irritant fluid into the empty cyst.
2. This causes an inflammation within the ganglion. A pressure bandage is then applied with the object of compressing the inflamed surfaces and thus obliterating the cyst.
3. **Please keep the bandage in place for 2 weeks.**
4. If it works loose, you may re-apply it firmly, but do not disturb the pressure-pad overlying the ganglion.
5. A the end of 2 weeks you may remove the pad and bandage, and normally no further follow-up visits are needed.
6. This treatment carries an 80% cure rate and has the advantage that there is no scar. If, however, you are in the 20% which recur, the same treatment can be offered again.
7. If you have any queries, please do not hesitate to contact the surgery.

The Surgery

5 Instructions Following Treatment with Liquid Nitrogen

1. Liquid nitrogen destroys tissues by freezing to –196°C. This results in ice forming inside the cells and, as this thaws, it causes cell death.
2. Immediately following treatment, apart from a slight discomfort, it will look as if nothing has happened to the skin.
3. Gradually, over the next few days, swelling, reddening and sometimes blistering will occur.
4. Following this stage, healing occurs, which is usually remarkably pain-free, and leaves only a very slight scar or none at all.
5. In dark skins there is usually an area of depigmentation following cryotherapy; this normally recovers over the following year.
6. Reaction to liquid nitrogen is very variable; in some patients quite alarming looking blisters can occur together with swelling of the surrounding tissues. Despite this, satisfactory healing occurs.
7. Keep the treated area dry for 6 days if at all possible – it does not need any dressing unless blistering occurs, in which case just a simple non-stick dressing may be applied.
8. More than one treatment is commonly required.
9. If you have any queries, please do not hesitate to contact the surgery.

The Surgery

6 Electrocautery: Postoperative Instructions

1. Many warts, moles, naevi and keratoses can be removed with a scalpel or curette, and the base cauterized with the electrocautery. This stops any bleeding.
2. Alternatively, the mole may be removed entirely with the electrocautery or a high-frequency electro-surgical unit. This cuts through the tissues and seals any bleeding points simultaneously, thus avoiding the need for any stitches and in many cases gives a neater scar.
3. After cautery, healing occurs over the next few weeks.
4. It is helpful to keep the area dry for 2 or 3 days.
5. When you remove any dressing you may find a reddened, weeping area which forms a dry crust. This will then separate leaving a bright pink area, and may even form another crust.
6. Try not to pick off any scabs or crusts, but allow them to come away naturally.
7. The bright pink area will slowly fade to match the surrounding skin over a period of 18 months to 2 years.
8. Where possible, every specimen is sent for routine examination under a microscope to establish an exact diagnosis. We normally receive the results back from the laboratory after 10 days. You can assume that if you have not heard from us the lesion was harmless, but we are happy to give you the result personally if you contact the surgery.
9. If you have any queries, please do not hesitate to contact the surgery.

The Surgery

7 Meibomian Cysts: Postoperative Instructions

1. A Meibomian cyst occurs inside the eye-lid and is caused by a blockage of one of the little lubricating glands.
2. Treatment consists of incising the cyst under local anaesthetic.
3. This is done from inside the lid so there will not be any visible scar.
4. After the operation eye-ointment is applied and a pad and bandage put on; this is to protect the eye against dust, etc. on the way home as the eye will still be anaesthetized.
5. The pad and bandage may be removed after 4 hours.
6. Do not be alarmed when you remove the pad – there will be a mixture of ointment, secretions and blood which can look alarming!
7. Gently clean the eye-lids with warm water and a face flannel.
8. Thereafter, apply the chloramphenicol eye-drops three times a day for 1 week.
9. It is not normally necessary to see you again, but if you have any queries please do not hesitate to contact the surgery.

The Surgery

8 Tongue-tie: Preoperative and Postoperative Instructions

1. The fibrous band holding down the tongue can usually be divided under a local anaesthetic.
2. One hour before your operation, apply the local anaesthetic solution on a dental cotton-wool roll to the area below the tongue. It is helpful to renew the anaesthetic solution three or four times until that part of the mouth feels completely 'numb'.
3. Do not have hot drinks from now on, until normal sensation returns as there would be a risk of burning the inside of the mouth. Likewise, avoid biting on the inside of the cheek with the teeth.
4. Following the operation, rinse the mouth out with warm water or mouth-rinse three or four times a day until healing has taken place.
5. Bleeding is unusual – however, should it occur, it may easily be controlled by applying a clean dressing or handkerchief and pressing firmly for at least **10 minutes by the clock**.
6. Normally, no follow-up is necessary. If you do have any queries, please do not hesitate to contact the surgery.

The Surgery

9 Hormone Implants

1. Most of the symptoms occurring at the menopause are due to a deficiency of oestrogens.
2. Hormone replacement therapy (HRT) consists of giving oestrogens to the patient and, in the majority of women, all the symptoms are relieved. As well as relieving symptoms, it has been shown to offer protection against osteoporosis (thinning of the bones), heart disease and stroke, and can even lower the levels of cholesterol.
3. Oestrogens may be given as tablets, adhesive patches, creams or implants.
4. A hormone implant consists of a small tablet of pure oestradiol (the naturally occurring hormone in the body) which is inserted just under the skin. This is done under local anaesthetic and the skin closed with either a single stitch or by skin closure adhesive Steri-strips.
5. The implant slowly dissolves, releasing the oestradiol over a period of six months.
6. If you have had a hysterectomy, hormone replacement is very simple as you will only need oestrogens. If, however, you still have a uterus, you will need additional progesterone and this can be given intermittently each month to bring on a period, or continuously when it may be possible to avoid having a period.
7. Some patients feel their implant has 'worn off" in less than six months and feel they would like another at shorter intervals. This is generally not advisable nor necessary as blood tests show the level of circulating oestradiol is still adequate, and another implant would raise the levels too much. Thus, unless your doctor has recommended otherwise, we suggest **one implant every six months** will give the best results.
8. After five months please would you make an appointment to see our Practice Nurse. This will enable us to offer a simple check-up, answer any questions about HRT, and at this visit we can give you a prescription for the next implant.
9. At this visit you can also make an appointment for your next implant.

The Surgery

10 Patient Information Leaflet: Basal Cell Carcinoma

1. A basal cell carcinoma (also known as a rodent ulcer or BCC) is a type of skin tumour which is increasing in frequency in this country.
2. It is thought to arise from previous repeated exposures to severe ultra violet light causing sun burn up to 40 years previously.
3. They are not malignant cancers (i.e. they do not spread to other parts of the body producing secondary tumours), but slowly grow and, if not treated, become larger and larger, slowly invading tissues beneath the surface.
4. Small basal cell cancers can be treated in a variety of ways – some are excised surgically and the wound stitched, others are treated with radiotherapy, some with liquid nitrogen cryotherapy, and others by removing with a steel spoon and cauterizing the base several times with a diathermy or electrocautery.
5. Whichever method is chosen, it is essential to have meticulous follow-up for several years – your doctor will let you know how this should be done in your case.
6. As a general guide, however, if there are no signs of any lumps re-appearing in the scar of the original tumour, all is well. If you think there may be a recurrence, please contact your doctor for advice.

The Surgery

11 Care of Wounds which have been Sutured

1. When suturing a wound the object is to obtain the neatest scar possible.
2. This is achieved at the time of the operation by inserting many fine sutures, rather than a few, widely-spaced, thick sutures.
3. It is also helped by designing the scar such that the minimum tension occurs on the skin edges.
4. As well as sutures we sometimes use sterile self-adhesive strips (Steri-strips) to support the edges of the wound while it is healing.
5. Where the wound is deep, we also insert absorbable sutures under the skin to give additional support during healing.
6. The timing of the removal of sutures is critical – if they are left in too long 'cross-hatching' can occur leaving permanent scars, whereas if they are removed too soon the edges of the wound can gape open.
7. Where there is little tension on the skin, e.g. the face, the sutures may be removed after only a few days, but where there is considerable tension, e.g. over the knee, shoulder or back, we need to leave them in for a much longer time.
8. You can help to achieve the neatest scar yourself by following the following simple rules:
   a) Where the wound is open to the air (e.g. on the face and scalp) keep it dry for at least 48 hours.
   b) Where the wound is covered, keep it dry and do not disturb the dressing – this will prevent any infection.
9. Please make an appointment with our nurse to have the stitches removed on

   ______________________ at ______________________

10. If the wound looks reddened or discharging, or you are at all concerned, please do not hesitate to contact the surgery.
11. We may apply Steri-strips to the wound after the stitches have been removed – this is to give external support; it helps to leave these in place for as long as possible.
12. In certain sites such as the arm and shoulder it is helpful to apply Steri-strip support for several weeks after the stitches have been removed.

The Surgery

12 Removal of Skin Lesions by Radio-surgery

1. Radio-surgery is a new method of treating many skin lesions using high-frequency radiowaves (4 million hertz) which both cuts through the skin and also seals off any small bleeding vessels.
2. This tends to give superior cosmetic results to conventional surgical excision or electrocautery.
3. At the end of the treatment a small plaster is usually applied – please keep this in place for 2 days.
4. After this time the plaster may be removed and the area cleaned gently with warm, soapy water.
5. Healing can take from 1 to 4 weeks depending on the size of the original lesion; during this time it helps to keep the wound clean and moist by regular washing with warm, soapy water – about six times a day using soft cotton-wool. Do not rub the area too vigorously or it may bleed. If bleeding does occur it may be stopped by covering with a small dressing and pressing firmly with the finger for 10 minutes.
6. Normally no other treatment is necessary, but if the area becomes very messy or inflamed or develops a reddened surrounding area which seems to be spreading, please contact the surgery for advice.
7. Initially the wound will be moist with a slight discharge. This will gradually dry and may form a thin scab on the surface. Try not to pick this off but leave to separate naturally.
8. At this stage the wound will appear bright red and dry.
9. Over the next few weeks the reddened area will gradually fade and eventually, after about 18 months, should match the surrounding skin.
10. The majority of all lesions are sent to the hospital for routine examination under a microscope, and we normally receive the full histological report after 10 days.
11. If you have any concerns, please do not hesitate to contact the surgery.

The Surgery

13 Advice about 'Moles' and 'Naevi'

1. Moles (naevi) occur on everyone.
2. The majority are harmless and remain harmless, but in recent years there has been a marked increase in three types of mole:
   (a) Basal cell carcinoma
   (b) Squamous cell carcinoma
   (c) Malignant melanoma
3. It is now realized that exposure to sunlight increases the chances of developing melanoma and skin cancers. There may be a delay of 10–40 years between exposure and the development of a skin tumour.
4. Basal cell cancers (rodent ulcers) and squamous cell cancers are thought to arise in people who have repeated exposure to strong sunlight (e.g. farm workers, etc.) They start as a small raised, circular lesion, slightly translucent with very small blood vessels crossing the surface, and are commonly seen on the face. Basal cell carcinomas are not malignant (i.e. don't spread to distant parts of the body), but just tend to get bigger and invade local tissues. Treatment is removal surgically.
5. Malignant melanoma is the most serious of the skin tumours. It is thought to arise following one episode of severe blistering sunburn many years previously. It can spread to glands and other parts of the body, so early diagnosis and treatment is essential. Treatment is by wide surgical excision.
6. The most important advice is to seek medical help for any mole which **has recently changed**, i.e. changed colour, changed size, or has started to bleed or itch.
7. Some facts about melanoma:
   1) They are commonly more than 1cm in diameter
   2) They are irregular in outline
   3) They are usually multi coloured, black, brown, pink and red
   4) The mole has recently changed size or colour
   5) It may itch
   6) They are common in fair-skinned people
   7) They are very rare before puberty
   8) They may be raised above the surface of the skin
   9) They are more common in people who already have more than 50 pre-existing moles.
8. IF IN DOUBT SEEK MEDICAL ADVICE
9. Prevention:
   (a) Although everyone likes a sun tan and enjoys the warmth of sunbathing, over-exposure to sunlight is definitely bad for you.
   (b) Therefore, avoid exposure to sun.
   (c) Avoid getting accidentally sun-burned.
   (d) Protect children from sunlight.
   (e) Use high factor sun barrier cream (Factor 15 or above).
   (f) Don't use sun beds.
   (g) Cover any dark moles before exposure to sunlight with total sunblock cream or clothing.

Other harmless skin lesions

Benign intradermal naevus – a raised, circular mole
Melanocytic naevus – a coloured mole
Juvenile melanoma – very dark, usually in children; harmless
Solar keratosis – flaky, warty lesion
Seborrhoeic wart – coloured, warty lesion, usually on trunk
Hand warts and verrucae – harmless but a nuisance; caused by a virus
Blue naevus – black/blue small circular raised spot
Kerato-acanthoma – rapidly growing warty lesion with rough centre
Molluscum contagiosum – small, pearly spots with dimple in centre; can spread
Histiocytoma (dermato-fibroma) – hard nodule in the skin; pale, harmless

Terminology

Solar – Related to exposure to sunlight
Actinic – also related to sunlight
Melanocytic – coloured
Benign – harmless
Intradermal – in the skin
Naevus – another name for a mole

The Surgery

14 Tennis Elbow

1. Tennis elbow is diagnosed by a very painful spot over the outer bony part of the elbow.
2. It is thought to be due to tearing of a few tendon fibres where they are attached to the bone at the elbow – usually as a result of repeated muscle strain (e.g. such as playing tennis).
3. If left to nature, all tennis elbows eventually recover, but it may take several years.
4. Various treatments have been suggested but none are very successful.
5. Injection with steroid and local anaesthetic gives about the best results when other treatments have failed.
6. The injection itself can be quite painful, and during the next two or three days the pain may be very severe and require strong pain killers.
7. After a few days, if the injection has been successful, the original pain disappears.
8. Unfortunately, if you are still overusing the arm a tennis elbow can recur.
9. Following an injection, it is helpful to rest the elbow for two days, avoiding any heavy lifting and repetitive movements.
10. Up to three injections can be given, but each becomes less effective, and if symptoms persist after three injections it is better to live with it, knowing that it will eventually clear on its own.
11. In very rare cases an operation can be offered if symptoms are extremely severe, but even this cannot guarantee a cure!

The Surgery

The Treatment of Piles (Haemorrhoids)

1. Piles are merely veins inside the anus.
2. They can bleed or even prolapse.
3. Bleeding, when it occurs, is usually painless and bright red.
4. Treatment is important to abolish any bleeding, otherwise more serious conditions such as tumours and ulcers may be missed.
5. Simple piles can be treated with creams and suppositories.
6. Where these measures fail, injections and/or banding may be offered.
7. Where injections are done, a small volume of oily phenol is injected above the pile, and this causes it to shrink over the next six weeks.
8. Where 'banding' is done, a small neoprene band is applied to the loose lining above the pile, and this pulls the pile away from the anus, preventing it prolapsing. The band eventually drops off.
9. Both injections and banding are remarkably pain-free. A slight discomfort may be experienced during the procedure, but this soon passes off.
10. Improvement occurs gradually over the following six weeks.
11. To help recovery, please note the following instructions:
    (a) Avoid becoming constipated.
    (b) Drink plenty of water (more than 6 glasses daily).
    (c) Do not sit for a long time on the toilet (i.e. do not take a library book in the 'loo'). Wait until you feel you need to have your bowels open and then go quickly. Sitting and straining makes piles worse.
    (d) Eat plenty of fruit and vegetables in your diet.
12. You may notice bleeding during the first six weeks following injections or banding – this is quite normal.
13. **Bleeding which occurs after six weeks should be reported**.
14. If you have any concerns, please do not hesitate to contact the surgery.

The Surgery

19 Information Sheet: Ganglion

1. A ganglion is a cyst filled with clear jelly.
2. They usually occur near an underlying joint, particularly at the wrist, and fingers, and can cause pain or discomfort.
3. It is possible they arise from a leak of lubricating jelly in the joint through the tissues, to the skin, where they appear as a smooth, tender swelling.
4. Many ganglia, if left alone, will eventually disappear on their own, but this may take many years.
5. An old-fashioned treatment used to be to hit it with the Family Bible in the hope of bursting it and releasing the jelly under the skin. Unfortunately, this treatment was never very successful, and there was a high recurrence rate!
6. Small ganglia on the fingers can be pricked with a sterile needle and the jelly squeezed out. If a firm tape is then applied around two-thirds of the finger for six weeks, this carries an 80% cure rate and can always be repeated if the first attempt fails.
7. Larger ganglia around the wrist can be cut out, but even this carries a 20% recurrence rate so is not always the preferred treatment unless everyone is desperate!
8. At this surgery we offer a treatment called 'Aspiration and sclerose' which involves putting a small amount of local anaesthetic in the skin, inserting a needle into the ganglion, and sucking out the jelly. We then inject a small quantity of sclerosant, which makes the inside of the cyst sticky, and then apply a firm compression bandage for the next two weeks.
9. The object of this bandage is to press the front and back walls of the cyst together in the hope that they will stick together and seal off the little hole through which the jelly has leaked.
10. This treatment also carries an 80% cure rate, but has the advantage that it does not leave a scar and, should the ganglion recur, we can always repeat the treatment.

The Surgery

20 Information Sheet: Warts

1. Warts are caused by a virus and therefore spread by contact.
2. Verrucae are warts on the sole of the foot.
3. If left alone, the majority of warts and verrucae will eventually disappear. This is because the body has built up a high enough level of immunity to the wart virus and at this stage the wart is destroyed.
4. When warts disappear spontaneously they do not leave a scar.
5. Treatments are many and varied! As with most conditions in medicine, where there are many different treatments available, it usually means none of them is particularly effective!
6. Simple remedies can be purchased from the chemists and consist of paints, ointments and plasters. It is important to follow the instructions.
7. Where there are large numbers of warts or verrucae, no treatment seems to be very good, and it probably means waiting patiently until they disappear on their own.
8. Large, single, stubborn warts can be treated either with liquid nitrogen or surgically. Liquid nitrogen destroys the wart by freezing to –196°C and is very effective in many cases.
9. If this fails we can remove the wart surgically or with a radiowave surgical instrument.
10. It is important to realize that no treatment can offer a 100% guarantee of cure. Even with very thorough treatment they can return, so you should be aware of this possibility.

51

Medicolegal aspects of minor surgery

(Based on the booklet of the same title by Dr Patrick Dando of the Medical Defence Union Ltd)

> *If a doctor fails to exercise the skill which he has, or claims to have, he is in breach of his duty of care. He is negligent*
>
> *Donaldson L.J.*

Many doctors contemplating minor surgery are worried about possible medicolegal implications, and even litigation. Fortunately, up to the present time, minor surgery in general practice has not been a 'high-risk' area as far as medicolegal problems are concerned. This chapter covers those aspects which will enable the doctor to offer a high standard of care, so that his technique will not be open to criticism, and to reduce the risk of harm to his patients.

51.1 SURGICAL SKILL

All doctors must evaluate their surgical proficiency before offering a minor surgery service to patients; to this end it is good practice to approach a local consultant surgical colleague to discuss any problems, to ask for guidance, and for support in the future. This is usually more than willingly given.

As experience grows, doctors may wish to extend their range of surgical skills; it is important always to ensure that they have received adequate instruction and supervised practice before embarking on any new minor operation.

51.2 PREOPERATIVE ASSESSMENT OF THE PATIENT

Careful preoperative assessment of the lesion and a patient's suitability for minor surgery is fundamental to safety. Where the doctor suspects a malignant melanoma, or basal-cell or squamous-cell carcinoma, the patient should be referred urgently to a specialist colleague for assessment.

Certain patients such as very young children, elderly, frail patients, and the psychiatrically disturbed may find difficulty coping with a procedure done under local anaesthesia, or may find difficulties with mobility during the postoperative period. It would, therefore, be wise to refer such patients.

Knowledge about the patient's past medical history and current medication is extremely important. Such conditions as diabetes, peripheral vascular disease, skin sepsis, and previous keloid scar formation would be possible contraindications to operation, as would treatment with anticoagulants and long-term steroids. Patients taking any medication which affects coagulation and haemostasis such as warfarin, aspirin, non-steroidal anti-inflammatory drugs, and the oral contraceptive pill should be given careful assessment; in certain circumstances stopping the medication one week prior to surgery may be advisable.

Certain lesions have predictable difficulties: sebaceous cysts on the back of the neck can be quite difficult to remove, or extremely vascular, and frequently difficult to anaesthetize adequately. Similarly, lipomata, particularly in the midline on the back, or large lipomata over the shoulder may be found to extend deeper than originally anticipated and are better referred.

Recurrent lesions may also be better referred, as fibrous scarring may make accurate dissection difficult. Keloid scars should never be revised as a larger keloid scar will certainly recur. The skin over the anterior tibial surface heals poorly, so care needs to be taken in removing any lesion in this site.

51.3 CONSENT

For most minor surgical procedures in general practice, informed oral consent is adequate. If the doctor feels a written consent form is necessary, this should be signed by both the patient and the doctor only after the whole procedure has been carefully explained to, and understood by the patient. Written consent should be obtained for vasectomy (Chapter 39). The fact that consent has been obtained should be recorded in the patient's notes, together with any warning about visible scars or risk of keloid formation. It is also important to explain to the patient what alternative treatments are available, what to expect at operation, that there will inevitably be a scar (it is surprising how many patients assume they can have an operation without a scar!), how much time off work may be needed, and to ensure they have adequate transport home. Keloid scarring is more likely on the anterior chest wall, deltoid, shoulder, and back of neck, particularly in patients of Afro-Caribbean origin.

51.4 HISTOLOGY

Because surprises can always occur, it is good practice to send every specimen for histological examination. Not only does this establish an accurate diagnosis, but also improves the doctors diagnostic acumen. Where a laboratory finds it cannot deal with all specimens, one of two alternative courses of action are possible:

1. Selected specimens should be fixed, mounted in paraffin wax, but filed away, only to be sectioned and examined if a subsequent query arises.
2. The consultant histopathologist should provide written criteria to define those lesions which do not need to be sent for routine examination.

The usual fixative is 10% formaldehyde in normal saline – remember this is toxic and should be kept away from young children. The specimen should be carefully labelled with the patient's name and address and the nature of the specimen.

It is not sufficient just to send every specimen for routine histological examination; it is essential that a foolproof system is evolved whereby every histology report is personally seen by the doctor. To this end, a 'Histology Book' can be recommended (Chapter 19) whereby the patient's name and address, specimen, clinical diagnosis and histological diagnosis are recorded. By putting a tick opposite each entry when the report is received and noted, any missing reports can easily be identified.

51.5 DANGER AREAS

Before making an incision, a thorough knowledge of the underlying anatomy is essential, particularly the surface markings of nerves, arteries, and tendons.

The axilla, femoral triangle, neck and wrist are complicated areas anatomically, and great caution needs to be exercised. If it pulsates – don't touch it! Incisions in the line of skin creases will give the neatest scars (Chapter 10), but beware of three areas where superficial nerves may be damaged:

1. The posterior triangle of the neck (spinal accessory nerve)
2. Lateral side of popliteal fossa (common peroneal nerve)
3. Side of the jaw (mandibular branch of the facial nerve).

Operations on the face, particularly for cosmetic reasons, should be given careful consideration, and if necessary referred to a plastic surgeon. Skin closure can be difficult on the tip of the nose, and pinna of the ear; similarly, beware of excising lesions near the eyes, particularly near the nasolachrymal ducts.

Before suturing lacerations following trauma, ensure that there are no foreign bodies still present, and that no vascular damage has occurred. If necessary arrange an X-ray, and check the patient's tetanus immunization status.

51.6 INFECTION

It is essential that all surgical instruments are properly sterilized [5, 57]; this requires the use of an autoclave or hot-air oven, or CSSD facilities (Chapter 6). Given this, infection rates for general practitioner minor surgery are very low.

For both patients' and doctors' safety, gloves should be worn, and hepatitis-B vaccine offered to both doctors and assistants. No doctor should operate if he has any infection, particularly one involving the hands.

It is worth considering giving prophylactic antibiotics to those patients with a past history of rheumatic fever, a pacemaker, artificial heart valves, or any artificial joint.

If electrocautery or diathermy is to be used, avoid any spirit-based antiseptics which may ignite. Joint injections and aspirations must be done under completely aseptic conditions.

51.7 ANAESTHETICS

As a general guide, local anaesthetics are remarkably safe, but the doctor should be aware of the maximum dose for each preparation used (see Chapter 8). Lignocaine should be used cautiously in patients with cardiac and hepatic disease. Lignocaine with added adrenaline should not be used on any digit, the tip of the nose, ear, penis, or scrotum.

Nerve blocks in experienced hands provide safe and efficient means of anaesthesia, but if the doctor is considering using an intravenous regional block (Bier's block), scrupulous attention to detail must be observed, an assistant should **always** be present to monitor the tourniquet, a double sphygmomanometer cuff employed, and full resuscitation facilities available (Chapters 8 and 49). Similar safeguards also apply where intravenous diazepam or midazolam is used, and the doctor should also be aware that benzodiazepines may cause not only amnesia, but also hallucinations.

51.8 PRODUCT LIABILITY

Under the Consumer Protection Act 1987, it is now necessary for a doctor to record the batch numbers and source of supply of all drugs, anaesthetics, and suture materials used for minor surgery. Also, all equipment used should be properly maintained and records kept that this has been done. Such records need to be kept for 11 years.

51.9 MISHAPS

In the unlikely event of a mishap, it is sensible to inform the patient immediately of the facts, with the simple courtesy of a sincere apology, and to ensure that arrangements can be set in hand to rectify the problem quickly. Such action should be recorded in the patient's notes, and advice sought from the doctor's medical defence organization.

Fortunately, with appropriate selection and care, such problems are exceedingly rare, and should not deter a doctor from offering a minor surgery service to his patients.

52

The general practitioner and the National Health Service

I hope the House will not hesitate to tell the British Medical Association that we look forward to this Act starting on 5th July 1948 and that we expect the Medical Profession to take their proper part in it because we are satisfied that there is nothing in it that any doctor should be otherwise than proud to acknowledge

Aneurin Bevan, 1897–1960

52.1 REMUNERATION

The remuneration of a general practitioner working within the National Health Service is derived from the number of patients registered on his or her 'list', together with additional item-of-service payments and allowances as follows [58]:

Basic practice allowance (Para 12)
Seniority payments (Para 16)
Employment of an assistant (Para 18)
Associate allowance (Para 19)
Deprivation payments (Para 20)
Standard capitation fees (Para 21)
Child health surveillance fees (Para 22)
Registration fees (Para 23)
Night visit fees (Para 24)
Target payment childhood immunizations (Para 25)
Target payment for pre-school boosters (Para 26)
Vaccinations and immunizations (Para 27)
Schedule of procedures eligible for a fee (Para 27)
Target payments for cervical cytology (Para 28)
Contraceptive services (Para 29)
Health promotion and chronic disease management (Para 30)
Maternity medical services (Para 31)
Temporary residents (Para 32)
Fees for emergency treatment (Para 33)
Fees for services of an anaesthetist (Para 34)
Fee for arrest of dental haemorrhage (Para 35)
Fee for immediately necessary treatment (Para 36)
Postgraduate education allowance (Para 37)

Trainee practitioner scheme (Para 38)
Doctors' retainer scheme (Para 39)
Fee for teaching undergraduate medical students (Para 40)
Fee for minor surgery (Para 42)
Rural practice payments (Para 43)
Supply of drugs and appliances (Para 44)
Education courses (Para 47)
GP computer reimbursement scheme (Para 58)
Drugs
DMO reports
Others

Before considering these paragraphs, it is important to clarify when a doctor may charge a fee. Under their terms of service, general practitioners are expressly forbidden from asking for, or receiving, payment for, or token in lieu of, the provision of any medical service for any patient registered with them under the National Health Service [57]. The only exceptions which are allowed are for certain documents, private certificates, and vaccination certificates. A GP is allowed to accept private fee-paying patients, provided they are not already registered with the GP or his or her partners under the National Health Service, and charges may be made to such patients for all medical services rendered.

In the past it was suggested that a general practitioner could request the removal of a NHS patient from his or her list for 3 months and treat the patient privately, in which case the charging of a fee is allowable. Although this is perfectly legal, most doctors would not be happy to do it, and it cannot be recommended.

An item-of-service fee is payable for a minor surgical operation performed on a patient receiving emergency medical treatment who is not registered with that general practitioner, nor any of his or her partners. In this case, form FP 32 is completed, provided the emergency was not caused by the use of a motor vehicle on the road! What constitutes a minor surgical operation is not defined in this section of the regulations.

Likewise, a separate item-of-service fee is payable for the administration of a general anaesthetic, provided a second qualified doctor (not a trainee general practitioner) is in attendance and personally administers the anaesthetic. This is claimed on form FP 31. Thus, although the numbers of general anaesthetics given in general practice outside hospital is decreasing, nevertheless, there is a recognition by the Department of Health that the administration of a general anaesthetic qualifies for an additional payment. No such item-of-service payment exists for the administration of any local anaesthetic, be it infiltration, nerve block, or epidural. It is possible, however, to obtain indirect reimbursement by careful use of the 'Red Book' utilizing paragraph 44.13 for all injections, anaesthetics, suture materials, intrauterine contraceptive devices, and skin closure strips, as follows:

1. The doctor personally purchases all injections, anaesthetics, sutures, coils, and skin closure strips.
2. For each patient where any of the above are used, and which the

doctor or their nurse personally administers, the doctor writes the items on a standard FP 10 prescription form.
3. The patient pays no prescription charge, irrespective of age or exemption category.
4. Once per month, all prescriptions are sent to the Central Prescription Pricing Bureau together with a claim form FP 34 duly signed.
5. The doctor is subsequently refunded as follows:
   (a) The basic price of the item used.
   (b) An 'on-cost' allowance.
   (c) A 'container' allowance.
   (d) A dispensing fee.

This results in a very small profit on each item prescribed. As an example, for the excision of a sebaceous cyst, the practitioner could submit prescriptions for three items used, namely local anaesthetic, suture materials, and Steri-strips.

In addition to utilizing paragraph 44.13, savings may be achieved by writing a prescription for certain drugs, dressings, and appliances used for any surgical procedure, giving it to the patient, who then brings it back for use by the doctor on that particular patient. However, it must not be overlooked that the general medical practitioner already receives a few pence each year included in the patient's capitation fee to take account of the occasional bandage and dressing.

Items which may be obtained on prescription include the following:

All bandages, whatever type and size
Elastoplast bandages
Eye pad and bandage
Triangular bandages
Cotton wool, lint, gamgee, gauze
Catheters, drainage bags
Self adhesive tapes
Povidone-iodine alcoholic solution
Any drugs, ointments, creams, drops
Injections and insufflations used.

52.2 1990 CONTRACT

Under the Government Contract introduced in 1990 minor surgery was recognized for the first time, and a limited payment scheme introduced (SFA 42.1–42.6). In order for a general practitioner to be able to claim the fees for minor surgical procedures he must apply to be included in the Family Health Services Authority's 'Minor Surgery List'. This usually entails an inspection of his premises and equipment, together with record-keeping, sterilization, histology, and resuscitation facilities, and suitable instruments and rooms. He may also have to demonstrate competence in the various procedures on the list.

52.3 MINOR SURGERY PROCEDURES

- Injections
  - Intra-articular
  - Periarticular
  - Varicose veins
  - Haemorrhoid
- Aspiration
  - Joints
  - Cysts
  - Bursae
  - Hydrocele
- Incisions
  - Abscesses
  - Cysts
  - Thrombosed piles
- Excisions
  - Sebaceous cysts
  - Lipoma
  - Skin lesions for histology
  - Intradermal naevi, papilloma, dermatofibroma and similar conditions
  - Removal of toe-nails (partial and complete)
- Curette, cautery and cryocautery
  - Warts and verrucae
  - Other skin lesions (e.g. molluscum contagiosum)
- Other
  - Removal of foreign bodies
  - Nasal cautery.

A fee will be payable where a general practitioner has performed 15 operations included in the above list in any quarter. Where more than 15 minor operations have been performed, no additional fee is payable.

A general practitioner in a group practice may delegate his minor surgery to a partner provided he is also on the 'Minor Surgery List'. Thus a practice of four doctors, where one partner chooses to do all the minor surgery can claim a fee for 60 minor operations in any one quarter.

52. 4 OFFERING A MINOR SURGERY SERVICE TO COLLEAGUES

52.4.1 To fund-holding GPs

Additional income can be generated by contacting neighbouring fund-holding general practitioners and giving them a list of minor surgical procedures that can be offered.

Fees can be based on the recommended BMA hourly rate plus costs of materials, histology and administration.

52.4.2 To non-fund-holding GPs

By approaching the Commissioning Health Authority it is possible for general practitioners to become 'providers' and to negotiate a contract to undertake a set number of minor operations per year for neighbouring non-fund-holding colleagues.

52.5 OBTAINING HELP FROM HEALTH AUTHORITIES

The majority of health authorities will welcome general practitioners undertaking their own minor surgery, and if approached, will generally be very willing to offer help. Advice about the choice and variety of surgical instruments can always be obtained by approaching the District Supplies Officer, the Operating Theatre Sisters, or the Central Sterile Supplies Department manager. The hospital will usually have favourable arrangements for bulk buying surgical instruments and will often be able to include the general practitioner in their scheme.

Similarly, the Hospital Supplies Officer may know of obsolete items such as operating theatre tables, lights, trolleys, and other such equipment which may be purchased by the general practitioner for a nominal sum.

If the practitioner intends using CSSD instrument packs, it is worth discussing with the hospital the possibility of using their autoclaves, particularly if the hospital is near the general practitioner's surgery. Some Health Districts make a small service charge for CSSD facilities – others waive this charge in recognition of the considerable financial savings resulting from the general practitioner undertaking minor surgery. Either way, prepacked presterilized instrument sets are invaluable and greatly increase the scope and safety of what can be done. Where the doctor is well known to the hospital, certain less-used instrument packs such as abdominal paracentesis, lumbar puncture, or chest aspiration sets may be loaned to save the practitioner having to purchase instruments.

52.6 COLLABORATION WITH CONSULTANT COLLEAGUES

It is always a good policy to obtain the support of local consultant surgeons should advice or help be required. Generally this is willingly given and improves relationships; assuming that general practitioners only tackle what they feel they can safely complete, the need for help seldom arises, but it is reassuring to know that it is there if required.

52.7 THE PRIVATE PATIENT

General practitioners are entitled to treat private patients as well as to accept National Health Service patients. Where a doctor has an exclusively private practice, and no NHS patients, arrangements are straightforward the doctor charges for all medical services rendered, and included in these may be fees for minor surgical operations; there is no set scale of fees – this is left entirely to the discretion of the doctor. Where a general practitioner has a predominantly National Health Service list of patients, he or she is still entitled to accept fee-paying patients but the overall earnings from private practice should not exceed 10% of the total practice income otherwise the GP will be liable to forfeit certain allowances.

If a patient is treated privately, he or she cannot be registered as a National Health Service patient with that doctor or any of his or her partners, neither can the patient be given a National Health Service prescription and the doctor cannot utilize paragraph 44.13 of the Statement of Fees and Allowances. Thus the fee for the operation must include the cost of all drugs, anaesthetics, suture materials, service charges and dressings used.

APPENDIX A

Surgical instrument and equipment suppliers

UK SUPPLIERS

Astra Pharmaceuticals Ltd, Home Park Estate, Kings Langley, Herts WD4 8DH Tel: 01923 266191 (local anaesthetics)

John Bell and Croyden, 50–54 Wigmore Street, London W1H 0AU Tel: 0171 935 5555. Telex 8955447 (surgical instruments)

Caterham Surgical Supplies Ltd, 89a Gloucester Road, Croydon, Surrey CR0 2DN Tel: 0181 683 1103. Fax: 0181 683 1105 (varicose vein forceps)

Chilworth Medicals, 19 Beach Road, Burton Bradstock, Dorset DT6 4RF Tel and Fax: 01308 898 150 (infrared coagulator)

Cryomedical Instruments Ltd, Cryo-tec House, Goods Road, Belper, Derbyshire DE56 1UU Tel: 01773 821515. Fax: 01773 821885 (cryosurgical equipment)

Doctors' Shop, Miller Freeman House, 30 Calderwood Street, London SE18 6QH Tel: 0181 855 7777 (general equipment)

Doherty Medical Hospital Equipment, 278 Alma Road, Enfield, Middlesex EN3 7BH Tel: 0181 804 1244

Eschmann Equipment Ltd, Peter Road, Lancing, West Sussex BN15 8TJ Tel: 01903 761122. Telex: 877075 (theatre equipment)

Ethicon Sutures Ltd, P.O. Box 408, Bankhead Avenue, Edinburgh EH11 4HE, Scotland. Tel: 0131 453 5555. Telex: 727222

Philip Harris Medical Ltd, Hazelwell Lane, Stirchley, Birmingham B30 2PS Tel: 0121 433 3030. Fax: 0121 433 4400

Henleys Medical Supplies Ltd, Brownfields, Welwyn Garden City, Herts AL7 1AN Tel: 01707 333164. Telex: 28942. Fax: 01707 334795

Hoechst Roussel Ltd, Broadwater Park, Dagenham, Uxbridge, Middlesex UB9 5HP Tel: 01895 834343. Fax: 01895 834479 (Norplant)

Kimberley Clark Ltd, Larkfield, Aylesford, Kent ME20 7PS Tel: 01622 717700. Telex: 93356 (paper towels and sheets)

Laerdal Medical Ltd, Laerdal House, Goodmead Road, Orpington, Kent BR6 0HX Tel: 01689 876634 (resuscitation equipment)

Ledu Lamps Ltd, 12 Barmeston Road, London SE6 3BF Tel: 0181 265 1681 (Lights)

Limbs and Things Ltd, Radnor Business Centre, Radnor Road, Horfield, Bristol BS7 8QS Tel: 01179 446 466. Fax: 01179 446 222

3-M United Kingdom, 3-M House, P.O. Box 1 Market Place, Bracknell, Berks RG12 1JU Tel: 01344 858 000 (Steri-strips and skin staplers)

Medinox International Ltd, Crown House, Hornbeam Square North, Harrogate, North Yorkshire HG2 8TD Tel: 01423 873 232 (Fern Cryosurgical Instruments)

Nova Instruments Ltd, Mill House, 127 Newgatestreet Road, Goffs Oak, Herts EN7 5RX Tel: 01707 875600 (chiropody instruments)

Practice Management Systems Ltd, The Clockhouse, 145B Hughenden Road, High Wycombe, Bucks HP13 5PN Tel: 01494 474811. Fax: 01494 474629 (cryosurgical equipment)

Prospect Medical Ltd, Prospect Centre, Prospect Way, Selby, North Yorkshire YO8 8BD Tel: 01757 213 373. Fax: 01757 213 491 (Ellman radio-surgical and general equipment)

Rimmer Bros Ltd, 18/19 Aylesbury Street, Clerkenwell, London EC1R 0DD Tel: 0171 251 6494 (electric cauteries)

Rocket of London, Imperial Way, Watford, Herts WD2 4XX Tel: 01923 239791. Telex: 922531 (surgical instruments)

Schuco International London Ltd, Lyndhurst Avenue, London N12 0NE Tel: 0181 368 1642. Telex: 893312 (Hyfrecator)

Seward Medical Ltd, 131 Great Suffolk Street, London SE1 1PP Tel: 0171 357 6527

S.T.D. Products Ltd, Field Yard, Plough Lane, Hereford HR4 0EL Tel: 01432 353 684. Telex: 35421 (sclerosants for varicose veins)

Chas Thackray Ltd, P.O. Box HP 171, 1 Shire Oak Street, Leeds LS6 2DP Tel: 01132 700 461 (instruments)

Warecrest Ltd, Unit D4, Cowdray Centre, Cowdray Avenue, Colchester, Essex CO1 1BW Tel: 01206 561404 (C28 rechargeable cautery)

NORTH AMERICA AND CANADA SUPPLIERS

Aaron Medical Industries, PO Box 261196, Tampa, Florida 33685, USA (Disposable electrocauteries)

American Hospital Services, 7080 River Road, Suite 131, Richmond, BC V6X lX5, Canada

Amsco Canada, 77 Hale Road, Brampton, Ontario L6W 3J9, Canada

Bard Canada Inc., 2345 Stanfield Road, Mississauga, Ontario, L4Y 3Y3, Canada

Birtcher Corporation, 4051 N. Arden Drive, El Monte, CA 91734, USA Tel: (213) 575 8144 TWX9105873445 (Hyfrecator)

Brymill Corporation, PO Box 2392, Veron, Connecticut 06066, USA Tel: (203) 875 2460. Fax: (203) 872 2371 (Cryosurgical equipment)

Clement Clarke Inc, 6947 Americana Parkway, Reynoldsburg, Columbus, Ohio 43068, USA

Cyanamid Canada Inc., Davis and Geck, 2255 Shepherd Avenue, Willowdale, Ontario M2J 4Y5, Canada

Downs Surgical Inc., 2500 Park Central Boulevard, Decatur GA, 30035 USA

Downs Surgical Canada, 5715 McAdam Road, Mississauga, Ontario L4Z 1PG, Canada

Electro-Med, 3278 Oak Street, Victoria, BC V8X lP7, Canada

Ellman International Inc., 1135 Railroad Avenue, Hewlett, NY11557, USA Tel: (516) 569-1482. Fax: (516) 569-0201 (radio-surgical instruments)

Ethicon Inc., Route No. 22, Somerville, New Jersey 08876, USA Tel: 201 524 0400. Telex 833487

Fern Medical, Suite 1500, 50 Milk Street, Boston, MA 02109, USA Tel: 617 338 6563. Fax: 617 451 2589 (Cryotherapy equipment)

Frigitronics of Connecticut Inc., 770 River Road, Shelton, CT 06484, USA Tel: 203/929-6321

Owen/Galderma, 6201 South Freeway, PO Box 6600, Fort Worth, Texas 76115, USA

Johnson and Johnson Inc., 2155 Pie IX Boulevard, Montreal, Quebec H1V 2E4, Canada

Keeler Instruments Ltd, 456 Parkway, Lawrence Park Industrial District, Broomhal PA 19008, USA Tel: 215 353 4350. Telex 831370.

Kimberley Clark Co., 1400 Holcomb Bridge Road, Roswell, Georgia 30076, USA

Laerdal Medical Corporation, 1 Labriola Court, Armonk, NY 10504, USA

Ledu Corporation, 25 Lindeman Drive, PO Box 358, Trumbull CT 06611, USA Tel: 203 371 5500 (Lamps)

3M, 3M Centre, St Paul, MN 55101, USA

Omnis Surgical Inc., 1425 Lake Cook Road, Deerfield, Illinois 60015, USA Tel: 312 480 5600

Physio Control International, 11811 Willows Road, Redmond, Washington 98052-1013, USA Tel: (206) 881-4000. Telex: 320166 PHYSIO RDMD (Cardiac monitors and defibrillators)

Roboz Surgical Instrument, 810 18th St, N.W. Washington DC 20006, USA

Scican, 260 Yorkland Boulevard, Toronto, Ontario M2J lR7, Canada Tel: 416 491 5000. Fax: 416 491 5040 (Cryotherapy equipment)

Chas F. Thackray (USA) Inc., 175-X New Boston Street, Woburn, Massachusetts 01801, USA Tel: (617) 935-6831

Wallach Surgical Devices Inc., 291 Pepe's Farm Road, Milford, CT 06460, USA Tel: (203) 783-1818. Fax: (203) 783-1825 (cryosurgical equipment)

APPENDIX B

Corresponding trade names for drugs named in the book

Drug	*United Kingdom*	*Canada*	*United States of America*
Lignocaine	Xylocaine	Xylocaine	Octocaine
Prilocaine	Citanest	Unavailable	Xylonest
Bupivacaine	Marcain	Marcaine	Marcain
Chlorhexidine	Hibitane	Hibitane	Hibiclens
Povidone-iodine	Betadine	Betadine	Isodine
Diazepam	Valium	Valium	Valium
Sodium tetradecyl	STD	Trombovar	Sotradecol
Glutaraldehyde	Cidex	Cidex	
Atropine	Atropine	Atropine	Atropine
Ethyl chloride	Ethyl chloride	Ethyl chloride	Ethyl chloride
Pethidine	Pethidine	Demerol	Demerol
Entonox	Entonox	Entonox	
Methylprednisolone	Depo-Medrone	Depo-Medrol	
Triamcinolone	Lederspan	Aristocort	
Chloramphenicol	Chloromycetin	Chloromycetin	Chloromycetin
Adrenaline	Adrenaline	Epinephrine	Epineprine

References

1. Brown JS. (1979) Minor operations in general practice. *Br Med J* **1** 1609–1610.
2. Robertson B. (1982) Minor surgery in general practice saves resources. *BMA News Review,* November, iv.
3. St John Ambulance; St Andrew's Ambulance Association; The British Red Cross Society. *First Aid Manual* (5th edn).
4. DHSS Booklet 3, AIDS – *Guidance for surgeons, anaesthetists, dentists and their teams dealing with patients infected with HTLV 111,* (1986).
5. Department of Health (Ref: HE1 No. 185 1988) *An Evaluation of Portable Steam Sterilisers for Unwrapped Instruments and Utensils.*
6. Langer K. (1861) Ueber die Spaltbarkeit der Cutis. S-B *Akad Wiss Wien Math-Nat* Kl **43** 23.
7. Froman S. (1939) *The Surgery of Injury and Plastic Repair.* Williams and Wilkins, Baltimore Md. 50.
8. Berson M. (1948) *Atlas of Plastic Surgery.* Grune and Stratton, New York, 3.
9. Barsky A. (1950) *Principles and Practice of Plastic Surgery.* Williams and Wilkins, Baltimore Md. 38.
10. Smith F. (1950) *Plastic and Reconstructive Surgery – A Manual of Management.* WB Saunders, London, 213.
11. Kraissl C. (1951) The selection of appropriate lines for elective surgical incisions. *Plast Reconstr Surg* **8** 1.
12. Eberhart NM. (1911) *A Working Manual of High Frequency Currents.* New Medicine Publishing, Chicago.
13. Morton ER. (1910) The use of solid carbon dioxide. *Lancet* **2** 1268–1270.
14. White AC. (1899) Liquid air in medicine and surgery. *Med Rec* 2899, **56** 109.
15. Lloyd Williams K, Holden HB. (1975) Cryosurgery in general and ENT surgery. *Br J Hosp Med* **14** 25.
16. Chamberlain, G. (1975) Cryosurgery in gynaecology. *Br J Hosp Med* **14** 26–37.
17. Hopkins P. (1982) *Proceedings of the Fifth meeting of the American College of Cryosurgery,* New Orleans, USA. 12.
18. Hopkins P. (1983) Cryosurgery by the general practitioner. *Practitioner* **227** 1861-1873.
19. Colver GB, Dawber RPR. (1989) Cryosurgery - the principles and simple practice. *Clin Exp Dermatol* **14** 1–6.
20. Holt PJA (1988) Cryotherapy for skin cancer. *Br J Dermatol* **119** 231-240.
21. Yates VM, Scott MM. Carter ED. (1988) Rupture of tendons after cryotherapy for hand wart. *Br Med J* **297** 1106.
22. Ruscoe MNJ (1990) Audit in general practice. *Br Med J* **300** 50.
23. Metcalfe DHH. (1989) Audit in general practice. *Br Med J* **299** 1293–1294.
24. Frost FA, Jessen B, Siggard Anderson (1980) A controlled, double blind comparison of mepivacaine injection versus saline injection for myofascial pain. *Lancet* **1** 499–500.
25. Nash JR. (1979) Sclerotherapy for hydrocele and epididymal cysts. *Br J Surg* **66** 289.
26. Haye KR, Maiti H. (1085) Self treatment of condylomata acuminata using 0.5% podophyllin resin. *Practitioner* **229** 37–39.

27. Dagnall JC. (1981) The history, development and current status of nail matrix phenolisation. *Chiropodist* 315.
28. Boll OF. (1945) Surgical correction of ingrowing toe-nails. *J Nat Assoc Chiropod* **35**(4)8.
29. Suppan RJ, Ritchilin JD. (1962) A non-debilitating procedure for ingrown toe-nail. *J Am Podiatr Assoc* **52** 900.
30. Barrish SJ. (1969) The phenol-alcohol technique. *Curr Podiatr* **18**(7)18.
31. Sykes PA, Kerr R. (1988) Treatment of ingrowing toe-nails by surgeons and chiropodists. *Br Med J* **297** 335–336.
32. Ellis H. (1984) Sigmoidoscopy. *Update* **1** 981–984.
33. Ellis H. (1984) Rectal bleeding and the general practitioner. *Cancer Care* **1**(4) 4.
34. Brown JS. (1983) Sigmoidoscopy in general practice. *R Coll Gen Pract* **33** 822.
35. Goligher JC. (1967) *Surgery of the Anus, Rectum, and Colon.* Bailliere Tindall and Cassell, London. 120.
36. Gabriel WB. (1956) Minor ano-rectal operations. In *Pye's Surgical Handicraft.* John Wright, Bristol. 426.
37. Lewis MI. (1972) Cryosurgical haemorrhoidectomy. *Dis Colon Rectum* 128.
38. Alexander-Williams J. (1982) The management of piles. *Br Med J* **285** 1137-1139.
39. Barron J. (1963) Office ligation of internal haemorrhoids. *Am J Surg* **105** 563-570.
40. Steinberg DM, Liegois H, Alexander-Williams J. (1975) Long term review of the results of rubber band ligation of haemorrhoids. *Br J Surg* **62** 144–146.
41. Panda AP *et al* (1975) Treatment of haemorrhoids by rubber band ligation. *Digestion* **12** 85.
42. Lord PH. (1975) Conservative management of haemorrhoids 2 – dilation treatment. *Clin Gastroenterol* **4** 601.
43. Fegan WG. (1983) Continuous compression technique of injecting varicose veins. *Lancet* **2** 109.
44. Fegan WG. (1967) *Varicose Veins, Compression Sclerotherapy.* Heinemann, London.
45. Feathers RS. (1981) Varicose veins in women. *Maternal and Child Health* **6** 318–324.
46. Studd J. (1986) A practical guide to HRT. *MIMS Magazine* **1** 21–22.
47. Yeates WK. (1984) Vasectomy. *Update* **28** 1229–1234.
48. McEvedy BV. (1962) Simple ganglia. *Br J Surg* **49** (218) 584–594.
49. Brett MS. (1977) Operations for ganglion. *In Operative Surgery – The Hand* (Ed Rob and Smith). Butterworth, London. 369.
50. Bier A. (1908) Ueber einen neuer weg Localanaesthesie an den Gliedmassen zu erzeugen. *Arch Klin Chir* **86** 1007.
51. Holmes C McK. (1963) Intravenous regional analgesia; a useful method of producing analgesia of the limbs. *Lancet* **1** 245–247.
52. Thorn-Alquist AM. (1971) Intravenous regional anaesthesia; a seven year survey. *Acta Anaesthesiol Scand* [Supplement] 40.
53. Ware RJ. (1975) *Anaesthesia* **30** 817.
54. Ware RJ. (1979) Intravenous regional anaesthesia using bupivacaine. *Anaesthesia* **34** 231–235.
55. Pattison CW. (1984) A review of the Bier's block technique. *Practitioner* **228** 235–237.
56. Mason MA. (1983) Regional anaesthesia with bupivacaine. *Lancet* **2** 1085.
57. *A Code of Practice for Sterilisation of Instruments and Control of Cross-Infection.* British Medical Association.
58. *The National Health Service (General Medical and Pharmaceutical Services)* Regulations SI 1982 no. 1283, Sch. I, Pt I, para 32–34.

Selected further reading for radio-surgery

Bisaccia E, Scarborough D. (1995) Blepharoplasty with radiosurgical instrumentation. *Cosmetic Dermatol* **8** 1207–1208.

Cresswell CC. (1992) Introduction to electro-surgery. *Br Podiatr Med* **47** (1) 11–14.

Garden JM, O'Banion MK, Shelnitz LS. *et al.* (1988) Papillomavirus in the vapor of carbon dioxide laser-treated verrucae. *JAMA* **259** 1199–1202

Henry F. (1989) Interet du bistouri haute frequence en chirurgie plastique. *Extrait Ann Cir Plast Esthet* **34** 65.

Hettinger D. (1995) Excision of plantar fibroma via radiowave technique. A review of the literature and a case report, Personal communication.

Hettinger D, Valinsky M, Nuccio G, Lim R. (1991) Nail matrixectomies using radio-wave technique. *J Am Podiatr Med Assoc* **81** (6) 317–321.

Hurwitz JJ, Johnson D, Howard D, Molgat YM. (1993) High frequency radiowave electrosection of full-thickness eyelid tissues, *Can J Ophthalmol* **28** 62–64.

Kendall MW. (1988) Radiosurgery: an advanced technique for performing nail matrixectomies. *Podiatr Management* 7 53.

McGlamry ED. (1987) *Comprehensive Textbook of Foot Surgery.* Vol II. Williams and Wilkins, Baltimore.

Pollack SV. (1991) Electrosurgery of the Skin. Churchill Livingstone, New York.

Pearce JA. (1986) *Electrosurgery.* John Wiley and Sons, New York.

Pfenninger JL, DeWitt DE. (1994) Radiofrequency surgery. In *Procedures for Primary Care Physicians.* Mosby, 91–101.

Saidi MH, Setzlter FD, Sadler RK, et al. (1994) Comparison of office loop electrosurgical conization and cold knife conization. *J Am Assoc Gynaecol Laparosc* **1** 135–139.

Sebben J. (1988) Electrosurgery: high frequency modulation. *J Dermatol Surg Oncol* **14** 367–371.

Sebben J. (1988) Electrosurgery principles: cutting current and cutaneous surgery – Part 1. *J Dermatol Surg Oncol* **14** 29–32.

Sebben JE. (1989) *Cutaneous Electrosurgery.* Year Book Medical Publishers, Chicago.

Sherman AJ. (1992) *Oral Electrosurgery, An Illustrated Clinical Guide.* Martin Dunitz, London.

Turjansky E, Stolar E. (1994) *Lesiones de Piel y Mucosas Tecnicas Terapeuticas.* EDAMA, Argentina.

Turner RJ, Cohen RA, Voet RL, et al. (1992) Analysis of tissue margins of cone biopsy specimens obtained with 'cold knife', and Nd:YAG lasers and a radiofrequency surgical unit. *J Reprod Med* **37** 607–610.

Valinsky M. (1990) Treatment of verrucae via radio-wave surgery. *J Am Podiatr Med Assoc* **80** 482–488.

Waldman SR. (1993) Management of superficial skin lesions in a cosmetic surgery practice. *Plastic and Reconstructive Surgery of the Head and Neck. Proceedings of the 5th International Symposium.* Chapter 120.

Waldman SR. (1994) Transconjunctival blepharoplasty minimising the risks of lower lid blepharoplasty. *Facial Plastic Surg* **10** 27–41.

White WF. (1986) Radiosurgery – an advancement over the scalpel in many procedures. *Podiatr Prod Rep* **3** 16.

Wyre HW. (1977) Extirpation of warts by a loop electrode and cutting current. *J Dermatol Surg* **3** 520–522.

Index

Page numbers appearing in **bold** refer to figures and page numbers appearing in *italic* refer to tables